2005

From Cancer Patient to Cancer Survivor

LOST IN TRANSITION

Committee on Cancer Survivorship: Improving Care and Quality of Life

National Cancer Policy Board

Maria Hewitt, Sheldon Greenfield, and Ellen Stovall, *Editors*

INSTITUTE OF MEDICINE *AND*
NATIONAL RESEARCH COUNCIL
OF THE NATIONAL ACADEMIES

THE NATIONAL ACADEMIES PRESS
Washington, D.C.
www.nap.edu

THE NATIONAL ACADEMIES PRESS 500 Fifth Street, N.W. Washington, DC 20001

NOTICE: The project that is the subject of this report was approved by the Governing Board of the National Research Council, whose members are drawn from the councils of the National Academy of Sciences, the National Academy of Engineering, and the Institute of Medicine. The members of the committee responsible for the report were chosen for their special competences and with regard for appropriate balance.

This study was supported by the National Cancer Institute, the Centers for Disease Control and Prevention, and the American Cancer Society. Any opinions, findings, conclusions, or recommendations expressed in this publication are those of the author(s) and do not necessarily reflect the view of the organizations or agencies that provided support for this project.

Library of Congress Cataloging-in-Publication Data

From cancer patient to cancer survivor : lost in transition / Committee on Cancer Survivorship: Improving Care and Quality of Life, National Cancer Policy Board ; Maria Hewitt, Sheldon Greenfield, and Ellen Stovall, editors.
p. ; cm.
Includes bibliographical references and index.
ISBN 0-309-09595-6 (hardcover)
1. Cancer—Patients—Rehabilitation—United States. 2. Cancer—Patients—Services for—United States. 3. Cancer—Treatment—United States. I. Hewitt, Maria Elizabeth. II. Greenfield, Sheldon. III. Stovall, Ellen. IV. National Cancer Policy Board (U.S.). Committee on Cancer Survivorship: Improving Care and Quality of Life.
[DNLM: 1. Neoplasms—psychology—United States. 2. Neoplasms—therapy—United States. 3. Continuity of Patient Care—United States. 4. Quality of Health Care—United States. 5. Survival Rate—United States. 6. Survivors—United States. QZ 266 F931 2005]
RC262.F76 2005
362.196′994—dc22

2005024963

Additional copies of this report are available from the National Academies Press, 500 Fifth Street, N.W., Lockbox 285, Washington, DC 20055; (800) 624-6242 or (202) 334-3313 (in the Washington metropolitan area); Internet, http://www.nap.edu.

For more information about the Institute of Medicine, visit the IOM home page at: **www.iom.edu.**

Printed in the United States of America

THE NATIONAL ACADEMIES

Advisers to the Nation on Science, Engineering, and Medicine

The **National Academy of Sciences** is a private, nonprofit, self-perpetuating society of distinguished scholars engaged in scientific and engineering research, dedicated to the furtherance of science and technology and to their use for the general welfare. Upon the authority of the charter granted to it by the Congress in 1863, the Academy has a mandate that requires it to advise the federal government on scientific and technical matters. Dr. Ralph J. Cicerone is president of the National Academy of Sciences.

The **National Academy of Engineering** was established in 1964, under the charter of the National Academy of Sciences, as a parallel organization of outstanding engineers. It is autonomous in its administration and in the selection of its members, sharing with the National Academy of Sciences the responsibility for advising the federal government. The National Academy of Engineering also sponsors engineering programs aimed at meeting national needs, encourages education and research, and recognizes the superior achievements of engineers. Dr. Wm. A. Wulf is president of the National Academy of Engineering.

The **Institute of Medicine** was established in 1970 by the National Academy of Sciences to secure the services of eminent members of appropriate professions in the examination of policy matters pertaining to the health of the public. The Institute acts under the responsibility given to the National Academy of Sciences by its congressional charter to be an adviser to the federal government and, upon its own initiative, to identify issues of medical care, research, and education. Dr. Harvey V. Fineberg is president of the Institute of Medicine.

The **National Research Council** was organized by the National Academy of Sciences in 1916 to associate the broad community of science and technology with the Academy's purposes of furthering knowledge and advising the federal government. Functioning in accordance with general policies determined by the Academy, the Council has become the principal operating agency of both the National Academy of Sciences and the National Academy of Engineering in providing services to the government, the public, and the scientific and engineering communities. The Council is administered jointly by both Academies and the Institute of Medicine. Dr. Ralph J. Cicerone and Dr. Wm. A. Wulf are chair and vice chair, respectively, of the National Research Council.

www.national-academies.org

COMMITTEE ON CANCER SURVIVORSHIP: IMPROVING CARE AND QUALITY OF LIFE

SHELDON GREENFIELD *(Chair)*, Director, Center for Health Policy Research, University of California–Irvine, Irvine, CA

ELLEN STOVALL *(Vice Chair)*, President and CEO, National Coalition for Cancer Survivorship, Silver Spring, MD

JOHN Z. AYANIAN, Associate Professor of Medicine and Health Care Policy, Harvard Medical School and Brigham and Women's Hospital, Boston, MA

REGINA M. BENJAMIN, Founder and CEO, Bayou La Batre Rural Health Clinic, Inc., Bayou La Batre, AL

HARRIS A. BERMAN, Dean of Public Health and Professional Degree Programs and Chair, Department of Public Health and Family Medicine, Tufts University School of Medicine, Boston, MA

SARAH S. DONALDSON, Catharine and Howard Avery Professor, Stanford University School of Medicine, Stanford, CA

CRAIG EARLE, Assistant Professor, Dana Farber Cancer Institute, Department of Health Policy and Management, Harvard University, Boston, MA

BETTY R. FERRELL, Research Scientist, Department of Nursing Research and Education, City of Hope National Medical Center, Duarte, CA

PATRICIA A. GANZ, Professor, UCLA Schools of Medicine and Public Health, Director, Division of Cancer Prevention & Control Research, Jonsson Comprehensive Cancer Center at UCLA, Los Angeles, CA

FRANK E. JOHNSON, Professor of Surgery, Saint Louis University Health Sciences Center, St. Louis, MO

MARK S. LITWIN, Professor of Health Services and Urology, UCLA School of Medicine, Los Angeles, CA

KAREN POLLITZ, Project Director, Georgetown University Health Policy Institute, Washington, DC

PAMELA FARLEY SHORT, Professor of Health Policy and Administration, Director of the Center for Health Care and Policy Research, Pennsylvania State University, University Park, PA

BONNIE TESCHENDORF, Director, Quality of Life Sciences, American Cancer Society, Atlanta, GA

MARY M. VARGO, Associate Professor, Department of Physical Medicine and Rehabilitation, Case Western Reserve University at MetroHealth Medical Center, Cleveland, OH

RODGER J. WINN, Clinical Consultant, National Quality Forum, Washington, DC
STEVEN H. WOOLF, Professor of Family Practice, Preventive Medicine, and Community Health, Virginia Commonwealth University, Richmond, VA

Staff

MARIA HEWITT, Study Director
ROGER HERDMAN, Director, National Cancer Policy Board
ELIZABETH J. BROWN, Research Associate
JAEHEE YI, Intern
ANIKE JOHNSON, Administrative Assistant

Reviewers

This report has been reviewed in draft form by individuals chosen for their diverse perspectives and technical expertise, in accordance with procedures approved by the NRC's Report Review Committee. The purpose of this independent review is to provide candid and critical comments that will assist the institution in making its published report as sound as possible and to ensure that the report meets institutional standards for objectivity, evidence, and responsiveness to the study charge. The review comments and draft manuscript remain confidential to protect the integrity of the deliberative process. We wish to thank the following individuals for their review of this report:

Diane Blum, CancerCare, Inc.
Cathy Bradley, Virginia Commonwealth University
Murray F. Brennan, Weill Medical College of Cornell University
Robert S. Galvin, General Electric
Eva Grunfeld, Cancer Care Nova Scotia
Sandra Horning, Stanford Cancer Center
Jon Kingsdale, Tufts Health Plan
Susan Leigh, Cancer Survivorship Consultant
Kevin Oeffinger, Memorial Sloan-Kettering Cancer Center
Barbara Schwerin, Cancer Legal Resource Center
Phyllis Torda, National Committee for Quality Assurance
LuAnn Wilkerson, David Geffen School of Medicine at UCLA

Although the reviewers listed above have provided many constructive comments and suggestions, they were not asked to endorse the conclusions or recommendations nor did they see the final draft of the report before its release. The review of this report was overseen by **Joseph P. Newhouse**, Harvard Medical School and Kennedy School of Government; and **Melvin Worth**, Scholar-in-Residence, Institute of Medicine. Appointed by the National Research Council and the Institute of Medicine, they were responsible for making certain that an independent examination of this report was carried out in accordance with institutional procedures and that all review comments were carefully considered. Responsibility for the final content of this report rests entirely with the authoring committee and the institution.

Acknowledgments

The committee was aided in its deliberations by the researchers, administrators, and health professionals who presented informative talks to the committee and participated in lively discussions at the open meetings, including:

Karen Antman, Deputy Director for Translational and Clinical Sciences, National Cancer Institute (NCI), who set the stage for the committee's first meeting by providing an overview, "The U.S. National Cancer Program from 60,000 Feet."

Noreen M. Aziz, Program Director, Office of Cancer Survivorship (OCS), NCI, reviewed for the committee at their first meeting the characteristics of U.S. cancer survivors and provided information about the OCS and its research portfolio and other survivorship activities within the NIH.

Peter Bach, Senior Adviser, Office of the Administrator, Centers for Medicare and Medicaid Services (CMS), at the committee's third meeting provided an overview of cancer-related activities at CMS with a particular focus on demonstration programs in the areas of quality of care, cancer navigation, and coordination of care.

Kevin Brady, Acting Director, Division of Cancer Prevention and Control, Centers for Disease Control and Prevention (CDC), at the committee's first meeting presented information on the public health implications of cancer survivorship, including the role of comprehensive cancer control planning.

He also described the effort co-sponsored by the CDC and the Lance Armstrong Foundation which resulted in the 2004 publication, *A National Action Plan for Cancer Survivorship: Advancing Public Health Strategies.*

Mark Clanton, Deputy Director, NCI, Office of Cancer Care Delivery Systems, addressed the committee at their third meeting and discussed survivorship-related strategic planning, priority setting, and implementation, and in addition, issues related to quality of cancer care.

Robert Hiatt, Director of Population Science and Deputy Director of the University of California, San Francisco Comprehensive Cancer Center, at the committee's second meeting, described progress on two initiatives related to information technology and data systems, that of C-Change and the National Committee for Quality Assurance (NCQA).

Margaret Kripke, member of the President's Cancer Panel (PCP), at the committee's first meeting reviewed recommendations of the PCP's 2004 report, *Living Beyond Cancer: Finding a New Balance,* and showed the Panel's video that was based on testimony presented at the PCP's public hearings.

Julia Rowland, Director, NCI's Office of Cancer Survivorship, at the committee's third meeting provided an update and overview of the federal research portfolio on cancer survivorship and discussed research opportunities (and challenges) in survivorship and examples of NCI-sponsored initiatives that are underway.

Jerome Yates, National Vice President for Research, American Cancer Society (ACS), at the committee's first meeting provided information about the ACS's survivorship research programs and, in particular, two large survivorship studies being conducted within the ACS's Behavioral Research Center.

The publishers of *Seminars in Oncology* generously agreed to provide to the committee copies of two of their issues focused on survivorship, "Post-treatment Surveillance for Potentially Curable Malignancies" (June 2003), and "Late Effects of Treatment and Survivorship Issues in Early-Stage Breast Carcinoma" (December 2003).

The committee also wishes to acknowledge with appreciation the assistance of many individuals committed to improving the lives of cancer survivors.

Wendy Demark-Wahnefried, Program of Cancer Prevention, Detection & Control Research, Duke Comprehensive Cancer Center, provided assistance in drafting the section of the report on lifestyle following cancer treatment.

Eric Feuer, Chief of NCI's Statistical Research and Applications Branch, Surveillance Research Program, provided the committee with estimates of conditional survival (these are included in chapter 2 of the report).

Ann M. Flores, Assistant Professor, Department of Obstetrics and Gynecology, Meharry Medical College School of Medicine, provided background information to staff about physical therapy and cancer rehabilitation.

Marshall Fritz, Statistician, Health Resources and Services Administration, provided special tabulations of the 2000 National Sample Survey of Registered Nurses and assisted staff in their understanding the oncology nursing workforce.

Barbara Hoffman, Rutgers University, provided a background paper to the National Cancer Policy Board on legal issues confronting cancer survivors and contributed to the chapter on employment, insurance, and financial issues.

Jimmie Holland, Chair, Department of Psychiatry and Behavioral Sciences, Memorial Sloan-Kettering Cancer Center, discussed with staff issues related to psychosocial distress in the context of cancer survivorship

Linda Jacobs, Living Well After Cancer at the University of Pennsylvania, **Joan Armstrong**, Breast Wellness Clinic at the University of Michigan, and **Rena Sellin**, Life After Cancer Care, M.D. Anderson Cancer Center, provided information to staff pertaining to their cancer survivorship clinics.

Susan Leigh, Cancer Survivorship Consultant, and **Pamela J. Haylock**, Oncology Consultant, helped staff and the committee understand the important roles of nurses in cancer survivorship care.

Mary McCabe and **Jennifer Ford**, Memorial Sloan-Kettering Cancer Center, provided information on new survivorship care initiatives at Sloan-Kettering.

Cindy Pfalzer, University of Michigan-Flint, discussed the role of physical therapists in cancer survivorship care with staff.

Paul J. Placek, Senior Statistician, Office of the Center Director, National Center for Health Statistics, Centers for Disease Control and Prevention (retired), and **John F. Hough**, Health Scientist Administrator, National

Institute on Alcohol Abuse and Alcoholism, National Institutes of Health, provided information on the World Health Organization's International Classification of Functioning, Disability and Health. This classification system was considered by the Committee to describe the late effects of cancer.

Margarette Shelton, M.D. Anderson Cancer, provided information to staff on the role of occupational therapists in cancer survivorship care.

Robert Villanueva, Executive Director of the Maryland State Council on Cancer Control, provided information on the survivorship component of the Maryland Comprehensive Cancer Control Plan.

Many individuals within the IOM provided invaluable guidance and assistance.

Hellen Gelband helped draft the report executive summary.

Roger Herdman through his dedication, effort, and commitment helped move this report from concept to reality in his role as Director of the National Cancer Policy Forum (formerly the National Cancer Policy Board). Dr. Herdman provided assistance throughout the committee process, participating in all meetings, reviewing drafts, and providing guidance to staff as the report progressed.

Linda Martin, Senior Scholar, provided staff with information on disability and health as it relates to survivorship issues.

Michael McGeary, Senior Program Officer, provided information to staff on the Supplemental Security Income and Social Security Disability Insurance programs of the Social Security Administration.

Wilhelmine Miller and **Dianne Wolman**, Senior Program Officers, reviewed sections of the draft pertaining to health insurance.

Thanks also to **Mark Chesnek** (Communications Officer), **Jennifer Otten** (Director, Communications), **Jennifer Bitticks** (Senior Editorial/Publication Project Manager), **Liesl Peters** (Report Review Associate), **Janice Mehler** (Associate Director, Report Review Committee), and the National Academies Press production staff.

This report was made possible by the generous support of the National Cancer Institute, Centers for Disease Control and Prevention, and the American Cancer Society.

Contents

Boxes, Figures, and Tables

Executive Summary

Chapter 2

Tables

Chapter 3

Boxes

Figures

Tables

Chapter 4

Boxes

Figures

Tables

Chapter 5

Boxes

Tables

Chapter 6

Boxes

Figures

Tables

Chapter 7

Boxes

Figures

Tables

Preface

A rather startling statistic opened the eyes of many on our committee when they were invited to undertake a study for the Institute of Medicine (IOM) on cancer survivorship. The eye-opening statistic describes a burgeoning population of cancer survivors who live among us today and who are more than 10 million strong. Cancer survivors swell the ranks of the many places where we live, work, and play, yet, as our committee concluded, they remain largely understudied and lost to follow-up by our scientific research and health services delivery communities, respectively. Although the concept of survivorship is not new, we have determined there are times when trends in medical science, health services research, and public health awareness converge to forge a new realization. Such may be happening with respect to survivorship research and cancer care with the publication of this report.

These three trends forecast how we believe the findings and recommendations of this report can have an impact on our health care delivery system for the majority of cancer survivors who suffer the long-term and late effects of their diagnosis and treatment for cancer. First, for many, cancer has become a chronic condition as a new generation of cancer survivors is living longer following improved access to effective screening, diagnosis, and treatments. Second, strides have been made in the science of health services research with models of care emerging for individuals with chronic conditions needing complex care. Third, a persistent and energetic consumer movement has demanded patient-centered quality of care across the entire cancer trajectory.

These trends dovetail nicely with the extensive review of peer-reviewed literature that was considered by the IOM Committee on Cancer Survivorship. The report by this committee builds on the large body of IOM's work to improve Americans' access to quality health care. By also reviewing reports that summarize the anecdotal and compelling stories of survivorship, we heard the voices of survivors who underwent a life-changing experience—learning that large numbers of them are dealing with a legacy of physical, psychological, social, vocational, spiritual, and economic consequences. Hearing about their experiences further opened our eyes to the unspoken and hidden disabilities that follow successful treatment for cancer.

The committee was composed of 17 members representing many disciplines with broad knowledge and expertise. Several committee members had a personal diagnosis of cancer, and others would be considered cancer survivors because they include the family, friends, and loved ones of individuals diagnosed with cancer.

Both of us have very personal reasons for wanting this report to find its voice with policy makers and all those who share responsibility for our health care financing and delivery systems. For one of us (Ellen Stovall), who is a 33-year survivor of two diagnoses of cancer, it represents a huge step in a dream come true for her and the founders of the National Coalition for Cancer Survivorship (NCCS): the recognition of cancer survivorship as a topic unto itself. Ellen currently leads NCCS, which began its efforts in the mid-1980s with few listening. For the other of us (Shelly Greenfield), it represents a rare victory, an endorsement of the recognition that the efforts of doctors alone, no matter how hard they are trying, are going to fall short if systemic issues such as care coordination, patient-centered care delivery, financing, informatics, and accountability for quality of care are not enjoined.

For all of us who have ever been diagnosed with cancer, for all of us who know someone with cancer, for all of us who have lost someone to cancer, for all of us who will be diagnosed with cancer in our lifetime, and the millions who will survive this diagnosis, we hope this report will forge a new era of cancer survivorship by raising awareness of the many concerns facing cancer survivors. Most importantly, we want to persuade the policy makers named in our recommendations of the imperative to assume the large tasks ahead and ultimately to improve the care and quality of life of individuals with a history of cancer.

On behalf of our committee, we want to extend our gratitude to the Institute of Medicine for giving us superb staff to guide our discussions and push us toward prioritizing what at times seemed to be an endless list of important issues on which to focus. With appreciation to all involved with this report, we are deeply indebted to Roger Herdman, Director, National Cancer Policy Board for his leadership. Maria Hewitt's organizational skills, her vast background in cancer activities, her rare ability to handle highly opinionated experts from diverse fields, and her wide perspective blending both the professional and public aspects of this complex topic made this report happen. We also thank Elizabeth Brown for the flawless management of the project. The dedication of both the committee and staff to excellence in research has made this report a document that will guide critical work in health care for cancer survivors for many years to come.

Shelly Greenfield, *Chair*
Ellen Stovall, *Vice Chair*

From Cancer Patient to Cancer Survivor

Executive Summary

With a risk of more than one in three of getting cancer over a lifetime, each of us is likely to experience cancer, or know someone who has survived cancer. Although some cancer survivors recover with a renewed sense of life and purpose, what has often not been recognized is the toll taken by both cancer and its treatment—on health, functioning, sense of security, and well-being. Long-lasting effects of treatment may be apparent shortly after its completion or arise years later. Personal relationships change and adaptations to routines and work may be needed. Importantly, the survivor's health care is forever altered.

The transition from active treatment to post-treatment care is critical to long-term health. If care is not planned and coordinated, cancer survivors are left without knowledge of their heightened risks and a follow-up plan of action. However, such a plan is essential so that routine follow-up visits become opportunities to promote a healthy lifestyle, check for cancer recurrence, and manage lasting effects of the cancer experience. The nature of these lasting effects and their long-term implications for survivors and their families is the subject of this report. There are now 10 million Americans alive with a personal history of cancer, all of whom are considered cancer survivors. Widespread adoption of cancer screening, successes in treating cancers, and the aging of the population will contribute to an even larger cohort of cancer survivors in the near future.

A committee was established at the Institute of Medicine (IOM) of the National Academies to examine the range of medical and psychosocial issues faced by cancer survivors and to make recommendations to improve their health care and quality of life. In effect, the committee took up the task identified by Fitzhugh Mullan, a physician and cancer survivor, who in 1985 said, "*The challenge in overcoming cancer is not only to find therapies that will prevent or arrest the disease quickly, but also to map the middle ground of survivorship and minimize its medical and social hazards*" (Mullan, 1985). **This report focuses on survivors of adult cancer during the phase of care that follows primary treatment.** The committee recognized the importance of addressing unmet needs of the large and growing number of cancer survivors during this phase of care. Previous IOM reports addressed the needs of childhood cancer survivors (IOM, 2003) and issues concerning care at the end of life (IOM, 1997, 2001b).

The committee reviewed the consequences of cancer and its treatment and concluded that they are substantial. Although the population of cancer survivors is heterogeneous, with some having few late effects of their cancer and its treatment, others suffer permanent and disabling symptoms that impair normal functioning. Psychological distress, sexual dysfunction, infertility, impaired organ function, cosmetic changes, and limitations in mobility, communication, and cognition are among the problems faced by some cancer survivors. The good news is that there is much that can be done to avoid, ameliorate, or arrest these late effects of cancer. To ensure the best possible outcomes for cancer survivors, the committee aims in this report to:

1. Raise awareness of the medical, functional, and psychosocial consequences of cancer and its treatment.
2. Define quality health care for cancer survivors and identify strategies to achieve it.
3. Improve the quality of life of cancer survivors through policies to ensure their access to psychosocial services, fair employment practices, and health insurance.

The committee's findings and recommendations that follow are directed to cancer patients and their advocates, health care providers and their leadership, health insurers and plans, employers, research sponsors, and the public and their elected representatives.

RAISING AWARENESS OF CANCER SURVIVORSHIP

There are many ways to define cancer survivorship, but for the purpose of this report, it is a distinct phase of the cancer trajectory which has been relatively neglected in advocacy, education, clinical practice, and research. Quality cancer survivorship care involves the provision of four essential components of care within a delivery system that facilitates access to comprehensive and coordinated care (Box ES-1). Raising awareness of the medi-

BOX ES-1
Essential Components of Survivorship Care

1. **Prevention** of recurrent and new cancers, and of other late effects;
2. **Surveillance** for cancer spread, recurrence, or second cancers; assessment of medical and psychosocial late effects;
3. **Intervention** for consequences of cancer and its treatment, for example: medical problems such as lymphedema and sexual dysfunction; symptoms, including pain and fatigue; psychological distress experienced by cancer survivors and their caregivers; and concerns related to employment, insurance, and disability; and
4. **Coordination** between specialists and primary care providers to ensure that all of the survivor's health needs are met.

cal and psychosocial needs that may follow cancer treatment will help both survivors and their health care providers to ensure that appropriate assessments are completed and available interventions employed. The constellation of cancer's long-term and late effects varies by cancer type, treatment modality, and individual characteristics, but there are common patterns of symptoms and conditions that must be recognized so that health and well-being can be improved.

Recommendation 1: Health care providers, patient advocates, and other stakeholders should work to raise awareness of the needs of cancer survivors, establish cancer survivorship as a distinct phase of cancer care, and act to ensure the delivery of appropriate survivorship care.

Cancer patients and their advocates can call attention to their survivorship experiences and the need for change. The leadership of organizations representing physicians, nurses, and psychosocial care providers can collaborate to improve care. Third-party payors of health care and health plans can improve access to needed services through reimbursement policies and improvements in systems of care. Employers can ensure fair workplace policies and accommodations. Sponsors of research can improve the opportunities to increase what we know about survivorship and appropriate care. Congress and state legislatures can enact policies and ensure the support needed to improve survivorship care and quality of life.

PROVIDING A CARE PLAN FOR SURVIVORSHIP

The recognition of cancer survivorship as a distinct phase of the cancer trajectory is not enough. A strategy is needed for the ongoing clinical care of cancer survivors. There are many opportunities for improving the care of cancer survivors—psychosocial distress can be assessed and support provided; cancer recurrences and second cancers may be caught early and treated; bothersome symptoms can be effectively managed; preventable conditions such as osteoporosis may be avoided; and potentially lethal late effects such as heart failure averted. Cancer survivors are often lost to systematic follow-up within our health care system and opportunities to effectively intervene are missed. Many people finish their primary treatment for cancer unaware of their heightened health risks and are ill-prepared to manage their future health care needs. Furthermore, recommended follow-up care is often not delivered and the psychosocial needs of cancer patients are often not addressed.

Recommendation 2: Patients completing primary treatment should be provided with a comprehensive care summary and follow-up plan that is clearly and effectively explained. This "Survivorship Care Plan" should be written by the principal provider(s) who coordinated oncology treatment. This service should be reimbursed by third-party payors of health care.

Such a care plan would summarize critical information needed for the survivor's long-term care:

- Cancer type, treatments received, and their potential consequences;
- Specific information about the timing and content of recommended follow-up;
- Recommendations regarding preventive practices and how to maintain health and well-being;
- Information on legal protections regarding employment and access to health insurance; and
- The availability of psychosocial services in the community.

These content areas, adapted from those recommended by the President's Cancer Panel (2004), are elaborated on in Chapter 3.

The content of the Survivorship Care Plan could be reviewed with a patient during a formal discharge consultation. Appropriate reimbursement would need to be provided, given the complexity and importance of the consultation. The member of the oncology treating team who would be responsible for this visit could vary depending on the exact course of treatment. The responsibility could be assigned either to the oncology specialist coordinating care or to the provider responsible for the last component of treatment. Oncology nurses could play a key role. The survivorship plan may help patients share in the responsibility for their health care. It could prompt survivors to raise questions with doctors and help ensure appropriate follow-up care.

Survivorship care plans have been recommended by the President's Cancer Panel and by the IOM committee, however, the implementation of such plans has not yet been formally evaluated. Despite the lack of evidence to support the use of survivorship care plans, the committee concluded that some elements of care simply make sense—that is, they have strong face validity and can reasonably be assumed to improve care unless and until evidence accumulates to the contrary. Having an agreed-upon care plan that outlines goals of care falls into this "common sense" area. Health services research should be undertaken to assess the impact and costs associated with survivorship care plans, and to evaluate their acceptance by both cancer survivors and health care providers.

DEVELOPING CLINICAL PRACTICE GUIDELINES FOR SURVIVORSHIP CARE

The Survivorship Care Plan would inform clinicians involved in the subsequent care of cancer survivors about treatment exposures and signs and symptoms of late effects, and, in some cases, would provide concrete steps to be taken. To carry out this plan, an organized set of clinical practice guidelines based on the best available evidence is needed to help ensure appropriate follow-up care. Some guidelines are available for certain aspects of survivorship care, but most are incomplete. Such guidelines would provide specific information on how to manage the complex issues facing survivors of adult cancers. Assessment tools and screening instruments for common late effects are also needed to help identify cancer survivors who have, or who are at high risk for, late effects and who may need extra surveillance or interventions.

Recommendation 3: Health care providers should use systematically developed evidence-based clinical practice guidelines, assessment tools, and screening instruments to help identify and manage late effects of cancer and its treatment. Existing guidelines should be refined and new evidence-based guidelines should be developed through public- and private-sector efforts.

Cancer survivors represent a very large at-risk population and without evidence-based clinical practice guidelines, health care providers will vary widely in their practices, leading to inefficiencies in care delivery (see Chapters 3 and 4). More than 60 percent of cancer survivors are aged 65 and older, so the Centers for Medicare and Medicaid Services (CMS) the administrators of the Medicare program, have a stake in developing clinical practice guidelines. The Agency for Healthcare Research and Quality (AHRQ) maintains a National Guideline Clearinghouse and supports Evidence-Based Practice Centers that review relevant literature on clinical, behavioral, organizational, and financial topics to produce evidence reports and technology assessments (AHRQ, 2001). Such reviews can form the foundation of evidence-based guidelines. Professional organizations (e.g., those representing oncology, primary care, nursing) also have a role to play in developing interdisciplinary guidelines. The guideline development process is a costly one, and public and private support is needed to improve and expedite the development process. Evaluations are needed of the impact of guidelines in the context of survivorship care.

DEFINING QUALITY HEALTH CARE FOR CANCER SURVIVORS

For certain types of cancer, some evidence-based measures of quality survivorship care exist. Survivors of breast cancer, for example, need to receive annual mammograms, survivors of prostate cancer need periodic testing with the prostate-specific antigen (PSA) test, and survivors of colon cancer require periodic colon examinations. Other measures could likely be developed with available evidence, for example, the need to monitor some individuals treated with certain chemotherapeutic agents for heart conditions and certain individuals treated by radiotherapy for thyroid conditions. In contrast to these disease-specific or treatment-specific measures, some evidence-based measures of quality apply broadly across all types of cancer. For example, routinely assessing cancer survivors for psychosocial distress is warranted because it often exists and effective interventions are available. Given the frequency of other common and treatable symptoms such as fatigue and sexual dysfunction, other measures of quality could likely be formulated with available evidence that would be broadly applicable to cancer survivors.

Recommendation 4: Quality of survivorship care measures should be developed through public/private partnerships and quality assurance programs implemented by health systems to monitor and improve the care that all survivors receive.

OVERCOMING DELIVERY SYSTEM CHALLENGES

The problems that cancer survivors face in getting comprehensive and coordinated care are common to those faced by others with chronic health conditions. Because cancer is a complex disease and its management involves the expertise of many specialists, often practicing in different settings, cancer illustrates well the "quality chasm" that exists within the U.S. health care system and the need for health insurance reforms and innovations in health care delivery. The committee endorses the conclusions and recommendations in the IOM report *Crossing the Quality Chasm* (IOM,

2001a). That report provided the rationale and a strategic direction for redesigning the health care delivery system. It concluded that fundamental reform of health care is needed to ensure that all Americans receive care that is safe, effective, patient centered, timely, efficient, and equitable. Needed is a health care environment that fosters and rewards improvement by (1) creating an infrastructure to support evidence-based practice, (2) facilitating the use of information technology, (3) aligning payment incentives, and (4) preparing the workforce to better serve patients in a world of expanding knowledge and rapid change.

Barriers facing cancer survivors and their providers in achieving quality survivorship care include (1) a fragmented and poorly coordinated cancer care system; (2) the absence of a locus of responsibility for follow-up care; (3) poor mechanisms for communication; (4) a lack of guidance on the specific tests, examinations, and advice that make up survivorship care; (5) inadequate reimbursement from insurers for some aspects of care; and (6) limited experience on the best way to deliver care.

Recommendation 5: The Centers for Medicare and Medicaid Services (CMS), National Cancer Institute (NCI), Agency for Healthcare Research and Quality (AHRQ), the Department of Veterans Affairs (VA), and other qualified organizations should support demonstration programs to test models of coordinated, interdisciplinary survivorship care in diverse communities and across systems of care.

Several promising models for delivering survivorship care are emerging, including:

1. A shared-care model in which specialists work collaboratively with primary care providers.
2. A nurse-led model in which nurses take responsibility for cancer-related follow-up care with oversight from physicians.
3. Specialized survivorship clinics in which multidisciplinary care is offered at one site.

There is limited evidence on which of these, or other delivery strategies, is feasible, cost-effective, or acceptable to survivors and clinicians (see Chapter 4). It is likely that different care models will be preferred and appropriate for different survivor groups and communities. Models for delivering survivorship care should address the fact that oncology specialists and primary care providers, facing an expanding population of cancer survivors, will become overburdened with follow-up care. The proposed demonstration programs could include assessments of methods to improve care with advanced information systems, such as electronic health records, virtual consultations, smart cards, and web-based approaches. CMS is the primary payor of care for cancer survivors and should therefore have a strong interest in identifying cost-effective models of care.

SURVIVORSHIP AS A PUBLIC HEALTH CONCERN

The Centers for Disease Control and Prevention (CDC) and the Lance Armstrong Foundation have developed a public health approach to survivorship care that may assist communities in identifying and addressing the survivorship needs of individuals, their families, and their health care providers (CDC, 2004; CDC and LAF, 2004). Among the public health capacities that could be addressed are:

- Population-based surveillance systems for survivorship care and quality of life;
- Areawide community-based resource guides for survivors and health care providers;
- Service needs assessments;
- A clearinghouse for health care provider education and training opportunities;
- Provision of primary and secondary prevention services (e.g., smoking cessation, cancer screening); and
- Program evaluation and identification of best practices.

Health departments have had a long tradition of managing cancer registries, offering health education, and providing community-based health promotion and disease prevention activities. Interventions for common chronic public health problems such as heart disease and diabetes could well be germane to cancer survivors and their families. These public health approaches are early in their development. Resources are needed to evaluate the effectiveness of community-based services and comprehensive cancer control plans in improving the care and quality of life of cancer survivors.

Recommendation 6: Congress should support Centers for Disease Control and Prevention (CDC), other collaborating institutions, and the states in developing comprehensive cancer control plans that include consideration of survivorship care, and promoting the implementation, evaluation, and refinement of existing state cancer control plans.

IMPROVING HEALTH CARE PROFESSIONAL CAPACITY

Few oncology and primary care health professionals have formal education and training regarding cancer survivorship. With the growing ranks of cancer survivors, it is likely that additional health personnel will be needed, particularly nurses with advanced oncology training. Online resources are increasingly available and appear to be an attractive means of reaching multiple provider audiences, but the effectiveness of this and other approaches needs to be assessed. Limited financial support has been available through public and private sectors for survivorship-related education and training.

> **Recommendation 7: The National Cancer Institute (NCI), professional associations, and voluntary organizations should expand and coordinate their efforts to provide educational opportunities to health care providers to equip them to address the health care and quality of life issues facing cancer survivors.**

Efforts are needed to update undergraduate and graduate curricula for those in training and to provide continuing education for practicing providers of survivorship care. Continuing education is needed across many disciplines, but in order to ensure the provision of quality survivorship care, it is especially important to reach (1) medical oncologists, hematologists, urologists, surgeons, and radiation oncologists who initially treat cancer patients; (2) primary care physicians; (3) nurses; and (4) social workers and other providers of psychosocial services.

To augment the supply of nurses who could provide survivorship care, the committee recommends increasing the number of nursing schools that provide graduate training in oncology, providing incentives to nurses who seek certification in oncology, and supporting general efforts to ease the nursing shortage. To ensure access to psychosocial services, continuing education opportunities are needed for social workers and other mental health providers. In addition, efforts are needed to maintain social services in cancer programs. Detailed recommendations on professional education by health care specialty are outlined in Chapter 5.

ADDRESSING EMPLOYMENT-RELATED CONCERNS

Most cancer patients who are working require some kind of accommodation to work throughout treatment, and some experience difficulties at work after treatment. Estimates of the impact of cancer on employment vary. The majority of cancer survivors who worked before their diagnosis return to work following their treatment. However, as many as one in five individuals who work at the time of diagnosis have cancer-related limitations in ability to work 1 to 5 years later. Half of those with limitations are unable to work at all.

All survivors are at risk of experiencing subtle, although not necessarily blatant, employment discrimination. Federal laws enacted in the 1990s have offered cancer survivors some protections from discriminatory practices such as firing or denial of benefits because of cancer. Such laws have clarified the responsibilities of employers to accommodate workers returning to work with health-related limitations. The most important of these laws, the Americans with Disabilities Act (ADA), continues to be interpreted by the courts. Although protections cover disabled cancer survivors, some survivors have not been fully protected from job loss and access to accommodations for cancer-related work limitations. Successful resolutions on the part of cancer survivors who have filed formal complaints against employers suggest that not all employers have yet fully complied with the law.

Recommendation 8: Employers, legal advocates, health care providers, sponsors of support services, and government agencies should act to eliminate discrimination and minimize adverse effects of cancer on employment, while supporting cancer survivors with short-term and long-term limitations in ability to work.

- Cancer providers, advocacy organizations, NCI, and other government agencies should continue to educate employers and the public about the successes achieved in cancer treatment, the improved prospects for survival, and the continuing productivity of most patients who are treated for cancer.
- Public and private sponsors of services to support cancer survivors and their families should finance programs offering education, counseling, support, legal advice, vocational rehabilitation, and referral for survivors who want to work.
- Providers who care for cancer survivors should become familiar with the employment rights that apply to survivors who want to work; make available information about employment rights and programs; and routinely ask patients who are cancer survivors if they have physical or mental health problems that are affecting their work
- Employers should implement programs to assist cancer survivors, for example, through short- and long-term disability insurance, return-to-work programs, accommodation of special needs, and employee assistance programs.
- Cancer survivors should tell their physicians when health problems are affecting them at work. Survivors should educate themselves about their employment rights and contact support organizations for assistance and referrals when needed.

Improving Access to Adequate and Affordable Health Insurance

The health insurance issues facing cancer survivors bring into sharp focus the gaps and limitations of health insurance in the United States. All Americans are at risk of becoming a cancer survivor and finding themselves without access to adequate and affordable health insurance. Cancer survivors, like other Americans with serious, chronic health conditions, face significant barriers to coverage because of their health status. In particular, access to individual health insurance may be denied to residents in many states if they have a history of cancer. Cancer survivors may also face surcharged premiums for coverage because of their cancer history, depending on where they live and the type of coverage they seek. The improvements in the care of cancer survivors envisioned by the committee can not be achieved without health insurance that is accessible, adequate, and affordable.

Health insurance provides protection from the very high costs of cancer care. Most cancer survivors have health insurance through the federal Medicare programs because they are aged 65 and older. Nevertheless, 11 percent of adult cancer survivors under the age of 65 are uninsured and, for these individuals, the costs of cancer care can be financially devastating. These younger uninsured cancer survivors report access to care problems due to concerns about cost—51 percent report delays in obtaining medical care; 44 percent report not getting needed care; and 31 percent report not getting needed prescription medicine. The financial problems posed by cancer loom larger, because even those with health insurance can have trouble paying for prescription drugs and other types of care.

The IOM Committee on the Consequences of Uninsurance, in its 2004 report, *Insuring America's Health*, recommended that the President and Congress develop a strategy to achieve universal insurance coverage and to establish a firm and explicit schedule to reach this goal by 2010 (IOM, 2004).

Recommendation 9: Federal and state policy makers should act to ensure that all cancer survivors have access to adequate and affordable health insurance. Insurers and payors of health care should recognize survivorship care as an essential part of cancer care and design benefits, payment policies, and reimbursement mechanisms to facilitate coverage for evidence-based aspects of care.

Cancer survivors need continuous access to health insurance that covers their health care needs. Policy makers should act to ensure that cancer survivors and others with serious chronic health conditions can obtain health insurance that is adequate and affordable. For example, policy makers could provide federal support to improve state high-risk pools—through premium subsidies, lower cost-sharing options (e.g., lowering copayments and deductibles), expanded coverage for prescription drugs, and elimination of preexisting condition exclusion periods. This could help such programs better serve the needs of people with serious and chronic health conditions. Federal programs that guarantee availability of coverage (e.g., those provided under the Consolidated Omnibus Budget Reconciliation Act [COBRA] and the Health Insurance Portability and Accountability Act [HIPAA]) could also be expanded to include premium subsidies. Because federal legislation generally covers only federal programs such as Medicare and Medicaid, many health insurance reforms must also be addressed at the state level.

Policy makers can also improve other existing programs aimed at improving health insurance coverage of cancer survivors. In 2000, Congress established a new eligibility category option in Medicaid for uninsured women with breast and cervical cancer. However, only women screened through CDC-funded programs are eligible for this Medicaid coverage, and CDC-funded programs today reach fewer than 15 percent of the program-eligible population. Policy makers could strengthen and build on this program, first by ensuring that more eligible women with breast and cervical cancer are reached by it, and second by expanding Medicaid eligibility to include other cancer patients and survivors who have no other coverage options.

All health insurance in the United States, including Medicare, Medicaid, employer-sponsored group health plans, and individually purchased policies, should cover effective cancer survivorship care. National coverage standards should be promulgated and include interventions for which there is good evidence of effectiveness (e.g., certain post-treatment surveillance strategies, treatments for late effects, interventions for symptom management, rehabilitative services). Importantly, coverage standards should include the development of a post-treatment plan of survivorship care (see Recommendation 2). National coverage standards should evolve with the development of clinical guidelines and evidence-based research into the quality and effectiveness of care. Congress has already taken preliminary steps to assure adequacy of some cancer survivorship care. The Women's Health and Cancer Rights Act requires health insurance to cover reconstructive surgery, prostheses, and care for complications following mastectomy, including lymphedema. This model could be expanded to assure minimum federal standards for all cancer survivorship care under all health insurance.

Making Investments in Research

Within the past decade, a focus for federally sponsored research has been organized within NCI's Office of Cancer Survivorship. Findings from this first era of dedicated research have informed much of this report. A greater investment in research is needed to learn more about late effects and their management. Cancer treatments are constantly evolving, and consequently, what is known about today's cancer survivors may not be relevant to future patients. Newer therapies hold the promise of limiting the late effects of cancer, but mechanisms to monitor long-term effects need to be put in place. Also needed are studies to determine how best to detect and treat cancer recurrence, new primary cancers, and other late effects. Providers responsible for follow-up need to know which tests to use, how often to use them, and the relative costs and benefits of alternative surveillance strategies. Investments are needed in the science on which clinical decisions must be based.

Among the challenges to conducting survivorship research are the difficulties and costs associated with long-term follow-up, the complexities of accruing sufficient sample sizes through multi-institutional research endeavors, and emerging problems associated with compliance with privacy provisions of the HIPAA. Survivorship research is funded at relatively modest levels within both public and private sectors, especially as contrasted to levels of support for treatment-related research.

Recommendation 10: The National Cancer Institute (NCI), Centers for Disease Control and Prevention (CDC), Agency for Healthcare Reseach and Quality (AHRQ), Centers for Medicare and Medicaid Services (CMS), Department of Veterans Affairs (VA), private voluntary organizations such as the American Cancer Society (ACS), and private health insurers and plans should increase their support of survivorship research and expand mechanisms for its conduct. New research initiatives focused on cancer patient follow-up are urgently needed to guide effective survivorship care.

Research is especially needed to improve understanding of:

- Mechanisms of late effects experienced by cancer survivors and interventions to alleviate symptoms and improve function;
- The prevalence and risk of late effects;
- The cost-effectiveness of alternative models of survivorship care and community-based psychosocial services; and
- Interventions to improve the quality of life of cancer survivors, their families, and caregivers.

To conduct research in these priority areas, large study populations are needed that represent the diversity of cancer survivors in terms of their type of cancer and treatment as well as their sociodemographic and health care characteristics. Existing research mechanisms need to be fully utilized and in some cases enhanced to provide better opportunities for cancer survivorship research. For example:

- More long-term follow-up studies should be conducted of individuals enrolled in clinical trials through the NCI-sponsored Cooperative Groups;
- Additional survivorship special studies should be conducted through population-based cancer registries;
- National household and health care surveys should be analyzed to capture information on survivorship;
- Opportunities should be sought to link data from cancer registries to administrative databases;
- The follow-up period of ongoing cancer health services research studies should be extended to yield more information on long-term survivorship; and
- Investigators should be encouraged to use existing primary care and health services research networks to conduct cancer survivorship research.

In addition to harnessing these existing mechanisms, the committee recommends that federal (e.g., CMS, AHRQ, NCI) and private (ACS, health plans) research sponsors support a large new research initiative on cancer patient follow-up. Answers to the following basic questions about survivorship care are needed:

- How frequently should patients be evaluated following their primary cancer therapy?
- What tests should be included in the follow-up regimen?
- Who should provide follow-up care?

A call for such research was made in IOM's *Ensuring Quality Cancer Care* report (1999), but it has not yet been conducted. In some cases large clinical trials will be needed to answer these questions. The committee concluded that improvements in cancer survivors' care and quality of life depend on a much expanded research effort.

REFERENCES

CDC (Centers for Disease Control and Prevention). 2004. *National Comprehensive Cancer Control Program.* [Online]. Available: http://www.cdc.gov/cancer/ncccp/ [accessed November 29, 2004].

CDC and LAF (Lance Armstrong Foundation). 2004. *A National Action Plan for Cancer Survivorship: Advancing Public Health Strategies.* Atlanta, GA: CDC.

IOM (Institute of Medicine). 1997. *Approaching Death: Improving Care at the End of Life.* Field MJ, Cassell CK, eds. Washington, DC: National Academy Press.

IOM. 1999. *Ensuring Quality Cancer Care.* Hewitt M, Simone JV, eds. Washington, DC: National Academy Press.

IOM. 2001a. *Crossing the Quality Chasm: A New Health System for the 21st Century.* Washington, DC: National Academy Press.

IOM. 2001b. *Improving Palliative Care for Cancer.* Foley KM, Gelband H, eds. Washington, DC: National Academy Press.

IOM. 2003. *Childhood Cancer Survivorship: Improving Care and Quality of Life.* Hewitt M, Weiner SL, Simone JV, eds. Washington, DC: The National Academies Press.

IOM. 2004. *Insuring America's Health: Principles and Recommendations.* Washington, DC: National Academies Press.

Mullan F. 1985. Seasons of survival: Reflections of a physician with cancer. *N Engl J Med* 313(4):270–273.

President's Cancer Panel. 2004. *Living Beyond Cancer: Finding a New Balance.* Bethesda, MD: National Cancer Institute.

1

Introduction

The ranks of cancer survivors in the United States are 10 million strong and growing, in large part because of advances in early detection and cancer treatment. Some cancers that were once uniformly fatal, such as testicular cancer, are now cured in nearly all cases. And many of those who get common cancers—cancers of the breast, colon and rectum, and prostate—become long-term survivors. Other people may be living with a cancer such as lymphoma that is controlled with ongoing or periodic treatment, but not cured. All of these individuals can be considered survivors of their disease, and also of their treatment. All major forms of treatment—surgery, chemotherapy, hormone therapy, and radiation therapy—can have unwanted, long-term effects on tissues and organ systems that impair a person's health and quality of life in small and large ways. Increasing the risks of these late effects are the use of multiagent and intensive administrations of therapies that improve survival, but are more toxic. Some anticancer drugs are taken for extended periods—years instead of months—obscuring the delineation of the end of cancer treatment.

Each phase of survivorship brings different concerns to the fore. For many of the 1.4 million individuals diagnosed with cancer each year, resuming the routines of work and family life after completing active treatment may be especially difficult.[1] Anxiety over the possibility of cancer recurrence may dominate at this time. Questions also arise about next steps

[1]All cancer statistics presented in this report exclude non-melanoma skin cancers.

to care: Who should I see? What tests should I have? How can I manage my cancer- and treatment-related symptoms? What services are available to help me and my family cope? Half of all men and one-third of women in the United States will develop cancer in their lifetime, so these are questions many of us will face. Today, 1 in 30 Americans has a history of cancer, and among those 65 and older, the figure is 1 in 7. A new paradigm of survivorship is emerging that addresses the needs of this group and the issues that face society in providing for them—for us, in the greater sense. This Institute of Medicine (IOM) report explores this new territory and offers a plan for moving ahead.

The committee's report focuses on adult survivors of cancer during the phase of care that follows primary treatment and (1) examines the medical and psychosocial consequences of cancer and its treatment; (2) defines quality care for cancer survivors and strategies to achieve it; (3) explores social and economic hardships facing cancer survivors related to, for example, problems in insurance coverage and employment discrimination, and proposes policies to ameliorate such problems; and (4) describes how we can improve what we know about the quality of care and quality of life for cancer survivors and their families.

This study could hardly be better timed to ensure both public and policy attention. The committee's report builds on a significant body of work. In particular, the President's Cancer Panel concluded a series of public meetings and in June 2004 released its report, *Living Beyond Cancer*, with policy recommendations for consideration (President's Cancer Panel, 2004). In addition, in April 2004 the Centers for Disease Control and Prevention (CDC) and the Lance Armstrong Foundation released *A National Action Plan for Cancer Survivorship* to advance public health strategies (CDC and LAF, 2004). Cancer has recently overtaken heart disease as the leading cause of death in the United States among those under age 85 (Jemal et al., 2005), and the public views cancer as the most important health problem facing the nation (Blendon et al., 2001). Consumer advocacy organizations have long been interested in improving the care provided to cancer patients and survivors (NCCS, 1996).

ORIGINS OF THE STUDY

The idea to embark on a major study of cancer survivorship within the National Academies originated with the National Cancer Policy Board (NCPB). The NCPB was established in 1997 in the IOM and the National Research Council's Division of Earth and Life Studies at the request of the National Cancer Institute (NCI), the National Institutes of Health, and the President's Cancer Panel. The NCPB identified emerging policy issues in the nation's effort to combat cancer, and prepared reports that address those issues, including a series of reports on topics ranging from cancer prevention to end-of-life care.

The Board's first major report, *Ensuring Quality Cancer Care* (IOM, 1999), recommended strategies to promote evidenced-based, comprehensive, compassionate, and coordinated care throughout the cancer care trajectory, but its focus was on primary treatment and it did not directly address the quality of care for cancer survivors. However, it noted that such issues needed attention. This report, then, is part of a Board initiative to address quality concerns for cancer survivors with an emphasis on what happens following the primary treatment of cancer. The Board report, *Improving Palliative Care for Cancer* (IOM, 2001), addressed the need for quality care at the end of life for those who die from cancer and symptom management throughout the care trajectory.

The NCPB decided to separate its exploration of cancer survivorship into three reports. The first report examined childhood cancer survivorship (IOM, 2003a). Some policy issues are common to both children and adults who have survived cancer (e.g., insurance and employment concerns); however, unique features of pediatric treatment and health care delivery systems led to the decision to pursue childhood and adult cancer survivorship issues independently. The second report addressed one particular aspect of survivorship, focusing on psychosocial needs of survivors, using female breast cancer as the best studied example (IOM, 2004). This third report is intended as a comprehensive look at the current status and future requirements of the large and growing cohort of adult survivors. The first two reports were carried out by the NCPB itself, but the Board decided to establish a separate and independent committee for this third report in order to assemble the large number of experts needed to consider the variety and importance of issues relevant to the diverse body of adult survivors who are increasingly coming to the attention of the public, cancer care providers, and policy makers.

In its deliberations, the committee has adopted the definition of cancer survivor used by NCI's Office of Cancer Survivorship, "An individual is considered a cancer survivor from the time of diagnosis, through the balance of his or her life. Family members, friends, and caregivers are also impacted by the survivorship experience and are therefore included in this definition" (NCI, 2004). In applying this definition, however, the committee decided to focus its attention on a relatively neglected phase of the cancer care trajectory, the period following first diagnosis and treatment and prior to the development of a recurrence of the initial cancer or death. The committee identified several areas of concern for individuals during this monitoring/surveillance period, for example, the lack of clear evidence on recommended follow-up care and the unique psychosocial needs of cancer survivors following treatment, a time when frequent contact with cancer care providers often abruptly ceases. This particular phase of care has been relatively unexamined. The committee also addressed the needs of those individuals with cancer living with disease on an intermittent or chronic basis. Given prior work of the IOM on palliative care (IOM, 2001) and care at the end of life (IOM, 1997, 2003b), the committee decided to exclude these broad areas from their consideration for the purposes of this report. Also, information on the impact of cancer survivorship on family members is just beginning to emerge and consequently this report focuses more on the experience of individuals with a history of cancer.

FRAMEWORK OF THE REPORT

This report considers cancer survivorship as a medical and social condition with major economic implications, and as such it examines the long-term medical and social consequences of cancer treatment and survival and assesses the quality of care provided to cancer survivors, individuals living beyond their primary cancer treatment.

Chapter 2 characterizes adult survivors of cancer and the trends in cancer incidence and mortality that have contributed to the growth of this population.

Chapter 3 reviews the long-term consequences of cancer and its treatment, and the need for services following treatment for cancer (includes recommendations 1, 2, and 3).

Chapter 4 defines optimal care for cancer survivors; identifies barriers to the delivery of such care; describes alternative models for the delivery of comprehensive, coordinated post-treatment care; reviews what is known about the existing U.S. infrastructure for delivering survivorship care; and proposes steps to improve the delivery of survivorship care (includes recomendations 4, 5, and 6).

Chapter 5 discusses the adequacy of professional education and training on cancer survivorship (includes recommendation 7).

Chapter 6 reviews employment, insurance, and economic issues of relevance to cancer survivors (includes recommendations 8 and 9).

Chapter 7 surveys ongoing clinical and health services research aimed at improving care and outlines research strategies to prevent and ameliorate the consequences of the late effects of cancer and its treatment (includes recommendation 10).

The committee met and deliberated at three meetings—in Woods Hole, MA (July 28 and 29, 2004), Irvine, CA (October 27, 28, and 29, 2004), and Washington, DC (March 24 and 25, 2005). The committee benefited from presentations from the following individuals at their meetings:

- Karen Antman, Deputy Director for Translational and Clinical Sciences, NCI
- Noreen Aziz, Program Director, Office of Cancer Survivorship, NCI
- Peter Bach, Senior Adviser, Office of the Administrator, Centers for Medicare and Medicaid Services
- Kevin Brady, Acting Director, Division of Cancer Prevention and Control, National Center for Chronic Disease Prevention and Health Promotion, CDC
- Mark Clanton, Deputy Director, NCI
- Robert Hiatt, Director of Population Science and Deputy Director of the University of California-San Franscisco (UCSF) Comprehensive Cancer Center
- Margaret Kripke, member, President's Cancer Panel member and Chief Academic Officer, M.D. Anderson Cancer Center
- Julia Rowland, Director, Office of Cancer Survivorship, NCI
- Jerome Yates, National Vice President for Research, American Cancer Society

The committee benefited from estimates of conditional survival produced by Eric Feurer and colleagues at the National Cancer Institute. The committee also benefited from analyses completed by Robert Friedland and colleagues at the Georgetown Center on an Aging Society on cancer-related medical expenditures as reported in the Medical Expenditure Panel Survey (see Chapter 6).

REFERENCES

Blendon RJ, Scoles K, DesRoches C, Young JT, Herrmann MJ, Schmidt JL, Kim M. 2001. Americans' health priorities: Curing cancer and controlling costs. *Health Aff (Millwood)* 20(6):222–232.

CDC and LAF (Centers for Disease Control and Prevention and the Lance Armstrong Foundation). 2004. *A National Action Plan for Cancer Survivorship: Advancing Public Health Strategies.* Atlanta, GA: CDC.

IOM (Institute of Medicine). 1997. *Approaching Death: Improving Care at the End of Life.* Field MJ, Cassell CK, eds. Washington, DC: National Academy Press.

IOM. 1999. *Ensuring Quality Cancer Care.* Hewitt M, Simone JV, eds. Washington, DC: National Academy Press.

IOM. 2001. *Improving Palliative Care for Cancer.* Foley KM, Gelband H, eds. Washington, DC: National Academy Press.

IOM. 2003a. *Childhood Cancer Survivorship: Improving Care and Quality of Life.* Hewitt M, Weiner SL, Simone JV, eds. Washington, DC: The National Academies Press.

IOM. 2003b. *Describing Death in America: What We Need to Know.* Lunney JR, Foley KM, Smith TJ, Gelband H, eds. Washington, DC: The National Academies Press.

IOM. 2004. *Meeting Psychosocial Needs of Women with Breast Cancer.* Hewitt M, Herdman R, Holland J, eds. Washington, DC: The National Academies Press.

Jemal A, Murray T, Ward E, Samuels A, Tiwari RC, Ghafoor A, Feuer EJ, Thun MJ. 2005. Cancer statistics, 2005. *CA Cancer J Clin* 55(1):10–30.

NCCS (National Coalition for Cancer Survivorship). 1996. *Imperatives for Quality Cancer Care: Access, Advocacy, Action, and Accountability*. Clark EJ, Stovall EL, Leigh S, Siu AL, Austin DK, Rowland JH. Silver Spring, MD: NCCS.

NCI (National Cancer Institute). 2004. *About Survivorship Research: Survivorship Definitions*. [Online]. Available: http://dccps.nci.nih.gov/ocs/definitions.html [accessed April 9, 2004].

President's Cancer Panel. 2004. *Living Beyond Cancer: Finding a New Balance*. Bethesda, MD: National Cancer Institute.

2

Cancer Survivors

Who are cancer survivors and what does cancer survivorship mean? The terms have different meanings to different people, and how to refer to this growing population has stirred some controversy. The recent report of the President's Cancer Panel describes some of the issues associated with the definition (Box 2-1).

This section of the report reviews the history and conceptual development of the terms "cancer survivor" and "survivorship." In addition, some of the clinical and sociodemographic characteristics of cancer survivors are described using epidemiological data from the National Cancer Institute (NCI). Some attention is paid to the definitions developed by the National Coalition for Cancer Survivorship (NCCS) and NCI's Office of Cancer Survivorship, for they have been adopted by the committee. While adopting these definitions, the committee decided to focus much of its attention on a particular period of survivorship—the period following first diagnosis and treatment and prior to the development of a recurrence of cancer or death. This period of survivorship represents a distinct phase of the cancer control continuum that has not been well described (Box 2-2). Chapter 4 discusses in further detail the trajectory of cancer care and provides more detail on the committee's rationale for focusing on this particular phase of survivorship.

DEFINING CANCER SURVIVORS AND SURVIVORSHIP

The NCI and the Centers for Disease Control and Prevention (CDC) estimate that as of 2002 there were 10.1 million living persons who had

BOX 2-1
Who Is a Cancer Survivor?

Among health professionals, people with a cancer history, and the public, views differ as to when a person with cancer becomes a survivor. Many consider a person to be a survivor from the moment of diagnosis; in recent years, this view has become increasingly prevalent. Some, however, think that a person with a cancer diagnosis cannot be considered a survivor until he or she completes initial treatment. Others believe a person with cancer can be considered a survivor if he or she lives 5 years beyond diagnosis. Still others believe survivorship begins at some other point after diagnosis or treatment, and some reject the term "survivor" entirely, preferring to think of people with a cancer history as fighters, "thrivers," champions, patients, or simply as individuals who have had a life-threatening disease. A considerable number of people with a cancer history maintain that they will have survived cancer if they die from another cause.

SOURCE: President's Cancer Panel (2004b).

BOX 2-2
The Cancer Control Continuum

Prevention	Early Detection	Diagnosis	Treatment	Survivorship	End-of-Life Care
-Tobacco control -Diet -Physical activity -Sun exposure -Virus exposure -Alcohol use -Chemoprevention	-Cancer screening -Awareness of cancer signs and symptoms	-Oncology consultations -Tumor staging -Patient counseling and decision making	-Chemotherapy -Surgery -Radiation therapy -Adjuvant therapy -Symptom management -Psychosocial care	-Long-term follow-up/surveillance -Late-effects management -Rehabilitation -Coping -Health promotion	-Palliation -Spiritual issues -Hospice

The cancer control continuum has been used at least since the mid-1970s to describe the various points from cancer prevention, early detection, diagnosis, treatment, survivorship, and end of life. The continuum has changed somewhat over time. Because survivors are now a large and growing population, survivorship has been added to the continuum. Rehabilitation was once a specific phase; now it is generally considered part of treatment and survivorship care.

Like many other useful concepts, the continuum is oversimplified. As modern biology has changed our understanding of cancer, it is now recognized that the categories are useful labels, but the processes are not so discrete. For example, colonoscopy is now recognized as both a screening test for colon cancer and a prevention strategy if polyps are found. Moreover, many topics are cross-cutting. For example, communication, decision making, quality of care, and health disparities are of concern at each point along the continuum.

SOURCE: Adapted from National Cancer Institute figure on the "Cancer Control Continuum" (NCI, 2005a).

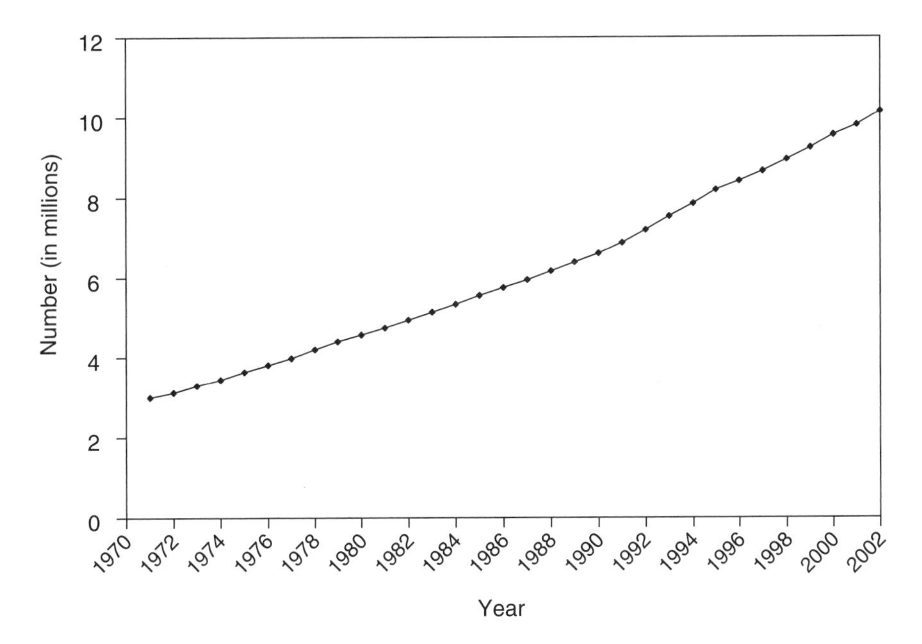

FIGURE 2-1 Estimated number of cancer survivors in the United States from 1971 to 2002.
DATA SOURCES: U.S. prevalence counts were estimated by applying U.S. population counts to SEER 9 Limited Duration Prevalence proportions and historical Connecticut Limited Duration Prevalence proportions and adjusted to represent complete prevalence (2004 submission). Complete prevalence is estimated using the completeness index method (Capocaccia and De Angelis, 1997; Merrill et al., 2000). Populations from January 2002 were based on the average of the July 2001 and July 2002 population estimates from the U.S. Census Bureau.
SOURCE: NCI (2005c).

ever received a diagnosis of cancer (NCI, 2005c). This represents a tripling of the number of survivors since 1971 (Figure 2-1). Much of this increase can be traced to the advent of widespread screening for breast, cervical, and prostate cancers, which identified many more cases of early disease. Advances in treatment also account for a portion of the increase, albeit to a lesser extent (Welch et al., 2000a,b).

Only since the mid-1970s have half of individuals diagnosed with cancer been expected to be alive 5 years following their diagnosis (Rowland et

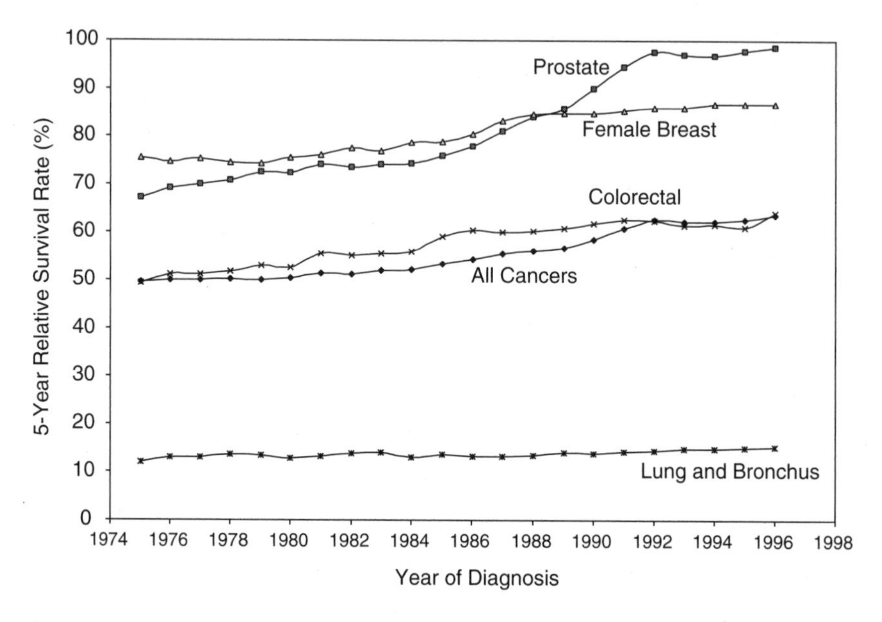

FIGURE 2-2 Five-year relative survival rates.
SOURCE: NCI (2004c).

al., 2004). By the late 1990s, the overall 5-year relative survival rate[1] had increased to 64 percent (Ries et al., 2004) (Figure 2-2). When cancer was considered incurable, the term "survivor" applied to the family members whose loved one died from the disease (Leigh, 2004). As improvements in treatment occurred in the 1960s, physicians began to refer to "cancer survivors" as those who had survived 5 years past their diagnosis or treatment, a time when the risk of a recurrent cancer had diminished substantially (Leigh, 2004).

The number of survivors of cancer is expected to balloon with the anticipated growth of the U.S. population and the aging of the baby boom cohort (individuals born between the years 1946 to 1964) (Yancik, 1997; Cheeseman Day, 2001). In 2011, the first members of this group will reach age 65, the age at which the risk of cancer steadily rises. From 2000 to

[1]For cancer, the relative survival rate is calculated by adjusting the survival rate to remove all causes of death except cancer. The rate is determined at specific time intervals, such as 5 years after diagnosis. Relative survival is defined as the ratio of the proportion of observed survivors in a cohort of cancer patients to the proportion of expected survivors in a comparable set of cancer-free individuals. The formulation is based on the assumption of independent competing causes of death.

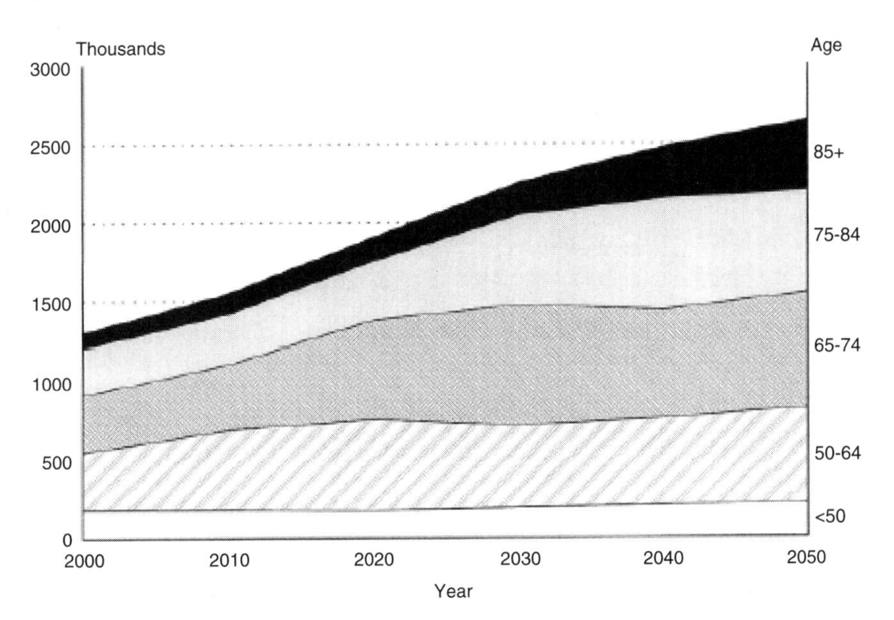

FIGURE 2-3 Projected number of cancer cases for 2000 through 2050. Projections based on (1) U.S. Census Bureau population projections (2000–2050) and (2) age-specific cancer incidence rates (1995–1999) from the Surveillance, Epidemiology, and End Results (SEER) Program and the National Program of Cancer Registries (NPCR), 1995–1999.
SOURCE: Edwards et al. (2002). Reprinted by permission of Wiley-Liss, Inc., a subsidiary of John Wiley & Sons, Inc. *Cancer* 94(10):2766–2792. Copyright © 2002. American Cancer Society.

2050, the absolute number of people aged 65 and older diagnosed with cancer is expected to double (Figure 2-3) (Edwards et al., 2002). This estimate is based on applying current cancer incidence rates to Census Bureau population projections. If accurate, these estimates would indicate that the number of cancer survivors will grow at an even greater rate than incident cancers, putting great demands on service providers and systems of care.

As the number of cancer survivors increased throughout the 1970s and 1980s, a cancer survivorship advocacy community emerged and identified medical, psychosocial, economic, and legal issues related to their history of cancer. The National Coalition for Cancer Survivorship (NCCS), a cancer advocacy group founded in 1986, defined cancer survivorship as "the experience of living with, through, and beyond a diagnosis of cancer" (NCCS, 1996). Full articulation of the concept of "cancer survivorship" can be traced to a 1985 article written by one of NCCS's founders, Fitzhugh

Mullan, in the *New England Journal of Medicine* (Mullan, 1985). It describes his personal experience as a cancer survivor.

> Actuarial and population-based figures give us survival estimates for various cancers, but those figures do not speak to the individual patient, whose experience is unique and not determined or described by aggregate data. Many patients are "cured" long before they pass the five-year mark, and others go well beyond the five-year point with overt or covert disease that removes them from the ranks of the "cured," no matter how well they feel. Survival is a much more useful concept, because it is a generic idea that applies to everyone diagnosed as having cancer, regardless of the course of the illness. Survival, in fact, begins at the point of diagnosis, because that is the time when patients are forced to confront their own mortality and begin to make adjustments that will be part of their immediate, and to some extent, long-term future (Mullan, 1985).

Mullan described three "seasons" of survival, each with unique sets of concerns:

1. **Acute survival** begins with the diagnosis of the illness and is dominated by diagnostic and therapeutic efforts. Fear and anxiety are important and constant elements of this phase.
2. **Extended survival** is a period during which a patient goes into remission or has terminated the basic, rigorous course of treatment and enters a phase of watchful waiting, with periodic examinations and "consolidation" or intermittent therapy. Psychologically, this time is dominated by fear of recurrence. This is usually a period of physical limitations since the tumor and treatment have exacted a corporal price. Diminished strength, fatigue, a reduced capacity for exercise, amputation of a body part, or hair loss may have occurred in the acute phase, but now they must be dealt with in the home, the community, and the workplace.
3. **Permanent survival** is roughly equated with "cure," but the person who has come through a cancer experience is indelibly affected by it. Problems with employment and insurance are common for persons who have been treated for cancer and are ready to resume a full life. The long-term, secondary effects of cancer treatment on health represent another area in which permanent survivors are at risk.

Welch-McCaffrey and colleagues (1989) further developed the concept of survivorship and described several potential cancer survival trajectories:

- Live cancer free for many years
- Live long cancer free, but die rapidly of late recurrence
- Live cancer free (first cancer), but develop second primary cancer

- Live with intermittent periods of active disease
- Live with persistent disease
- Live after expected death

This new focus on both the short- and long-term consequences of cancer represented a radical departure from earlier conceptualizations of survivorship. These consequences include changes in self-concepts and personal horizons, modifications in social relationships, and considerations of costs of treatment and follow-up.

NCI established an Office of Cancer Survivorship in 1996. The Office of Cancer Survivorship adopted the NCCS definition of a cancer survivor (NCI, 2004b):

> An individual is considered a cancer survivor from the time of diagnosis, through the balance of his or her life. Family members, friends, and caregivers are also impacted by the survivorship experience and are therefore included in this definition.

While adopting this broad definition, the Office of Cancer Survivorship decided to focus its research on the post-acute diagnosis and treatment phase of cancer care.

> Cancer Survivorship research encompasses the physical, psychosocial, and economic sequelae of cancer diagnosis and its treatment among both pediatric and adult survivors of cancer. It also includes within its domain, issues related to health care delivery, access, and follow up care, as they relate to survivors. Survivorship research focuses on the health and life of a person with a history of cancer beyond the acute diagnosis and treatment phase. It seeks to both prevent and control adverse cancer diagnosis and treatment-related outcomes such as late effects of treatment, second cancers, and poor quality of life, to provide a knowledge base regarding optimal follow-up care and surveillance of cancers, and to optimize health after cancer treatment (NCI, 2004b).

Even if survivorship is defined to begin with the post-treatment period, advances in treatment have obscured when this phase of care begins (Marcus, 2004). Although some have considered cancer survivors to be those who have completed the traditional treatments for cancer—radiation, chemotherapy, or surgery—adjuvant care and treatments such as tamoxifen may now be given to patients for years.

Further complicating the definition of survivors are the consequences of cancer screening. Among those counted as "survivors" are people treated for cancers that would never have come to light clinically, but were diagnosed after a positive screening test (so-called "latent disease"). Men with early-stage prostate cancer diagnosed following prostate-specific antigen (PSA) screening are probably the largest and fastest growing such group today. In addition, mammography leads to the identification of many cases of ductal carcinoma in situ (DCIS), a cancer that typically remains indolent if left untreated. In both cases, it is difficult at the diagnosis stage to separate which cancers will progress and which will not.[2] Physicians are likely to recommend treatment for everyone in these categories, and most will elect to be treated. As "survivors," they may be at a very different risk for certain events—particularly recurrences—but at equal risk for adverse effects of treatment. Until better diagnostic and prognostic tools become available, these "survivors" of treatment for cancers identified through screening programs will continue to join the ranks of the larger survivor pool.

Aside from the inherent clinical vagaries associated with survivorship, some so-called cancer survivors find the term objectionable because it is so closely associated with the Holocaust or victims of violent crime such as rape (Marcus, 2004). Some people may not want to be labeled as a survivor, and reject the notion that they are different than anyone else. "Survivor" in the context of cancer may be an American construct. The President's Cancer Panel found in its report, *Living Beyond Cancer: A European Dialogue*, that Europeans rarely use the term "survivor" to refer to life beyond a cancer diagnosis (President's Cancer Panel, 2004a). Having cancer still carries a heavy social stigma in Europe and so may not be discussed at all. Europeans and others, however, are increasingly viewing survivorship as an important topic for research and health care.

CHARACTERISTICS OF CANCER SURVIVORS

For statistical purposes, cancer survivors are "prevalent cases"[3] and estimates of the number and characteristics of cancer survivors are derived using incidence and survival information from cancer registries overseen by NCI, called the Surveillance, Epidemiology, and End Results (SEER) Program.[4]

---

[2]Improvements in presymptomatic diagnosis can be expected from many quarters, particularly the Human Genome Project. It is likely that the definition of cancer itself will change. The diagnosis of cancer has always been based on the appearance of the tissue under a microscope, but with improved understanding of the genetic changes in a given cancer, diagnosis and treatment planning could potentially be individualized and thus optimized for each patient.

[3]Prevalent cases are the number of existing cases of a particular disease at a point in time, as opposed to the number of new cases diagnosed in a period of time (incident cases) (Mausner and Kramer, 1985).

[4]NCI's SEER Program is an authoritative source of information on cancer incidence and survival in the United States. The SEER Program currently collects and publishes cancer incidence and survival data from 14 population-based cancer registries and 3 supplemental registries covering approximately 26 percent of the U.S. population (NCI, 2004a).

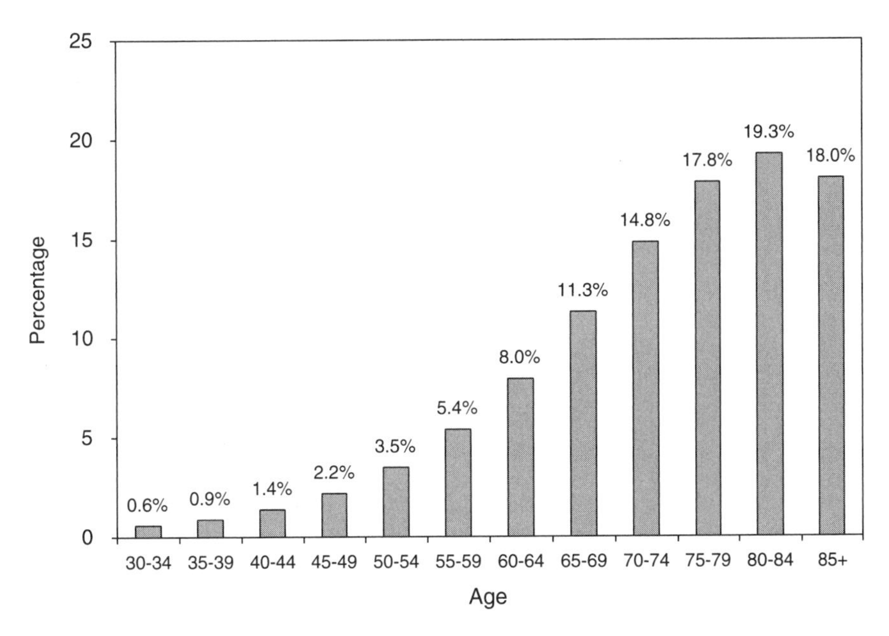

FIGURE 2-4 Cancer prevalence by age, 2002.
SOURCE: NCI (2005b).

The prevalence of cancer is calculated as the number of prevalent cases per total population. Cancer prevalence rises sharply with age as is shown in Figure 2-4. By age 40 to 44, an estimated 1.4 percent of the U.S. population has a history of cancer. This rises steadily by age, and by age 80 to 84, the prevalence of cancer is 19.3 percent (prevalence is 15 percent for those aged 65 and older; 3.5 percent for the total U.S. population). These estimates are limited to prevalent cases diagnosed within the past 27 years.

Type of Cancer

According to the most recent estimates for 2002, the most frequent sites for invasive primary cancer among survivors were breast cancer among women (22 percent), prostate cancer among men (18 percent), and colorectal cancer (10 percent) (Figure 2-5). Half (50 percent) of cancer survivors had a history of one of these cancers. Figures 2-6 and 2-7 show the distribution of prevalent cases by type of cancer and by gender. Among male cancer survivors the three leading types of cancer are prostate cancer (41 percent), colorectal cancer (11 percent), and cancer of the urinary bladder (8 percent). Among female cancer survivors the three leading types of cancer are

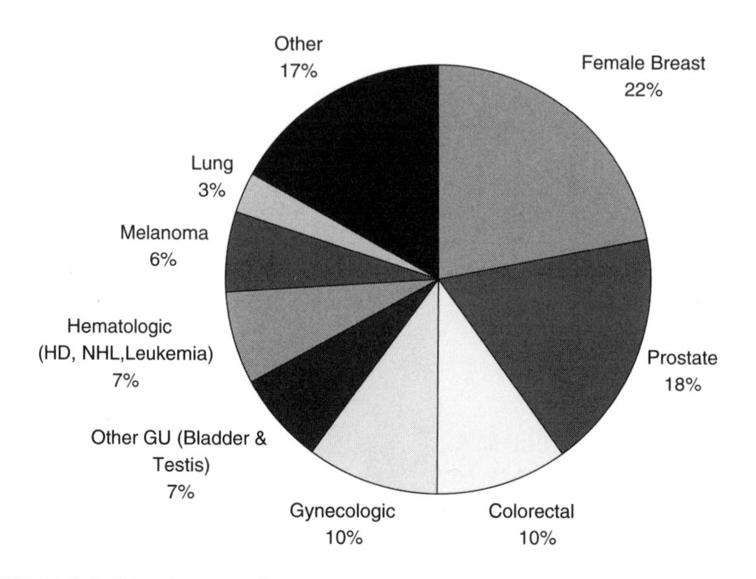

FIGURE 2-5 Distribution of cancer survivors in the U.S. by site, 2002.
DATA SOURCE: U.S. prevalence counts were estimated by applying U.S. population counts to SEER 9 and historical Connecticut Limited Duration Prevalence proportions and adjusted to represent complete prevalence (2004 submission). Complete prevalence is estimated using the completeness index method (Capocaccia and De Angelis, 1997; Merrill et al., 2000). Populations from January 2002 were based on the average of the July 2001 and July 2002 population estimates from the U.S. Census Bureau. The size of the survivorship population was 10.1 million. HD = Hodgkin's disease, NHL = non-Hodgkin's lymphoma, GU = genital or urinary. Gynecologic includes cancer of the cervix, corpus uteri, and ovary.
SOURCE: NCI (2005c).

breast cancer (40 percent), cancers of the corpus and uterus (excluding the cervix, 10 percent), and colorectal cancer (10 percent).

Age

As of 2002, more than one-third (38 percent) of survivors were of working age (ages 20 to 64), and 5 percent were in their primary reproductive years (ages 20 to 39) (Figure 2-8). Most (61 percent) cancer survivors were over the age of 65 and therefore eligible for Medicare coverage. Survivors of childhood cancer who are under age 20 make up a small fraction of all cancer survivors (1 percent).

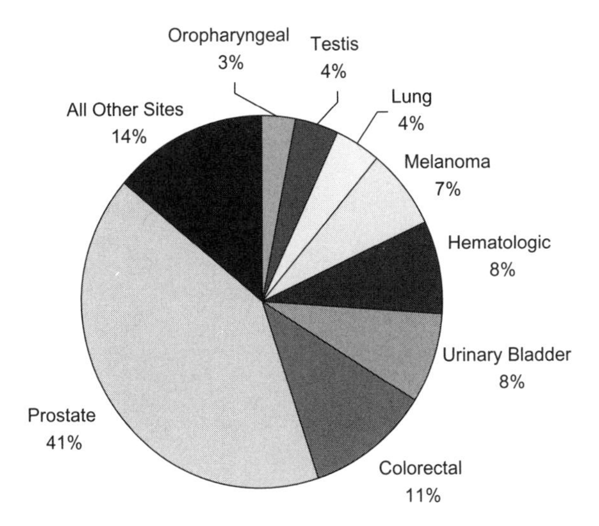

FIGURE 2-6 Distribution of male cancer survivors in the U.S. by site, 2002.

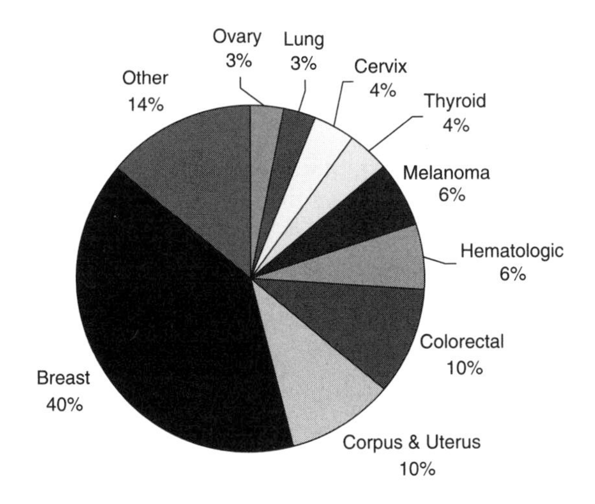

FIGURE 2-7 Distribution of female cancer survivors in the U.S. by site, 2002.
DATA SOURCES: U.S. prevalence counts were estimated by applying U.S. population counts to SEER 9 and historical Connecticut Limited Duration Prevalence proportions and adjusted to represent complete prevalence (2004 submission). Complete prevalence is estimated using the completeness index method (Capocaccia and De Angelis, 1997; Merrill et al., 2000). Populations from January 2002 were based on the average of the July 2001 and July 2002 population estimates from the U.S. Census Bureau. The estimated size of the survivorship population in 2002 was 10.1 million (men: N = 4.5 million; women: N = 5.6 million).
SOURCE: NCI (2005c).

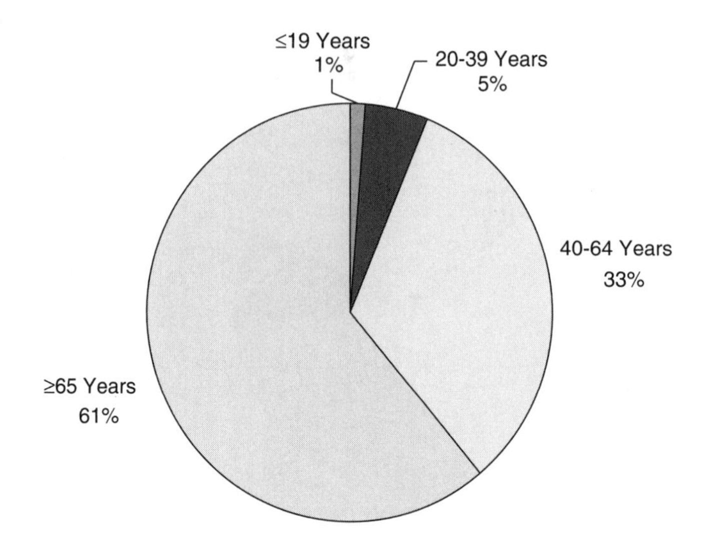

FIGURE 2-8 Estimated percentage of persons alive in the U.S. diagnosed with cancer by current age, 2002.
DATA SOURCES: U.S. prevalence counts were estimated by applying U.S. population counts to SEER 9 and historical Connecticut Limited Duration Prevalence proportions and adjusted to represent complete prevalence (2004 submission). Complete prevalence is estimated using the completeness index method (Capocaccia and De Angelis, 1997; Merrill et al., 2000). Populations from January 2002 were based on the average of the July 2001 and July 2002 population estimates from the U.S. Census Bureau. Includes invasive/first primary cases only. The estimated size of the survivorship population in 2002 was 10.1 million.
SOURCE: NCI (2005c).

Years Since Diagnosis

Most cancer survivors (62 percent) had their cancer diagnosed within the previous 10 years (Figure 2-9). Females are more likely to be long-term cancer survivors, with 19 percent diagnosed 20 or more years ago. Among male survivors, 8 percent were diagnosed 20 or more years ago.

Racial, Ethnic, and Economic Characteristics

Individuals who are poor and members of medically underserved groups are less likely to be represented among cancer survivors. When diagnosed with cancer, such individuals are more likely to be diagnosed at later cancer stages, to have worse treatment outcomes, and to experience a shortened period of survival (IOM, 2003). Health disparities arise from a

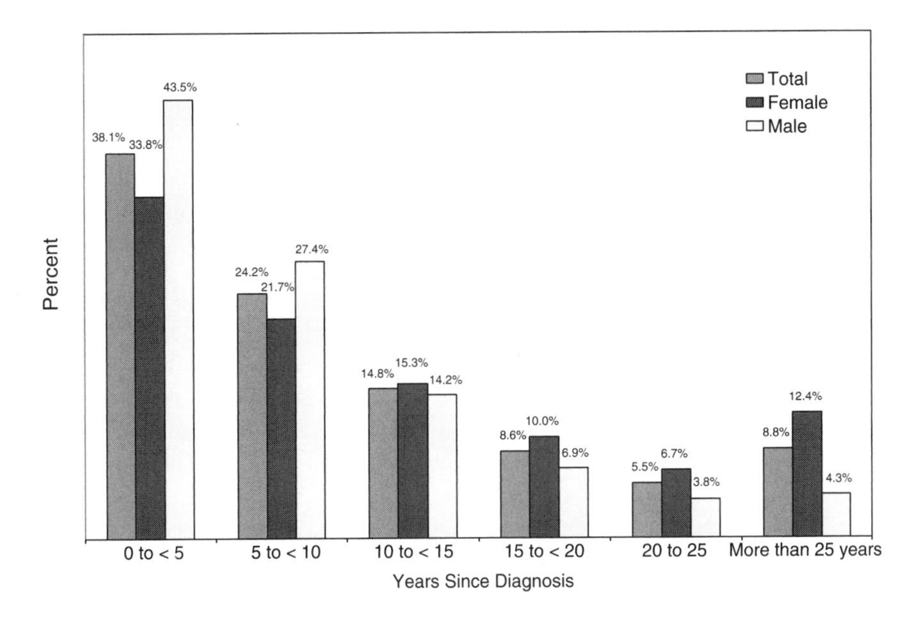

FIGURE 2-9 Distribution of cancer survivors by year since diagnosis, 2002.
DATA SOURCES: U.S. prevalence counts were estimated by applying U.S. populations to SEER 9 and historical Connecticut Limited Duration Prevalence proportions and adjusted to represent complete prevalence (2004 submission). Complete prevalence is estimated using the completeness index method (Capocaccia and De Angelis, 1997; Merrill et al., 2000). Populations from January 2002 were based on the average of the July 2001 and July 2002 population estimates from the U.S. Census Bureau. Includes invasive/first primary cases only. The estimated size of the survivorship population in 2002 was 10.1 million.
SOURCE: NCI (2005c).

complex interplay of economic, social, and cultural factors, with poverty being a key determinant of poor outcomes (Freeman, 2003). In general, when compared to non-Hispanic whites, members of racial and ethnic minority groups are more likely to be poor, have lower education levels, lack health insurance coverage, and have no source of primary care (ACS, 2004a). Cultural factors, including language, values, traditions, and trust in providers, can influence underlying risk factors, health behaviors, beliefs about illness, and approaches to medical care. Social inequities and racial discrimination can also influence the interactions between patients and physicians (IOM, 2003). Racial and ethnic disparities in the receipt of cancer treatment have been documented that could not be completely explained by racial/ethnic variation in clinically relevant factors (Shavers and Brown, 2002). The consequences of these treatment disparities include more frequent recurrence, shorter disease-free survival, and higher mortality rates. The unequal burden of cancer has been widely recognized and efforts are underway to reduce the gaps in access to care that often contribute to the resultant excess cancer morbidity and mortality (ACS, 2004a). These efforts include interventions to reduce cancer risk factors, improve screening, and improve access to state-of-the-art medical care, including diagnosis and cancer treatment.

This section of the chapter summarizes information on survival for certain racial and ethnic groups provided by the American Cancer Society (Ward et al., 2004; ACS, 2004a).[5] Compared to whites and other racial ethnic groups, African-American men and women have the highest mortality rates for all cancer sites combined (Figure 2-10). African Americans have the highest overall incidence rates among men but, among women, whites have the highest incidence rates.

As a group, African Americans are underrepresented in the cancer survivor population—they made up approximately 13 percent of the U.S. population in 2000 (Grieco and Cassidy, 2001; Ingram et al., 2003), but only 8 percent of the survivor population. Furthermore, among cancer survivors in 2000, African Americans are less likely than whites to be long-term survivors (29 percent versus 38 percent had survived 10 years or more).

Cancer registries do not routinely collect information on an individual's educational attainment, income, and other socioeconomic characteristics, so it is not possible to use registry data to analyze cancer statistics by individual socioeconomic status. However, the relationship between cancer survival and the areawide poverty level of an individual's residence has been examined (Singh et al., 2003). Across all racial and ethnic groups, the 5-year survival rate is more than 10 percent higher for persons who live in affluent census tracts (tracts with less than 10 percent of the population below the poverty line) than for persons who live in poorer census tracts (tracts with more than 20 percent of the population below the poverty line) (Figures 2-11 and 2-12). Racial and ethnic differences persist, however, when county poverty level is accounted for, especially for African Americans.

---

[5]This summary focuses on the implications of health disparities on the makeup of the cancer survivor population. For a more complete review of cancer-related disparities, see the reviews cited.

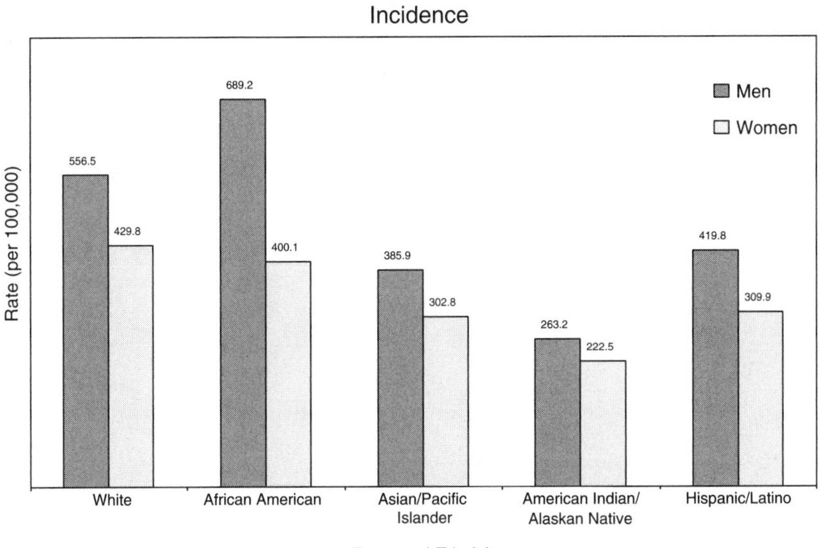

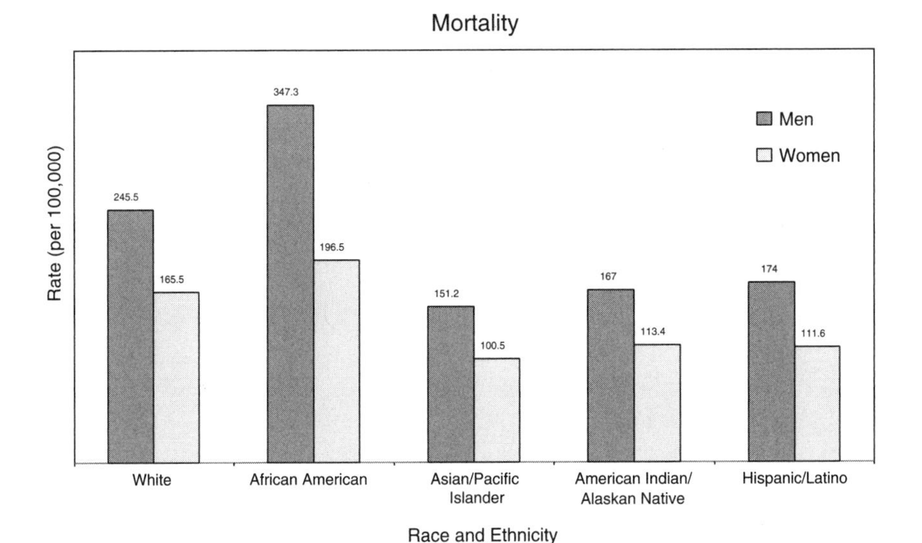

FIGURE 2-10 Age-standardized incidence and death rates, by race and ethnicity, U.S., 1997 to 2001. Rates are age adjusted to the 2000 U.S. standard population. Hispanics/Latinos are not mutually exclusive from whites, African Americans, Asian/Pacific Islanders, and American Indians/Alaskan Natives.
SOURCE: Jemal et al. (2005).

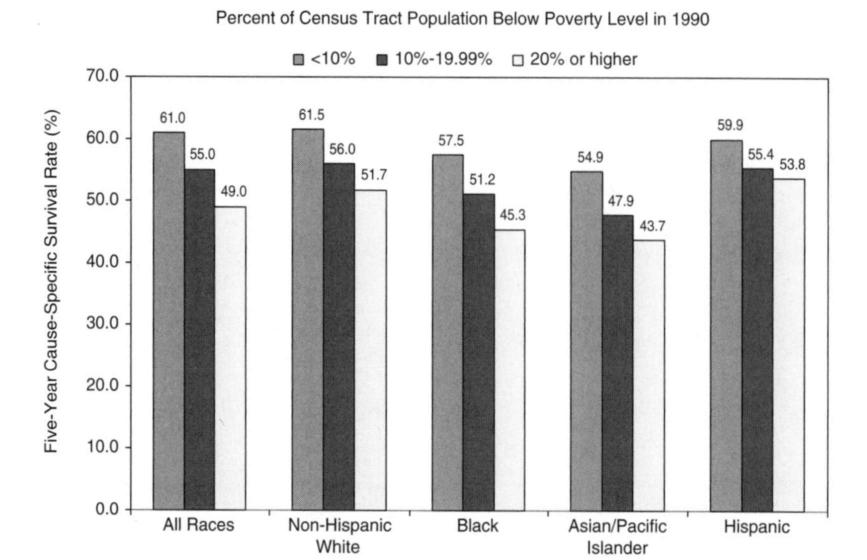

FIGURE 2-11 Cancer survival among men, all sites combined, 1988–1994. Based on data from 11 SEER registries.
SOURCE: Singh et al. (2003).

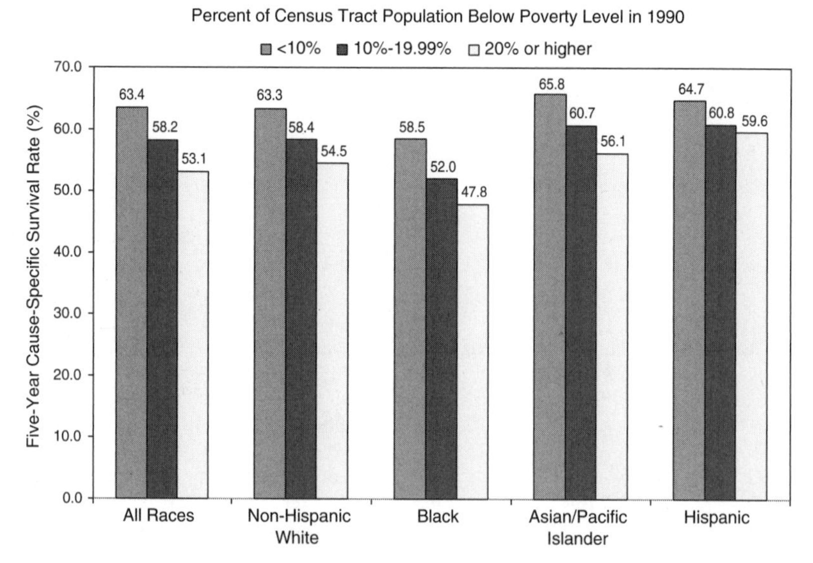

FIGURE 2-12 Cancer survival among women, all sites combined, 1988–1994. Based on data from 11 SEER registries.
SOURCE: Adapted from Singh et al. (2003).

Disability

Disability among older adults is now caused primarily by chronic disease (Ostir et al., 1999). In large studies of physical disability in the community setting, self-report has traditionally been employed to assess the degree of difficulty individuals face in self-maintenance and active involvement in the community (Ostir et al., 1999). The Activities of Daily Living (ADLs) and Instrumental Activities of Daily Living (IADLs) scales are the two most commonly used measures to assess physical disability. ADL items cover basic mobility and activities required for community living (e.g., bathing, dressing, using the toilet, transferring from bed to chair, feeding, walking). Difficulty in performing ADLs can reflect serious health problems, and ADLs are the most frequently used indicators of the ability to live independently. IADLs are intended to identify individuals who are having difficulty performing important activities of living and who may be at risk for loss of independence. The items shown in Box 2-3 are activities that are frequently measured IADLs.

Information on the health and disability status of cancer survivors is available from the National Health Interview Survey (NHIS). However, only those residing in households and well enough to participate in the Survey are interviewed for important components of the Survey. Another limitation of the NHIS is that cancer cases are self-reported and not validated with medical records or cancer registry data. A strength of these data are that they provide estimates that are population based and nationally representative. Analyses of the 1998–2000 NHIS provide information on the prevalence of disability among those reporting a history of cancer (Hewitt et al., 2003). According to these national survey data, adults who

BOX 2-3
Instrumental Activities of Daily Living Items

- Using the telephone
- Driving a car or traveling alone on a bus or taxi
- Shopping
- Preparing meals
- Doing light housework
- Taking medicine
- Handling money
- Doing heavy housework
- Walking up and down stairs
- Walking half a mile without help

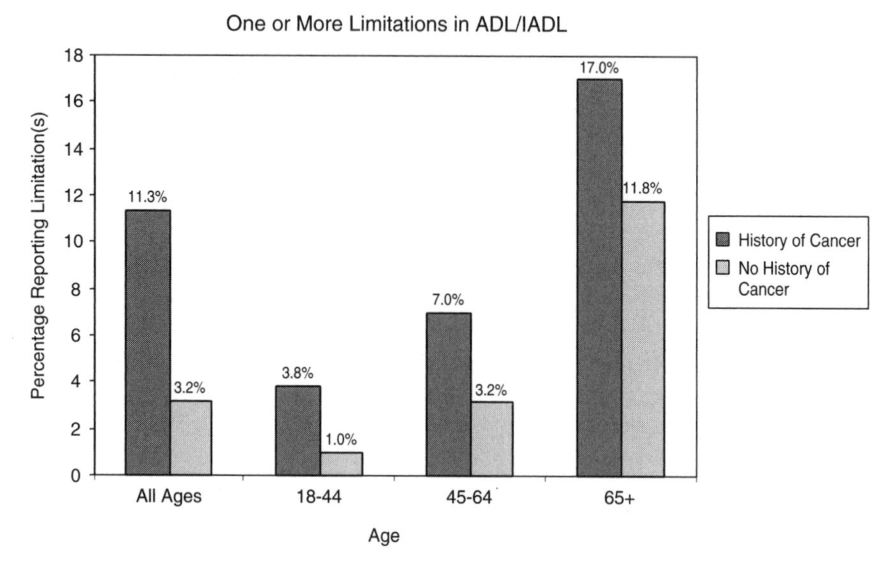

FIGURE 2-13 Limitations in ADL/IADL in cancer survivors versus those with no history of cancer. Data include individuals reporting one or more limitations in ADL/IADL. Individuals with limitations in ADLs include those who reported needing the help of other persons with personal care needs, such as eating, bathing, dressing, or getting around inside the home because of a physical, mental, or emotional problem. Limitations in IADLs included needing the help of other persons in handling routine needs, such as everyday household chores, doing necessary business, shopping, or getting around for other purposes because of a physical, mental, or emotional problem.
SOURCE: Hewitt et al. (2003).

report a history of cancer have higher levels of disability relative to the general population (Figures 2-13 and 2-14). By age group, they are more likely to report having limitations in ADLs (e.g., personal care needs) and functional limitations (e.g., walking, participating in social activities) (see Chapter 6 for a description of work limitations).

Results from other large, nationally representative surveys also associate a history of cancer with relatively high rates of disability (McNeil and Binette, 2001). In 1999, 2 percent of individuals with a history of cancer reported cancer as a main cause of disabilities, including ADL/IADLs, functional limitations, and work limitations. This finding came from the Census Bureau's Survey of Income and Program Participation in which 36,700 households were represented. Cancer ranked 13th of the conditions most associated with disability (the leading causes of disability were arthritis or rheumatism, back or spine problems, and heart trouble).

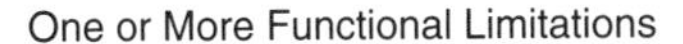

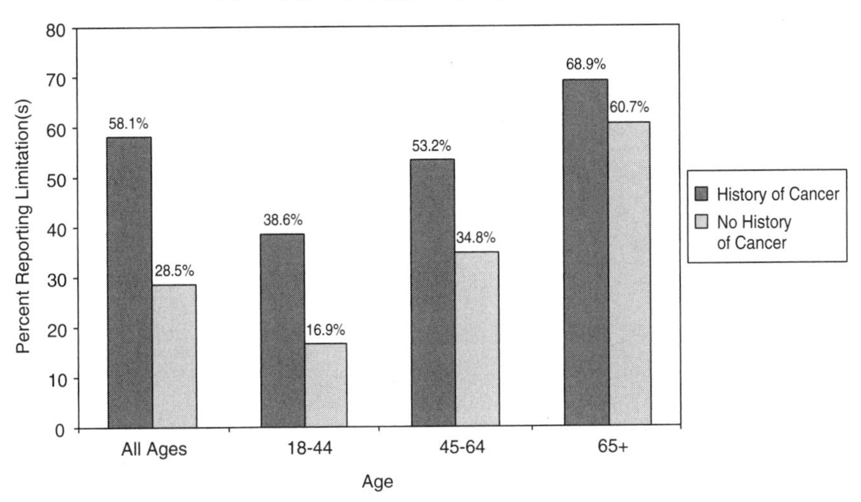

FIGURE 2-14 Functional limitations in cancer survivors versus those with no history of cancer. Data include individuals reporting one or more functional limitations. Functional limitations include those having any degree of difficulty without using any special equipment with walking a quarter of a mile; walking up 10 steps without resting; standing or being on your feet for about 2 hours; sitting for about 2 hours; stooping, bending, or kneeling; reaching up over head; using fingers to grasp or handle small objects; lifting or carrying something as heavy as 10 pounds; pushing or pulling large objects; going out to do things such as shopping, movies, or sporting events; participating in social activities, such as visiting friends, attending clubs and meetings, going to parties, and relaxing at home or for leisure.
SOURCE: Hewitt et al. (2003).

Comorbidity

The term "comorbidity" refers to the co-occurrence of two disorders or syndromes (not symptoms) in the same patient (Yates, 2001; Krishnan et al., 2002). Comorbidities are causally unrelated to the primary diagnosis and so exclude complications of the primary diagnosis or its treatment. The presence of comorbid conditions can affect treatment options, survival, and risk of late effects. In some cases, the factor contributing to the development of cancer (e.g., smoking, obesity) can contribute as well to comorbid disorders (e.g., heart disease).

Cancer survivors often report having comorbid chronic illnesses, in part because many are elderly (Yates, 2001; Yancik et al., 2001a). To learn more about the prevalence of comorbid illness among individuals with cancer and to the assess the implications of comorbidity on cancer out-

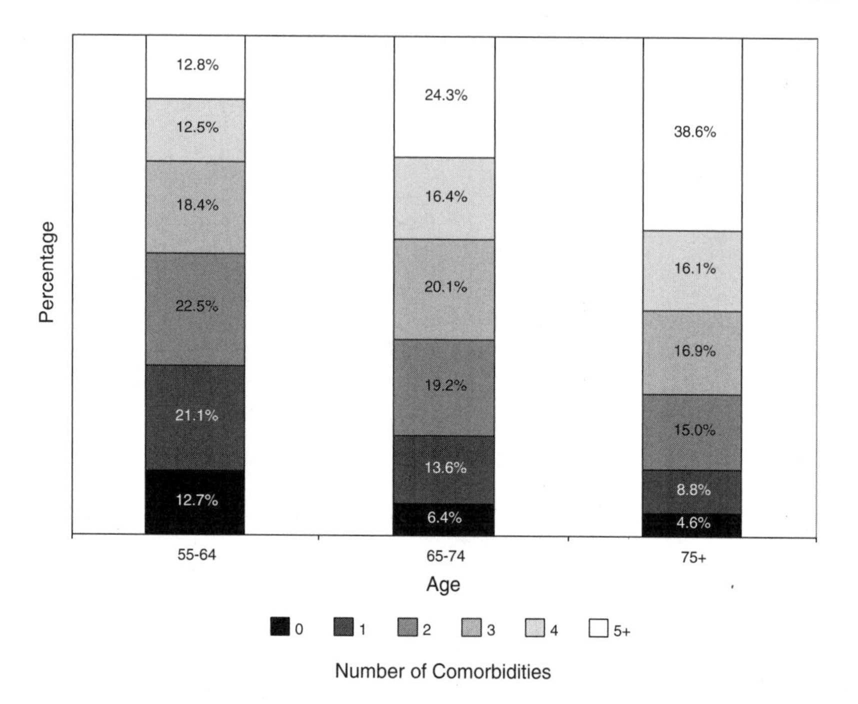

FIGURE 2-15 Number and percentage of chronic conditions among cancer patients, by age group.
SOURCE: Adapted from Yancik (1997).

comes, the National Institute on Aging (NIA) and NCI co-sponsored the SEER Collaborative Study on Comorbidity and Cancer in the Elderly (Yancik, 1997).[6] As expected, the prevalence and number of chronic comorbid conditions among cancer patients increases with age (Figure 2-15).

Information regarding the severity of comorbidity is available from a large cohort of 17,712 cancer patients seen at two teaching hospitals in St. Louis, MO, from 1995 to 2001 (Piccirillo et al., 2004).[7] Although this

[6]The NIA/NCI study included a random sample of 7,638 cancer patients diagnosed in 1992 and identified through SEER registries. Information on comorbidity was obtained from the SEER registry and from hospital and medical records.

[7]The certified tumor registrars at these hospitals were trained to code 27 different comorbid ailments from their review of the medical record during the usual chart abstraction process (see information about the comorbidity training course at http://cancercomorbidity.wustl.edu) (Washington University School of Medicine, 2004). The research group has validated a comorbidity index for use with cancer patients (called Adult Comorbidity Evaluation 27 or ACE-27).

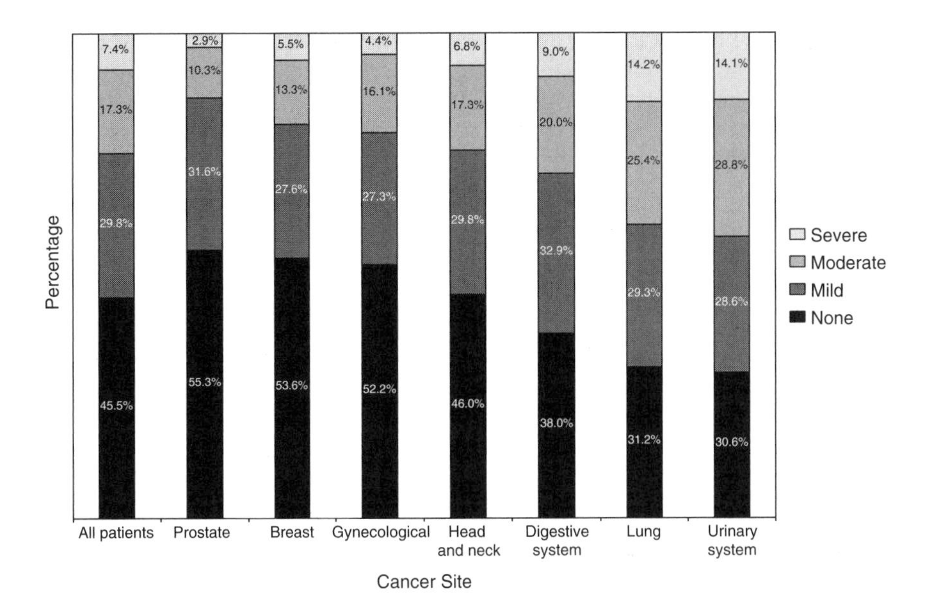

FIGURE 2-16 Severity of comorbidity for all patients and each tumor site.
SOURCE: Piccirillo et al. (2004).

cohort of cancer patients is not representative of the larger population of patients with cancer, it does provide some information on the widespread prevalence and severity of comorbid conditions among patients cared for at selected institutions. Prostate and breast cancer patients were least likely to have comorbid conditions, and individuals with urinary system and lung cancer were most likely to have severe comorbid conditions (Figure 2-16). Severity was graded according to information on diseases and conditions in patients' medical charts.

SITE-SPECIFIC EPIDEMIOLOGY

Summary statistics by cancer site/type—the numbers of survivors, incident cases, and deaths, and the rates of incidence, mortality, and 5-year relative survival—are shown for 2002 in Table 2-1. Another useful statistic for cancer survivors is the "conditional" relative survival rate (Henson et al., 1995; Merrill et al., 1998). The commonly reported survival statistics shown in Table 2-1 provide information that is pertinent to cancer patients at the time of their diagnosis. Once individuals have survived for a period of time, however, they are more interested in how their subsequent prospects for survival have changed. Cancer patients who have already survived 1

TABLE 2-1 Estimated Number of Cancer Survivors, Incident Cases, and Deaths as Well as Age-Adjusted Incidence and Mortality Rates, and 5-Year Relative Survival Rates, United States, 2002

	Numbers		
Site	Survivors	New Cases	Deaths
All sites	10,146,324	1,284,900	555,500
Female breast	2,278,269	203,500	39,600
Prostate	1,831,929	189,000	30,200
Colorectal	1,051,682	148,300	56,600
Corpus and uterus, NOS[c]	571,854	39,300	6,600
Melanoma	629,822	53,600	7,400
Urinary bladder	499,199	56,500	12,600
Lung and bronchus	350,679	169,400	154,900
Non-Hodgkin's lymphoma	347,039	53,900	24,400
Cervix uteri	223,441	13,000	4,100
Leukemia	189,865	30,800	21,700
Testes	164,009	7,500	400
Hodgkin's disease	145,501	7,000	1,400

NOTE: Includes invasive cancers only, except urinary bladder, which includes invasive and in situ cancers.

[a]Rates per 100,000 and age-adjusted to the 2000 U.S. standard population by 5-year age groups (1997–2002).

[b]Five-year relative survival rates expressed as percentages (1997–2002). For cancer, the relative survival rate is calculated by adjusting the survival rate to remove all causes of death

year after diagnosis usually have a better chance of surviving the next 5 years than during the first 5 years after diagnosis.

What follows are several figures showing, for selected cancers, the 5-year relative survival rates at diagnosis, and then the 5-year conditional survival rates at 1, 2, and 3 years following diagnosis. Differences in conditional survival are most pronounced among those with late-stage disease. For example, a person with Stage IV colorectal cancer has an estimated 7 percent chance of surviving 5 years from the time of diagnosis, but a 23 to 25 percent chance of surviving 5 additional years if he or she has already survived 2 years beyond diagnosis (Figures 2-17 to 2-19). These estimates were based on analyses of SEER cancer registry data for cases diagnosed from 1993 to 2000 and provided to the committee by NCI (see source information in Figures 2-17 to 2-19).

The next section of the chapter provides more detailed statistics to describe people who are newly diagnosed (the incident population) and

Rates		
Age-Adjusted Incidence[a]	Age-Adjusted Mortality[a]	5-Year Relative Survival[b]
471.4	193.5	64.8
132.9	25.5	88.5
176.3	28.1	99.7
51.9	19.6	63.1
24.5	4.2	84.9
18.3	2.6	90.4
20.7	4.4	80.7
62.1	54.9	15.4
19.3	7.6	61.0
7.2	2.5	72.1
11.7	7.5	48.4
5.6	0.3	95.0
2.9	0.5	88.1

except cancer. Relative survival is defined as the ratio of the proportion of observed survivors in a cohort of cancer patients to the proportion of expected survivors in a comparable set of cancer-free individuals. The formulation is based on the assumption of independent competing causes of death. If age, race, sex, or year information is missing, that individual is excluded from the analysis (NCI, 2004d).

[c]NOS = not otherwise specified.

SOURCES: ACS (2002); Ries et al. (2005).

those who are cancer survivors living with a history of cancer (the prevalent population). Information specific to four types of cancer are provided: female breast cancer, prostate cancer, colorectal cancer, and Hodgkin's disease (HD). Together, these cancers account for more than half of the survivorship population. These four cancer sites will be used to illustrate the variable nature of survivorship discussed in Chapter 3.

Characteristics of the incident population, such as cancer stage and age at diagnosis, can significantly affect disease prognosis, treatment options, insurance status, and other circumstances, as well as emotional responses to cancer. The makeup of the survivorship population is determined by the dynamics of who is diagnosed with cancer (and at what age), and who dies from cancer (and the length of their lives). Well represented in the survivorship population are people who are diagnosed at an early age with cancers with a good prognosis (e.g., early-stage breast and prostate cancer). Not well represented in the survivorship population are people with cancers that

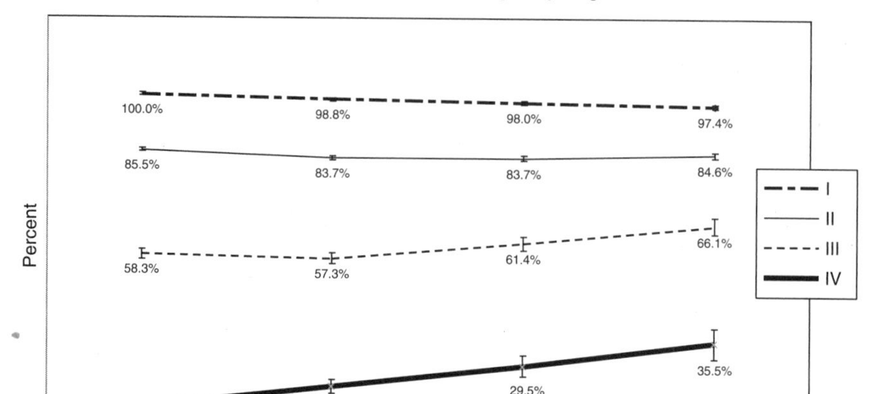

FIGURE 2-17 Conditional 5-year relative survival rates, breast cancer, by stage (modified American Joint Committee on Cancer [AJCC] staging).
NOTE: For Figures 2-17 to 2-19, bars around the point estimates indicate 95 percent confidence intervals.
SOURCE: Estimates based on NCI analyses of Surveillance, Epidemiology, and End Results (SEER) cancer registry data for cases diagnosed from 1993 to 2000 using SEER*Stat software and SEER 12 registries. Software: Surveillance Research Program, NCI SEER*Stat software (www.seer.cancer.gov/seerstat), version 6.0.0-beta. Data: SEER Program SEER*Stat database: Incidence—SEER 11 Regs + AK, Public Use Nov 2003 Sub (1973-2001 varying), NCI, Division of Cancer Control and Population Sciences, Surveillance Research Program, Cancer Statistics Branch, released April 2004, based on the November 2003 submission.

are diagnosed at older ages and those with late-stage disease (e.g., pancreatic and lung cancer). The availability of screening tests for certain cancers has changed the composition of the survivorship population, increasing greatly the number of survivors living long term with preclinical and treatable early-stage disease. Differential use of these tests has contributed to an underrepresentation of certain groups in the survivorship population, for example, those with poor access to health care. Because there is unequal access to health care in the United States, significant disparities arise in cancer survivorship. This section will describe the nature of some of these

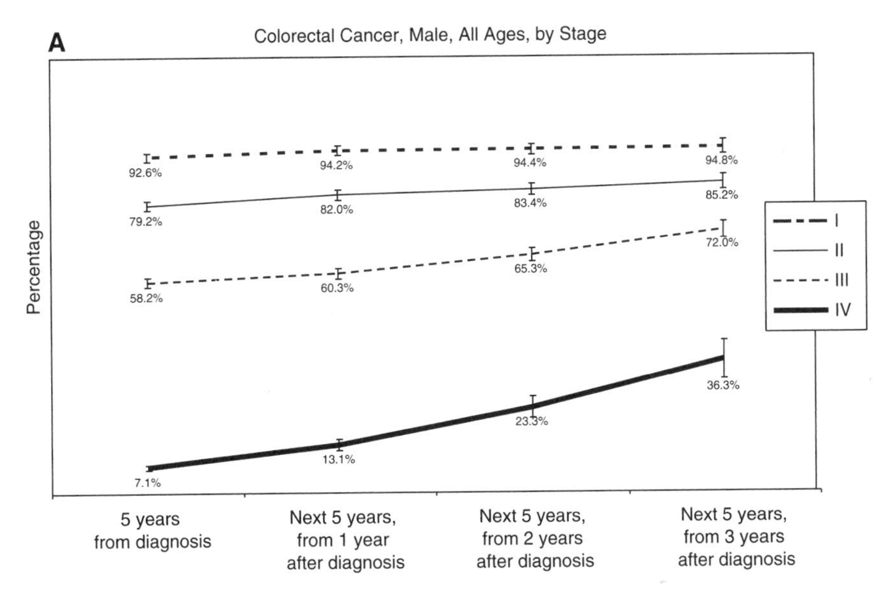

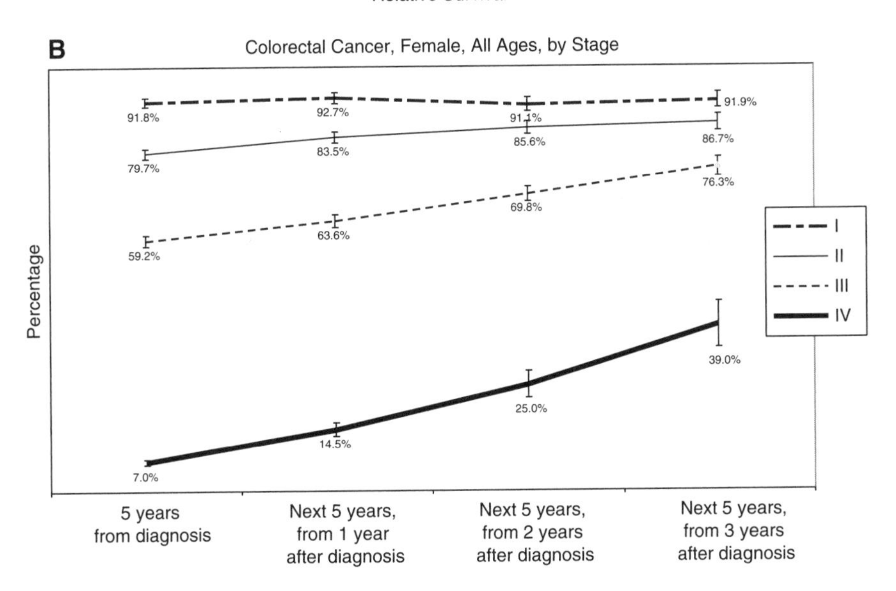

FIGURE 2-18 Conditional 5-year relative survival rates, colorectal cancer, by sex and stage (modified AJCC staging).

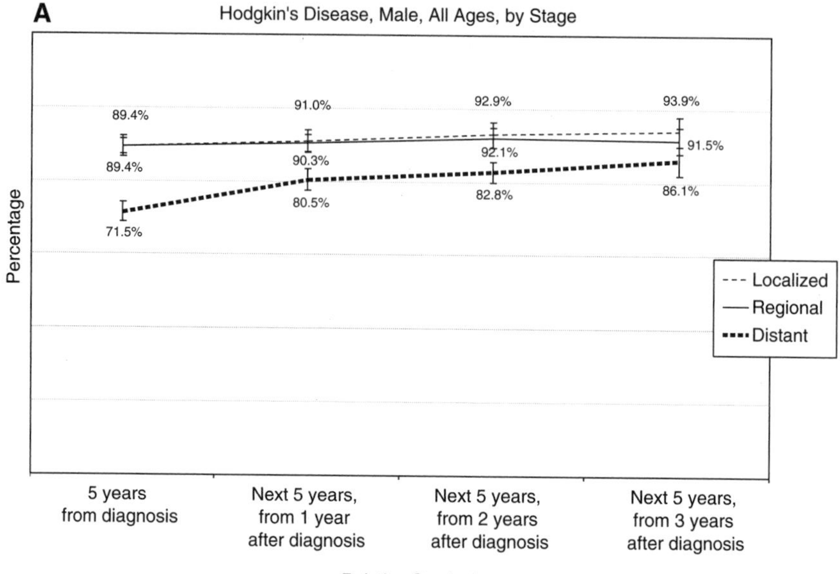

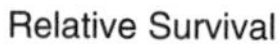

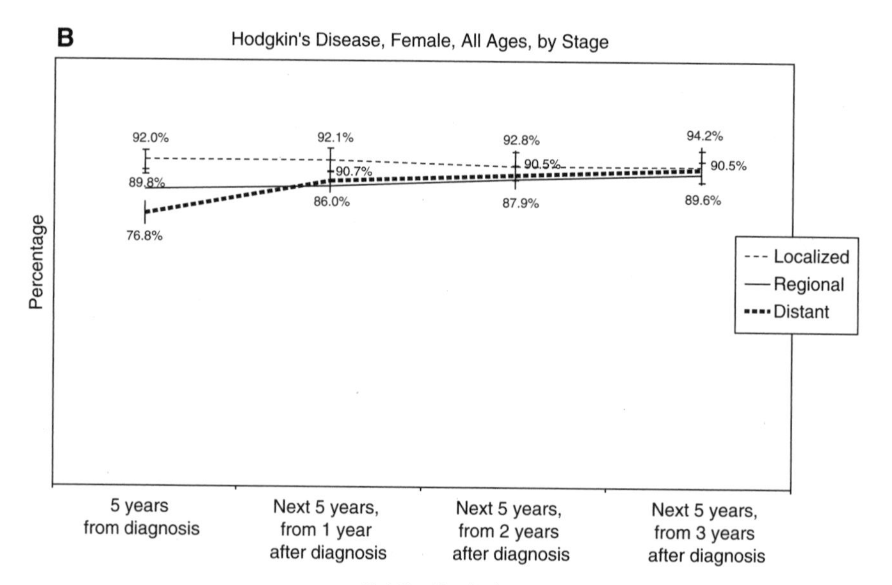

FIGURE 2-19 Conditional 5-year relative survival rates, Hodgkin's disease, by sex and age (historical stage).

disparities and highlight some important distinctions between the incident and prevalent populations that have policy implications, for example, different age distributions that affect health insurance coverage.

Female Breast Cancer

Breast cancer is the most common invasive cancer among women in the United States, and 211,240 new cases will be diagnosed in 2005 (ACS, 2005a). There is a one in seven probability for women to develop breast cancer in their lifetime (ACS, 2005a). The incidence of breast cancer among women increased on average 0.5 percent per year during the period 1987 to 2001, while mortality declined an average of 2.3 percent per year during the period 1990 to 2001 (Jemal et al., 2004; Ries et al., 2004). This has resulted in a 12.8 percent increase in 5-year survival (from 74.9 percent in 1975–1979 to 87.7 percent in 1995–2000) (Figure 2-20). In 2005 the number of deaths from breast cancer is expected to be 40,410.

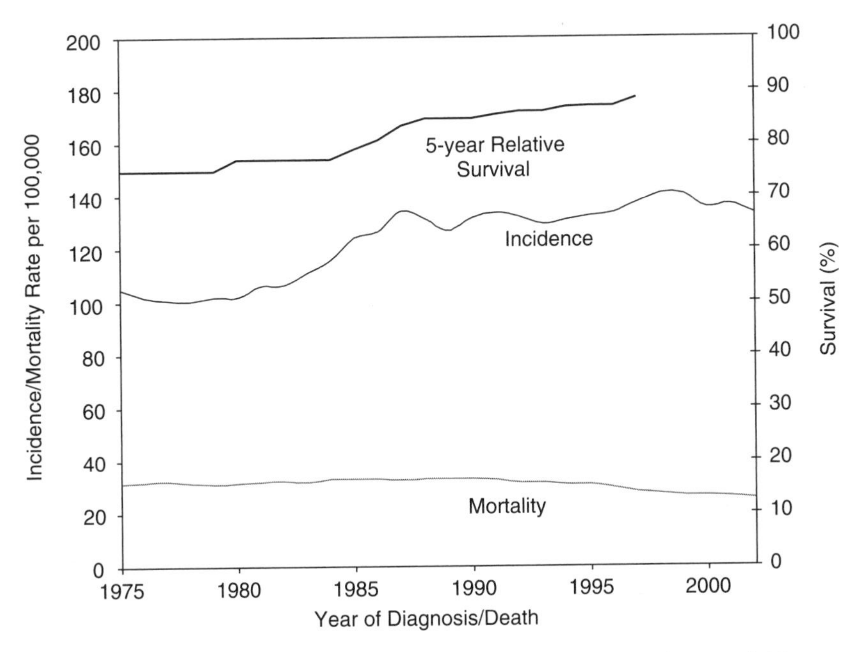

FIGURE 2-20 Trends in breast cancer incidence, mortality, and survival. Five-year relative survival is reported as an average for diagnosis years 1975–1979 and 1980–1984.
SOURCE: Ries et al. (2005).

Mammography is effective in the early diagnosis of breast cancer, and it is recommended that women age 40 and older have a mammogram every 1 to 2 years (USPSTF, 2002). Most (70 percent) women aged 40 and older reported in 2000 that they had a mammogram in the past 2 years (ACS, 2004b). The widespread use of mammographic screening has resulted in diagnosis at younger ages and with smaller tumors. The 20 to 30 percent decrease in mortality associated with mammographic screening (among women aged 50 and older) has also contributed to the growing population of breast cancer survivors, estimated at 2.3 million as of 2002 (NCI, 2005b). High screening rates have also resulted in more women being diagnosed with DCIS, a type of noninvasive breast cancer of uncertain clinical significance (IOM, 2005). In 2005, an estimated 58,490 women will be diagnosed with DCIS (ACS, 2005a). These women were not counted among the 211,240 cases of invasive breast cancer but, because women with DCIS usually receive the same treatment as women with invasive early breast cancer, the rise in DCIS detection has increased the use of breast-cancer-related services and created a new cohort of women who are worried about their future risk of invasive disease but for whom clear prognostic guidance is lacking.

Lower rates of use of screening among certain groups result in certain women being diagnosed at later stages when treatment is less effective. Rates of mammography use in 2000, for example, was significantly lower among American Indians and Alaskan Natives relative to women who are white (37 percent versus 57 percent, respectively) (ACS, 2004a). This lower rate of screening likely accounts for the relatively low percentage of American Indians and Alaskan Natives diagnosed with localized breast cancer as compared to whites (56 versus 66 percent, respectively) (Figure 2-21).

African-American women, despite having rates of mammography use similar to white women (53 versus 57 percent) and lower incidence rates, have higher rates of breast cancer death (Table 2-2) (ACS, 2005a). This anomaly persists even when adjusting for age, socioeconomic status, and disease stage. Recent research suggests that African-American women are more likely to be diagnosed at a younger age with aggressive breast cancer than are white women (Cross et al., 2002; Porter et al., 2004; Jones et al., 2004; Chlebowski et al., 2005).

African-American women are more likely to have later stage tumors (larger tumors and/or positive lymph nodes), tumors with higher histological and nuclear grades, and genetic characteristics that are associated with a poor outcome. While African-American women have tumors that are more aggressive biologically, socioeconomic status is also consistently associated with poor outcomes and is a better predictor of outcomes than race (Bradley et al., 2002). Breast cancer strikes African-American women at

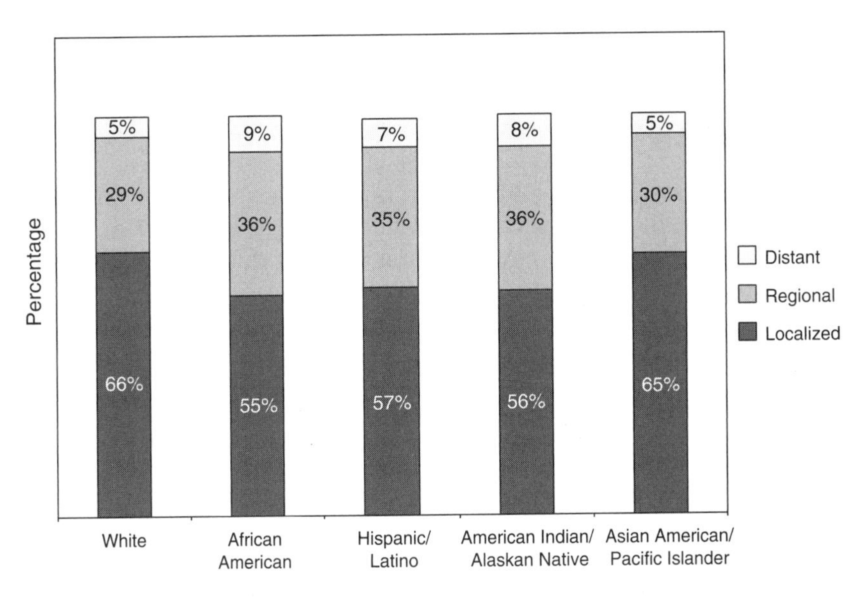

FIGURE 2-21 Percentage distribution of stage at diagnosis of breast cancer, by race and ethnicity, 1996 to 2000. Hispanics/Latinos are not mutually exclusive from whites, African Americans, Asian/Pacific Islander, and American Indians/Alaskan Natives.
SOURCE: ACS (2004a).

TABLE 2-2 Age-Standardized Incidence and Death Rates[a] for Breast Cancer (Female) by Race and Ethnicity, U.S., 1997 to 2001

Race/Ethnicity	Incidence	Mortality
White	141.7	26.4
African American	119.9	35.4
Asian/Pacific Islander	96.8	12.6
American Indian/ Alaskan Native	54.2	13.6
Hispanic/Latino[b]	89.6	17.3

[a]Rates are per 100,000 and age-adjusted to the 2000 U.S. standard population.
[b]Hispanics/Latinos are not mutually exclusive from whites and other groups shown.
SOURCE: ACS (2005a).

younger ages, at a median age of 57 as compared to age 63 for white women (Ries et al., 2004).

Women with newly diagnosed breast cancer tend to be younger than women who are breast cancer survivors. As many as two-thirds (66 percent) of incident cases of breast cancer occur under age 65 and roughly one-third (35 percent) occur before age 55. Given this relatively young age distribution, many of these women would be expected to be working and have responsibilities as mothers with school-age children, caregivers to aging parents, and spouses. In contrast, breast cancer survivors as a group are older with most (55 percent) women being aged 65 and older. This older age distribution of prevalent as compared to incident cases of breast cancer is illustrated in Figure 2-22. With this age distribution, most breast cancer survivors are of retirement age, are likely to be facing other chronic illnesses associated with aging, and are eligible for Medicare health insurance coverage.

Many women with breast cancer have other chronic illnesses at the time of their diagnosis. Such comorbid conditions can affect treatment

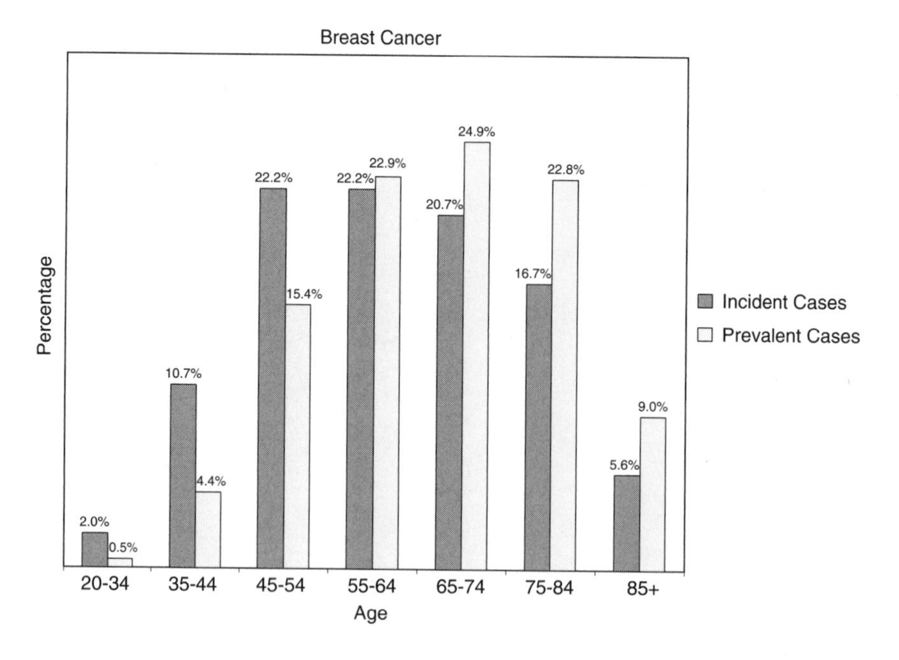

FIGURE 2-22 Age distribution of incident and prevalent cases of breast cancer. Incidence figures are for 1998–2002; prevalence figures are for SEER 2002 and are limited to individuals diagnosed within the past 27 years.
SOURCES: Ries et al. (2005); NCI (2005b).

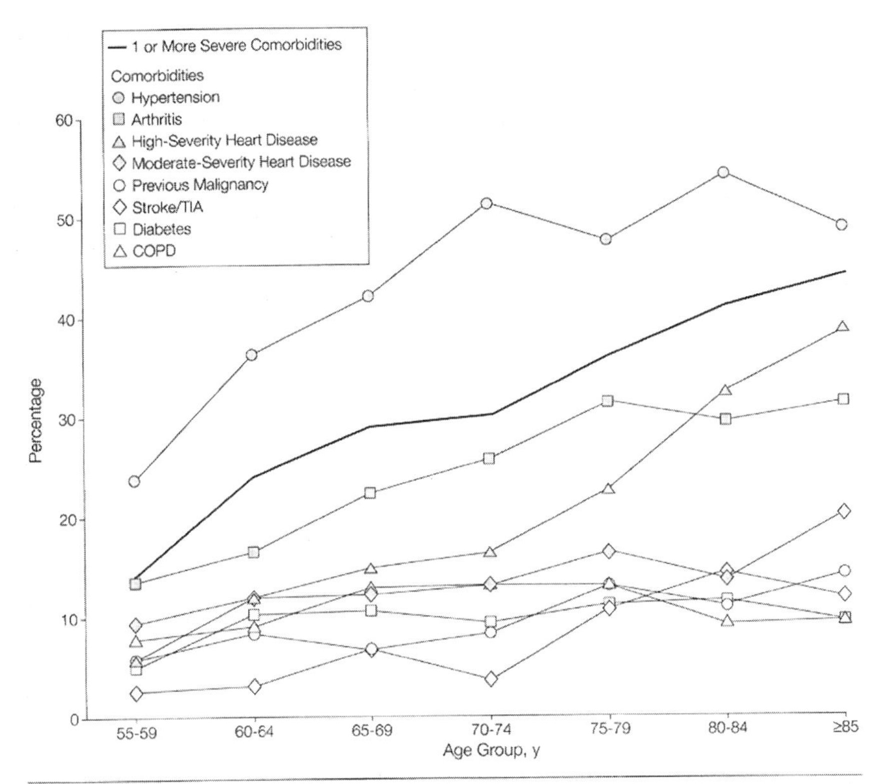

TIA indicates transient ischemic attack; COPD, chronic obstructive pulmonary disease. All trends were significant at the $P<.05$ level except for diabetes and COPD.

FIGURE 2-23 Prevalence of selected comorbidities among postmenopausal women with breast cancer, by age.
SOURCE: Yancik et al. (2001b).

choices and outcomes. In a population-based sample of 1,800 breast cancer patients diagnosed in 1992, the prevalence of one or more comorbid conditions increased from roughly 15 percent at ages 55 to 59 to more than 40 percent among women aged 85 and older (Figure 2-23) (Yancik et al., 2001b). The most prevalent condition in all age groups was hypertension. Arthritis ranked second or third across all age groups. The proportion of patients with previous cancers increased by age: 11 percent for those aged 55 to 64 years, 14 percent for those aged 65 to 74 years, and 20 percent for patients aged 75 and older.

Prostate Cancer

Prostate cancer is the most common invasive cancer diagnosed among men; in 2005 an estimated 232,090 cases will be diagnosed. One in six men develop prostate cancer in their lifetimes (ACS, 2005a). Between 1988 and 1992, prostate cancer incidence rates increased dramatically; this is probably due to earlier diagnosis through PSA blood testing (Figure 2-24). Prostate cancer incidence rates subsequently declined and have increased at a less rapid rate since 1995. This trend could reflect a decline in true incidence, lower use of PSA testing, or a combination of these factors.

It is recommended that PSA testing be offered annually, beginning at age 50, to men who have a life expectancy of at least 10 years. Men at high risk (African-American men and men with a strong family history of prostate cancer) should begin testing at age 45 (ACS, 2005b). In 2002, an estimated 54 percent of men over age 50 (who did not have prostate cancer) had a PSA test in the past year (ACS, 2004b). Despite its popularity, there is insufficient evidence to recommend for or against early prostate cancer testing using PSA. Definitive answers regarding the value of PSA screening

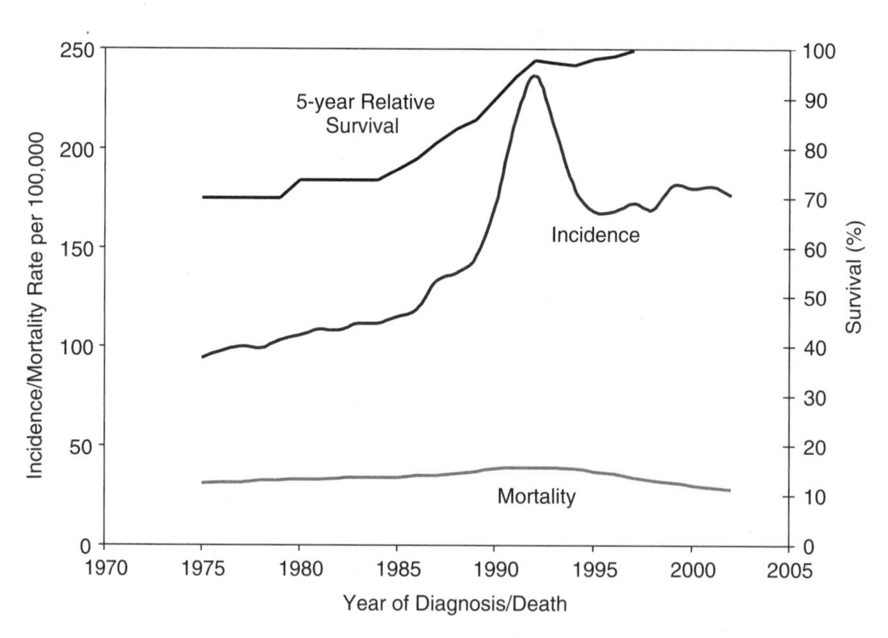

FIGURE 2-24 Trends in prostate cancer incidence, mortality, and survival. Five-year relative survival is reported as an average for diagnosis years 1975–1979 and 1980–1984.
SOURCE: Ries et al. (2005).

TABLE 2-3 Age-Standardized Incidence and Death Rates[a] for Prostate Cancer by Race and Ethnicity, U.S., 1997 to 2001

Race/Ethnicity	Incidence	Mortality
White	167.4	28.8
African American	271.3	70.4
Asian/Pacific Islander	100.7	13.0
American Indian/ Alaskan Native	51.2	20.2
Hispanic/Latino[b]	140.0	23.5

[a]Rates are per 100,000 and age-adjusted to the 2000 U.S. standard population.

[b]Hispanics/Latinos are not mutually exclusive from whites and other groups shown.

SOURCE: ACS (2005a).

from clinical trials may be available by 2008 (Brenner and Arndt, 2005). According to recommendations, men at average or high risk should be given information about the benefits and limitations of testing so they can make informed decisions about testing. Men diagnosed with prostate cancer tend to be better educated, in part because they are more likely to use (and be aware of recommendations for) PSA screening (Steenland et al., 2004).

Prostate cancer death rates declined an average of 4.1 percent per year from 1994 to 2001 (Jemal et al., 2004) (Figure 2-24). The majority of men diagnosed with prostate cancer in the PSA screening era do not have excess mortality compared to the general population under current patterns of medical care (Wilding and Remington, 2005; Brenner and Arndt, 2005). This finding does not suggest that PSA screening is either beneficial or ineffective, but it is reassuring information that can be provided to individuals recently diagnosed with prostate cancer.

With an estimated 30,350 deaths in 2005, prostate cancer is the second leading cause of cancer death in men (after lung cancer) (ACS, 2005a). Although death rates have been declining among white and African-American men since the early 1990s, rates in African-American men remain more than twice as high as rates in white men (Table 2-3). It is unclear what accounts for the marked racial differences in incidence and mortality among men with prostate cancer, but explanations include differences in biological and environmental factors, disparities in treatment, or combinations of these factors (Moul et al., 1996; Horner, 1998; Hsing and Devesa, 2001; Hsieh and Albertsen, 2003). Prostate cancer occurs at younger ages in African-American men and recommendations are that they begin screening earlier than white men.

Men who are American Indians and Alaskan Natives are much more likely than white men to have their prostate cancer detected at a more advanced stage (12 versus 5 percent) (Figure 2-25). African-American men are somewhat more likely than white men to have advanced disease at diagnosis (7 versus 5 percent).

In one recent study, comorbidity at the time of diagnosis explained some of the increased mortality among African Americans. However, men without any comorbid conditions at the time of diagnosis had higher mortality (Freeman et al., 2004). Investigators speculate that these men may have had more limited contact with the health care system and therefore failed to have their cancer detected at an early stage. Other research has indicated that men with less than a high school education have much lower survival rates from prostate cancer, even after controlling for stage and

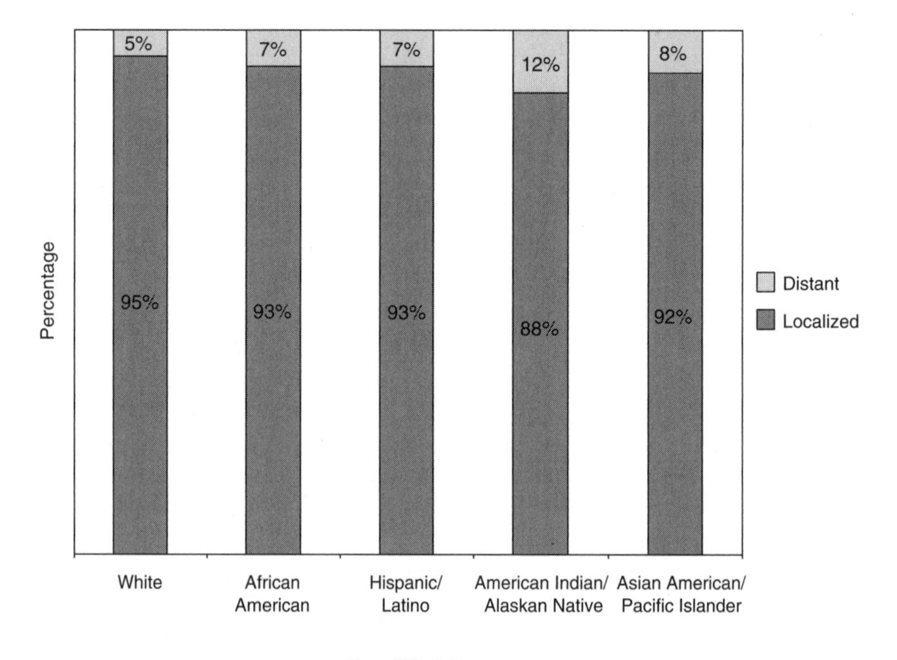

FIGURE 2-25 Stage at prostate cancer diagnosis, by race and ethnicity, U.S., SEER 1996 to 2000.
SOURCE: Ward et al. (2004).

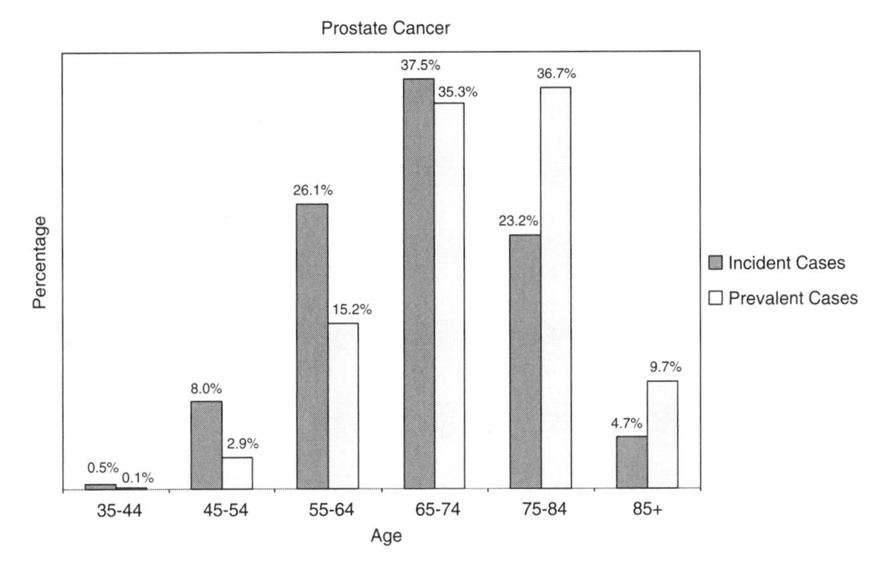

FIGURE 2-26 Age distribution of incident and prevalent cases of prostate cancer. Incidence figures are for 1998–2002; prevalence figures are for SEER 2002 and are limited to individuals diagnosed within the past 27 years.
SOURCES: Ries et al. (2005); NCI (2005b).

grade at diagnosis (Steenland et al., 2004). This finding may reflect disparities in diagnosis and treatment by educational attainment.

One-third of prostate cancer cases are diagnosed in men under the age of 65, but because men tend to live a long time with prostate cancer, the age distribution of prevalent cases is shifted to older ages, and 82 percent of prevalent cases are among men aged 65 and older (Figure 2-26). Issues related to the health care provided to survivors of prostate cancer should be of great concern to the Centers for Medicare and Medicaid Services, as four in five prostate cancer survivors are likely Medicare beneficiaries.

Colorectal Cancer

Colorectal cancer is the third most common invasive cancer overall (ACS, 2005c). There is a 1 in 17 probability for men and a 1 in 18 probability for women to develop colorectal cancer in their lifetimes (ACS, 2005a). In 2005 about 145,290 people will be diagnosed with colorectal cancer and about 56,290 people will die of the disease. Colorectal cancer is the second leading cause of cancer death after lung cancer. The great majority of these cancers and deaths could be prevented by applying existing knowledge about cancer prevention and by wider use of established screening tests. Although recommendations are for adults aged 50 and older to be screened for colorectal cancer, only 39 percent of people aged 50 or older in the United States have had a fecal occult blood test within the past year or endoscopy (i.e., either sigmoidoscopy or colonoscopy) within the past 5 years. Screening rates are lower among those without health insurance, recent immigrants, people with lower educational attainment, and Hispanics/Latinos (ACS, 2005c). Individuals at higher risk for colorectal cancer include those with a family history of colorectal cancer, those with a history of inflammatory bowel disease, and those with certain lifestyle risk factors (e.g., obesity, cigarette smoking, high alcohol use, physical inactivity).

Mortality rates from colorectal cancer continued to decline in both men and women from 1984 to 2001, at an average of 1.8 and 1.4 percent per year, respectively (Jemal et al., 2004). This decline reflects the decreasing incidence rates since the mid-1980s and improvements in survival. The decreases in incidence may reflect detection and removal of precancerous polyps during endoscopic screening. They may also reflect the increased use of hormone replacement therapy in women and anti-inflammatory drugs, both of which appear to reduce the risk of colorectal cancer.

Colorectal cancer incidence and mortality rates are highest in African-American men and women (Table 2-4). African Americans and American Indians and Alaskan Natives are more likely than whites to be diagnosed after the disease has spread beyond the bowel wall (Figure 2-27). The higher incidence rates, later stages at diagnosis, and higher mortality rates among certain racial and ethnic group members results in their

TABLE 2-4 Age-Standardized Incidence and Death Rates[a] for Colorectal Cancer by Race and Ethnicity, U.S., 1997 to 2001

	Incidence		Mortality	
Race/Ethnicity	Males	Females	Males	Females
White	63.1	45.9	24.8	17.1
African American	72.9	56.5	34.3	24.5
Asian/Pacific Islander	56.3	38.6	15.8	10.8
American Indian/ Alaskan Native	38.3	32.7	17.1	11.7
Hispanic/Latino[b]	49.6	32.5	18.0	11.6

[a]Rates are per 100,000 and age-adjusted to the 2000 U.S. standard population.

[b]Hispanics/Latinos are not mutually exclusive from whites and other groups shown.

SOURCE: ACS (2005c).

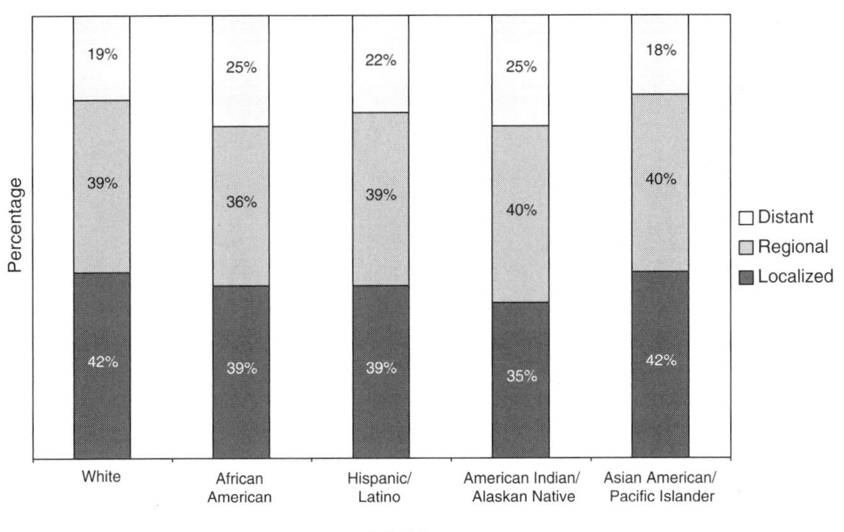

FIGURE 2-27 Stage at colorectal cancer diagnosis, by race and ethnicity, U.S., SEER 1996 to 2000.
SOURCE: Ward et al. (2004).

underrepresentation among cancer survivors. Efforts are needed to improve screening for colorectal cancer within these groups.

As is the case for other cancer sites, prevalent cases of colorectal cancer are more likely than incident cases to be aged 65 and older (76.7 versus 68.1 percent) (Figure 2-28).

Hodgkin's Disease

In 2005, there will be about 7,350 new cases of Hodgkin's disease and 1,410 HD deaths in the United States. Epidemiologic evidence suggests that HD results from a complex of related conditions that are in part mediated by infectious diseases, immune deficits, and genetic susceptibilities (Cartwright and Watkins, 2004). Death rates have fallen more than 60 percent since the early 1970s because of better diagnosis and treatment. There are no recommended screening tests for HD. Improvements in treatment have increased the size of the survivorship population, estimated at 145,501 in 2002.

HD is an unusual cancer in that as many as 64 percent of new cases of HD and 60 percent of survivors of HD are under age 45 (Figure 2-29).

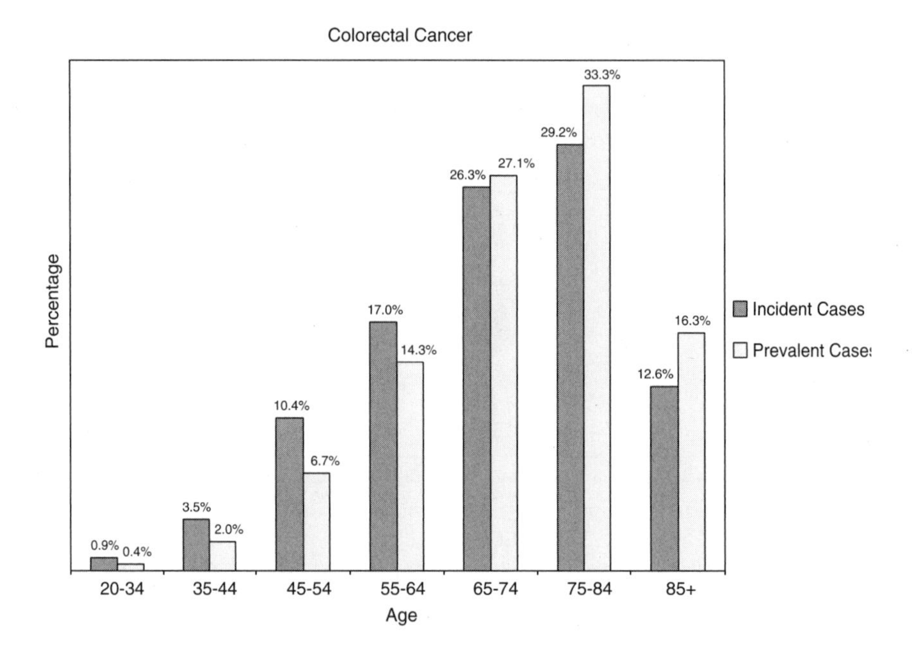

FIGURE 2-28 Age distribution of incident and prevalent cases of colorectal cancer. Incidence figures are for 1998–2002; prevalence figures are for SEER 2002 and are limited to individuals diagnosed within the past 27 years.
SOURCES: Ries et al. (2005); NCI (2005b).

Because HD is a rare cancer, relatively little has been published to describe the sociodemographic characteristics of the HD survivor population.

SUMMARY

It has been 20 years since Fitzhugh Mullan described survivorship as a unique phase of the cancer trajectory and spoke of the need to minimize its medical and social hazards. The concept of survivorship has evolved and to some extent continues to stir controversy. But for many, an accepted definition of cancer survivors includes all of those who are living with a history of cancer. In this report, the committee decided to focus on the phase of survivorship that follows primary treatment and lasts until cancer recurrence or end of life. This period represents largely uncharted territory in terms of evidence-based guidance for providers of survivorship care. The psychosocial issues that arise during this phase have also been relatively unexamined.

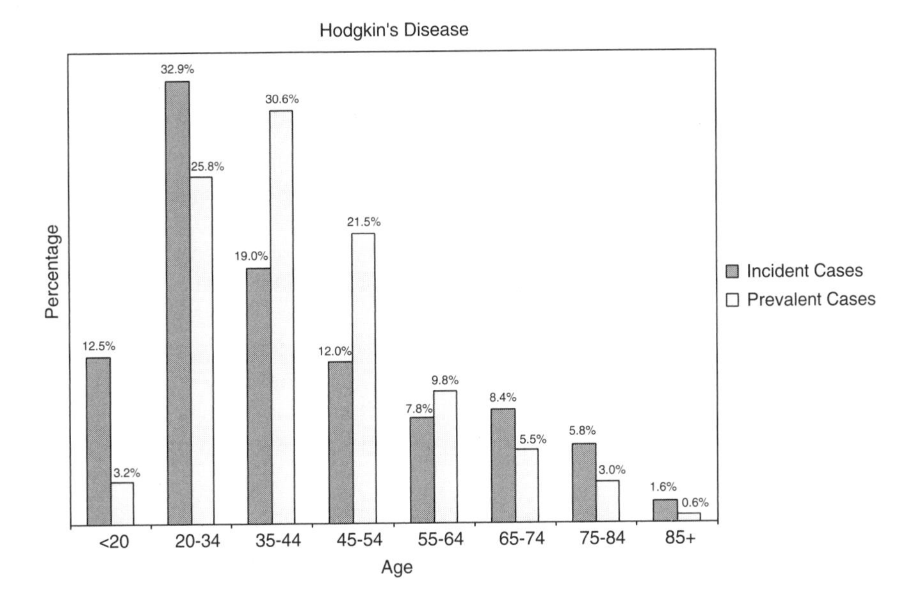

FIGURE 2-29 Age distribution of incident and prevalent cases of Hodgkin's disease. Incidence figures are for 1998–2002; prevalence figures are for SEER 2002 and are limited to individuals diagnosed within the past 27 years.
SOURCES: Ries et al. (2005); NCI (2005b).

There are about 10 million cancer survivors in the United States, representing 3.5 percent of the population. Prevalence rises steadily with age so that by age 80 to 84, prevalence is 19 percent. Although most cancer survivors are over age 65, more than one-third are young to late-middle-age adults and facing cancer-related concerns regarding reproduction, child rearing, employment, and the care of their aging parents. Factors that will continue to drive the increase in the number of survivors include the aging of the baby boom cohort, increased use of effective cancer screening, and improvements in treatment. Survival has improved as individuals with cancer are increasingly being diagnosed at younger ages with early-stage disease. The probability of long-term survival depends on many factors, including age, type of cancer, stage of illness, and comorbidity, but estimates of "conditional" survival provided to the committee by NCI generally show that cancer patients who have already survived 1 year after diagnosis have a better chance of surviving the next 5 years than the first 5 years after diagnosis.

Cancer survivors are likely to have comorbid illnesses, ADL limitations, and functional limitations. The relatively high prevalence of these conditions and limitations poses challenges to those providing survivorship care and points to the need for the integrated delivery of chronic health care and rehabilitation services.

Half of cancer survivors in the United States have been diagnosed with cancers of the breast, prostate, colon, and rectum. An examination of the epidemiology of these cancers reveals consistent disparities in incidence, mortality, and survival by race and ethnicity. The sources of the disparities have not been completely explained, but an important reason that African Americans and other members of minority groups are underrepresented among cancer survivors is their relatively poor access to primary health care and effective screening tests and treatments for cancer. To increase the number of long-term, disease-free cancer survivors and ensure that the full cross-section of Americans with cancer live beyond their cancer, efforts are needed to improve access to cancer prevention and health care services.

REFERENCES

ACS (American Cancer Society). 2002. *Cancer Facts & Figures, 2002*. Atlanta, GA: ACS.

ACS. 2004a. *Cancer Facts & Figures 2004*. Atlanta, GA: ACS.

ACS. 2004b. *Cancer Prevention & Early Detection Facts & Figures 2004*. Atlanta, GA: ACS.

ACS. 2005a. *Cancer Facts & Figures 2005*. Atlanta, GA: ACS.

ACS. 2005b. *Can Prostate Cancer Be Found Early?* [Online]. Available: http://www.cancer. org/docroot/CRI/content/CRI_2_4_3X_Can_prostate_cancer_be_found_early_36.asp [accessed April 28, 2005].

ACS. 2005c. *Colorectal Cancer Facts and Figures Special Edition 2005*. Atlanta, GA: ACS.

Bradley CJ, Given CW, Roberts C. 2002. Race, socioeconomic status, and breast cancer treatment and survival. *J Natl Cancer Inst* 94(7):490–496.

Brenner H, Arndt V. 2005. Long-term survival rates of patients with prostate cancer in the prostate-specific antigen screening era: Population-based estimates for the year 2000 by period analysis. *J Clin Oncol* 23(3):441–447.

Capocaccia R, De Angelis R. 1997. Estimating the completeness of prevalence based on cancer registry data. *Stat Med* 16(4):425–440.

Cartwright RA, Watkins G. 2004. Epidemiology of Hodgkin's disease: A review. *Hematol Oncol* 22(1):11–26.

Cheeseman Day J (U.S. Census Bureau). 2001. *National Population Projections*. [Online]. Available: http://www.census.gov/population/www/pop-profile/natproj.html [accessed August 4, 2004].

Chlebowski RT, Chen Z, Anderson GL, Rohan T, Aragaki A, Lane D, Dolan NC, Paskett ED, McTiernan A, Hubbell FA, Adams-Campbell LL, Prentice R. 2005. Ethnicity and breast cancer: Factors influencing differences in incidence and outcome. *J Natl Cancer Inst* 97(6):439–448.

Cross CK, Harris J, Recht A. 2002. Race, socioeconomic status, and breast carcinoma in the U.S: What have we learned from clinical studies? *Cancer* 95(9):1988–1999.

Edwards BK, Howe HL, Ries LA, Thun MJ, Rosenberg HM, Yancik R, Wingo PA, Jemal A, Feigal EG. 2002. Annual report to the nation on the status of cancer, 1973–1999, featuring implications of age and aging on U.S. cancer burden. *Cancer* 94(10):2766–2792.

Freeman HP. 2003. Commentary on the meaning of race in science and society. *Cancer Epidemiol Biomarkers Prev* 12(3):232s–236s.

Freeman VL, Durazo-Arvizu R, Keys LC, Johnson MP, Schafernak K, Patel VK. 2004. Racial differences in survival among men with prostate cancer and comorbidity at time of diagnosis. *Am J Public Health* 94(5):803–808.

Grieco EM, Cassidy RC. 2001. *Overview of Race and Hispanic Origin: Census 2000 Brief.* Washington, DC: U.S. Census Bureau.

Henson DE, Ries LA, Carriaga MT. 1995. Conditional survival of 56,268 patients with breast cancer. *Cancer* 76(2):237–242.

Hewitt M, Rowland JH, Yancik R. 2003. Cancer survivors in the United States: Age, health, and disability. *J Gerontol A Biol Sci Med Sci* 58(1):82–91.

Horner RD. 1998. Racial variation in cancer care: A case study of prostate cancer. *Cancer Treat Res* 97:99–114.

Hsieh K, Albertsen PC. 2003. Populations at high risk for prostate cancer. *Urol Clin North Am* 30(4):669–676.

Hsing AW, Devesa SS. 2001. Trends and patterns of prostate cancer: What do they suggest? *Epidemiol Rev* 23(1):3–13.

Ingram DD, Parker JD, Schenker N, Weed JA, Hamilton B, Arias E, Madans JH. 2003. *United States Census 2000 Population With Bridged Race Categories. Vital Health Stat* 2(135). Hyattsville, MD: National Center for Health Statistics, Centers for Disease Control and Prevention.

IOM (Institute of Medicine). 2003. *Unequal Treatment: Confronting Racial and Ethnic Disparities in Health Care.* Washington, DC: The National Academies Press.

IOM. 2005. *Saving Women's Lives: Strategies for Improving Breast Cancer Detection and Diagnosis.* Joy JE, Penhoet EE, Petitti DB, eds. Washington, DC: The National Academies Press.

Jemal A, Clegg LX, Ward E, Ries LA, Wu X, Jamison PM, Wingo PA, Howe HL, Anderson RN, Edwards BK. 2004. Annual report to the nation on the status of cancer, 1975–2001, with a special feature regarding survival. *Cancer* 101(1):3–27.

Jemal A, Murray T, Ward E, Samuels A, Tiwari RC, Ghafoor A, Feuer EJ, Thun MJ. 2005. Cancer statistics, 2005. *CA Cancer J Clin* 55(1):10–30.

Jones BA, Kasl SV, Howe CL, Lachman M, Dubrow R, Curnen MM, Soler-Vila H, Beeghly A, Duan F, Owens P. 2004. African-American/white differences in breast carcinoma: p53 alterations and other tumor characteristics. *Cancer* 101(6):1293–1301.

Krishnan KR, Delong M, Kraemer H, Carney R, Spiegel D, Gordon C, McDonald W, Dew M, Alexopoulos G, Buckwalter K, Cohen PD, Evans D, Kaufmann PG, Olin J, Otey E, Wainscott C. 2002. Comorbidity of depression with other medical diseases in the elderly. *Biol Psychiatry* 52(6):559–588.

Leigh S. 2004. Cancer survivorship: Defining our destiny. In: Hoffman B, ed. *A Cancer Survivor's Almanac.* 3rd ed. Hoboken, NJ: John Wiley & Sons.

Marcus AD. 2004, March 24. Debate heats up on defining a cancer survivor. *Wall Street Journal.* P. D4.

Mausner JS, Kramer S. 1985. *Epidemiology—An Introductory Text.* 2nd ed. Philadelphia, PA: W.B. Saunders.

McNeil JM, Binette J. 2001. Prevalence of disabilities and associated health conditions among adults—United States, 1999. *MMWR* 50(7):120–125.

Merrill RM, Capocaccia R, Feuer EJ, Mariotto A. 2000. Cancer prevalence estimates based on tumour registry data in the Surveillance, Epidemiology, and End Results (SEER) Program. *Int J Epidemiol* 29(2):197–207.

Merrill RM, Henson DE, Ries LA. 1998. Conditional survival estimates in 34,963 patients with invasive carcinoma of the colon. *Dis Colon Rectum* 41(9):1097–1106.

Moul JW, Douglas TH, McCarthy WF, McLeod DG. 1996. Black race is an adverse prognostic factor for prostate cancer recurrence following radical prostatectomy in an equal access health care setting. *J Urol* 155(5):1667–1673.

Mullan F. 1985. Seasons of survival: Reflections of a physician with cancer. *New England Journal of Medicine* 313(4):270–273.

NCCS (National Coalition for Cancer Survivorship). 1996. *Imperatives for Quality Cancer Care: Access, Advocacy, Action, and Accountability.* Clark EJ, Stovall EL, Leigh S, Siu AL, Austin DK, Rowland JH. Silver Spring, MD: NCCS.

NCI (National Cancer Institute). 2004a. *About SEER.* [Online]. Available: http://seer.cancer.gov/about/ [accessed December 13, 2004].

NCI. 2004b. *About Survivorship Research: Survivorship Definitions.* [Online]. Available: http://dccps.nci.nih.gov/ocs/definitions.html [accessed April 9, 2004].

NCI. 2004c. *Cancer Progress Report—2003 Update.* [Online]. Available: http://progressreport.cancer.gov/index.asp [accessed May 31, 2004].

NCI. 2004d. *Relative Survival.* [Online]. Available: http://seer.cancer.gov/seerstat/WebHelp/Relative_Survival.htm [accessed May 10, 2004].

NCI. 2005a. *Cancer Control Continuum.* [Online]. Available: http://cancercontrol.cancer.gov/od/continuum.html [accessed April 19, 2005].

NCI. 2005b. *Cancer Query System: Cancer Prevalence Database.* [Online]. Available: http://srab.cancer.gov/prevalence/canques.html [accessed June 2, 2005].

NCI. 2005c. *Estimated U.S. Cancer Prevalence.* [Online]. Available: http://cancercontrol.cancer.gov/ocs/prevalence/prevalence.html [accessed May 31, 2005].

Ostir GV, Carlson JE, Black SA, Rudkin L, Goodwin JS, Markides KS. 1999. Disability in older adults. Prevalence, causes, and consequences. *Behav Med* 24(4):147–156.

Piccirillo JF, Tierney RM, Costas I, Grove L, Spitznagel EL Jr. 2004. Prognostic importance of comorbidity in a hospital-based cancer registry. *JAMA* 291(20):2441–2447.

Porter PL, Lund MJ, Lin MG, Yuan X, Liff JM, Flagg EW, Coates RJ, Eley JW. 2004. Racial differences in the expression of cell cycle-regulatory proteins in breast carcinoma. *Cancer* 100(12):2533–2542.

President's Cancer Panel. 2004a. *Living Beyond Cancer: A European Dialogue.* Bethesda, MD: National Cancer Institute.

President's Cancer Panel. 2004b. *Living Beyond Cancer: Finding a New Balance.* Bethesda, MD: National Cancer Institute.

Ries LAG, Eisner MP, Kosary CL, Hankey BF, Miller BA, Clegg L, Mariotto A, Feuer EJ, Edwards BK, eds. 2004. *SEER Cancer Statistics Review, 1975–2001.* Bethesda, MD: National Cancer Institute. [Online]. Available: http://seer.cancer.gov/csr/1975_2001/ [accessed April 29, 2004].

Ries LAG, Eisner MP, Kosary CL, Hankey BF, Miller BA, Clegg L, Mariotto A, Feuer EJ, Edwards BK, eds. 2005. *SEER Cancer Statistics Review, 1975–2002.* Bethesda, MD: National Cancer Institute. [Online]. Available: http://seer.cancer.gov/csr/1975_2002/, based on November 2004 SEER data submission [accessed June 7, 2005].

Rowland J, Mariotto A, Aziz N, Tesauro G, Feuer EJ, Blackman D, Thompson P, Pollock LA. 2004. Cancer survivorship—United States, 1971–2001. *MMWR* 53(24):526–529.

Shavers VL, Brown ML. 2002. Racial and ethnic disparities in the receipt of cancer treatment. *J Natl Cancer Inst* 94(5):334–357.

Singh GK, Miller BA, Hankey BF, Edwards BK. 2003. *Area Socioeconomic Variations in U.S. Cancer Incidence, Mortality, Stage, Treatment, and Survival, 1975–1999.* NCI Cancer Surveillance Monograph Series, No. 4. Bethesda, MD: National Cancer Institute.

Steenland K, Rodriguez C, Mondul A, Calle EE, Thun M. 2004. Prostate cancer incidence and survival in relation to education (United States). *Cancer Causes Control* 15(9):939–945.

USPSTF (United States Preventive Services Task Force). 2002. *Screening for Breast Cancer.* [Online]. Available: http://www.ahrq.gov/clinic/uspstf/uspsbrca.htm [accessed April 13, 2005].

Ward E, Jemal A, Cokkinides V, Singh GK, Cardinez C, Ghafoor A, Thun M. 2004. Cancer disparities by race/ethnicity and socioeconomic status. *CA Cancer J Clin* 54(2):78–93.

Washington University School of Medicine. 2004. *Comorbidity Coding Course.* [Online]. Available: http://cancercomorbidity.wustl.edu [accessed September 13, 2004].

Welch HG, Schwartz LM, Woloshin S. 2000a. Are increasing 5-year survival rates evidence of success against cancer? *JAMA* 283(22):2975–2978.

Welch HG, Schwartz LM, Woloshin S. 2000b. Do increased 5-year survival rates in prostate cancer indicate better outcomes? *JAMA* 284(16):2053–2055.

Welch-McCaffrey D, Hoffman B, Leigh SA, Loescher LJ, Meyskens FL Jr. 1989. Surviving adult cancers. Part 2: Psychosocial implications. *Ann Intern Med* 111(6):517–524.

Wilding G, Remington P. 2005. Period analysis of prostate cancer survival. *J Clin Oncol* 23(3):407–409.

Yancik R. 1997. Epidemiology of cancer in the elderly. Current status and projections for the future. *Rays* 22(1 Suppl):3–9.

Yancik R, Ganz PA, Varricchio CG, Conley B. 2001a. Perspectives on comorbidity and cancer in older patients: Approaches to expand the knowledge base. *J Clin Oncol* 19(4):1147–1151.

Yancik R, Wesley MN, Ries LA, Havlik RJ, Edwards BK, Yates JW. 2001b. Effect of age and comorbidity in postmenopausal breast cancer patients aged 55 years and older. *JAMA* 285(7):885–892.

Yates JW. 2001. Comorbidity considerations in geriatric oncology research. *CA Cancer J Clin* 51(6):329–336.

3

The Medical and Psychological Concerns of Cancer Survivors After Treatment

The medical and psychological effects of cancer and its treatment have been recognized for many years, but it is only recently that survivorship is coming to be recognized as a distinct phase of the cancer trajectory. Findings from research studies that have tracked the health and well-being of individuals long after cancer treatment has ended have identified risks that both the survivors and their health care providers should recognize. Advances in knowledge of how to manage conditions that arise in the post-treatment period have led to the development of some guidelines for health care providers to follow. The survivorship period provides many opportunities to improve the health and quality of life of cancer survivors. This chapter begins with a general overview of the potential medical and psychological consequences of cancer and its treatment. Brief descriptions are then provided on the late effects associated with four cancer types (breast, prostate, colorectal, and Hodgkin's disease) as well as information on the need for services to ameliorate them. Lifestyle issues of interest to cancer survivors are reviewed—smoking cessation, physical activity, nutrition and diet, healthy weight, and the use of complementary and alternative medicine. The chapter concludes with a review of the committee's findings and recommendations.

OVERVIEW

The meaning of health and life itself can be altered following a diagnosis of cancer (Herold and Roetzheim, 1992; Muzzin et al., 1994; Vachon, 2001). Cancer survivors report ongoing struggles to achieve a balance in their lives and a sense of wholeness and life purpose after a life-altering experience (Ferrell, 2004). Individuals may reappraise their lives following a diagnosis of cancer and search for a sense of control and meaning. Survivors of cancer, although free of the cancer for which they were treated, may be immobilized by fears of recurrence and have difficulties making life decisions, for example, proceeding with vocational plans or marriage. Existential and spiritual issues may also arise related to concerns about death and dying, having a new orientation to time and future, and changed values and goals. The survivorship experience is dynamic, changing over time, with particular moments of stress being transitions, such as the transition from treatment to long-term follow-up. Cancer survivors face these psychosocial concerns and worries about the physical effects of their treatment across the continuum of cancer care (Ganz, 2000).

Cancer's effects are not isolated to an individual. Instead, it has an impact on the entire family, and the needs of children, spouses, partners, and other loved ones all need to be considered. Family members routinely provide personal care and emotional support for the duration of the cancer experience. Financial concerns may also arise because family income, insurance status, and employment can all be profoundly affected by cancer (see Chapter 6). Caregivers and family members often require, but do not receive, the respite, health care, psychosocial, and financial assistance they need in meeting the many needs of cancer survivors in their lives.

Quality of life (QOL) is a term used widely to describe an individual's assessment of his or her own general well-being. There is no one agreed-on conceptual model or definition for health-related QOL, and investigators continue to work on developing ways to measure outcomes that matter to patients (Ganz, 2002a; Zebrack et al., 2003). Central to the concept of QOL, however, is the importance of capturing the perspective of the patient across multiple "domains" or areas of well-being. Standardized, self-administered questionnaires are generally used to assess symptoms and functioning in physical, psychological, social, and spiritual domains (Mandelblatt and Eisenberg, 1995; Cella, 1995; Dow et al., 1996; Montazeri et al., 1996; Ferrell et al., 1997a,b, 1998; Ferrans, 2005).[1] An example of a conceptual model of QOL is shown in Figure 3-1.

This chapter reviews what is known about these various dimensions of quality of life for cancer survivors. The recognition of these health effects of

[1]Some QOL instruments are generic in nature and are used in general population studies (e.g., Medical Outcomes Study Short Form 36 or SF-36), while others have been developed specifically for use among cancer patients or survivors (e.g., Cancer Rehabilitation Evaluation System or CARES).

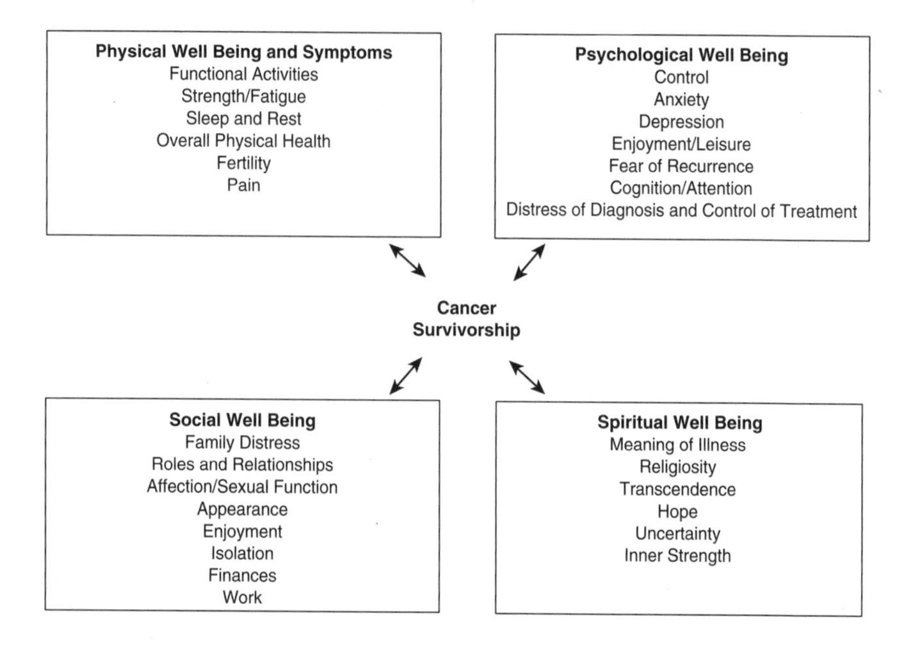

FIGURE 3-1 Quality of life: conceptual model.
SOURCE: City of Hope Beckman Research Institute (2004). Reprinted with permission from Betty R. Ferrell, PhD, FAAN; and Marcia Grant, DNSc, FAAN, City of Hope National Medical Center.

cancer and its treatment, sometimes referred to as "the price of survival," follows investments in cancer survivorship research directed to better understand the long-term consequences of cancer (Ganz, 2002b). Because most of the research conducted to assess QOL of cancer issues among survivors involves individuals with certain types of cancer (or certain treatments), descriptions of the cancer survivorship experience are provided by selected cancer site. What follows are brief reviews of the quality of life literature for individuals with a history of cancer of the breast, prostate, and colon and rectum, and Hodgkin's disease. The terms "late effects" and "long-term effects" can be used to distinguish health effects according to their onset (Box 3-1). However, in this report, the general term "late effects" is used to describe the consequences of cancer and its treatment, regardless of their date of onset.

There is limited information on the prevalence of late effects, but there is a general recognition that they have become more common, largely as a result of the more frequent use of complex cancer interventions,

BOX 3-1
Defining Late- and Long-Term Effects of Cancer Treatment

Late effects refer specifically to unrecognized toxicities that are absent or subclinical at the end of therapy and become manifest later with the unmasking of hitherto unseen injury because of any of the following factors: developmental processes, the failure of compensatory mechanisms with the passage of time, or organ senescence.

Long-term effects refer to any side effects or complications of treatment for which a cancer patient must compensate; also know as persistent effects, they begin during treatment and continue beyond the end of treatment. Late effects, in contrast, appear months to years after the completion of treatment.

SOURCE: Aziz and Rowland (2003).

often combinations of surgery, chemotherapy, radiation, and hormone treatments.

Of particular concern for cancer survivors are psychological effects. There may be cancer-specific concerns, such as fear of recurrence, to more generalized symptoms of worry, fear of the future, fear of death, trouble sleeping, fatigue, and trouble concentrating (Box 3-2). The pervasive uncertainty associated with cancer survival has been labeled the "Damocles syndrome" (Smith and Lesko, 1988; Quigley, 1989; Herold and Roetzheim, 1992). In Greek mythology, Damocles was invited to the king's banquet for dinner. Once there, he found himself seated beneath a sword suspended over his head by a single horsehair. Damocles was happy to be at the king's feast, but any movement he made while reaching for food or drink might knock the sword loose and spell a quick death. For cancer survivors, fears of recurrence can result in persistent anxiety and difficulties in planning for the future (Lee-Jones et al., 1997).

Individuals with cancer may also experience a mental disorder as a result of cancer or treatment, or they may experience an exacerbation of a prior psychiatric disorder (e.g., recurrent depression). Major depression and depressive symptoms occur frequently in cancer patients (Massie, 2004). According to a recent review of the literature, prevalence rates varied from 10 to 25 percent for major depressive disorders, a rate at least four times higher than in the general population (AHRQ, 2002). The timing and method of the assessment, concurrent treatment, medical morbidity, pain, gender, and age of subjects contributed to the wide range of estimates. The higher rates are usually seen in patients with more advanced illness and uncontrolled pain or other physical symptoms.

The term "psychosocial distress" has been coined to reflect a broader

BOX 3-2
Psychosocial Concerns of Cancer Survivors

Negative
- Fear of recurrence, concerns about future and death
- Depression, sadness
- Inability to make plans
- Adjustment to physical compromise, health worries, sense of loss for what might have been (e.g., loss of fertility)
- Uncertainty and heightened sense of vulnerability
- Alterations in social support
- Fears regarding accomplishment of adult developmental tasks
- Existential and spiritual issues
- Psychosocial reorientation
- Sexuality, fertility, and intimate relationships
- Parenting
- Employment and insurance problems
- Relationship with the treatment team

Positive
- Feelings of gratitude and good fortune
- Sense of self-esteem and mastery

SOURCE: Ganz (2002c).

set of concerns (NCCN, 1999). As conceived, distress is a "multi-factorial unpleasant emotional experience of a psychological (cognitive, behavioral, emotional), social, and/or spiritual nature that may interfere with the ability to cope effectively with cancer, its physical symptoms, and its treatment. Distress extends along a continuum, ranging from common normal feelings of vulnerability, sadness, and fears to problems that can become disabling, such as depression, anxiety, panic, social isolation, and existential and spiritual crisis" (NCCN, 1999). Distress may be experienced as a reaction to the disease and its treatment and also as a result of the consequences of the disease on employment, health insurance, and social functioning, including family relationships (McEvoy and McCorkle, 1990; Kornblith, 1998) (see Chapter 6 for a discussion of employment and insurance issues).

Brief screening tools can be used to identify individuals with symptoms of distress so that clinical assessment by the primary oncology team and referral to psychosocial providers can take place (Trask, 2004). The Distress Thermometer, for example, is a visual analogue scale that the National Comprehensive Cancer Network (NCCN) guidelines suggest for the screening of psychosocial distress (NCCN, 1999).

Many survivors function at high levels and do not report excess depressive symptoms. Importantly, not all of the psychological effects are negative. Cancer survivors are often grateful to be alive and have an enhanced appreciation of life. Their self-esteem and sense of mastery may also be enhanced. Social late effects may be negative (alienation and isolation) or positive (affinity and altruism). Socioeconomic concerns may arise following treatment, particularly financial concerns related to costs of care, access to health insurance, and the ability to return to work or school (see Chapter 6). Recent evidence suggests that there are income-related disparities in the QOL of cancer survivors that cannot be explained by the effect of health on earnings. High-income patients are not only more likely to survive cancer, but they enjoy better QOL as survivors (Short and Mallonee, in press).

Aside from psychosocial distress, there are two main categories of late effects. First, cancer survivors are at increased risk for cancer, either a recurrence of the cancer for which they were initially treated, or the independent development of a second cancer (either of the same type or a different type from the original cancer).[2] The increased risk of developing a second cancer may be due to cancer treatment (e.g., chemotherapy-induced leukemia and bladder cancer), genetic or other susceptibility, or some interaction between treatment and an inherent susceptibility. In addition to concerns about the risk of cancer following treatment, cancer survivors are at increased risk for a wide range of treatment-related problems notable for their variability and unpredictability. Their variability can be traced, in part, to the complexity of cancer itself (e.g., the type of tumor and stage of disease), the wide array of therapies that can be employed, the intensity of treatment (e.g., doses of chemotherapy or radiation, the extent of surgery needed), and the age and underlying health status of the individual at the time of treatment.

A number of tissues and body systems can potentially be impaired as a consequence of cancer and its treatment, as illustrated in Tables 3-1 and 3-2. Some of the late effects associated with certain chemotherapeutic agents, for example, can result in significant changes in physical functioning, leading to effects such as post-treatment fatigue or sexual or urinary problems. Clinicians, in designing initial treatment plans, consider the potential for late effects and attempt to be as conservative as guidelines warrant to maximize treatment effectiveness while minimizing late effects. Late effects will likely be reduced in the future with the advent of therapies that are tailored to the characteristics of an individual and their cancer. In addition, advances in methods to assess individuals risk for late effects (e.g., their DNA repair mechanisms related to radiation-induced DNA damage) and to personalize treatments will improve the outlook for cancer survivors.

---

[2]A National Cancer Institute (NCI) monograph on the risks of second cancers is forthcoming by early 2006.

TABLE 3-1 Examples of Possible Late Effects of Radiation Therapy, Chemotherapy, and Hormonal Therapy Among Survivors of Adult Cancers

		Chemotherapy/Hormonal Therapy	
Organ System/ Tissue	Radiation Therapy Late Effects	Late Effects	Agent Responsible
All tissues	Second cancers	Second cancers	Steroids, alkylating agents, nitrosureas, topoisomerase inhibitors, anthracyclines
Bone and soft tissue	Atrophy, deformity, fibrosis, bone death	Bone death and destruction, risk of fractures	Steroids
Cardiovascular	Scarring or inflammation of the heart, coronary artery disease; scarring of heart sac (pericardium)	Inflammation of the heart, congestive heart failure	Anthracylines, high-dose cyclophosphamide, cisplatin, herceptin, taxanes
Dental/oral health	Dental caries, dry mouth	—	—
Endocrine-pituitary	Various hormone deficiencies	Diabetes	Steroids
Endocrine-thyroid	Low thyroid function, thyroid nodules	—	—
Endocrine-gonadal	Men: Sterility, testosterone deficiency Women: Sterility, premature menopause	Men: Sterility, testosterone deficiency Women: Sterility, premature menopause	Alkylating agents, Procarbazine hydrochloride, nitrosureas
Gastrointestinal	Malabsorption, intestinal stricture	Motility disorders	Vinca drugs
Genitourinary	Bladder scarring, small bladder capacity	Hemorrhagic cystitis (symptoms include urinary frequency, urgency, bleeding, and pain)	Cyclophosphamide, ifosfamide, transplant therapy

Hematologic	Low blood counts, myelodysplastic syndrome and acute leukemia	Myelodysplastic syndrome and acute leukemia	Alkylating agents, nitrosureas, topoisomerase inhibitors, purine analogs, any high-dose therapy with autologous transplantation
Hepatic	Abnormal liver function, liver failure	Abnormal liver function, cirrhosis, liver failure	Methotrexate, carmustine (BCNU)
Immune system	Impaired immune function, immune suppression	Impaired immune function, immune suppression	Steroids, anti-thymocyte globulin (ATG), methotrexate, rituximab, alemtuzumab, purine analogs, and any high-dose therapy with autologous transplantation
Lymphatic	Lymphedema	—	—
Nervous system	Problems with thinking, learning, memory; structural changes in the brain; bleeding into the brain	Problems with thinking, learning, memory; structural changes in the brain; paralysis; seizure	Methotrexate, multiagent chemotherapy, bortezomib
		Numbness and tingling, hearing loss	Cisplatin
		Numbness and tingling	Vinca alkaloids, taxanes. oxaliplatin
Ophthalmologic	Cataracts, dry eyes, visual impairment	Cataracts	Steroids
Pulmonary	Lung scarring, decreased lung function	Lung scarring, inflammation	Bleomycin sulfate, carmustine (BCNU), methotrexate
		Potentiation of radiation therapy effects (gemcitabine)	Actinomycin D/ doxorubicin (Adriamycin)
Renal	Hypertension, impaired kidney function	Impaired kidney function, delayed-onset renal failure	Cisplatin, methotrexate, nitrosoureas

TABLE 3-2 Examples of Possible Late Effects of Surgery Among Survivors of Adult Cancers

Procedure	Late Effect
Any procedure	Pain, cosmetic, psychosocial, impaired wound healing
Surgery involving neurologic structures (brain, spinal cord)	Impairment of cognitive function, motor sensory function, vision, swallowing, language, bowel and bladder control
Head and neck surgery	Difficulties with communication, swallowing, and breathing; cosmetic; damage to muscles affecting movement
Removal of lymph nodes	Lymphedema, retrograde ejaculation in testicular cancer
Abdominal surgery	Risk of intestinal obstruction, hernia, altered bowel function
Pelvic surgery	Sexual dysfunction, incontinence, hernia, risk of intestinal obstruction
Removal of spleen	Impaired immune function, increased risk of sepsis, hernia
Amputation; limb-sparing procedures	Functional changes; cosmetic deformity; psychosocial impact; accelerated arthritis in other joints; post-surgical, phantom, and/or neuropathic pain
Lung resection	Difficulty breathing, fatigue, generalized weakness
Prostatectomy	Urinary incontinence, sexual dysfunction, poor body image
Oophorectomy	Premature menopause and infertility
Orchiectomy	Infertility, testosterone deficiency
Ostomy	Bowel obstruction, constipation, nausea, vomiting, loss of appetite, fatigue, poor body image

Second cancers are perhaps the most frequent life-threatening late effect, but other disabling conditions may occur. Some of these are identified early in follow-up and resolve without consequence (e.g., treatment-related fatigue). Other late effects may persist, become chronic problems, and influence the progression of other diseases associated with aging (e.g., radiation-induced changes in the lung called "radiation pneumonitis," renal failure). Some late effects may only become evident years after treatment (e.g., congestive heart failure, graft versus host disease, neurological syndromes).

Certain late effects are easy to identify because they are visible or have direct effects on function. Examples include major paralysis from brain or spine neoplasms, communication and swallowing problems from head and neck cancers, and limb loss or deformity due to osteosarcoma or another type of sarcoma. Many affected individuals, in addition to their medical surveillance needs, require expensive equipment, such as wheelchairs or prostheses, to maintain functional independence and quality of life. Such equipment requires maintenance and often replacement over the lifespan.

Other effects, however, can be subtle and apparent only to the trained observer (e.g., change in posture secondary to osteoporosis) or are not directly observable and identified only through diagnostic tests (e.g., for hypothyroidism, infertility). It is sometimes difficult to distinguish among cancer-related changes, age-related changes, and those caused by comorbid conditions (see Chapter 2 for a description of the survivor population by age and comorbidity). Cancer can be considered a chronic disease, in part because of the serious consequences and persistent nature of some of cancer's late effects.

The limited empirical evidence on the late effects of adult cancer treatment is primarily confined to small case series that are not population-based. There are relatively few longitudinal cohort studies available to understand the link between specific treatment regimens and late physical and psychological effects, making it difficult to describe the natural history of late effects for patients and their health care providers. Unfortunately, absent data from longitudinal studies, the degree of risk of late effects to individual patients cannot be predicted.

To illustrate the range of late effects and the diversity of the cancer survivor population, one could consider the individual who had an early-stage melanoma successfully removed, leaving an inconspicuous scar, to have had cancer with minimum late effects and impact on life. Such a person would have concerns regarding subsequent risk of cancer, but likely would not suffer serious long-term health effects of treatment. At the other extreme might be an individual with a hematological cancer undergoing intensive chemotherapy followed by a bone marrow transplant. Such a person would face substantial long-term health problems associated with treatment. This variation in survivorship experience is more fully described in the next section, where late effects and interventions to ameliorate them are more fully described for four cancer types: cancer of the breast, prostate, and colon and rectum, and Hodgkin's disease. These sites were selected because more than half of all cancer survivors have had these types of cancer. In addition, they were selected because investigators have focused research on these cancers and there is an extensive survivorship literature available. Other cancer sites, while not covered at length in this review, also have potential for major, varied, and often lifelong disabling effects. For example, individuals with brain or spine tumors may develop severe neurologic deficits (Mukand et al., 2001); survivors of head and neck cancer may have impaired eating, communication, and musculoskeletal functions of the neck and shoulder (Hammerlid and Taft, 2001); and individuals with bone cancers may require amputations or limb-sparing procedures that interfere with mobility (Hoffman et al., 2002).

SITE-SPECIFIC REVIEW

The following brief site-specific summaries of late effects of cancer and its treatment are based on selected reviews and literature to which the reader is referred for more detailed information. Information on interventions that are available to ameliorate these health effects are also described, as are available clinical practice guidelines (CPGs) for the management of late effects. CPGs are "systematically developed statements to assist practitioner and patient decisions about appropriate health care for specific clinical circumstances" (IOM, 1990).

Female Breast Cancer[3]

The experience of survivors of breast cancer has been the most extensively researched. Women with a history of breast cancer are the largest group of cancer survivors, representing 22 percent of the survivorship population (see Chapter 2 for a description of breast cancer survivors). The evolving nature of breast cancer treatment has generated a heterogeneous group of breast cancer survivors (Box 3-3). Elderly survivors treated 20 to 30 years ago, for example, had fewer treatment options and likely experienced mastectomy. The issues of concern to those women were often linked to late effects of surgery such as lymphedema and body image. Younger cohorts of women, in contrast, have benefited from a wider range of options, but may be concerned about a broader set of late effects related to their treatment.

Quality of Life

At the conclusion of primary treatment for breast cancer, women generally report good emotional functioning, but decreased physical function-

[3]Much of this section is based on recent comprehensive reviews relating to breast cancer treatment and late effects (Burstein and Winer, 2000; Shapiro and Recht, 2001; Partridge et al., 2001, 2003; Emens and Davidson, 2003; Hurria and Hudis, 2003; Kattlove and Winn, 2003; Harris et al., 2004; Mrozek and Shapiro, 2005). Literature was identified by searching PubMed for articles published in English since 1994 with the MeSH heading "breast neoplasms" and an additional search term, including "survivors" [MeSH], "lymphedema" [MeSH], "menopause" [MeSH], "heart diseases" [MeSH], "weight gain," "cognitive impairment," "fatigue," and "late effects." Articles relating to childhood cancer survivors were excluded.

ing, especially those women who have had a mastectomy or receive chemotherapy (Ganz et al., 2004a). Persistent symptoms one year following either lumpectomy or mastectomy to treat early-stage breast cancer can include numbness in the chest wall or axilla, tightness, pulling or stretching in the arm or axilla, less energy or fatigue, difficulty in sleeping, and hot flashes (Shimozuma et al., 1999). Despite these symptoms most women report high levels of functioning and quality of life, with no relationship between the type of surgery and quality of life. By 2 to 3 years following surgery, breast cancer survivors in one study rated their quality of life more favorably than outpatients with other common medical conditions, and they identified many positive aspects from the cancer experience (Ganz et al., 1996). However, some aspects of quality of life (e.g., sexual function and interest, body image) and rehabilitation problems (e.g., physical functioning) worsened after that time. Among the factors that have been associated with poorer ratings of quality of life among breast cancer survivors are impaired physical functioning, poor body image, a lack of social support, coping strategies, and aspects of care such as poor communication with physicians (Mandelblatt et al., 2003; Ganz et al., 2003b, Avis et al., 2005).

Several studies of the long-term consequences of breast cancer and its treatment have been conducted. The largest of these assessed the quality of life of disease-free survivors of Stage I or II breast cancer at 1 to 5 years (baseline) and then at 5 to 10 years following their diagnosis (Ganz et al., 1998b, 2002).[4] At baseline, breast cancer survivors were found to function at a high level, similar to healthy women without cancer. However, compared to survivors with no adjuvant therapy, those who received chemotherapy had significantly more sexual problems, and those treated with tamoxifen experienced more vasomotor symptoms such as hot flashes and night sweats (Ganz et al., 1998b). At the 5- to 10-year follow-up, physical well-being and emotional well-being were excellent. The minimal changes between the baseline and follow-up assessments reflected expected age-related changes. Complaints at baseline of hot flashes, night sweats, vaginal discharge, and breast sensitivity were reported less frequently at follow-up. However, symptoms of vaginal dryness and urinary incontinence were increased. In this study, survivors with no past systemic adjuvant therapy had a better quality of life than those who had received systemic adjuvant therapy (chemotherapy, tamoxifen, or both) (Ganz et al., 2002). The asso-

[4]Stage I: primary tumor is 2 cm or less, with no spread to the lymph nodes. Stage II: primary tumor is 2-5 cm with spread to the lymph nodes, or larger than 5 cm with no spread to the lymph nodes.

BOX 3-3
Advances in Breast Cancer Treatment: Implications for Late Effects

Research that demonstrated that breast-conserving therapy followed by radiation is an efficacious alternative to mastectomy in most women has contributed to less disfigurement and reduced morbidity among women (Fisher et al., 2002). In research conducted over the past three decades, clinical trials have demonstrated that chemotherapy given to women shortly after their primary surgery and/or radiation treatment (called adjuvant therapy) reduces the risk of recurrence by 20 to 40 percent and reduces mortality by 10 to 30 percent at 10 years following treatment (NIH, 2000; Shapiro and Recht, 2001; Early Breast Cancer Trialists' Collaborative Group, 2004a). For women whose tumors are hormone receptor positive (with either estrogen or progesterone receptor expression), which includes about 70 percent of breast cancer patients, endocrine therapies (e.g., aromatase inhibitors, tamoxifen, surgical removal of the ovaries) have been found to reduce recurrence rates by nearly 50 percent and death rates by more than 25 percent (Early Breast Cancer Trialists' Collaborative Group, 2004b; Mrozek and Shapiro, 2005). Adjuvant chemotherapy, endocrine therapy, or both are widely recommended for women with invasive breast tumors greater than 1 cm in diameter, irrespective of whether axillary lymph nodes are involved (NIH, 2000; NCCN, 2004b). Although these interventions are beneficial, they can lead to late effects, and decision making about the approach to adjuvant therapy can be complex (Langer, 2001; Ganz, 2001a). During the 1990s, many women with metastatic breast cancer underwent high-dose chemotherapy and bone marrow transplantation, which was later shown not to be more effective than standard-dose chemotherapy alone for advanced disease. Women who survived this treatment experienced not only the late effects, but also the financial costs of this expensive procedure. Most women alive today

ciation of lower quality of life among women treated with systemic chemotherapy as compared to local therapy has been observed in more recent studies (Ahles et al., 2005).

Information on the long-term consequences of breast cancer are also available from the longitudinal Nurses' Health Study, a study that began in 1976 and has prospectively followed 121,700 female nurses ages 30 to 55 (Michael et al., 2000). The unique contribution of this study is that information on functional health status is available about women both before and after their diagnosis of cancer. In addition, the study was able to control for age-related changes in functional status by comparing women with a history of breast cancer to the large cohort of women in the Nurses' Health Study without breast cancer. In this study, there were greater than expected declines in physical function and role function due to physical and emotional problems, vitality, social function, and increased bodily pain among the breast cancer survivors relative to the control population. Risk after transplantation received it for extensive nodal disease without distant metastases.

Contemporary treatment for breast cancer usually involves various combinations of surgery, radiation therapy, cytotoxic chemotherapy, and hormone therapy. Selection of therapy is influenced by the age and menopausal status of the patient, stage of the disease, and certain characteristics of the tumor (e.g., its histologic and nuclear grade,[a] presence of estrogen and progesterone receptors, measures of proliferative capacity, and genetic characteristics such as overexpression of some growth factor receptors such as human epidermal growth factor receptor 2, or HER2/neu) (NCI, 2004a).

The effectiveness of adjuvant chemotherapy can be improved by administering a higher dose of drug per unit time (called dose density). In a recent study, for example, women with node-positive breast cancer were more likely to survive when a given dose of adjuvant chemotherapy was administered over a period of 22 weeks instead of 33 weeks (Citron et al., 2003; Stearns and Davidson, 2004). This intensification in dose increases the drugs' toxicity, but data are not yet available to determine if the risk of late effects is increased.

Genetic profiling methods are becoming available that can help predict which women will benefit most from chemotherapy and adjuvant therapies. As such methods become part of the standard initial evaluation of patients, treatment of late effects may decline as therapies are tailored to individual risk (Paik et al., 2004; Mrozek and Shapiro, 2005).

[a]Nuclear grade is an evaluation of the size and shape of the nucleus in tumor cells and the percentage of tumor cells that are in the process of dividing or growing. Cancers with low nuclear grade grow and spread less quickly than cancers with high nuclear grade.

of decline was attenuated with increasing time since diagnosis, but remained significant for some domains of function up to 4 years after diagnosis. Prediagnosis level of social integration is an important factor in future health-related QOL among breast cancer survivors, pointing to the need for adequate social support (Michael et al., 2002). In a subsequent study of breast cancer survivors participating in the Nurses' Health Study (NHS I and II), investigators found significant functional declines among breast cancer survivors who had been diagnosed at age 40 or younger (Kroenke et al., 2004). Relative to their peers, these women experienced declines in physical roles, bodily pain, social functioning, and mental health. Declines observed among breast cancer survivors aged 65 and older were those expected with age.

Younger breast cancer survivors (under age 50) have reported good quality of life and high levels of functioning when assessed 5 to 10 years after their diagnosis (Bloom et al., 2004; Casso et al., 2004). Mild impairment, however, has been observed in the area of sexual functioning.[5] Recent evidence suggests that among women of reproductive age, concerns about reproduction lower ratings of quality of life (Schover, 2005; Wenzel et al., 2005).

There is limited information on racial or ethnic differences in quality of life among women diagnosed with breast cancer. One study that compared outcomes of African-American and white breast cancer survivors found that differences in reported quality of life were attributable to socioeconomic and life-burden factors and not to race/ethnicity (Ashing-Giwa et al., 1999). African-American women demonstrated better quality of life outcomes as compared to white women in a study of younger breast cancer survivors (aged 50 years or younger) who were also disease-free survivors for 2 to 10 years (Ganz et al., 2003a). African-American women found more meaning in life as a result of having had breast cancer, while Hispanic women reported more physical symptoms, according to a study of breast cancer survivors followed up within 5 years of their diagnosis (Giedzinska et al., 2004).

Table 3-3 summarizes specific late effects found among breast cancer survivors. These late effects are described more fully below.

Cancer Recurrence

Women with recurrent disease in the breast or regional lymph nodes can be treated and potentially cured. Disease that has metastasized to distant organs, however, is not curable, but some women live years or even decades after such metastases are discovered. Most recurrences in the breast are detected within 5 years of diagnosis with a peak rate of recurrence during the second year following diagnosis (Burstein and Winer, 2000; Emens and Davidson, 2003). There is not a defined time at which breast cancer survivors can be considered definitively cured of their disease because recurrences can occur more than 20 years after primary therapy. More than three-quarters of recurrences are identified through symptoms (e.g., shortness of breath, bone pain) or by physical examination (e.g., feeling a mass). Recommendations for follow-up include routine history, physical examination, and annual mammogram.

[5] The presence of breast-related symptoms at baseline, use of adjuvant therapy, having lower income, and type of breast surgery (mastectomy) were significantly associated with lower quality of life at follow-up.

Second Primary Cancer

Women with a history of breast cancer, in addition to being at risk for a recurrence of their original cancer, are at risk of developing another cancer, independent of the first occurrence. The risk of developing these so-called "second primary cancers" depends not only on an individual's inherent predisposition, but also on the treatments used for the initial cancer. The underlying risk of developing a second primary cancer in the contralateral breast is estimated to be 0.5 to 1 percent per year and is greater in women whose first cancer was diagnosed at a younger age and women with heritable or familial breast cancer (Burstein and Winer, 2000). Radiation therapy contributes to a higher risk of cancer in exposed areas (e.g., soft-tissue sarcomas of the thorax, shoulder, and pelvis; lung cancer) (Matesich and Shapiro, 2003; Levi et al., 2003). Adjuvant chemotherapy, including alkylating agents and topoisomerase II inhibitors (e.g., anthracyclines), can increase the risk for acute myelogenous leukemia (Mrozek and Shapiro, 2005). Little is known about long-term side effects of a class of drugs called taxanes (i.e., paclitaxel, docetaxel)[6] due to their relatively recent introduction into standard practice in the adjuvant setting (Mrozek and Shapiro, 2005).

Tamoxifen is usually administered for 5 years to women with estrogen receptor- (ER-) positive tumors.[7] While providing survival benefits, serious medical risks associated with tamoxifen include endometrial cancer, strokes, and blood clots. Women taking tamoxifen have a two- to threefold increase in the risk of developing endometrial cancer (about 80 excess cases per 10,000 treated women at 10 years) (Matesich and Shapiro, 2003). This increase occurs primarily in women over the age of 50. Most of the endometrial cancers that develop are early-stage and low-grade tumors that can be successfully treated (Burstein and Winer, 2000). Women taking tamoxifen are advised to undergo an annual pelvic examination while taking tamoxifen, and to see a gynecologist if they have irregular bleeding (Shapiro and Recht, 2001).[8]

Two small groups of breast cancer survivors face relatively high risks of

[6]Taxanes are effective when used to treat women with metastatic breast cancer. More recently taxanes have been shown to improve outcomes when used in addition to other adjuvant chemotherapy for women with node-positive breast cancer (Henderson et al., 2003; Stearns and Davidson, 2004).

[7]Tamoxifen is a drug that acts like estrogen on some tissues, but blocks the effect of estrogen on other tissues (it is in a class of drugs called selective estrogen receptor modulators).

[8]Routine endometrial surveillance using biopsy or transvaginal ultrasound is not warranted, according to findings from clinical trials of their effectiveness in identifying early uterine cancer among breast cancer survivors (Emens and Davidson, 2003).

TABLE 3-3 Possible Late Effects Among Breast Cancer Survivors

Late Effect	Population at Risk	Risk	Interventions
Cancer recurrence	All women with a history of breast cancer	Varies by stage and tumor characteristics	Mammography, physical examination
Second primary cancer	All women with a history of breast cancer	Varies by treatment, age, and genetic predisposition (women with BRCA[a] mutations are at higher risk)	Mammography, pelvic examination, general physical examination, patient education
Psychosocial distress	All women with a history of breast cancer	Approximately 30 percent experience distress at some point; distress declines over time	Assessment for distress Some psychosocial interventions are effective in reducing distress
Arm lymphedema	Women who had axillary dissection and/or radiation therapy	Across treatments and time since treatment, approximately 12 to 25 percent of women develop lymphedema	Massage and exercise (manual lymphatic drainage), use of elastic compression garments, complex decongestive therapy
Premature menopause and related infertility and osteoporosis	Women who received adjuvant chemotherapy (e.g., alkylating agents such as cyclophosphamide) Women with BRCA mutations who elect oopherectomy	Risk depends on the chemotherapy regimen, the cumulative dose, and patient age (see details below)	New reproductive technologies for infertility Diagnostic and preventive strategies for osteoporosis Assessment of sexual function
Symptoms of estrogen deprivation (e.g., hot flashes, sweats, vaginal discharge)	Women taking endocrine therapy	More than half report symptoms, although mild in most cases	Promising nonhormone treatments include antidepressants, dietary changes. and exercise

Weight gain (associated with poorer prognosis)	Women who had adjuvant chemotherapy and experience menopause	Roughly half report weight gain of 6 to 11 pounds; one-fifth report weight gain of 22 to 44 pounds	Diet/exercise interventions
Cardiovascular disease	Women receiving specific therapies (e.g., anthracycline chemotherapy, trastuzumab [Herceptin]) Premenopausal women with ovarian failure following chemotherapy	Congestive heart failure develops in 0.5 to 1 percent of women Increased risk of atherosclerosis	Symptomatic women should have a symptom-directed cardiac work-up; routine screening of cardiac function is not recommended Preventive strategies for heart disease
Fatigue	Women with breast cancer	Reported in one-third of survivors 1 to 5 years after diagnosis. Prevalence similar to that seen in women in the general population of same age. A subgroup of survivors has more severe and persistent fatigue.	Exercise programs appear promising
Cognitive impairment	Women who received adjuvant chemotherapy	Estimates vary, but up to one-third of women with impairments. New evidence suggests onset may precede chemotherapy treatment.	Evidence lacking
Risk to family members	All survivors	An estimated 5 to 10 percent of women with breast cancer have a hereditary form of the disease	Genetic counseling

[a]BRCA genes (e.g., BRCA1 and BRCA2) are genes that normally help to suppress cell growth. A person who inherits an altered version of the BRCA genes has a higher risk of getting breast, ovarian, or prostate cancer.

second cancers. First, women with BRCA mutations (5 to 10 percent of women with breast cancer) are at increased risk of ovarian cancer, non-colonic gastrointestinal cancers, and second primary breast cancer. Women with BRCA1 and BRCA2 mutations who do not undergo prophylactic surgery have a risk of breast cancer of 45 to 84 percent by age 70 (Ford et al., 1998; Antoniou et al., 2003; King et al., 2003; Easton et al., 2004). Such women may benefit from genetic counseling, breast cancer early detection tools (i.e., breast self-examination, clinical breast examinations, annual mammograms, magnetic resonance imaging (MRI) examinations) (Warner et al., 2004), and ovarian cancer detection tools (e.g., transvaginal ultrasound, annual pelvic examination) (Isaacs et al., 2004). Counseling can be provided regarding prophylactic measures such as mastectomy and tamoxifen use to reduce the risk of breast cancer, and oophorectomy to minimize the risk of ovarian cancer. A second small group of women at significantly higher risk of second cancer are those treated with intensive-dose chemotherapy (Fisher et al., 1999). These women are at higher risk of myelodysplasia and acute myelogenous leukemia, and if symptomatic can be evaluated with blood counts.

Psychosocial Distress[9]

Most of the literature on the psychosocial aspects of breast cancer suggests that the vast majority of women adjust well to the diagnosis of breast cancer, and manage the complex and sometimes aggressive treatments associated with primary treatment and recurrent disease (Maunsell et al., 1992; Schag et al., 1993; Ganz et al., 1996; Dorval et al., 1998; Ganz et al., 1998a; Hanson Frost et al., 2000; Ganz et al., 2002). When cancer-related distress occurs, it generally dissipates with time for the majority of individuals diagnosed with breast cancer.

The frequency and patterns of psychosocial distress that occur among women with breast cancer depend greatly on which concerns are included in the operational definition of distress and how it is measured. The highest distress levels appear to occur at transition points in treatment: at the time of diagnosis, awaiting treatment, during and on completion of treatment, at follow-up visits, at time of recurrence, and at time of treatment failure (Box 3-4). Taken overall, around 30 percent of women show significant distress at some point during the illness. At higher risk for psychosocial distress are

[9]This section of the report is based primarily on the Institute of Medicine report *Meeting the Psychosocial Needs of Women with Breast Cancer* (IOM, 2004) and a recent review of the psychosocial literature pertaining to breast cancer (Kornblith and Ligibel, 2003).

BOX 3-4
Psychosocial Issues Related to Transition Points in Treatment

"After my very last radiation treatment for breast cancer, I lay on a cold steel table hairless, half-dressed, and astonished by the tears streaming down my face. I thought I would feel happy about finally reaching the end of treatment, but instead, I was sobbing. At the time, I wasn't sure what emotions I was feeling. Looking back, I think I cried because this body had so bravely made it through 18 months of surgery, chemotherapy, and radiation. Ironically, I also cried because I would not be coming back to that familiar table where I had been comforted and encouraged. Instead of joyous, I felt lonely, abandoned, and terrified. This was the rocky beginning of cancer survivorship for me."

SOURCE: McKinley (2000).

women who are relatively young, have a history of preexisting depression or psychological distress, have other serious comorbid conditions, and have inadequate social support (Maunsell et al., 1992; Ganz et al., 1992, 1993; Schag et al., 1993; Mor et al., 1994; Schover, 1994; Maunsell et al., 1995; Wenzel et al., 1999; Leedham and Ganz, 1999; Shimozuma et al., 1999). The specific type of breast cancer surgery or taking tamoxifen does not influence the level of distress (Maunsell et al., 1989; Ganz et al., 1992, 1993, 1998a,b; Omne-Ponten et al., 1994; Schover et al., 1995; Day et al., 1999, 2001; Rowland et al., 2000; Fallowfield et al., 2001).

Functional status, sense of well-being, and self-perceived health reported by disease-free breast cancer survivors were found to be similar or more positive than those from healthy women of comparable ages in a large cross-sectional study (Figure 3-2) (Ganz et al., 1998a). This and other studies have shown that marital relationships are generally maintained and are often reported to have strengthened following breast cancer treatment (Kornblith and Ligibel, 2003; Schover, 2004; Dorval et al., 2005). Assessing the factors that contribute to resilience, effective coping with cancer, and positive psychological outcomes associated with the cancer experience is of increasing interest to researchers (Petrie et al., 1999; Justice, 1999; Cordova et al., 2001; Brennan, 2001; Tomich and Helgeson, 2002).

For a minority of women, however, a diagnosis of breast cancer contributes to significant psychosocial distress that can interfere with functioning and well-being (Massie and Holland, 1991). In a review of the literature on depression in patients with cancer, Massie found breast cancer to be among the sites that had especially high prevalence, ranging from 2 to 46 percent, in the studies reviewed (Massie, 2004). This range of estimates is in part due to variation in assessment procedures (Trask, 2004). In terms of

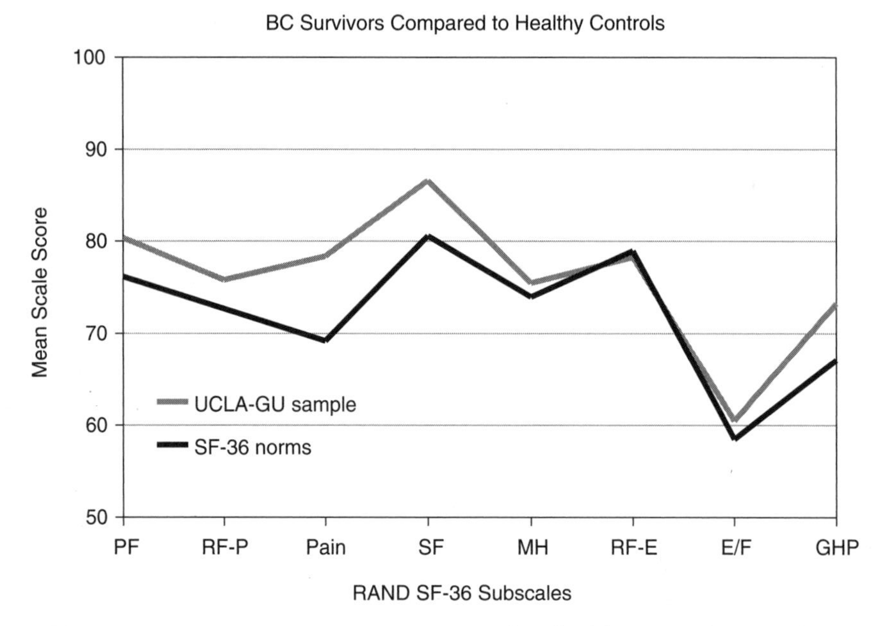

FIGURE 3-2 Breast cancer survivors compared to healthy controls. BC = breast cancer; PF = physical functioning; RF-P = role limitations attributed to physical problems; SF = social functioning; MH = mental health; RF-E = role limitations attributed to emotional problems; E/F = energy and fatigue; GHP = general health perception; UCLA-GU sample = University of California-Los Angeles and Georgetown University sample of breast cancer survivors; SF-36 norms = healthy controls. SOURCE: Reprinted with permission from the American Society of Clinical Oncology. Ganz PA, Rowland JH, Desmond K, Meyerowitz BE, Wyatt GE. 1998a. Life after breast cancer: Understanding women's health-related quality of life and sexual functioning. *J Clin Oncol* 16(2):501–514.

extreme psychiatric morbidity, some evidence points to breast cancer as potentially leading to the development of post-traumatic stress disorder (PTSD).[10] For example, in one study that assessed breast cancer survivors 20 years after treatment, relatively few women (5 percent) had clinical

[10]Diagnostic criteria for post-traumatic stress disorder include (1) experiencing or witnessing an event that is perceived as a threat to life or the bodily integrity of self or loved one, with an accompanying reaction of intense fear, horror, or helplessness; (2) persistent reexperiencing of the event; (3) avoidance of things, events, or people that remind one of the event or numbing of responsiveness; and (4) persistent symptoms of increased arousal. The disturbance lasts for more than 1 month and causes clinically significant distress or impairment (American Psychiatric Association, 1994).

levels of distress, but 15 percent reported two or more symptoms of PTSD that were moderately to extremely bothersome (Kornblith et al., 2003).

Beneficial effects of a range of psychosocial interventions have been found in randomized trials in women with breast cancer (IOM, 2004). Notably, there is evidence for the benefit of individual interventions and relaxation/hypnosis/imagery for women with early-stage breast cancer. Group interventions are effective for women with both early and metastatic breast cancer. According to a recent clinical trial, relatively simple interventions (e.g., a videotape on issues related to reentry transitions, sessions with a cancer educator) helped to reduce common symptoms experienced by women during the transition from active treatment to survivorship (Stanton et al., 2004). Another recent clinical trial suggests that psychological interventions have immunological benefits in addition to relieving distress and improving health behaviors (Andersen et al., 2004). Although it needs strengthening, this body of evidence supports the conclusion that psychosocial interventions can be expected to reduce psychiatric symptoms and improve quality of life in routine clinical care of breast cancer (IOM, 2004). (See Chapter 4, Appendix 4D for a description of the delivery of psychosocial services for women with breast cancer.)

Lymphedema[11]

Lymphedema is a relatively common late effect of surgery and radiation therapy for breast cancer. Surgery to remove lymph nodes for biopsy and radiation treatment both contribute to an interruption of the flow of fluid within the axillary lymphatic system. When impeded, fluid accumulates in subcutaneous tissue in the arm. Lymphedema and related long-term chronic inflammatory changes can be painful, limit function, increase the risk of infection, and diminish quality of life. In addition to the discomfort associated with lymphedema, women may suffer arm pain and numbness following their treatment.

No large population-based studies of the incidence of lymphedema have been carried out using standardized procedures for diagnosis, measurement, and follow-up time. Consequently, there are no precise estimates of its risk (Erickson et al., 2001; Sparaco and Fentiman, 2002). Available evidence suggests that across treatments and time since treatment, approximately 12 to 25 percent of women develop arm edema after treatment for breast cancer. The onset of lymphedema following breast

---

[11]This section of the report is based on literature reviews of Kligman et al. (2004), Erickson et al. (2001), and Sparaco and Fentiman (2002).

cancer treatment varies. For most women it develops within 1 year of treatment, but for others it can occur up to 4 years or more following treatment (Mortimer et al., 1996). The risk appears to vary by extent of treatment with surgery and radiotherapy; however, the relative contributions of these interventions to the development of lymphedema is not clearly understood. Prospective studies of lymphedema are needed that use consistent definitions and measures.[12]

Lymphedema frequently occurs among women who have lymph nodes removed to determine the extent of cancer spread. Until the late 1990s, most women with early breast cancer had a procedure called axillary dissection, where some or all of the lymph nodes in the armpit area near the affected breast were removed. In 1994, a procedure called sentinel lymph node biopsy was tested on women with breast cancer in an effort to reduce the morbidity associated with axillary dissection while preserving the diagnostic utility of examining lymph nodes for evidence of cancer (Posther et al., 2004).[13] Evidence of the effectiveness of sentinel lymph node biopsy will be available toward the end of the decade at the conclusion of clinical trials now underway (National Surgical Adjuvant Breast and Bowel Project, 2004; White and Wilke, 2004; Krag et al., 2004; Posther et al., 2004).[14] In the meantime, sentinel lymph node biopsy is widely used in the United States, especially at major cancer centers. Estimates are that sentinel lymph node biopsy, if proven effective, could save 70 percent of women with negative findings at physical examination and negative pathology results following sentinel lymph node biopsy from the morbidity of immediate, complete axillary dissection (Schwartz, 2004). Some descriptive studies suggest that sentinel lymph node biopsy significantly reduces the occurrence of arm lymphedema among women with breast cancer (Blanchard et al., 2003b).

---

[12]Variability in study design and lymphedema assessment in available studies make it difficult to draw firm conclusions regarding lymphedema's etiology, natural history, and risk factors. Many of the studies are retrospective and may underestimate incidence because of a lack of documentation in the medical record or a failure on the part of clinicians to check for lymphedema. Other studies rely on patient self-reports, which may reflect different impressions of lymphedema.

[13]Sentinel node biopsy relies on techniques to identify the "sentinel" node, the first node likely to be invaded by cancer. This technique involves injecting substances into the breast that enter the lymph system and concentrate in what is thought to be the sentinel node. This node can be identified and removed to test for cancer. If no cancer is detected, the remainder of the lymph nodes are spared.

[14]Two cooperative groups sponsored by the National Cancer Institute, the National Surgical Adjuvant Breast and Bowel Project and the American College of Surgeons Oncology Group, initiated three multicenter clinical trials in 1999. Accrual of patients for two of the trials was completed in 2003 and 2004. With endpoints including 5-year survival, final results of the trials will not be available until the end of this decade (Posther et al., 2004).

BOX 3-5
Case Study: Lymphedema

Shop owner Catherine Pascucci had three lymph nodes removed and a lumpectomy and radiation treatment for breast cancer 3 years ago. After her surgery, she returned to her fragrance shop, lifting boxes and ringing sales, never knowing that she was at risk for lymphedema. About 3 months after cancer surgery, she noticed her bracelet was tight, but her breast surgeon attributed her swollen arm to a reaction to a bug bite. Months later, another doctor told her about lymphedema, and she sought treatment. She now undergoes regular physical therapy treatments and wears compression bandages to control the swelling.

SOURCE: Adapted from Parker-Pope (2004).

There have been relatively few well-designed, randomized trails to test the range of therapies that are available to treat lymphedema (Badger et al., 2004a,b,c). Nonpharmacologic treatments, such as massage and exercise (manual lymphatic drainage), use of elastic compression garments, and a technique called complex physical therapy or complex decongestive therapy, appear to be effective therapies for lymphedema (Kligman et al., 2004). These complex therapies involve skin care, manual lymphatic drainage, and low-stretch compression bandaging followed by a fitted compression garment when the edema has plateaued (Sparaco and Fentiman, 2002). Pharmacologic interventions (e.g., anticoagulants, diuretics) have not been shown to be effective in treating lymphedema itself (Loprinzi et al., 1999; Sparaco and Fentiman, 2002; Kligman et al., 2004), but certain medications may help alleviate discomfort, infection, or other side effects associated with lymphedema (Erickson et al., 2001). Avoidance of activities and factors known to trigger lymphedema (e.g., having blood pressure checked or blood drawn) can reduce its development (NCCN, 2004a) (Box 3-5). The role of exercise and prevention (e.g., use of low-pressure sleeve at specified times of arm use) in reducing the occurrence of lymphedema among women with breast cancer is being examined (Paskett, 2003). Obesity is a risk factor for lymphedema, and maintenance of a healthy weight is recommended (Johansson et al., 2002). Areas in need of further research include assessments of the value of prevention, early diagnosis, surveillance strategies, and treatment (Erickson et al., 2001). (See Chapter 4, Appendix 4D for a description of the delivery of rehabilitation services, including lymphedema services.)

Reproductive/Sexual Function[15]

Adjuvant chemotherapy improves the survival of women with breast cancer, but is associated with late effects of the reproductive system and in turn sexual function. Menopause can be precipitated among premenopausal women who were treated with certain types of chemotherapy that are directly toxic to the ovaries. Issues related to fertility and lactation are of particular concern to younger breast cancer survivors who may have delayed childbearing and not completed their families.

Premature menopause The risk of amenorrhea (either temporary or permanent) after common adjuvant treatments for breast cancer varies by the agent used, its dose, and the patient's age (Figure 3-3) (Goodwin et al., 1999b; Burstein and Winer, 2000). Most women over age 40 who receive chemotherapy can expect permanent or prolonged menstrual dysfunction. For example, more than 70 percent of women over age 40, and 40 percent of younger women treated with the chemotherapy regimen CMF, will develop permanent ovarian failure (Mrozek and Shapiro, 2005).[16] Younger women are likely to have a transient period of amenorrhea and then resume menses.

Roughly one-third (35 percent) of women newly diagnosed with breast cancer are under age 55. Given that the average age of menopause in North American women is 51 years, many of these women will be subject to immediate menopause, and those who continue to menstruate after chemotherapy are at risk for premature menopause. More than half of all women taking tamoxifen experience hot flashes, sweats, and vaginal discharge; however, in most cases, symptoms are mild and subside over time (Fallowfield et al., 2001; Ganz, 2001a).

Premenopausal women who elect to have their ovaries removed (oophorectomy) as a part of their breast cancer treatment, such as women with BRCA mutations, will also experience premature menopause. Women with ER-positive tumors may have an oophorectomy or have the function of their ovaries temporarily suppressed through treatments with hormones (e.g., luteinizing hormone-releasing hormone analogues such as goserelin).

---

[15]This section of the report is largely based on several comprehensive reviews of reproductive, gynecological, and sexual consequences of breast cancer and its treatment (Burstein and Winer, 2000; Ganz, 2001b; Chlebowski et al., 2003; Kornblith and Ligibel, 2003; Friedlander and Thewes, 2003).

[16]CMF is a regimen that contains cyclophosphamide, methotrexate, and fluorouracil. The risk of ovarian failure is lower with a regimen of doxorubicin and cyclophosphamide than with CMF. Paclitaxel-containing adjuvant chemotherapy does not appear to increase the risk of ovarian failure (Mrozek and Shapiro, 2005).

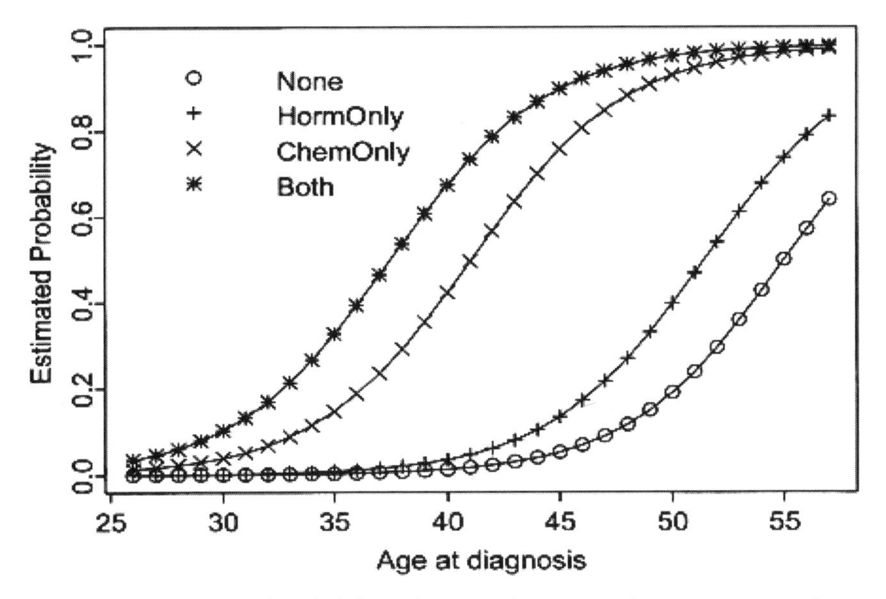

FIGURE 3-3 Estimated probability of amenorrhea among breast cancer survivors, by age at diagnosis and treatment modality.
SOURCE: Reprinted with permission from the American Society of Clinical Oncology. Goodwin PJ, Ennis M, Pritchard KI, Trudeau M, Hood N. 1999b. Risk of menopause during the first year after breast cancer diagnosis. *J Clin Oncol* 17(8):2365–2370.

The short-term effects of diminished circulating levels of estrogen that occur with menopause include:

- Hot flashes, sweats, and palpitations (referred to as "vasomotor symptoms")
- Vaginal dryness and sexual changes, including pain with sexual intercourse
- Urinary incontinence
- Musculoskeletal complaints such as joint pains and skin changes
- Sleep disturbance
- Mood changes

Because chemotherapy causes an abrupt change in menopausal status, symptoms can be more severe than those associated with the usual transition that with normal aging lasts from 5 to 10 years (Burstein and Winer, 2000; Ganz, 2001b; Crandall et al., 2004).

Menopausal symptoms are very prevalent among breast cancer survivors, according to the Cancer and Menopause Study, a study designed to evaluate the quality of life and health outcomes of younger survivors of breast cancer (aged 50 or younger at diagnosis and disease-free for 2 to 10 years) (Ganz et al., 2003a; Crandall et al., 2004). Hot flashes, for example, occurred in 17 percent, 51 percent, and 71 percent of pre-, peri-,[17] and post-menopausal breast cancer survivors, respectively. Nearly three-fourths of women had received some form of adjuvant therapy, and amenorrhea frequently resulted. Some have noted the unique menopausal experience of breast cancer survivors and have called for longer term monitoring of the severity and duration of their menopausal symptoms (Fiorica, 2004).[18]

How to best manage menopausal symptoms among breast cancer survivors is uncertain. Results of the Women's Health Initiative trial reaffirmed the small but significant increased risk of breast cancer associated with hormone replacement therapy (HRT). Long-term estrogen use is contraindicated among women with a history of breast cancer, but other non-hormonal strategies are available (Chlebowski et al., 2003; Hoda et al., 2003). For example, treatment of menopausal symptoms with antidepressants (selective serotonin reuptake inhibitors or SSRIs), vitamin E, dietary changes, and exercise appears to be promising (Friedlander and Thewes, 2003). The antidepressant fluoxetine modestly improved hot flashes among women with breast cancer when tested as part of a randomized clinical trial (Loprinzi et al., 2002).

A comprehensive menopausal assessment intervention program delivered by a nurse practitioner succeeded in reducing symptoms and improving sexual functioning among post-menopausal breast cancer survivors with at least one severe menopausal symptom (Ganz et al., 2000; Zibecchi et al., 2003). The program, evaluated through a randomized controlled trial, involved symptom assessment, education, counseling, and, as appropriate, specific pharmacologic and behavioral interventions.

There is much interest in alternative or natural therapies to treat the symptoms of menopause among all women, including those with a history of breast cancer (DiGianni et al., 2002; Canales and Geller, 2003; Sparreboom et al., 2004; Navo et al., 2004). Products on the market range from soy protein in powder form, to evening primrose oil and yam creams

[17]Perimenopause is the transitional period from normal menstrual periods to no menstrual periods. In this study, perimenopausal was defined as irregular periods, or periods that stopped for 3 months or more and then resumed.

[18]Emerging findings from clinical trials suggest that more premenopausal breast cancer patients will receive therapies that result in premature menopause and/or ovarian suppression (e.g., goserelin), and that more post-menopausal patients will receive hormone-based therapies (e.g., aromatase inhibitors) that exacerbate estrogen deficiency symptoms for longer periods of time (Chlebowski et al., 2003).

(a source of natural progesterone). A few of these substances have been tested among breast cancer survivors in randomized controlled trials, but have not been found to be effective (Jacobson et al., 2001; Van Patten et al., 2002; Amato et al., 2002; Tice et al., 2003).

Sexual function Understanding sexual functioning following treatment of breast cancer is difficult because there is a general decline in libido and an increase in vaginal dryness with normal aging. These problems are, however, often exacerbated as a result of breast cancer treatment (Ganz, 2001b). Many women who are treated with adjuvant chemotherapy report loss of libido, body image concerns, decreased breast sensitivity, and a decline in sexual activity. However, sexual functioning among a large cohort of breast cancer survivors when assessed on average 3 years after their breast cancer diagnosis was found to be very similar to that of healthy women (Ganz et al., 1998a; Meyerowitz et al., 1999). Predictors of sexual dysfunction in breast cancer survivors include being younger at diagnosis, a history of chemotherapy, and having treatment-induced amenorrhea (Ganz et al., 1998a, 1999). There is little evidence of a link between type of surgical treatment (e.g., lumpectomy versus mastectomy) and sexual functioning, but women who have had a mastectomy report poorer body image (Rowland et al., 2000; Thors et al., 2001). Tamoxifen does not appear to adversely affect sexual functioning among breast cancer survivors (Fallowfield et al., 2001; Ganz, 2001a). Few differences in sexual function between African-American and white breast cancer survivors have been reported; however, studies generally have been limited to women who are well educated, high income, and highly functional (Wyatt et al., 1998). The American Cancer Society's (ACS's) website has information on sexuality for women and their partners (ACS, 2004b). Cognitive and behavioral sexual rehabilitation interventions are available to assist persons with cancer in understanding and adjusting to the physical changes caused by cancer treatment (Gallo-Silver, 2000).

Pregnancy and lactation Reproductive-age women making treatment decisions need to be apprised of the benefits and adverse effects of treatment on reproductive function to aid in their decision making (Friedlander and Thewes, 2003). Patients are often advised to wait 2 years after diagnosis before becoming pregnant because of the higher rate of recurrence of breast cancer in this period. Women under age 35 may have a higher likelihood of relapse than older patients, which may affect reproductive decision making. For older women, a decision to delay pregnancy may diminish their chances of becoming pregnant. Evidence on the consequences of breast cancer for the estimated 3 to 7 percent of survivors who become pregnant is limited, but reassuring. To date, most studies have not shown increases in cancer recurrence among women who bear children and no increase in birth defects among offspring has been observed.

While on tamoxifen, menstrual function may be disrupted and continuous tamoxifen use is believed to suppress ovulation in most women. Women can, however, become pregnant while taking tamoxifen, but its effect on fetal development is not known. It is therefore recommended that women who wish to become pregnant discontinue tamoxifen therapy several months before conceiving (Burstein and Winer, 2000). Because tamoxifen is recommended for 5 years, women with ER-positive tumors wanting to have children must consider delaying childbearing for more than 5 years.

Assisted reproductive techniques are an option to overcome fertility problems (Oktay, 2001; Oktay et al., 2003; Oktay and Sonmezer, 2004; Oktay et al., 2005; Partridge and Winer, 2005). The reproductive strategies typically require exposure to high levels of exogenous steroidal hormones, raising a concern regarding increased risk of recurrence or second cancer, especially for women with ER-positive tumors.[19] Some promising approaches to preserve ovarian function have been suggested, but more research is needed (Friedlander and Thewes, 2003). The recent report of a live birth after the transplantation of cryopreserved ovarian tissue from a woman with Hodgkin's lymphoma holds promise for younger women diagnosed with cancer (Donnez et al., 2004).

The extent and nature of breast-conserving surgery affect the likelihood of successful lactation in the affected breast. An estimated 25 to 30 percent of women are able to lactate after breast-conserving surgery and irradiation, but the majority of women continue to report difficult and inadequate lactation in the affected breast (Burstein and Winer, 2000).

Weight Gain[20]

At least half of women receiving adjuvant chemotherapy report gaining weight, with mean gains of 2.5 to 5 kg (5.5 to 11 pounds). More significant weight gain, as much as 10 to 20 kg (22 to 44 pounds), has been reported in as many as 20 percent of women. The exact cause of weight gain is uncertain, but it may be explained in part by decreased levels of physical

[19] However, there is no evidence of an increased incidence of new cases of breast cancer among women undergoing in vitro fertilization, as compared with either the population at large or women with infertility who have not undergone in vitro fertilization. It is not known how reliably these findings apply to women who have already had breast cancer.

[20] This section is based on the review of Partridge et al. (2001).

activity during therapy and changes in metabolic rate that are associated with the menopause transition. Use of adjuvant therapy and onset of menopause are the strongest clinical predictors of weight gain when assessed 1 year from treatment (Goodwin et al., 1999a). Recent evidence suggests that obesity prior to diagnosis and decreased current physical activity, but not adjuvant treatment, were associated with obesity among breast cancer survivors when assessed approximately 6 years from the time of diagnosis (Herman et al., in press). Obesity can have serious health consequences and also impair psychosocial adaptation. Of great concern is the suggestion by some studies that weight gain may increase a woman's risk of disease recurrence and death (Chlebowski et al., 2002a; Carmichael and Bates, 2004; Dignam and Mamounas, 2004; Kroenke et al., 2005). Exercise and dietary interventions may help alleviate weight gain among women receiving adjuvant breast cancer chemotherapy (Rock and Demark-Wahnefried, 2002; Demark-Wahnefried and Rock, 2003).

Osteoporosis

Estrogen is known to contribute to the risk of breast and endometrial cancer, but to be protective against osteoporosis. Women with breast cancer, who are more likely to have had relatively high exposure to estrogens, have a significantly lower risk of osteoporosis, according to both epidemiologic and clinical research (Lamont and Lauderdale, 2003; Lamont et al., 2003). Premenopausal women who experience ovarian failure following chemotherapy are, however, at much higher risk for accelerated bone density loss.

Osteoporosis is characterized by a reduction in bone density and strength, which predisposes individuals to an increased risk of fractures (Box 3-6). Post-menopausal women average a decline in bone mineral density of about 1 to 2 percent per year, but in one study of 35 premenopausal

BOX 3-6
Case Study: Osteoporosis

A 53-year-old woman with a 13-year history of breast cancer was seen for multiple fractures that were not related to any trauma she had sustained. The fractures were determined to be due to a marked reduction in bone mineral density following premature menopause, which was secondary to her adjuvant chemotherapy.

SOURCE: Ganz (2004).

breast cancer patients who experienced ovarian failure following chemotherapy, there was an 8 percent loss in bone density after 12 months of treatment (Shapiro et al., 2001). Recent evidence suggests that post-menopausal women are also at increased risk for fractures relative to their peers (Chen et al., 2005). Tamoxifen preserves bone mineral density in post-menopausal women, but may increase bone loss in premenopausal women (Ramaswamy and Shapiro, 2003). Available evidence indicates that women treated with anastrazole (e.g., post-menopausal women with early-stage, ER-positive breast cancer) are at increased risk for fractures relative to those treated with tamoxifen (Ramaswamy and Shapiro, 2003). Aromatase inhibitors may also increase osteoporosis and lead to more bone fractures (NCCN, 2004i; Mackey and Joy, 2005).

A guideline for patient management to help maintain bone health has been published by the American Society of Clinical Oncology (ASCO). Recommended are regular monitoring of bone density, adequate dietary intake of calcium and vitamin D, exercise, and smoking cessation (Hillner et al., 2003; Friedlander and Thewes, 2003; Chlebowski, 2005b). Clinical trials are underway to prospectively monitor bone mineral density and test interventions to reduce or ameliorate the impact of treatment-related bone loss (Hillner et al., 2003).

Musculoskeletal Complaints

There is an emerging role for aromatase inhibitors (e.g., anastrozole, letrozole, exemestane) in post-menopausal women either as primary therapy or after several years of tamoxifen (Winer et al., 2005). This class of drugs completely blocks the production of estradiol in post-menopausal women, and as a result these drugs may lead to an increased risk of fractures, as well as some musculoskeletal complaints and vaginal dryness (Campos, 2004). The late effects of this class of drugs may not be life threatening, but can be very troubling (Box 3-7).

Cardiovascular Disease

One of the most serious and life-threatening late complications of chemotherapy is congestive heart failure, which develops in 0.5 to 1 percent of women treated with standard anthracycline-based chemotherapy regimens (e.g., doxorubicin) (Box 3-8) (Burstein and Winer, 2000). The cardiac dysfunction associated with anthracycline is potentially irreversible, long term, and capable of appearing years or decades following therapy (Ewer and Lippman, 2005).

Although congestive heart failure is the most extreme manifestation of anthracycline cardiotoxicity, a range of problems may arise, from mild

BOX 3-7
Case Study: Aromatase Inhibitors' Late Effects

E-mail from a patient, 3 months after starting aromatase inhibitor therapy after 5 years of tamoxifen:

"It has been several months since I started taking Femara. Although I do want to continue taking it and not take any chances with a cancer recurrence, I have encountered some problems. I am experiencing constant pain in my muscles, joints, etc., as if my body was continuously sore from strenuous exercise. The hardest times are in the morning and in the late afternoon, and I am usually very tired in the afternoon as well. I feel much better after exercise, but often I do not have enough energy or willpower after work to go to the gym. Instead I go to my bedroom and sleep. Altogether, this is not me and I want to do something to change it."

SOURCE: Ganz (2004).

BOX 3-8
Case Study: Cardiovascular Late Effects

Nearly 10 years ago, Mrs. O'Donnell found a lump in her breast. At first, she wasn't worried. A routine mammogram a month earlier showed no signs of a tumor. The lump grew so quickly during a 2-week vacation that Mrs. O'Donnell went to see her doctor days after returning home. The doctor ordered an immediate biopsy. The 42-year-old mother of three boys was diagnosed with advanced breast cancer and told she had only a 5 percent chance of surviving the next year. She proved the doctors wrong. In 1995 Mrs. O'Donnell began chemotherapy treatments, underwent two surgeries, including a mastectomy, and is now considered cancer free. Her survival came at a price. Mrs. O'Donnell, now 51, has chronic health problems arising from her cancer treatment. Just 6 weeks after her last chemotherapy session, her heart failed—a side effect of the chemotherapy. She underwent a heart transplant in 1996. That, in turn, caused other problems (e.g., medication-caused spinal deterioration, kidney disease, blood clots), which have resulted in hospitalizations and physical limitations.

SOURCE: Marcus (2004).

blood pressure changes to thrombosis and myocardial infarction (Theodoulou and Seidman, 2003). Of some concern is the observation that women treated with an anthracycline have subclinical signs of heart trouble (e.g., systolic dysfunction) that may portend later heart disease or cardiac compromise with subsequent cardiac stressors, such as hypertension

(Partridge et al., 2001). Risk factors for cardiac toxicity following anthracycline exposure include older age, preexisting heart disease, higher dose of anthra-cycline, and radiation treatment that includes the heart. Symptoms of heart disease usually develop within several months after chemotherapy, but may develop years after completion of therapy (Theodoulou and Seidman, 2003).

Other chemotherapies can cause long-term heart problems: alkylating agents (e.g., cisplatin) can cause ischemia, hypertension, and congestive heart failure; trastuzumab (Herceptin) can cause myocardial depression;[21] and paclitaxel (Taxol) is associated with arrhythmias (Yeh et al., 2004). Tamoxifen has been associated with an increased risk of stroke, but the absolute risk is small, according to a recent meta-analysis (Bushnell and Goldstein, 2004). Some research suggests that tamoxifen may protect against the development of heart disease (Bradbury et al., 2005).

The early onset of menopause precipitated by cancer treatment can also place women at increased risk of atherosclerotic cardiovascular disease. This increased risk has not been well quantified, but is related to the declining levels of estrogen and subsequent increases in cholesterol levels and changes to the circulatory system (Ganz, 2001b). Reassuring data on cardiovascular risk factors among breast cancer survivors come from a cohort study in which women were followed approximately 6 years after the time of diagnosis. The cardiovascular lipid levels and blood pressure among this cohort of breast cancer survivors were within the normal range for women of comparable age and other sociodemographic characteristics (Herman et al., in press).

When radiation therapy is administered even in the absence of anthracyclines, clinically important heart damage can occur, particularly if the dose of radiation therapy is high and administered to the left breast. In their review of the evidence regarding the cardiac effects of radiation therapy, Theodoulou and Seidman note that post-operative radiation therapy increases the risk of cardiac mortality, but this mortality is offset by a reduced number of deaths from breast cancer. With new techniques, machines, and planning, these authors conclude that radiation therapy is safer today than in the past (Theodoulou and Seidman, 2003). Some evidence of this lowering of risk comes from a recent study that found differences in heart disease mortality between women diagnosed with left-sided and right-sided breast cancer in the period 1973 to 1979, but not during the period 1980 to 1984 (Giordano et al., 2005; Cuzick, 2005).

[21]The effects of trastuzumab on cardiac function appear to be largely reversible and short lived, according to a recent review (Singh et al., 2003). Trastuzumab substantially increased cardiac dysfunction in patients treated concurrently with anthracycline.

Given the increased risk of cardiotoxicity from various treatments, women with breast cancer need to be carefully monitored for risk factors such as hypertension and hypercholesterolemia (Theodoulou and Seidman, 2003). Routine screening of cardiac function is not recommended, although patients with symptoms suggestive of heart disease should be evaluated with electrocardiography and echocardiography (Burstein and Winer, 2000).

Fatigue

Fatigue is a common symptom of cancer and its treatment, and as many as one-third of breast cancer survivors report fatigue by 1 to 5 years after diagnosis. However, this level of fatigue is comparable to age-matched controls in the general community (Bower et al., 2000). A subgroup of survivors appear to have more severe and persistent fatigue. Co-occurring depression and pain are the strongest predictors of fatigue. Other factors potentially contributing to fatigue include menopausal symptoms, changes in weight, difficulties in coping, and a lack of social support (de Jong et al., 2002). Cancer-related fatigue can be a consequence of other treatment-related effects and so is difficult to diagnose (Box 3-9).

Identifying and treating underlying causes of fatigue is the first step in fatigue management. Depression, anemia, pain, and hypothyroidism can all contribute to fatigue and can be treated. Therapies for fatigue include pharmacologic interventions (e.g., psychostimulant and antidepressant medications) as well as nonpharmacologic interventions (e.g., stress management training and energy conservation and restoration) (Sadler and Jacobsen, 2001; Rao and Cohen, 2004). Controlled clinical trials of many of these interventions are underway. Some evidence suggests that exercise is a useful strategy to overcome post-treatment fatigue (Pinto and Maruyama,

BOX 3-9
Case Study: Fatigue

A 38-year-old survivor of breast cancer treated with high-dose chemotherapy and radiation for Stage III breast cancer suffered from chronic anxiety and depression for the first 4 to 5 years following her treatment, but her mental health symptoms improved with medications. Six years following her treatment, she went to the doctor with a new complaint of debilitating fatigue. Following a careful examination, it was determined that she had radiation-induced hypothyroidism.

SOURCE: Ganz (2004).

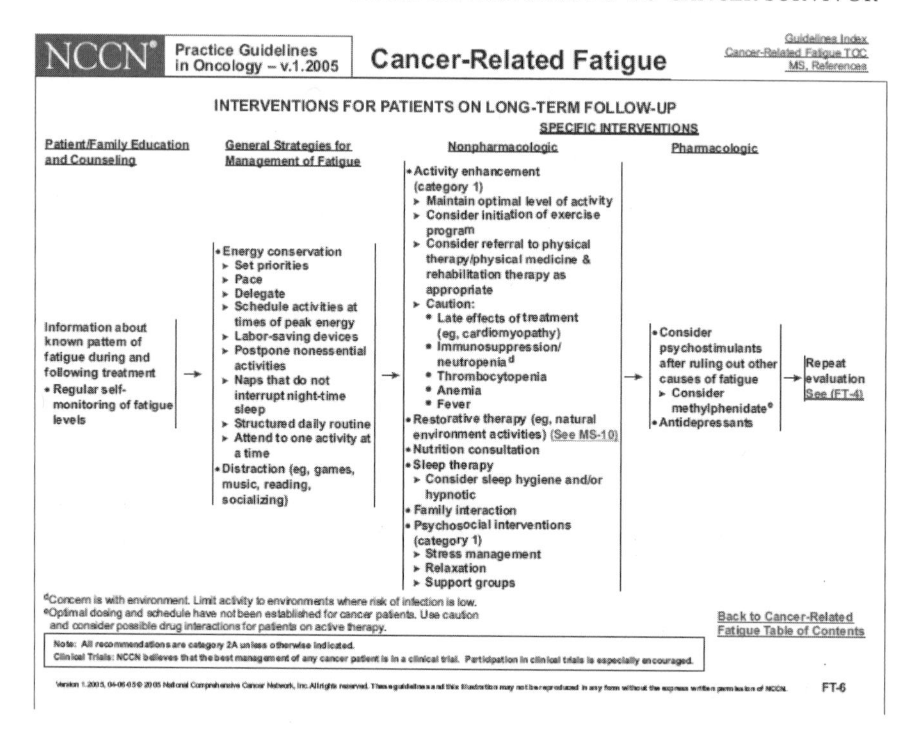

FIGURE 3-4 NCCN practice guideline on cancer-related fatigue.
NOTE: These Guidelines are a work in progress that will be refined as often as new significant data becomes available.

The NCCN Guidelines are a statement of consensus of its authors regarding their views of currently accepted approaches to treatment. Any clinician seeking to apply or consult any NCCN guideline is expected to use independent medical judgment in the context of individual clinical circumstances to determine any patient's care or treatment. The National Comprehensive Cancer Network makes no warranties of any kind whatsoever regarding their content, use or application and disclaims any responsibility for their application or use in any way.

SOURCE: NCCN (2005). Reprinted with permission from the NCCN 2.2005 Cancer-Related Fatigue Clinical Practice Guideline in Oncology. Available at: http: //nccn.org. Accessed July 22, 2005. To view the most recent and complete version of the guideline, go online to www.nccn.org.

1999). The NCCN (2005) has published guidelines on cancer-related fatigue in clinical practice (Figure 3-4).

Cognitive Effects

Cognitive dysfunction has been observed among breast cancer survivors treated with adjuvant chemotherapy (Ganz, 1998; Meyers, 2000; Brezden et al., 2000; Ahles and Saykin, 2002; Rugo and Ahles, 2003; Saykin et al., 2003; Phillips and Bernhard, 2003; Tannock et al., 2004; Wefel et al., 2004a,b). The cognitive dysfunction, sometimes called "chemobrain," includes deficits in memory, concentration, and executive functioning.[22] Such dysfunction can impede attainment of work, education, and general quality of life goals. Underlying mechanisms are unknown, but recent evidence indicates that some degree of cognitive impairment exists prior to chemotherapy, suggesting that the disease itself rather than the treatment may be responsible (Wefel et al., 2004a). In their review of baseline measurements taken as part of three clinical trials, Wefel and colleagues found that 35 percent of women exhibit cognitive impairment before the start of systemic therapy for breast cancer. According to this review, distress was found to be significantly related to cognitive impairment. Other preliminary studies suggest there may be a genetic predisposition to susceptibility to chemotherapy-associated cognitive decline (Ahles et al., 2003). In order to understand its onset and underlying mechanisms, longitudinal studies of cognitive function are needed as well as studies of interventions designed to alleviate such dysfunction.

Risk to Family Members

Approximately 5 to 10 percent of breast cancer is hereditary and accounted for by mutations in the BRCA1 and BRCA2 genes. The likelihood that a woman with breast cancer has a BRCA mutation is estimated at 1 in 50 in women who are not Ashkenazi Jewish, and 1 in 10 in Ashkenazi Jewish women (NCI, 2004b). Only women with family histories or a personal history of breast cancer at a young age are candidates for BRCA testing (NCCN, 2004e). ASCO guidelines recommend that genetic testing only be offered to selected patients with personal or family histories suggestive of a hereditary syndrome, in the context of pre- and post-test counseling to discuss the risks and benefits of genetic testing and cancer early detection and prevention methods, and only when the test results can be

[22]Executive functioning refers to the brain's supervisory or regulatory functions.

adequately interpreted and will aid in diagnosis or care management (ASCO, 2003). (See Chapter 4, Appendix 4D for a description of the delivery of cancer-related genetic counseling services.)

Breast Cancer Clinical Practice Guidelines

Table 3-4 lists 24 breast cancer clinical practice guidelines that were identified in the committee's review of survivorship-related CPGs.[23,24] These CPGs were evaluated in terms of their coverage of the following domains:

1. Surveillance for recurrent disease
2. Monitoring/prevention of second primary cancer
3. Management of late sequelae of disease
4. Management of late complications of treatment
5. Management of psychological, social, and spiritual issues
6. Management of genetic issues
7. Management of sexuality and fertility issues
8. Locus of care

Twelve of the guidelines address follow-up and include schedules and recommendations regarding testing. The four most comprehensive guidelines, those covering five or more of the eight domains assessed, were promulgated by government-sponsored guidelines groups in Australia, Canada, and Scotland. Eleven of the guidelines were very focused, addressing only one of the specific domains. A few of the guidelines addressed the appropriate use of a particular modality, such as radiotherapy or surgery, but these treatment-related CPGs included some recommendations or discussion that could apply to survivors.

---

[23]Several guidelines were identified as containing information that could guide the care of survivors, but did not specifically mention survivors or people who have been treated previously for cancer (e.g., some guidelines on chemoprevention of cancer and genetic predisposition). Those guidelines were not included in this review as survivorship guidelines. Most general guidelines for the management of menopause, hormone replacement therapy, and osteoporosis did not provide relevant recommendations specific to cancer survivors, according to the committee's review. Similarly, general psychological guidelines for the management of depression did not include recommendations that were directly relevant for the management of depression in the cancer survivor.

[24]Although Cancer Care Ontario has published a comprehensive review of treatment options for lymphedema, it is considered an evidence summary, not a guideline, and therefore was not included in this review. Other Cancer Care Ontario breast cancer guidelines were treatment focused. A guideline on depression in cancer patients is in development (Cancer Care Ontario, 2005).

The depth of coverage on survivorship issues varies markedly among guidelines, with some CPGs including both guidance on follow-up and extensive coverage of specific issues such as lymphedema and hormone replacement therapy (e.g., National Breast Cancer Center of Australia, British Columbia Cancer Agency, Steering Committee on Clinical Practice Guidelines for the Care and Treatment of Breast Cancer of Canada). Others cover only one or two topics, with little detail. Some guidelines describe potential late effects of treatment, but have little information on how to manage symptoms.

Only one guideline, from the National Breast Cancer Center of Australia, touches on all of the topics reviewed, although it does not cover each of them with equal depth. The Steering Committee on Clinical Practice Guidelines for the Care and Treatment of Breast Cancer covers nearly all of the topics; however, the lymphedema and hormone replacement therapy guidelines are published separately from the general breast cancer follow-up guideline. The clinician seeking comprehensive recommendations would be able to find them if multiple sources were searched, however, some of the guidelines are not easily identified. Of note, some major guidelines such as the Australian National Breast Cancer Center guidelines and those of the National Comprehensive Cancer Network were not included in the National Guideline Clearinghouse (NGC) that can be searched at the website of the U.S. Department of Health and Human Services (AHRQ, 2004b).[25]

All guidelines that address the issue of testing for recurrence advise against routine imaging, and blood and marker testing. The contraindication for such testing comes from randomized trials demonstrating no benefit from these procedures (Rosselli Del Turco et al., 1994; GIVIO, 1994; Liberati, 1995; Palli et al., 1999; Rojas et al., 2005). In terms of frequency of follow-up visits, all guidelines advise that visits occur on more than an annual basis, although one randomized trial assessing visit frequency showed no difference in outcomes or satisfaction for women seen on an annual or more frequent basis (Gulliford et al., 1997). The frequencies of visits in the CPGs reviewed varied within narrow limits from every 3 to 4 months to every 6 months in the first 2 years, and every 6 or 12 months in subsequent years.

Most of the guidelines offer similar schedules for follow-up visits, but recommendations for the content of follow-up visits varies. All reviewed guidelines that address surveillance recommend follow-up mammography. The strength of the mammography recommendations vary markedly, as shown in Table 3-5. Thus, depending on the guideline used, the clinician

[25]These guidelines may not have been submitted for inclusion in the NGC or they may not have met Agency for Healthcare Research and Quality criteria for inclusion (AHRQ, 1998).

TABLE 3-4 Breast Cancer Clinical Practice Guidelines

Clinical Practice Guideline	Follow-up Schedule and Testing	Monitoring for Second Primary Tumors; Chemoprevention for Second Primary Tumors
1. National Breast Cancer Center (NBCC) (Australia). Clinical Practice Guidelines for the Management of Early Breast Cancer. Follow-up, Radiotherapy, Surgery (NBCC, 2001).	•	•
2. Scottish Intercollegiate Guidelines Network (SIGN). Breast Cancer in Women: A National Clinical Guideline. Follow-up, Psychosocial Aspects, Rehabilitation, Menopausal Symptoms, and Complications of Local Treatment (1998) (SIGN, 1998).	•	•
3. British Columbia Cancer Agency. Breast Cancer. Follow-up, Lymphedema, Hormone Replacement, Pregnancy, Contraception (British Columbia Cancer Agency, 2004a).	•	•
4. Steering Committee on Clinical Practice Guidelines for the Care and Treatment of Breast Cancer (Canadian). 9. Follow-up After Treatment for Breast Cancer (2005 update). (Grunfeld et al., 2005).	•	•
5. American College of Radiology (ACR), American College of Surgeons (ACoS), College of American Pathology (CAP), Society of Surgical Oncology (SSO). Standard for Breast Conservation Therapy in the Management of Invasive Breast Carcinoma (Morrow et al., 2002a).	•	•
6. ACR, ACoS, CAP, SSO. Standard for the Management of Ductal Carcinoma in Situ of the Breast (DCIS) (Morrow et al., 2002b).	•	•

Late Effects of Disease/Treatment							
Treatment Complications	Reconstruction/ Post Surgery	Lymphedema	Sexuality/ Fertility	Menopause/ Hormone Replacement	Genetics	Psychosocial Issues	Locus of Care
•	•	•	•	•	•	•	•
		•		•		•	•
		•	•	•			
•			•				•
	•						
	•						

Continued

TABLE 3-4 Continued

Clinical Practice Guideline	Follow-up Schedule and Testing	Monitoring for Second Primary Tumors; Chemoprevention for Second Primary Tumors
7. American Society of Clinical Oncology (ASCO). Post-mastectomy Radiotherapy (Recht et al., 2001).		
8. National Comprehensive Cancer Network (NCCN). 2004 Breast Cancer Treatment Guidelines (NCCN, 2004b).	•	•
9. ASCO. 1998 Update of Recommended Breast Cancer Surveillance Guidelines[a] (Smith et al., 1999).	•	•
10. Canadian Task Force on Preventive Health Care (CTFPHC). Preventive Health Care, 1999 Update: 3. Follow-up after breast cancer (Temple et al., 1999).	•	•
11. Institute for Clinical Systems Improvement (ICSI). Breast Cancer Treatment (ICSI, 2003).	•	•
12. American Association of Clinical Endocrinology (AACE). AACE Medical Guidelines for Clinical Practice for Management of Menopause (AACE, 1999).		
13. ASCO. 2003 Update on the Role of Bisphosphonates and Bone Health Issues in Women with Breast Cancer (Hillner et al., 2003).		
14. ASCO. Technology Assessment of Pharmacologic Interventions for Breast Cancer Risk Reduction Including Tamoxifen, Raloxifene, and Aromatase Inhibition (Chlebowski et al., 2002b).		•

Late Effects of Disease/Treatment							
Treatment Complications	Reconstruction/ Post Surgery	Lymphedema	Sexuality/ Fertility	Menopause/ Hormone Replacement	Genetics	Psychosocial Issues	Locus of Care
•		•					•
							•
				•			
				•			

Continued

TABLE 3-4 Continued

Clinical Practice Guideline	Follow-up Schedule and Testing	Monitoring for Second Primary Tumors; Chemoprevention for Second Primary Tumors
15. ASCO. 2000 Update of Recommendations for the Use of Tumor Markers in Breast and Colorectal Cancer (Bast et al., 2001).	•	
16. European Society for Medical Oncology (ESMO). Minimum Clinical Recommendations for Diagnosis, Adjuvant Treatment, and Follow-up of Primary Breast Cancer (ESMO, 2003).	•	
17. European Society of Mastology (EUSOMA). Guidelines on Endocrine Therapy of Breast Cancer (Blamey, 2002).		
18. NBCC, National Cancer Control Initiative (Australia). Clinical Practice Guidelines for the Psychosocial Care of Adults with Cancer (NBCC and NCCI, 2004).		
19. NCCN. Genetic/Familial High Risk Assessment: Breast and Ovarian (NCCN, 2004e).		
20. NCCN. Distress Management (NCCN, 2004d).		
21. Society of Obstetricians and Gynaecologists of Canada (SOGC). Breast Cancer, Pregnancy, and Breast Feeding (Helewa et al., 2002).		
22. SOGC. Use of Hormonal Replacement Therapy after Treatment of Breast Cancer (Lea et al., 2004).		

Late Effects of Disease/Treatment							
Treatment Complications	Reconstruction/ Post Surgery	Lymphedema	Sexuality/ Fertility	Menopause/ Hormone Replacement	Genetics	Psychosocial Issues	Locus of Care
				•			
						•	
					•		
						•	
			•				
				•			

Continued

TABLE 3-4 Continued

Clinical Practice Guideline	Follow-up Schedule and Testing	Monitoring for Second Primary Tumors; Chemoprevention for Second Primary Tumors
23. Steering Committee on Clinical Practice Guidelines for the Care and Treatment of Breast Cancer (Canada). Clinical practice guidelines for the care and treatment of breast cancer: 14. The role of hormone replacement therapy in women with a previous diagnosis of breast cancer (Pritchard et al., 2002).		
24. The Steering Committee on Clinical Practice Guidelines for the Care and Treatment of Breast Cancer (Canada). Clinical practice guidelines for the care and treatment of breast cancer: 11. Lymphedema (Harris et al., 2001).		

[a]Although guideline was published in 1998, it was included because ASCO reviews literature an

may interpret the need for post-operative mammography differently. Other interventions are recommended by only a few guidelines. For example, the Institute for Clinical Systems Improvement Breast Cancer Treatment guideline pointedly addresses the increased risk of cataracts in women taking tamoxifen, and recommends that patients on tamoxifen should have annual eye exams. Few of the other guidelines mention the increased risk of cataracts, much less recommend annual eye exams. Recent evidence from a case control study suggests that tamoxifen does not increase the risk for cataracts (Bradbury et al., 2004).

In terms of the management of menopausal symptoms and the use of HRT to treat them, the recommendations vary (Table 3-6). These guidelines all agree that there is some leeway in the use of HRT, but provide different rationales for the recommendation's flexibility. There has been considerable controversy regarding the use of HRT since the publication of results of the Women's Health Initiative study in 2003 (Wassertheil-Smoller et al., 2003). This illustrates the importance of systems to keep guidelines

Late Effects of Disease/Treatment							
Treatment Complications	Reconstruction/ Post Surgery	Lymphedema	Sexuality/ Fertility	Menopause/ Hormone Replacement	Genetics	Psychosocial Issues	Locus of Care
				•			
	•						

ses guideline updates when necessary.

up to date. In general, it is recommended that CPGs be updated at least every 3 years (Shekelle et al., 2001). Some of the survivorship-related CPGs reviewed here have been updated since their original publication (e.g., American College of Radiology guidelines), but others were published 7 or more years ago and have not been updated (e.g., ASCO).

Prostate Cancer[26]

Men with a history of prostate cancer make up the second largest group of cancer survivors, representing 17 percent of the survivorship population (see Chapter 2 for a description of prostate cancer survivors). The advent of early detection with prostate-specific antigen (PSA) screening in the early

[26]Much of the information in this section is based on the following reviews: Eton and Lepore (2002); Litwin (2003); Penson and Litwin (2003a,b); Penson et al. (2004).

TABLE 3-5 Examples of Breast Cancer CPG Recommendations on Follow-up Mammography

Clinical Practice Guideline	Recommendation
British Columbia Cancer Agency	Baseline, post-treatment bilateral mammograms should be performed approximately 6 months after all treatment has been completed and repeated annually thereafter.
ASCO 1998 Update of Recommended Breast Cancer Surveillance Guidelines	It is prudent to recommend that all women with a prior diagnosis of breast cancer have yearly mammographic evaluation.
Canadian Task Force on Preventive Health Care 1999 Update: 3. Follow-Up After Breast Cancer	There is no evidence to suggest that mammography decreases mortality by detecting ipsilateral disease in the conservatively treated breast; however there is indirect evidence that it may be beneficial (grade C recommendation).[a] There is no direct evidence to suggest that physical examination or mammography, or both, should be used to detect contralateral breast cancer, however there is indirect evidence that it may be beneficial (grade C recommendation).[a]

[a]Grade C recommendation: Insufficient evidence regarding inclusion or exclusion of the condition or manuvere in a periodic health exam, but recommendations may be made on other grounds.
SOURCE: Adapted from Winn (2002).

1990s has contributed to an increase in the number of men diagnosed with localized prostate cancer at younger ages. Nearly all of these men will survive at least 5 years past diagnosis (Ries et al., 2004). With this high level of survival, the late effects of treatment on quality of life become of central importance to this group of cancer survivors. This section of the report will focus on the treatment and late effects associated with localized prostate cancer, but because some men with recurrent disease can live many years with cancer, the late effects of recurrent disease are also discussed. Varying approaches to prostate cancer treatment have resulted in a heterogeneous group of prostate cancer survivors (Box 3-10).

Quality of life is the primary outcome of interest for many men selecting among the available options for the treatment of localized prostate cancer. All of the treatments for localized prostate cancer have side effects that can profoundly affect patients' sexual, urinary, and bowel function

TABLE 3-6 Examples of Breast Cancer CPG Recommendations on Menopausal Symptom Management

Clinical Practice Guideline	Recommendation
British Columbia Cancer Agency Breast Cancer. Follow-up; Lymphedema; Hormone Replacement; Pregnancy; Contraception	Does not recommend HRT. If there are symptoms that interfere significantly with a woman's quality of life and there are no other therapeutic options, HRT should be considered.
American Association of Clinical Endocrinology (AACE) Medical Guidelines for Clinical Practice for Management of Menopause	A history of breast cancer or uterine cancer is still the main contraindication to HRT, except in special circumstances (e.g., investigational studies). The conventional prohibition against HRT in survivors of breast cancer and endometrial cancer is currently being reexamined.
Scottish Intercollegiate Guidelines Network (SIGN). Breast Cancer in Women: A National Clinical Guideline: Follow-up; Psychosocial Aspects; Rehabilitation, Menopausal Symptoms, and Complications of Local Treatment	Although HRT is widely advocated for the treatment of menopausal symptoms, its use in the treatment of women with a personal or family history of breast cancer remains controversial and alternative methods of coping with menopause have not been fully explored.

SOURCE: Adapted from Winn (2002).

and, in turn, their quality of life (Penson and Litwin, 2003a). Men who receive combination therapy for early-stage prostate cancer generally experience additional decrements in health-related quality of life (Litwin, 2003). Although most late effects associated with prostate cancer relate to aggressive treatment, studies of men who choose watchful waiting have shown that prostate cancer itself can contribute to late effects such as urinary incontinence (Penson and Litwin, 2003b). Table 3-7 summarizes certain late effects found among prostate cancer survivors. These late effects are described more fully below.

Cancer Recurrence

There is limited information on cancer recurrence among men with prostate cancer. In one study, 15 percent of men with localized disease who were treated with prostatectomy developed elevated PSA levels indicative of recurrence by 15 years of follow-up (Pound et al., 1999). Among these men, 34 percent developed metastatic disease within the 15-year study period.

BOX 3-10
Approaches to Localized Prostate Cancer Treatment: Implications for Late Effects

The most common treatments for localized prostate cancer are surgical removal of the prostate (prostatectomy), external beam radiation therapy, or brachytherapy (implanting radioactive "seeds"). These modalities may be used singly or in combination in the case of men considered to be at higher risk. Because prostate cancer is usually a slow-growing cancer, providing none of these therapies and instead monitoring the course of the disease for signs of progression (called "watchful waiting") is another option, especially for men who are elderly or suffer from other major health problems. Evidence from clinical trials on the relative effectiveness of these approaches is not yet available, and it is recommended that clinicians provide men with information about alternative treatments and their side effects and be supportive as decisions about treatment are made. In one study of national practice patterns, about half of men with low-risk prostate cancer had elected prostatectomy (Cooperberg et al., 2004).

Many men (approximately 20 percent over 5 years) treated for localized prostate cancer require follow-up cancer treatments such as radiation therapy, cryosurgery (freezing malignant areas of the prostate with cooled metal probes), prostatectomy (after the cancer has not responded to other treatments), or androgen deprivation therapy (Lu-Yao et al., 1996; Grossfeld et al., 1998). Additional treatment may be given prophylactically to men at high risk for disease recurrence (e.g., those with positive surgical margins, high-grade tumors, or positive lymph nodes) or therapeutically following biochemical (i.e., based on rising or elevated PSA levels) or clinical disease recurrence.

For locally advanced disease or recurrent prostate cancer that is localized, prolonged disease control is often possible with radiation and/or hormonal therapy. For disseminated recurrent disease, hormone therapy may be used along with palliative radiation therapy.

Practice guidelines are available for surveillance for prostate cancer recurrence. The National Comprehensive Cancer Network, for example, recommends that clinicians measure PSA every 6 months for 5 years after initial definitive therapy and then every year (NCCN, 2004g). An annual digital rectal examination (DRE) is also recommended. These guidelines are not supported by high-quality evidence from randomized clinical trials.

Second Primary Cancer

Rates of bladder cancer appear to be higher than expected among men with prostate cancer (Chun, 1997). According to a large Swedish study, rates of second primary cancers among men with prostate cancer were increased in the first 6 months of follow-up, most likely due to increased surveillance (Thellenberg et al., 2003). An increased risk of endocrine-related second primary cancers such as male breast cancer was observed in this study. A recent study indicates that prostate irradiation increases the risk of rectal cancer (Grady and Russell, 2005; Baxter et al., 2005). The authors recommend that endoscopic evaluation for rectal cancer begin 5 years after prostate cancer radiotherapy.

Psychosocial Distress

Relatively little is known about the psychologic effects of prostate cancer on men and their family members. Concerns about having cancer, fears of recurrence, and the effects of post-treatment symptoms on quality of life may all contribute to psychosocial distress (Bacon et al., 2002). Excess levels of anxiety and depression have been found among prostate cancer survivors and their wives (Manne, 2002). Spouses and partners play an integral role in the adjustment to prostate cancer and some research has shown that having a partner positively effects quality of life (Gore et al., 2005; Soloway et al., 2005).

Younger men appear to have more trouble with psychological adjustment following treatment for prostate cancer. This could be explained if older men have accommodated to preexisting urinary and sexual problems or if they are more inclined to expect that physical health problems would occur with treatment (Eton et al., 2001). The implications of prostate cancer among men according to their age, race and ethnicity, socioeconomic status, and sexual orientation are not well understood (Visser and van Andel, 2003; Pierce et al., 2003; Blank, 2005).

Undergoing treatment for prostate cancer can decrease fears that the cancer will recur but, according to one study, significant levels of fear remained after treatment, and the fear persisted even 2 years after treatment (Mehta et al., 2003). Some men express regret about their treatment decisions. In one study, 16 percent of men treated for early-stage prostate cancer regretted their treatment decisions. Men most likely to feel regret were those with less than a college education and those who had lower quality of life ratings (Hu et al., 2003).

Groups that provide education and support—such as "Man-to-Man" and "Us TOO!"—are available to men with prostate cancer, but few such groups have been evaluated (Manne, 2002). An exception is a university-based group education and support intervention for men recently diagnosed with prostate cancer. It was evaluated through a randomized controlled trial. Group education and support were found to be successful in enhancing quality of life, especially for men with less formal education (Lepore et al., 2003). Increased knowledge about prostate cancer, adoption of healthy behaviors, improvements in general physical functioning, greater employment stability, and improved QOL related to sexual dysfunction

TABLE 3-7 Possible Late Effects Among Prostate Cancer Survivors

Late Effect	Population at Risk	Risk	Interventions
Cancer recurrence	All men	Varies by stage and tumor characteristics	PSA testing every 6 months, annual digital rectal exam; bone scans only indicated if PSA level rises
Second primary cancer	All men	Possible increase in risk of bladder, rectal, and male breast cancer	Surveillance
Psychosocial distress	All men	Increased anxiety and depression, but prevalence is not well documented	Assessment for distress Support groups can be helpful
Sexual dysfunction	All men	Rates of erectile dysfunction vary by patient age, cancer characteristics, and treatment	Assessment for sexual function Oral agents: sildenafil, tadalafil, and vardenafil
		Men treated with prostatectomy at highest risk	External mechanical devices
		Men treated with testosterone-suppressing hormones may have reduced libido	Penile injection therapy Penile prostheses
Bladder dysfunction	All men	Varies by treatment	Assessment for urinary function
		Stress incontinence more common among men who had a prostatectomy	Medication for urge incontinence (e.g., oxybutynin, tolterodine)
		Irritative voiding symptoms and urge incontinence are more common among men who had radiation therapy	Diet and fluid intake (e.g., reduction in fluid intake; avoidance of substances that irritate the bladder such as coffee, tea, acid juices; treatment of constipation)

		Both symptoms tend to improve with time	Pelvic floor rehabilitation (e.g., pelvic muscle exercise)
			Supportive interventions (e.g., good skin care, use of absorbent pads)
			Surgical interventions (e.g., prosthetic urethral sphincters) are available for men with persistent or severe post-prostatectomy incontinence
Bowel dysfunction	All men	Varies by treatment	Assessment for bowel function
		Rates of fecal incontinence low after prostatectomy	Prescription antispasmotics (e.g., Levsin) or over-the-counter Anusol suppositories
		Risk among brachytherapy patients lower than for those with external beam radiotherapy	Surgery for rectal necrosis (includes colostomy)
		Most symptoms decline over the course of 1 to 2 years	
Osteoporosis, fatigue, muscle wasting	Men treated with testosterone-suppressing hormones	Degree of symptoms related to dose and duration of treatment	Preventive measures (e.g., calcium, vitamin D, weight-bearing exercise)
			Assessment of mineral bone density, consider treatment of osteoporosis with bisphosphonates
Cognitive function	Men treated with testosterone-suppressing hormones	When therapy is used less than 1 year, the effects are mostly reversible; mental deficits may become persistent with treatment over 2 years	Interventions to ameliorate the effects have not been evaluated

were among the benefits of the intervention. The results of a randomized controlled trial conducted to assess the impact of a psychoeducational intervention aimed at wives of men with prostate cancer suggest that group interventions targeting spouses may benefit both members of the couple (Manne, 2002).

Sexual Dysfunction

Significant sexual dysfunction can occur after all three therapies commonly used to treat localized prostate cancer. Reported rates of erectile dysfunction at 1 year after therapy are 66 percent for nerve-sparing prostatectomy, 75 percent for non-nerve-sparing prostatectomy, 24 percent for brachytherapy, 40 percent for those who received brachytherapy plus external beam radiotherapy, and 40 percent for those receiving external beam radiotherapy alone (Robinson et al., 2002). Improvement in sexual function usually occurs during the first year after treatment, but further improvement into the second year appears to be more likely for men treated with radical prostatectomy as compared to external beam radiotherapy. In a recent study of long-term outcomes among localized prostate cancer survivors, sexual function and urinary and bowel symptoms were similar when evaluated at a median of 2.6 years and then 6.2 years following radical prostatectomy (Miller et al., 2005). Some symptoms improved while others worsened (e.g., urinary incontinence) for men who had undergone external radiation and brachytherapy.

The effect of erectile dysfunction on patients' quality of life is variable and highly idiosyncractic—some men with severe dysfunction are troubled very little while others with modest levels of dysfunction view it as a significant problem (Stanford et al., 2000). Clinicians need to assess both sexual function and how men feel their sexual function has affected their quality of life. When asked about their perceptions, a significant portion reported dissatisfaction with their sexual function following treatment. In one study, 42 percent of men reported that their sexual function was a moderate to big problem at 2 years following radical prostatectomy (Stanford et al., 2000). The use of nerve-sparing techniques has modestly improved sexual function following this procedure. In a study of men undergoing external beam radiotherapy for localized prostate cancer, half reported that their overall quality of life had decreased much, or very much, as a direct result of decreased erectile function. Aggressive treatment for early prostate cancer may confer confidence in cancer control, yet be countered by sexual dysfunction, which can diminish intimate relationships and feelings of masculinity (Clark et al., 2003).

Interventions to improve sexual function following prostate cancer include use of a vacuum erection device, oral medications (e.g., sildenafil), penile injection therapy, and penile prostheses. There are no clinical practice guidelines specific to the management of sexual dysfunction among men with prostate cancer,[27] but a review article is available that describes treatment options (Teloken, 2001). Some investigators have tested a progressive local treatment protocol, trying interventions sequentially and moving on to the next intervention only if they failed the previous one (Baniel et al., 2001). In this study, nearly all of the men (94 percent) were treated sucessfully and continued to respond well after one year of follow-up. Not all men who are bothered by sexual dysfunction seek medical help, and one large survey of men with erectile dysfunction after prostate cancer suggests that interventions to overcome men's negative beliefs about seeking help for sexual dysfunction could potentially increase help-seeking behavior (Schover et al., 2002, 2004).

Bladder Dysfunction

Urinary dysfunction is seen in nearly all men with prostate cancer in the immediate post-therapy period, but function improves for most men during the first 2 years after therapy. Men who have radical prostatectomies are more likely to report urinary leakage when they cough or strain, whereas men undergoing either external beam radiotherapy or brachytherapy often experience significant pain, frequency, or urgency with urination. Although the type of urinary dysfunction differs among treatments, the impact on quality of life is considerable with both surgery and radiotherapy and represents a significant burden of disease for patients. In a study of men who had undergone external beam radiotherapy for prostate cancer, 54 percent (as compared to 31 percent of controls) reported urinary problems 8 years after treatment (Fransson and Widmark, 1999). A study of men treated with brachytherapy found that at 6 months after treatment, 40 percent reported urinary frequency and 17 percent reported pain upon urination (Arterbery et al., 1997). Even without aggressive treatment, men with localized prostate cancer can have lower urinary tract symptoms. Like sexual dysfunction, the significance of urinary dysfunction is highly individualized: not all men are bothered by it. In one study of men following radical prostatectomy, 2 percent had no urinary control, 7 percent reported frequent leakage, 40 percent reported occasional leakage, and 32 percent reported total urinary control 2 years after surgery. When questioned as to

[27]Clinical practice guidelines available on male sexual dysfunction do not specifically cover the management of men with prostate cancer (Guay et al., 2003).

how big a problem their incontinence was, 38 percent said it was no problem, 34 percent said it was a small problem, and 9 percent said it was a moderate to big problem.

A number of interventions are available to treat the urinary problems associated with prostate cancer treatment:

- Medication for urge incontinence (e.g., oxybutynin, tolterodine)
- Diet and fluid intake (e.g., reduction in fluid intake; avoidance of substances that irritate the bladder such as coffee, tea, and acid juices; treatment of constipation)
- Pelvic floor rehabilitation (e.g., pelvic muscle exercise)
- Supportive interventions (e.g., good skin care, use of absorbent pads, condom catheters)
- Surgical interventions (e.g., urethral sphincters) are available for men with persistent or severe post-prostatectomy incontinence

There are no clinical practice guidelines specific to the management of urinary dysfunction for men with a history of prostate cancer, but a review article is available that describes these treatment options (Grise and Thurman, 2001).

Bowel Dysfunction

Radiotherapy, either external beam or brachytherapy, can lead to significant bowel dysfunction, including bowel necrosis and symptoms such as rectal urgency or diarrhea (Penson and Litwin, 2003b). While many gastrointestinal problems were viewed as minor following treatment with external beam radiotherapy, a small proportion of men (10 percent or less) have reported severe bowel symptoms, including fecal soiling. For men treated with brachytherapy, bowel necrosis can occur, and it is estimated that problematic diarrhea may occur for 12 percent of men at 9 months following surgery (Krupski et al., 2000). Bowel dysfunction is fairly uncommon after prostatectomy. Interventions for bowel dysfunction include medication for cramping and diarrhea. Surgery, including colostomy, may be required for severe problems such as bowel necrosis.

Osteoporosis

Osteoporosis is a potentially serious complication of androgen deprivation therapy for prostate cancer (Smith, 2003). Such therapy may be used for men with advanced disease or recurrent prostate cancer. Androgen deprivation therapy either by bilateral orchiectomies (i.e., surgical removal of the testicles) or by treatment with a gonadotropin-releasing hormone agonist/antagonist decreases bone mineral density and increases the risk of fracture (Krupski et al., 2004). Lifestyle modification should be encouraged, including smoking cessation, moderation of alcohol consumption, and regular weight-bearing exercise. Recommended also are preventive measures such as taking supplemental calcium and vitamin D. Treatment with bisphosphonates may be warranted for men with osteoporosis, fractures, or high rates of bone loss during androgen deprivation therapy.

Cognitive Dysfunction

Androgen deprivation therapy for prostate cancer may be associated with impaired memory, attention, and executive functions (i.e., the brain's supervisory or regulatory functions) (Green et al., 2002a; Koupparis et al., 2004). In a recent study of men with prostate cancer treated with androgen deprivation therapy, cognitive effects were mostly reversible when therapy was used less than 1 year. However, mental deficits persisted with treatment that lasted more than 2 years (Salminen et al., 2005). Interventions to improve cognitive function by administering estrogen replacement therapy have not been shown to be effective (Taxel et al., 2004).

Clinical Practice Guidelines

Available prostate cancer CPGs focus on surveillance for recurrence and do not provide information on management of late effects (Finnish Medical Society Duodecim, 2002; Villers et al., 2003; British Columbia Cancer Agency, 2004b; NCCN, 2004g). All guidelines recommend routine surveillance with digital rectal examination and PSA testing, but the frequency of recommended follow-up vary somewhat. For example, the NCCN CPG recommends an annual DRE and PSA testing every 6 months for 5 years, and then every year thereafter. The British Columbia CPG recommends DRE and PSA testing at regularly scheduled intervals (e.g., every 3 months in the first year, increasing to every 6 months thereafter). The CPGs for follow-up of patients with prostate cancer are not based on clinical trials. Such trials are needed to test the effectiveness of the various follow-up measures and strategies.

In summary, prostate cancer treatment can result in high rates of urinary, sexual, and bowel dysfunction that can adversely affect quality of life. Treating physicians should actively inquire about these adverse effects and provide early treatment to maximize quality of life (Penson and Sokoloff, 2004). Validated questionnaires are available to assist clinicians in the ascertainment and documentation of complications such as urinary and fecal incontinence, erectile dysfunction, and intestinal inflammation, and effective treatments are available (Yao and Dipaola, 2003; Litwin et al.,

2004). Evidence-based clinical practice guidelines are needed to assist clinicians in the management of late effects of prostate cancer treatment.

Colorectal Cancer

Individuals with a history of colorectal cancer make up the third largest group of cancer survivors, representing 11 percent of the survivorship population. As a group, survivors of colorectal cancer are elderly, with 76 percent aged 65 and older (see Chapter 2 for a description of colorecal cancer survivors). Box 3-11 summarizes the most common treatments for colon and rectal cancers. Fortunately, 80 percent of people with colorectal cancer have local or locally advanced cancer and curative-intent surgery is performed (Meyerhardt and Mayer, 2003). However, up to 40 percent of these patients will subsequently develop recurrent disease.

Most long-term survivors of colorectal cancer report very good quality of life following their treatment, but certain deficits are still observed in some patients (Ramsey et al., 2002; Trentham-Dietz et al., 2003). According to one study, individuals who had survived colorectal cancer for at least 5 years reported a relatively uniform and high quality of life, irrespective of stage at diagnosis and time from diagnosis (Ramsey et al., 2002). Compared to age-matched individuals, however, cancer survivors reported higher

BOX 3-11
Approaches to Colorectal Cancer Treatment: Implications for Late Effects

Colon cancer: Surgical removal of the cancer and nearby lymph nodes is the standard treatment for patients with colon cancer. Sometimes a temporary colostomy is needed. Some very early-stage cancers may be removed endoscopically, with good results. 5-fluorouracil-based adjuvant chemotherapy is considered standard for patients with Stage III colon cancer, and an option for some with Stage II disease. Newer regimens incorporating oxaliplatin may be used. Adjuvant radiation therapy is sometimes given for patients with locally advanced colon cancer, but its use is controversial.

Rectal cancer: Surgery alone is often sufficient for individuals with low-stage rectal cancer. When the tumor is in the low rectum, the rectum and anus are removed and a permanent colostomy is necessary. In men, such surgery can damage genital nerves and impair bladder and sexual function. Sphincter-preserving surgery is feasible for patients with a tumor located in the upper or middle part of the rectum. Some of these procedures, however, may also damage the pelvic nerves involved in sexual function. For those with Stage II or III rectal cancer, radiation and chemotherapy are recommended. Radiation is increasingly being given preoperatively to increase the local control rate.

rates of depression and nearly half reported frequent bowel movements or chronic diarrhea. Long-term, disease-free survivors of rectal cancer have reported good quality of life, but residual pain and constipation sometimes negatively affected quality of life (Rauch et al., 2004). Table 3-8 summarizes some of the late effects associated with colorectal cancer and its treatment. Details regarding these late effects and their management are described below.

Cancer Recurrence and Second Primary Cancer

Up to 40 percent of individuals treated for local or locally advanced colorectal cancer will have their disease recur. Following treatment, periodic evaluations can lead to the earlier identification and management of recurrent disease, but the impact of such monitoring on overall mortality is limited by the relatively small proportion of patients in whom localized, potentially curable metastases or local recurrences are found. Survivors of colorectal cancer are also at risk of developing a second primary colorectal cancer. In a follow-up study of individuals with localized colon cancer, the incidence of a second primary colorectal cancer remained high (1.5 percent at 5 years) (Green et al., 2002b). The risk of other cancers developing is also higher among survivors of colorectal cancer, including cancers of the small intestine, cervix, uterus, and ovary (Evans et al., 2002).

The optimal regimen and frequency of follow-up examinations to detect cancer recurrence and second primary cancers are not well defined. No large-scale randomized trials have been completed to document the efficacy of any overall post-operative monitoring program (i.e., involving carcinoembryonic antigen (CEA) testing, imaging studies, office visits). Two such trials are now in progress, but the results will not be available for several years (Johnson et al., 2004; FACS, 2005). Guidelines concerning colonoscopy in high-risk groups such as those who have completed treatment are fairly consistent and supported by high-quality data (Table 3-9). However, there is variation in recommendations on other follow-up tests. In the area of routine CEA[28] testing for the early detection of recurrence, for example, several guidelines[29] recommend that patients who would be candidates for resection of metastases receive regular CEA testing. Other evidence suggest it is of no value (Moertel et al., 1993; Northover, 2003).

[28]Carcino-embryonic antigen is a serum glycoprotein that can be detected in the blood of individuals with colon cancer.

[29]Guidelines making this recommendation include those of The Finnish Medical Society Duodecim, British Columbia Cancer Agency, ASCO, American Society of Colon and Rectal Surgeons and NCCN (see Table 3-10).

TABLE 3-8 Possible Late Effects Among Colorectal Cancer Survivors

Late Effect	Population at Risk	Risk	Interventions
Cancer recurrence	All survivors	40 percent among those treated with local or locally advanced cancer	Follow-up imaging recommended. Periodic testing for carcino-embryonic antigen (CEA) may be indicated for some survivors in the first few years after diagnosis.
Second primary cancer	All survivors	Increased risk of cancers of the colon, rectum, small intestine, cervix, uterus, and ovary	Follow-up colonoscopy recommended
Psychosocial distress	All survivors	Higher rates of depression have been reported	Assessment for distress Evidence on the effectiveness of psychosocial interventions among survivors of colorectal cancer is limited
Bowel dysfunction: diarrhea and fecal leakage/incontinence, constipation, bowel obstruction, pain	Variable	Hemicolectomy can lead to loose stools that usually improve over time. Surgery can also lead to adhesions. Rectal cancer patients are at higher risk of fecal incontinence. Radiation may lead to small bowel scarring and bowel obstruction.	Dietary counseling, use of over-the-counter medications (e.g., fiber laxative, stool softeners, antidiarrheals), and anal sphincter biofeedback training

Colostomy	Rectal cancer survivors who had tumors located in the lower part of the rectum	Approximately 15 to 25 percent of survivors will have permanent colostomies	Enterostomal nurses provide education, training, and counseling
Sexual function	Rectal cancer survivors	Erectile dysfunction and ejaculatory difficulties in men. Painful coitus in women. Infertility, especially among women. Abnormal bowel function can affect sexual functioning.	Assessment for sexual function: For men, drugs for erectile dysfunction (e.g., sildenafil citrate); for women, vaginal dilatation, over-the-counter lubricants. For infertility, men can bank sperm. Effective options for fertility preservation in women are limited. Ovarian pexy, pinning the ovaries up out of the radiation field at the time of surgery, may preserve ovarian function, but the uterus will be damaged.
Peripheral neuropathy	Survivors who received oxaliplatin	Numbness or painful sensations	Prescription medications (i.e., vitamin B6, amitriptyline, gabapentin)
Risk to family members	All survivors	Most colorectal cancer is sporadic and relatives are not at higher risk. Family history and clinical characteristics of the cancer may suggest a genetic etiology.	Genetic counseling; in addition, those at high risk are counseled to begin colonoscopy 10 years before the earliest colorectal cancer in the family (or age 50, whichever comes first). Genetic tests are commercially available for some genetic disorders (e.g., hereditary nonpolyposis colorectal cancer [HNPCC], familial adenomatous polyposis [FAP]).

TABLE 3-9 Examples of Colorectal Cancer CPG Recommendations on Follow-up Colonoscopy

Clinical Practice Guideline	Recommendation
The American Society of Colon and Rectal Surgeons (ACSRS), Practice Parameters for the Detection of Colorectal Neoplasms	Pre-operative colonoscopy; repeat colonoscopy in 1-3 years, then 3 years , and then every 5 years if free of disease. If no pre-operative exam, colonoscopy 3 to 6 months post-surgery
American Society of Clinical Oncology (ASCO), 2000 Update of American Society of Clinical Oncology Colorectal Cancer Surveillance Guidelines	If polyp free, colonoscopy every 3 to 5 years.
British Columbia Council on CPGs, Protocol for Follow-Up of Patients After Curative Resection of Colorectal Cancer	Pre-operative colonoscopy; repeat once every 3 years; if free of disease, repeat every 5 years

SOURCE: Adapted from Winn (2002).

Several other guidelines[30] say that evidence is insufficient to make any recommendation regarding regular CEA testing. None of the guidelines recommend regular computed tomography (CT) scanning, although one guideline (i.e., Management of Colorectal Cancer, Scottish Intercollegiate Guidelines Network) says that regular scanning may be beneficial. Surveillance methods including CEA immunoscintigraphy and positron-emission tomography (PET) scan are under evaluation (NCI, 2005b).

Psychosocial Distress

There have been relatively few studies of the psychosocial impact of colorectal cancer, however, in one study, depression was more prevalent among survivors of colorectal cancer than expected in the general population (14 percent versus 10 percent) (Ramsey et al., 2002). Higher levels of psychosocial distress have been reported among individuals with perma-

[30]These guidelines include Scottish Intercollegiate Guidelines Network, Cancer Care Ontario, and British Society of Gastroenterology/Association of Coloproctology for Great Britain and Ireland (see Table 3-10).

nent colostomies (Sprangers et al., 1995). Among female survivors of colorectal cancer, contacts with relatives and friends and other measures of the extent of social networks appeared to improve mental health (Sapp et al., 2003). Another study of female survivors of colorectal cancer found health-related quality of life comparable with that of similarly aged women in the general population (mean follow-up was 9 years) (Trentham-Dietz et al., 2003).

Bowel Dysfunction

Some individuals with colon cancer experience bowel symptoms. Among rectal cancer patients, permanent colostomies represent a major life adjustment. For most colon cancer patients, there are often frequent bowel movements, but few disabling problems. Whether or not quality of life differed between those survivors who had had a permanent colostomy and those who hadn't was the subject of a review of the literature (Sprangers et al., 1995). According to this review, many patients are troubled by frequent or irregular bowel movements and diarrhea. Some patients, however, are not troubled (e.g., those who had constipation prior to surgery), and many individuals with colostomies are able to adapt very successfully. Patients with very early-stage cancer treated with polypectomy may have no change in bowel function.

Sexual Function

Survivors of colorectal cancer can have poor sexual functioning, in part as a consequence of the irregular bowel function that may occur. Most of what is known about sexual function in this group of survivors relates to rectal cancer. For women surviving rectal cancer, age at surgery and characteristics of the surgery are predictive of sexual functioning. For men, dry ejaculate and erectile dysfunction may occur among 25 to 45 percent of men following rectal surgery. Sexual function was consistently more impaired among survivors who had lost sphincter control following their surgery for rectal cancer than among patients with intact sphincters, according to a review of quality of life among colorectal survivors (Sprangers et al., 1995). For men with erectile dysfunction, prescription medications (e.g., sildenafil citrate) and devices (e.g., prostheses) are available. For women, vaginal dilatation[31] is an option as are over-the-counter vaginal lubricants.

---

[31]Vaginal dilatation involves the use of a device to expand the vagina.

Risk to Family Members[32]

About 70 percent of cases of colorectal cancer occur sporadically, with no evidence of familial or inherited predisposition (Calvert and Frucht, 2002). An inherited polyposis syndrome[33] accounts for fewer than 10 percent of individuals with colorectal cancer. For up to 25 percent of cases, the cancer is considered familial, meaning there is a family history of colorectal cancer, but it cannot be accounted for by the known inherited syndromes. Genetic testing is becoming more available, but its clinical indications are still limited. The testing should be limited to persons whose family history suggests an inherited syndrome or who exhibit specific features of an inherited cancer syndrome (e.g., colon cancer before age 50). If the genetic test results of the individual with colorectal cancer identify a specific mutation, phenotypically unaffected first-degree relatives can then be tested. However, if the results of a particular test are negative, unaffected first-degree relatives should not be tested for that genetic disorder because the test will be uninformative. When genetic testing is indicated, it should be preceded by a pretest counseling session detailing the limitations of the test and the potential psychological, ethical, legal, and societal implications for the individual with cancer and his or her family members.

Clinical Practice Guidelines

The committee identified and reviewed 15 CPGs that include recommendations on the follow-up care of colorectal cancer survivors (Table 3-10).[34] Despite the wide range of late effects associated with colorectal cancer, most of these CPGs address only two domains of survivorship: (1) surveillance testing, especially colonoscopy, and (2) the screening issues related to monitoring the genetic variants of colorectal carcinoma, which account for a small fraction of all disease. Notably absent is guidance regarding the functional sequelae that may follow surgical interventions (e.g., colostomy, bowel dysfunction, sexual dysfunction). Only one guide-

[32]This section is based on a review article, *The Genetics of Colorectal Cancer*, by Calvert and Frucht (2002).

[33]The polyposis syndromes include familial adenomatous polyposis and the hamartomatous polyposis syndromes. The nonpolyposis predominant syndromes include hereditary nonpolyposis colorectal cancer (Lynch syndrome I) and the cancer family syndrome (Lynch syndrome II) (Calvert and Frucht, 2002).

[34]Several of the generic guidelines that would be applicable to survivors of colorectal cancer, such as the NCCN Management of Distress Guideline described earlier, are not listed. Guidelines for general population colorectal screening are listed when they include recommendations for follow-up surveillance for cancer survivors.

line mentions enterostomal therapy (i.e., care for colostomy) and it provides little detail. Of the 15 colorectal cancer guidelines, 7 are specifically targeted to follow-up, 5 are oriented to screening or genetics, and 3 are part of general treatment guidelines.

The guidelines currently available are not uniform, and the possible reasons for variability among guidelines are numerous. The most important is probably the absence of adequately powered, well-controlled trials of high-intensity versus low-intensity follow-up after potentially curative initial therapy. As mentioned earlier, two such trials are now in progress, but the results will not be available for several years (Johnson et al., 2004; FACS, 2005). Funding agencies such as the U.K. Medical Research Council support the Follow-up After Colorectal Surgery (FACS) trial.

Hodgkin's Disease[35]

Survivors of Hodgkin's disease (HD) make up a small fraction (about 1 percent) of the population of cancer survivors (see Chapter 2 for a description of HD survivors). However, most individuals diagnosed with HD are relatively young and will be long-term survivors of their disease. Late effects of HD treatment have been recognized for many years due to the high survival rates, and are among the first to be well documented. Long-term follow-up studies have shown higher than expected death rates among HD survivors. Second cancers and cardiovascular disease attributable to HD treatment account for much of this excess mortality (Ng and Mauch, 2004). Modification of HD therapies have been made to reduce the serious late effects of treatment (Donaldson et al., 1999). Changes in therapy that have maintained good survival while minimizing late effects have included: elimination of the use of surgical staging with splenectomy; minimizing radiation doses and large volumes of the body irradiated; shifting to chemotherapy drugs that are less toxic and delivered over shorter periods of time; and therapy adapted to the patient's risk of recurrence. Box 3-12 outlines the main strategies for initial treatment for HD.

Quality of Life

Reductions in the toxicity of treatment for HD have improved survivors' quality of life. A recent prospective study assessed the quality of life of

---

[35]Much of this section is based on information provided in the Physician's Data Query, an online service of the National Cancer Institute (NCI, 2005a); review articles in *Seminars in Oncology* (Wooldridge and Link, 2003) and *Current Hematology Report* (Ng and Mauch, 2004); and the section on late effects in the textbook *Hodgkin's Disease* (Mauch et al., 1999).

TABLE 3-10 Colorectal Cancer Clinical Practice Guidelines

Clinical Practice Guideline	Follow-up Schedule and Testing: Colonoscopy	Imaging	CEA
1. Scottish Intercollegiate Guidelines Network Management of Colorectal Cancer (SIGN, 2003)	•	•	•
2. The Finnish Medical Society Duodecim Evidence-based Medicine Guidelines: Postoperative Follow-up of Colorectal Cancer (Finnish Medical Society Duodecim, 2001)	•	•	•
3. British Columbia Cancer Agency Colon: Follow-up (British Columbia Cancer Agency, 2002a)	•	•	•
4. American Society of Clinical Oncology (ASCO) 2000 Update of American Society of Clinical Oncology Colorectal Cancer Surveillance Guidelines (Benson et al., 2000)	•	•	•
5. Cancer Care Ontario Program in Evidence-Based Care Follow-up of Patients with Curatively Resected Colorectal Cancer: Practice Guideline (Figueredo et al., 2003)	•	•	•
6. National Comprehensive Cancer Network (NCCN) Colon Cancer Version 2.2004 (NCCN, 2004h)	•	•	•
7. American Society of Colon and Rectal Surgeons (ASCRS) Practice Parameters for the Surveillance and Follow-Up of Patients with Colon and Rectal Cancer (Anthony et al., 2004)	•	•	•
8. ASCRS Practice Parameters for the Detection of Colorectal Neoplasms (Simmang et al., 1999)	•		
9. British Columbia Guidelines and Protocols Advisory Committee Follow-up of Patients After Curative Resection of Colorectal Cancer (British Columbia Guidelines and Protocols Advisory Committee, 2004)	•		•

Late Effects of Disease/Treatment						
Bowels/Stoma	Sexuality/ Fertility	Post - Radiotherapy	Menopause/ Hormone Replacement	Genetics	Psychosocial Issues	Locus of Care
•				•		•
				•		•
						•
				•		

Continued

TABLE 3-10 Continued

Clinical Practice Guideline	Follow-up Schedule and Testing		
	Colonoscopy	Imaging	CEA
10. British Society of Gastroenterology (BSG), Association of Coloproctology for Great Britain and Ireland (ACPGBI) Guidelines for Follow-up After Resection of Colorectal Cancer (Scholefield and Steele, 2002)	•	•	
11. U.S. Multisociety Task Force on Colorectal Cancer Colorectal Cancer Screening and Surveillance: Clinical Guidelines and Rationale—Update Based on New Evidence (Winawer et al., 2003)	•		
12. ASCO 2000 Update of Recommendations for the Use of Tumor Markers in Breast and Colorectal Cancer (Bast et al., 2001)			•
13. ASCRS Practice Parameters for the Treatment of Patients with Dominantly Inherited Colorectal Cancer (Church and Simmang, 2003)			
14. BSG, ACPGBI Guidance on Gastrointestinal Surveillance for Hereditary Non-Polyposis Colorectal Cancer, Familial Adenomatous Polyposis, Juvenile Polyposis, and Peutz-Jeghers Syndrome (Dunlop, 2002)			
15. NCCN Colorectal Screening Version 1.2004 (NCCN, 2004c)			

247 survivors of early-stage HD treated as part of a clinical trial (Ganz et al., 2003c). Short-term decrements in quality of life were observed, but the scores at 1 year were similar to baseline scores before treatment, without further improvement at the 2-year assessment. HD survivors perceived that their health had declined following treatment. The adverse consequences of treatment are greater for those with more advanced disease. In one study of survivors of Stage III or IV HD assessed an average of 5 years after their treatment, nearly one-quarter (23 percent) of survivors had problems directly related to HD therapy (e.g., hypothyroidism, peripheral neuropathy)

Late Effects of Disease/Treatment						
Bowels/Stoma	Sexuality/ Fertility	Post – Radiotherapy	Menopause/ Hormone Replacement	Genetics	Psychosocial Issues	Locus of Care
				•		
				•		
				•		
				•		

(Kornblith et al., 1998). Table 3-11 provides information on some of the late effects experienced by HD survivors. These are described more fully below.

Cancer Recurrence

A minority of long-term survivors of HD will have their cancer recur. The risk is related to the effectiveness of the initial therapy. In one study 22

BOX 3-12
Approaches to Hodgkin's Disease Treatment: Implications for Late Effects

The majority of patients are treated with risk-adapted therapy. For those with early stage disease, the standard is combined modality therapy with radiation directed to initially involved sites and a brief course of chemotherapy selected to reduce late effects. Recent studies suggest that chemotherapy alone may be an alternative to combined modality therapy for select early-stage HD but the mature results of randomized trials are needed to compare late effects with these approaches.

High dose therapy and autologous transplantation represents a potentially curative option for HD patients with recurrence after initial therapy.

percent of patients had experienced a relapse at a median of 1.9 years (Torrey et al., 1997). Only 15 percent of relapses occurred after 5 years. Treatment of recurrent HD is often successful. Given the time course of recurrence, it is recommended that post-treatment surveillance for recurrence be concentrated in the first few years after primary treatment.

Second Cancers

At 15 years of follow-up, the risk of second solid tumors (cancers of the lung, breast, thyroid, bone/soft tissue, stomach, esophagus, uterine cervix, and head and neck) is approximately 13 percent, and at 25 years, approximately 22 percent (Dores et al., 2002). The risk of lung cancer is increased among HD survivors, especially among those who smoke and were treated at an older age (Travis et al., 2002). The risk of breast cancer is high among women treated with chest radiation before age 30, and the incidence increases substantially after 15 years of follow-up (Hancock et al., 1993). Women with therapy-related premature menopause have a lower risk of subsequent breast cancer (Travis et al., 2003). The risk of skin cancer is also increased and routine skin examinations are recommended. Counseling regarding healthy lifestyle, including smoking cessation, is recommended along with follow-up physical examination and selected laboratory and imaging studies (e.g., mammograms for females).

Psychosocial Distress

Survivors of HD often report post-treatment fatigue that can affect work and leisure activities and in turn contribute to psychological distress

(Fobair et al., 1986; Loge et al., 2000). One French study that compared psychosocial outcomes of HD survivors to those among healthy controls (matched for sex, age, and residency) found HD survivors to have more physical, role, and cognitive functioning impairments than their peers, but to report good overall health and psychologic status (Joly et al., 1996). Survivors of aggressively treated HD have been found to be at increased risk for psychological distress (Cella and Tross, 1986), and in one study, 22 percent of advanced HD survivors met the criterion suggested for a psychiatric diagnosis (Kornblith et al., 1992, 1998).

Infertility and Gonadal Dysfunction

Infertility can be a problem for HD survivors as a result of treatment with either chemotherapy or radiation therapy. Some survivors retain or regain fertility after treatment. In one study of 391 adult patients of reproductive age, female patients who attempted conception had pregnancy rates similar to those observed in the general population (81 percent versus 85 percent). The female partners of male patients, however, had a much lower frequency of pregnancy (49 percent) (Aisner et al., 1993). In this study, there was no apparent increase in complications of pregnancy, spontaneous abortions, or congenital abnormalities after treatment compared with pregnancies in this patient group before treatment or with pregnancies in the general population. Counseling regarding reproduction is advised.

Hypothyroidism

According to one study of 177 survivors of HD, more than one-quarter (27 percent) had developed hypothyroidism when examined after an average follow-up of 6 years (Bethge et al., 2000). Only those treated with radiotherapy were at risk. Patients who received radiation to the region of the thyroid gland should be evaluated by physical examination and have periodic thyroid function tests.

Cardiovascular Disease

HD survivors treated with radiation or cardiotoxic chemotherapy may experience cardiovascular effects, and aggressive risk reduction is warranted. Cardiovascular conditions that have been observed among HD survivors include pericarditis, coronary artery disease, heart valve damage, cardiomyopathy, pancarditis, and conduction abnormalities. The use of modern radiation techniques and low radiation doses can reduce the risk of cardiovascular late effects. Recommended risk reduction strategies for HD survivors at risk of cardiovascular disease include: smoking cessation; avoid-

TABLE 3-11 Possible Late Effects Among Survivors of Hodgkin's Disease

Late Effect	Population at Risk	Risk	Interventions
Cancer recurrence	All HD survivors	Risk highest within first few years of primary therapy	Post-treatment surveillance (physical examination, including skin examination) Prevention strategies (e.g., smoking cessation) For women: routine breast self-examination, mammography
Second primary cancer	Individuals receiving certain chemotherapies Individuals receiving radiation therapy	Increased risk of leukemia and lymphoma Increased risk of cancers of the lung, breast, thyroid, bone/soft tissue, gastrointestinal tract, and skin	
Psychosocial distress	All survivors	Not well understood	Not well investigated
Infertility and gonadal dysfunction	Individuals receiving pelvic irradiation and those receiving high cumulative doses of alkylating agent chemotherapy drugs	High cumulative alkylating agent exposure sterilizes nearly all males, and females over age 25 undergo menopause. Sexual dysfunction may occur with sex hormone deficiency	Pretreatment reproductive counseling, semen and embryo cryopreservation, and referral to specialists Hormone replacement therapy counseling based upon treatment received
Hypothyroidism	Individuals receiving high-dose neck radiation	Risk varies by radiation dose and area exposed	Routine physical examination of the thyroid; periodic thyroid function testing
Cardiovascular disease	Individuals receiving radiation to the heart or cardiotoxic chemotherapy	Patients treated with a lower radiation dose are at lower risk	Aggressive risk reduction (e.g., management of lipids, glucose intolerance, and hypertension;

	Individuals receiving radiation to the head and neck (vascular arterial changes)	Risk related to cumulative dose of anthracycline	smoking cessation)
Impaired pulmonary function	Individuals receiving high doses of radiation; bleomycin increases the risk	Worsening lung function depends on dose of radiation therapy and bleomycin	Smoking cessation, avoidance of other pulmonary toxins Annual influenza vaccine Steroid and antibiotic therapy
Increased risk of infection	Individuals who have undergone splenectomy or splenic radiation; patients exposed to intensive chemotherapy	Infection risk (e.g., sepsis) increases in asplenic patients, and with higher degree of immunosuppression	Pretreatment and periodic immunization; prophylactic antibiotics
Fatigue	All survivors	Some HD survivors have fatigue; it may be related to aspects of the disease rather than to treatment	Exercise may be beneficial
Nerve damage	Individuals receiving neurotoxins: vinca alkaloids and platinum compounds	Peripheral neuropathy and autonomic neuropathy	Avoid other neurotoxins: heavy metals, radiation, drugs
Osteoporosis; avascular necrosis	Individuals receiving corticosteroid therapy	Risk reduced through radiation shielding of the femoral head, minimizing prednisone exposure	Assessments and preventive strategies for osteoporosis (e.g., bone density examinations, calcium, and vitamin D) Orthopedic surgery
Musculoskeletal atrophy	Individuals receiving radiation to the head and neck	Risk related to dose of radiation and age at therapy	Rehabilitation if severe loss of muscle mass
Dental caries	Individuals receiving salivary gland radiation	Risk reduced through radiation shielding of the salivary glands	Dental prophylaxis (e.g., fluoride)

ance of obesity; and management of lipids, glucose intolerance, and hypertension. Unusual symptoms (e.g., chest or arm pressure, unexpected, profound exertional fatigue) should prompt careful cardiologic assessment (Hancock, 1999).

Impaired Pulmonary Function

HD survivors may experience damage to the lung if they are treated with radiation therapy that is of high dose and involves large volumes of the chest area or if they receive certain chemotherapy agents, such as bleomycin. Smoking cessation programs are very important. Severe pneumonitis may require steroid therapy.

Increased Risk of Infection

Individuals with HD are at increased risk of infection if they had a splenectomy, splenic radiation, or were treated with high-dose therapy and autologous transplantation. Such individuals should be immunized with Haemophilus influenza type B conjugate, meningococcal, and pneumococcal vaccines before treatment. Reimmunization with all three vaccines 2 years after completion of treatment and with pneumococcal vaccine every 6 years thereafter has also been recommended. Patients exposed to aggressive immunosuppressive treatment programs may benefit from antibiotic use. Patient education is important to alert HD survivors to the importance of medical attention during episodes of fever.

Fatigue

Fatigue has been observed among HD survivors in several studies (Bloom et al., 1993; Loge et al., 1999; Knobel et al., 2001; Flechtner and Bottomley, 2003), but according to a recent prospective study conducted by Ganz and colleagues, increased fatigue was evident prior to treatment. This suggests that an underlying disease process may be responsible (Ganz et al., 2003c). Further analyses of this study cohort found pretreatment fatigue not to be associated with medical factors related to disease or to hematologic status (Ganz et al., 2004b). Instead, fatigue was significantly associated with patient-reported symptoms and physical and psychosocial well-being. Post-treatment fatigue was related to depressed pretreatment vitality. Exercise may help cancer survivors who experience fatigue (Holtzman et al., 2004).

Nerve Damage

Those with preexisting neuropathies and those who receive neurotoxic drugs or radiation are at risk for nerve damage. The risk depends on dosages of radiation and certain chemotherapies. Survivors with nerve damage should avoid further exposure to neurotoxins.

Bone Damage

Chemotherapy programs using prolonged and high doses of steroids predispose to osteopenia and osteoporosis. Measures to reduce the risk of osteoporosis include using prescription medications (e.g., alendronate), performing bone density examinations, recommending the use of calcium and vitamin D supplements, and counseling survivors about the benefits of regular exercise, weight-bearing exercise, and a healthy weight. High radiation doses to bone, especially the mandible and femoral heads, has been associated with bone necrosis. However, these late effects are rarely seen with modern treatment programs.

Dental Caries

Radiation to large areas including the salivary glands can decrease the amount of saliva and change its quality so that it is less effective in cleansing normal oral bacteria from the mouth. This sets the stage for possible dental caries. People who get radiotherapy to the neck and mouth areas should have dental care pretreatment. After therapy, survivors need to take good care of their teeth. Regular dental visits, use of fluoride mouth washes, drinking fluorinated water, and use of dental floss are recommended. Antibiotic therapy may be needed before a tooth extraction. Pulling teeth after radiation therapy increases the risk of necrosis of the mandible and maxilla, and some patients elect to get all of their teeth pulled prior to radiation to avoid this. There are dentists available who specialize in the care of the mouth following radiation.

Clinical Practice Guidelines

The committee identified two clinical practice guidelines that describe management strategies for HD survivors.[36] The NCCN Hodgkin's disease CPG provides a visit schedule, vaccination recommendations, and sugges-

[36]The guideline developed by the Children's Oncology Group for survivors of childhood, adolescent, and young adult cancers was not included in this review (Children's Oncology Group, 2005).

BOX 3-13
NCCN CPG: Follow-up After Completion of Treatment for Hodgkin's Disease

Interim health visit and physical examination:

- Every 2–3 months for 1–2 years, then every 3–6 months for next 3–5 years, then annually
- Pneumococcal and meningococcal revaccination every 6 years, if patient treated with splenic radiation therapy (RT)
- Annual influenza vaccine (especially if patient treated with bleomycin or chest RT)

Laboratory studies:

- Complete blood count, platelets, erythrocyte sedimentation rate, chemistry profile every 2–4 months for 1–2 years, then every 3–6 months for next 3–5 years, then annually
- TSH at least annually if RT to neck

Chest imaging:

- Chest x-ray or computerized tomographic (CT) scan every 3–6 months during first 2–3 years, then annually thereafter depending on clinical circumstances[a]

Abdominal/pelvic CT:

- Every 6–12 months for first 2–3 years, then annually for next 2 years

Annual mammographic screening:

- Initiate 8 years post-therapy, if RT above diaphragm

Counseling:

- Reproduction, health habits, psychosocial, cardiovascular, breast self-exam, skin cancer risk, end-of-treatment discussion

Recommend written follow-up instructions for the patient

---

[a]Chest imaging optional after 5 years if patient treated with a non-alkylating agent, no radiation therapy to the chest and no other risk factors are present.

NOTE: The frequency and types of tests may vary depending on clinical circumstances; age and stage at diagnosis, social habits, treatment modality, etc.

SOURCE: NCCN (2004f).

tions for laboratory studies, including those for thyroid function, imaging, mammograms for women, and counseling (Box 3-13) (NCCN, 2004f). Somewhat more comprehensive coverage of survivorship issues can be found in the HD CPG of the British Columbia Cancer Agency (British Columbia Cancer Agency, 2002b). Included in this CPG is a follow-up schedule for visits, tests, and immunizations, as well as information on cancer relapse, second cancers, dental caries, hypothyroidism, and infertility. None of the CPGs for the follow-up of patients with HD are based on clinical trials. Such trials are needed to test the worth of high-intensity versus low-intensity strategies, assess quality of life prospectively, and measure the effectiveness of various follow-up measures.

Summary

There are many late effects associated with the treatment of breast cancer, prostate cancer, colorectal cancer, and Hodgkin's disease. CPGs exist for all of these sites, but they are incomplete and do not cover most of the essential elements of survivorship care. There have been relatively few population-based, longitudinal studies to accurately assess the prevalence of late effects among cancer survivors. Little is known regarding appropriate follow-up because few large clinical trials of specific strategies have been conducted, even for common cancers.

LIFESTYLE FOLLOWING CANCER TREATMENT

Cancer survivors are at increased risk for developing a second cancer and, depending on their treatment, may be at increased risk for cardiovascular disease, osteoporosis, and other chronic illnesses. If lifestyle behaviors that may have contributed to the onset of cancer, such as smoking and unhealthy diet, persist, they can continue to threaten survival and quality of life. Given this heightened level of risk, cancer survivors represent a large and important target population for health promotion interventions (Demark-Wahnefried et al., 2000; Blanchard et al., 2003a; Demark-Wahnefried et al., 2005; Ganz, 2005). After a diagnosis of cancer, individuals are often motivated to change their diet, exercise habits, and other lifestyles (Satia et al., 2004). Many are also interested in learning more about dietary supplements and nutritional complementary therapies to manage persistent symptoms of disease or treatment. This section of the chapter reviews evidence on some common issues of interest to cancer survivors regarding smoking cessation, physical activity, diet and nutrition, and the use of complementary and alternative medicine.

Smoking Cessation

Nearly one-third of cancers are caused by smoking. Declines in smoking prevalence in the United States have reduced deaths from lung and other respiratory cancers. Many cancer patients and survivors, however, continue to smoke after their diagnosis and providers may not encourage smoking cessation because they believe it is "too late," "it doesn't matter," or "it is too difficult" for their patients to quit (Dresler, 2003). However, smoking cessation has benefits even after cancer has developed. Effective behavioral therapy and pharmacotherapy are available to help smokers quit (Cox et

TABLE 3-12 Prevalence of Smoking by Self-Reported History of Cancer, by Age, United States, 1999–2000

Self-Reported History of Cancer and Age	Smoking Status		
	Current	Former	Never
History of Cancer			
All ages	20	38	42
18-44	41	17	43
45-64	24	38	38
65+	9	46	45
No History of Cancer			
All ages	24	22	54
18-44	27	13	60
45-64	24	30	46
65+	11	39	50

SOURCE: Hewitt et al. (2003).

al., 2003; McBride and Ostroff, 2003). Guidelines of the U.S. Preventive Services Task Force recommend that clinicians screen all adults for tobacco use and provide tobacco cessation interventions for those who use tobacco products (USPSTF, 2003). The committee believes that oncology providers' encounters with cancer patients represent "teachable moments," and a failure to routinely assess smoking status and provide smoking cessation counseling is a lost opportunity. According to two large surveys of cancer survivors, roughly 65 to 70 percent of individuals who reported that they smoked said their physician recommended they quit smoking (Demark-Wahnefried et al., 2000; Blanchard et al., 2003a). Evidence that physician smoking cessation advice is not provided routinely at each visit comes from national surveys of the content of ambulatory care (i.e., non-hospitalized) visits. Physicians are providing smoking cessation counseling for fewer than one in five cancer-related ambulatory care visits made by patients who use tobacco, according to national surveys of ambulatory care providers (see Chapter 4, Table 4-1).

The problem of smoking among cancer survivors appears to be substantial. As many as 20 percent of cancer survivors report that they currently smoke, a rate only slightly lower than the rate among individuals without a history of cancer (Table 3-12). Smoking rates are alarmingly high among young cancer survivors (ages 18 to 44), substantially higher than among their counterparts without a cancer history (41 versus 27 percent)

BOX 3-14
Counseling to Prevent Tobacco Use: Clinical Considerations

Brief tobacco cessation counseling interventions, including screening, brief counseling (3 minutes or less), and/or pharmacotherapy, have been proven to increase tobacco abstinence rates, although there is a dose-response relationship between quit rates and the intensity of counseling. Effective interventions may be delivered by a variety of primary care clinicians.

The "5-A" behavioral counseling framework provides a useful strategy for engaging patients in smoking cessation discussions:

1. *Ask* about tobacco use.
2. *Advise* to quit through clear personalized messages.
3. *Assess* willingness to quit.
4. *Assist* to quit.
5. *Arrange* follow-up and support.

Helpful aspects of counseling include providing problem-solving guidance for smokers to develop a plan to quit and to overcome common barriers to quitting, and providing social support within and outside of treatment. Common practices that complement this framework include motivational interviewing, the "5 R's" used to treat tobacco use (*relevance, risks, rewards, roadblocks, repetition*), assessing readiness to change, and more intensive counseling and/or referrals for quitters needing extra help. Telephone "quit lines" have also been found to be an effective adjunct to counseling or medical therapy.

SOURCE: Agency for Healthcare Policy and Research (USPSTF, 2003).

(Table 3-12). Many (38 percent) cancer survivors are former smokers and so are at considerable risk for relapse of their smoking habit.

Persistent smoking following diagnosis contributes to poor long-term outcomes (Dresler, 2003). Cessation of cigarette smoking has been associated with a reduction in treatment complications, improved survival, and a decrease in risk for second cancers (Dresler, 2003; Cox et al., 2003; Garces and Hays, 2003; McBride and Ostroff, 2003). Benefits of smoking cessation following a diagnosis of cancer also include reductions in the risk for cardiovascular and pulmonary disease.

Guidance on how to provide smoking cessation counseling is available and has been shown to be effective, in combination with pharmacotherapy, to help smokers quit (Box 3-14) (Carter et al., 2001). Smoking cessation interventions that have been evaluated in cancer patient populations have generally been associated with relatively high rates of cessation in the short term. However, relapse rates are high, suggesting that sustained and/or repeated cessation efforts are needed (Pinto et al., 2000, 2002; Cox et al., 2003; McBride and Ostroff, 2003). The studies to date have generally been limited to hospitalized cancer patients and have been of insufficient size to detect significant effects of interventions. The results of a recent clinical trial to test physician-initiated smoking cessation interventions in oncology settings are discouraging (Schnoll et al., 2003). According to this trial, training physicians to provide smoking cessation treatment to cancer patients enhanced physician adherence to clinical practice guidelines, but the physician interventions failed to yield significant gains in long-term quit rates among cancer patients.

Barriers to smoking cessation among cancer patients can include a strong nicotine dependence because of a long history of heavy tobacco use, fatalistic beliefs, psychological distress, and social influences (McBride and Ostroff, 2003). Building smoking cessation counseling into important cancer transitions has been suggested as a way to promote smoking cessation. Teachable moments for smoking cessation counseling and relapse prevention include the time of diagnosis, time of active treatment, and time of transition from inpatient to outpatient care and follow-up visits. In each of these clinical settings, involvement of family members is important given the likelihood that smoking is common among the family members of cancer patients (McBride and Ostroff, 2003).

The provision and acceptance of smoking prevention services are enabled when they are covered by insurance. However, smoking cessation counseling and pharmacotherapies are not consistently covered as paid services by Medicaid, health insurance plans, and managed care organizations (IOM, 2003). Medicare has recently added coverage of smoking and other tobacco use cessation services for certain beneficiaries (CMS, 2005). Coverage of cessation services is limited to beneficiaries who have an illness caused or complicated by tobacco use and to those who take any of the many medications whose effectiveness is complicated by tobacco use (e.g., agents to treat hypertension, thrombosis, and depression, as well as insulin to treat diabetes).

Research is needed to identify specific strategies for smoking cessation that are tailored to the specific needs of cancer survivors. How smoking cessation effects risks of recurrence and quality of life and the effectiveness of family-oriented interventions are issues that have not been extensively explored, but are worthy of future research (Cox et al., 2003).

Physical Activity

Many cancer patients reduce their levels of activity during treatment and do not resume activity at their prediagnosis levels (Irwin et al., 2003;

Blanchard et al., 2003a). The effectiveness of behavioral interventions to modify physical activity behaviors among cancer survivors was the subject of a 2004 Agency for Healthcare Research and Quality (AHRQ) evidence report (Holtzman et al., 2004).[37] According to this review, controlled trials of behavioral interventions to increase physical activity among cancer survivors show positive and consistent effects of physical activity on the following outcomes:

- Vigor and vitality
- Cardiorespiratory fitness
- Quality of life
- Depression
- Anxiety
- Fatigue/tiredness

Similar findings come from a recent systematic review of randomized controlled clinical trials (Knols et al., 2005; Pinto et al., 2005). The exercise prescription associated with these positive outcomes in cancer survivors was generally moderate- to vigorous-intensity aerobic activity on 3 or more days per week, for 10 to 60 minutes per session. The findings for many of these outcomes parallel the results in generally healthy populations. The effect of physical activity on cancer recurrence or survival is unknown, but physical activity might improve prognosis through beneficial effects on cardiovascular disease (McTiernan, 2004) or through hormonal mechanisms (Holmes et al., 2005). Resistance training has beneficial effects on muscle and bone and may counteract some of the side effects of cancer treatment (e.g., bone and muscle loss) and help improve survivors' physical function and quality of life (Galvao and Newton, 2005).

For physical activity to be recommended for cancer survivors, it must be safe and not associated with adverse outcomes. The results of the studies reviewed by AHRQ generally indicate that it is safe for cancer survivors to be physically active. Questions about the safety of physical activity remain, however. For example, one concern is that exercise by breast cancer survivors could induce or exacerbate lymphedema. Most studies have reported no adverse effects of upper body exercise on breast cancer survivors at risk for lymphedema. However, current clinical guidelines from multiple sources

[37]This section of the report is based almost entirely on the AHRQ evidence review (AHRQ, 2004). Additional randomized trials of exercise among survivors have been published that were not included in the AHRQ review. Their results are consistent with the review's findings of beneficial effects of exercise on cardiovascular fitness and/or quality of life (Courneya et al., 2003a,b; Thorsen et al., 2005).

(NCI, ACS, National Lymphedema Network, Susan G. Komen Foundation) include recommendations to breast cancer survivors to avoid ever lifting anything heavier than 5 to 15 pounds. This recommendation has negative health promotion and quality of life implications. According to the AHRQ review, "There is too little research on this topic thus far to appropriately and safely prescribe physical activity for breast cancer survivors at risk for (or with a diagnosis of) lymphedema." Further research on this topic is needed to guide the more than 2 million American breast cancer survivors.

There is an additional concern that too-vigorous physical activity could depress the immune system and promote the spread of cancer. In generally healthy adults, moderate-intensity physical activity is associated with overall improvement in immune parameters, while high-intensity, high-volume physical activity is associated with a temporary worsening of immune function. According to the AHRQ review, additional studies are needed to clarify the effects on certain immune parameters, with specificity as to timing across the cancer experience as well as physical activity mode, frequency, intensity, and duration (Holtzman et al., 2004).

There is limited evidence regarding the extent to which physicians are providing guidance regarding exercise to their patients who are cancer survivors. According to two relatively large surveys, 20 to 35 percent of cancer survivors reported that their physician recommended changes in their exercise behavior. One study included a sample of cancer survivors with several types of cancer (Blanchard et al., 2003a) while the other study was limited to survivors of breast and prostate cancer (Demark-Wahnefried et al., 2000). An oncologist's recommendation to exercise may increase exercise behavior, according to a randomized trial that involved breast cancer survivors (Jones et al., 2004). One study suggests that cancer survivors prefer that their oncologist initiate a discussion about exercise (Jones and Courneya, 2002).

A framework for examining physical activity across the cancer experience (Framework PEACE) has been proposed based on the cancer control perspective (Courneya and Friedenreich, 2001). The framework includes six possible cancer control outcomes after the point of cancer diagnosis, including buffering prior to treatment (i.e., building up physical condition before treatment), coping during treatment, rehabilitation immediately after treatment, health promotion and survival for those with positive treatment outcomes, and palliation for those without positive treatment outcomes. The AHRQ review concludes that additional research is needed on the effects of physical activity on pretreatment outcomes, health promotion, survival, and palliation.

Nutrition and Diet

A limited but growing body of evidence shows that nutritional interventions for cancer survivors reduce the risk of recurrence (Chlebowski et al., 2005). It is therefore reasonable to recommend that cancer survivors follow dietary guidelines established for primary prevention of cancer as well as other diseases (e.g., cardiovascular disease, osteoporosis, and diabetes). Cancer survivors can obtain information and guidance on nutrition and diet from the ACS and the American Institute for Cancer Research (AICR) (Brown et al., 2003; AICR, 2004; ACS, 2004a). In general, these guidelines for cancer survivors are similar to general recommendations for the primary prevention of cancer. The rationale for this guidance for cancer survivors is that the same factors that increase cancer incidence might also be important in promoting cancer recurrence after treatment. Data are most compelling for breast cancer, where the risk of recurrence might be increased by obesity and perhaps by diets high in fat and low in fruits and vegetables (Holmes and Kroenke, 2004; Chlebowski et al., 2005).[38] Prostate cancer recurrence might also be increased by a high saturated fat intake, with increased intakes of meat and dairy products associated with more aggressive cancers (Brown et al., 2003). Adherence to these dietary guidelines may also be the most effective method for preventing the growth of second primary cancers and to improve overall health. AICR's dietary recommendations for cancer survivors are shown in Box 3-15.

Most cancer survivors make at least some dietary changes following their diagnosis. In one survey of a general survivorship population, 51 percent of survivors said they had reduced their fat intake, 44 percent increased their fiber intake, and 43 percent reduced their red meat intake. More than one-quarter (28 percent) indicated their physician recommended that they reduce their fat intake, and 15 percent reported that their physician suggested they increase their fiber intake (Blanchard et al., 2003a). Findings from a survey of breast and prostate cancer survivors were similar, with 29 percent reporting that their doctor recommended that they reduce fat intake and 16 percent reporting a recommendation to increase their fruit and vegetable intake (Demark-Wahnefried et al., 2000).

Healthy Weight

There is convincing evidence that obesity is associated with an increased risk of several cancers, including cancers of the colon, breast, and

[38]Clinical trials are underway to examine the effects of dietary patterns on the risk for recurrence and on survival after diagnosis among women with early-stage breast cancer (e.g., The Women's Healthy Eating and Living (WHEL) Study, The Women's Intervention Nutrition Study (WINS) (Holmes and Kroenke, 2004; Chlebowski et al., 2005).

BOX 3-15
Nutritional Guidelines for Cancer Survivors from the American Institute for Cancer Research

1. Choose predominantly plant-based diets rich in a variety of vegetables and fruits.
2. If eaten at all, limit intake of red meat to less than 3 ounces daily.
3. Limit consumption of fatty foods, particularly those of animal origin. Choose modest amounts of appropriate vegetable oils.
4. Limit consumption of salted foods and use of cooking and table salt. Use herbs and spices to season foods.
5. Limit alcoholic drinks to less than two drinks a day for men and one for women.
6. Do not eat charred food. Consume the following only occasionally: meat and fish grilled in direct flame, and cured and smoked meats.
7. Avoid being overweight and limit weight gain during adulthood. Take an hour's brisk walk or similar exercise daily.

SOURCE: AICR (2004).

endometrium (IOM, 2003). In some cases, being overweight has been shown to reduce survival. Overweight and obese women with breast cancer, for example, have poorer survival compared with thinner women (Kroenke et al., 2005; Chlebowski, 2005a). Diminished survival among obese women with breast cancer may be caused by higher concentrations of tumor-promoting hormones found in association with higher degrees of adiposity (McTiernan et al., 2003). Obesity also has been found to be a poor prognostic factor for prostate cancer (Freedland et al., 2004; Amling et al., 2004). To date, relatively little research on interventions to help cancer survivors lose weight has been conducted, and much of it has been confined to survivors of breast cancer (Djuric et al., 2002; Jenkins et al., 2003; Jen et al., 2004). Interventions to improve self-confidence may be needed because some research suggests that low self-esteem among overweight and obese breast cancer survivors interferes with their ability to adopt healthy lifestyles (Pinto et al., 2002). As in healthy populations, exercise also has been found to play a major role in weight management of cancer survivors (Goodwin et al., 1998).

Complementary and Alternative Medicine

Complementary and alternative medicine (CAM) is a group of diverse medical and health care systems, therapies, and products that are not currently considered to be part of conventional medicine (NCCAM, 2002). The use of CAM is very common among the general population. In 2002 an estimated 62 percent of adults used some form of CAM therapy during the past year when the definition of CAM therapy included prayer specifically for health reasons (Barnes et al., 2004). When prayer was excluded from the definition, 36 percent of adults used some form of CAM therapy during the past year.

Individuals with cancer frequently use CAM products with the belief that their use will arrest their disease, alleviate symptoms, promote well-being, and increase their sense of control over their health (Burstein, 2000; Richardson et al., 2000; Antman et al., 2001). Common categories of CAM therapies used by cancer survivors include dietary modification and supplementation, herbal products and other biological agents, acupuncture, massage, exercise, and psychological and mind-body therapies (Weiger et al., 2002). In their review of the effectiveness and safety of such products, Weiger and colleagues found several CAM therapies that offer potential benefits for patients with cancer. For CAM therapies intended for palliation of symptoms associated with cancer or side effects of conventional treatment, the authors advised physicians to consider recommending and monitoring massage for anxiety or pain, moderate exercise, and psychological and mind-body therapies (e.g., support groups, relaxation training, imagery). Other CAM therapies, however, may be ineffective, and many present risks to cancer survivors (e.g., phytoestrogens for breast cancer survivors taking tamoxifen). The authors recommend that physicians communicate openly with patients about CAM use. Recent studies suggest, however, that many cancer patients do not discuss their use of CAM with their physicians (Lee et al., 2000; Navo et al., 2004). Such discussions are especially important given the association in some studies between the use of CAM and greater psychosocial distress (Burstein et al., 1999; DiGianni et al., 2002).

Cancer survivors can obtain comprehensive information about CAM from the American Cancer Society's *Guide to Complementary and Alternative Cancer Methods* (ACS, 2000) and from the NCI's Office of Cancer Complementary and Alternative Medicine (NCI and NCCAM, 2004).

Summary

Clinical encounters with cancer survivors provide "teachable moments" for health prevention and promotion (Demark-Wahnefried et al., 2005; Ganz, 2005). The adoption of healthy lifestyle behaviors provides an opportunity for cancer survivors to assume control of some aspects of their health and improve outcomes from cancer and other chronic illnesses. There are opportunities to intervene to help cancer survivors quit smoking, exercise, and adopt healthy diets. As many as 20 percent of cancer survivors smoke, and evidence suggests that not all are receiving assistance with smoking cessation during routine clinical visits. Moderate exercise has many benefits for cancer survivors, including improved vigor and vitality, cardiorespiratory fitness, quality of life, and mental health. Questions remain regarding the safety of exercise for some cancer survivors, for example, breast cancer survivors with, or at risk for, lymphedema, but for most cancer survivors, moderate exercise is beneficial. A healthy diet low in saturated fat and rich in fruits and vegetables is recommended for the general public to prevent cancer, but also for cancer survivors to reduce their risk for subsequent cancer. Data are limited, but physicians do not appear to be routinely counseling cancer survivors regarding diet and nutrition. Obesity is a risk factor for several cancers, and researchers are beginning to test interventions to help overweight and obese cancer survivors lose weight.

CAM interventions are used frequently by cancer survivors and, when tested, some CAM interventions have been shown to be beneficial. Among CAM therapies that can be recommended for cancer survivors are massage for anxiety or pain, moderate exercise, and psychological and mind-body therapies (e.g., support groups, relaxation training, imagery). Cancer survivors are sometimes reluctant to discuss CAM therapies with their providers. It is recommended that physicians openly discuss these therapies because some have been shown to be harmful, to interfere with cancer treatment, or to be ineffective.

FINDINGS AND RECOMMENDATIONS

Cancer survivorship, as defined in this report, is a distinct phase of the cancer trajectory, but has been relatively neglected in advocacy, education, clinical practice, and research. Raising awareness of the medical and psychosocial needs that may follow cancer treatment will help both survivors and their health care providers to ensure that appropriate assessments are completed and available interventions employed. The constellation of cancer's long-term and late effects varies by cancer type, treatment modality, and individual characteristics, but there are common patterns of symptoms and conditions that must be recognized so that health and well-being can be improved.

Recommendation 1: Health care providers, patient advocates, and other stakeholders should work to raise awareness of the needs of cancer survivors, establish cancer survivorship as a distinct phase of cancer care, and act to ensure the delivery of appropriate survivorship care.

Cancer patients and their advocates can call attention to their survivorship experiences and the need for change. The leadership of organizations representing physicians, nurses, and psychosocial care providers can collaborate to improve care. Third-party payors of health care and health plans can improve access to needed services through reimbursement policies and improvements in systems of care. Employers can ensure fair workplace policies and accommodations. Sponsors of research can improve the opportunities to increase what we know about survivorship and appropriate care. Congress and state legislatures can enact policies and ensure the support needed to improve survivorship care and quality of life.

Providing a Care Plan for Survivorship

The recognition of cancer survivorship as a distinct phase of the cancer trajectory is not enough. A strategy is needed for the ongoing clinical care of cancer survivors. There are many opportunities for improving care—psychosocial distress can be assessed and support provided; cancer recurrences and second cancers may be caught early and treated; bothersome symptoms can be effectively managed; preventable conditions such as osteoporosis may be avoided; and potentially lethal late effects such as heart failure averted.

> **Recommendation 2: Patients completing primary treatment should be provided with a comprehensive care summary and follow-up plan that is clearly and effectively explained. This "Survivorship Care Plan" should be written by the principal provider(s) that coordinated oncology treatment. This service should be reimbursed by third-party payors of health care.**

Such a care plan would summarize critical information needed for the survivor's long-term care:

- Cancer type, treatments received, and their potential consequences;
- Specific information about the timing and content of recommended follow-up;
- Recommendations regarding preventive practices and how to maintain health and well-being;
- Information on legal protections regarding employment and access to health insurance; and
- The availability of psychosocial services in the community.

These content areas, adapted from those recommended by the President's Cancer Panel (President's Cancer Panel, 2004), are elaborated upon in Box 3-16.

The content of the survivorship care plan could be reviewed with a

BOX 3-16
Survivorship Care Plan

Upon discharge from cancer treatment, including treatment of recurrences, every patient should be given a record of all care received and important disease characteristics. This should include, at a minimum:

1. Diagnostic tests performed and results.
2. Tumor characteristics (e.g., site(s), stage and grade, hormone receptor status, marker information).
3. Dates of treatment initiation and completion.
4. Surgery, chemotherapy, radiotherapy, transplant, hormonal therapy, or gene or other therapies provided, including agents used, treatment regimen, total dosage, identifying number and title of clinical trials (if any), indicators of treatment response, and toxicities experienced during treatment.
5. Psychosocial, nutritional, and other supportive services provided.
6. Full contact information on treating institutions and key individual providers.
7. Identification of a key point of contact and coordinator of continuing care.

Upon discharge from cancer treatment, every patient and his/her primary health care provider should receive a written follow-up care plan incorporating available evidence-based standards of care. This should include, at a minimum:

1. The likely course of recovery from treatment toxicities, as well as the need for ongoing health maintenance/adjuvant therapy.
2. A description of recommended cancer screening and other periodic testing and examinations, and the schedule on which they should be performed (and who should provide them).

patient during a formal discharge consultation. Clinicians would likely have discussed some aspects of the survivorship care plan before or during treatment, for example, short- and long-term treatment effects and their implications for work and quality of life.[39] However, during acute treatment, much time is spent dealing with the acute toxicities of treatment that little emphasis is given to the post-treatment care plan. A substantial amount of information needs to be communicated during this consultation and then documented in an end-of-treatment consultation note. Examples of such consultation notes are provided in Appendix 3A of this chapter. Appropri-

[39]Providing a survivorship care plan may prove difficult for those individuals who cease treatment prematurely and do not return for the remainder of their care. Primary care physicians involved in subsequent care of such patients may need to contact oncology providers to obtain a survivorship care plan.

3. Information on possible late and long-term effects of treatment and symptoms of such effects.

4. Information on possible signs of recurrence and second tumors.

5. Information on the possible effects of cancer on marital/partner relationship, sexual functioning, work, and parenting, and the potential future need for psychosocial support.

6. Information on the potential insurance, employment, and financial consequences of cancer and, as necessary, referral to counseling, legal aid, and financial assistance.

7. Specific recommendations for healthy behaviors (e.g., diet, exercise, healthy weight, sunscreen use, immunizations, smoking cessation, osteoporosis prevention). When appropriate, recommendations that first-degree relatives be informed about their increased risk and the need for cancer screening (e.g., breast cancer, colorectal cancer, prostate cancer).

8. As appropriate, information on genetic counseling and testing to identify high-risk individuals who could benefit from more comprehensive cancer surveillance, chemoprevention, or risk-reducing surgery.

9. As appropriate, information on known effective chemoprevention strategies for secondary prevention (e.g., tamoxifen in women at high risk for breast cancer; aspirin for colorectal cancer prevention).

10. Referrals to specific follow-up care providers (e.g., rehabilitation, fertility, psychology), support groups, and/or the patient's primary care provider.

11. A listing of cancer-related resources and information (e.g., Internet-based sources and telephone listings for major cancer support organizations).

SOURCE: Adapted from the President's Cancer Panel (2004).

ate reimbursement should be provided for such a visit, given the complexity and importance of the consultation.

The member of the oncology treating team who would be responsible for this visit could vary depending on the exact course of treatment. The responsibility could be assigned either to the oncology specialist coordinating care or to the provider responsible for the last component of treatment. Oncology nurses could play a key role. The survivorship care plan may need revision as new knowledge concerning late effects and interventions to ameliorate them, genetic disorders, and surveillance methods is identified. Cancer survivors can help to ensure that the plan is followed. The consultation at the conclusion of primary treatment could serve as a teaching event for survivors and their family members and provide opportunities to discuss with clinicians their prognosis, concerns, lifestyle issues, and follow-up schedules. The plan could be used by survivors subsequently to raise questions with doctors and prompt appropriate care during follow-up visits.

Agencies that accredit health plans and other providers could build compliance with the recommended consultation into their evaluation criteria (see discussion of quality measures in chapter 4). With 61 percent of cancer survivors aged 65 and older, the Medicare program could play a key role in ensuring that the survivorship care plan is written, communicated, and reimbursed. A formal assessment of survivorship care planning should be undertaken to assess its value.

Survivorship care plans have been recommended by the President's Cancer Panel and by the IOM committee, however, the implementation of such plans has not yet been formally evaluated. Despite the lack of evidence to support the use of survivorship care plans, the committee concluded that some elements of care simply make sense—that is, they have strong face validity and can reasonably be assumed to improve care unless and until evidence accumulates to the contrary. Having an agreed-upon care plan that outlines goals of care falls into this "common sense" area. Health services research should be undertaken to assess the impact and costs associated with survivorship care plans, and to evaluate their acceptance by both cancer survivors and health care providers.

Developing Clinical Practice Guidelines for Survivorship Care

The "Survivorship Care Plan" would inform clinicians involved in the subsequent care of cancer survivors about treatment exposures, signs and symptoms of late effects, and, in some cases, would provide concrete steps to be taken. To carry out this plan, an organized set of clinical practice guidelines based on the best available evidence is needed to help ensure appropriate follow-up care. Guidelines should be derived by a formal process and, depending on the predominant methodology used to develop them, CPGs may be characterized as evidence based or consensus derived (Woolf, 1992). Because the goal is to assist in clinical decision making, the guideline should reflect the major clinical decisions that must be made as the disease entity is managed (Winn and Botnick, 1997). Furthermore, the interventions recommended in a CPG must be appropriate, that is, the expected benefits must outweigh the expected risks and harms by a sufficient amount to make the intervention worthwhile (Park et al., 1986).

Unfortunately, the status of cancer-related guidelines falls far short of these ideals. Deficiencies exist both in the availability and content of the guidelines. Relatively few cancer-related CPGs are available to clinicians, and of those that are available, most focus on the most common cancers (Smith and Hillner, 2001). Many of the tumor-specific guidelines are limited to one phase of the care trajectory (e.g., screening, primary treatment, therapy with limited chance for cure), or are modality oriented and address issues related to a particular oncologic intervention (e.g., surgery, radiotherapy, adjuvant therapy).

Evidence-based guidelines would provide specific information on how to manage the complex issues facing survivors of adult cancers. Assessment tools and screening instruments for common late effects are also needed to help identify cancer survivors who have, or who are at high risk for, late effects and who may need extra surveillance or interventions.

> **Recommendation 3: Health care providers should use systematically developed evidence-based clinical practice guidelines, assessment tools, and screening instruments to help identify and manage late effects of cancer and its treatment. Existing guidelines should be refined and new evidence-based guidelines should be developed through public- and private-sector efforts.**

Cancer survivors represent a very large at-risk population, and without evidence-based clinical practice guidelines, health care providers will vary widely in their practices, leading to inefficiencies in care delivery. Evidence suggests that some tests are being overused in the context of routine surveillance care after cancer treatment (Elston Lafata et al., 2005). The critical need for more rational, consistent, and efficient cancer follow-up practices has been widely recognized (Johnson and Virgo, 1997; Schwartz et al., 2000). As a nation, we have not invested in the research on cancer survivors on which such clinical practice guidelines would be based. Without high-quality evidence on the benefits, harms, and relative cost-effectiveness of follow-up strategies, cancer survivors face the health and financial hazards of overuse, underuse, and misuse of resources. The adoption of evidence-based guidelines has the potential to reduce this variation, improve patient outcomes, and reduce health care costs. Health services research is needed to evaluate the impact of such guidelines in the context of survivorship care.

The most comprehensive CPGs included in the committee's review were created under the auspices of regional or national health policy organizations (e.g., Australia; British Columbia, Canada; Scotland). Similar support from appropriate bodies in the United States would facilitate guideline development. Public and private support of studies to generate evidence for guideline development is needed. The Centers for Medicare and Medicaid Services is the primary payor of care for cancer survivors and therefore have a stake in developing clinical practice guidelines. The Agency for Healthcare Research and Quality maintains a National Guideline Clearinghouse and supports Evidence-Based Practice Centers that review relevant scientific literature on clinical, behavioral, organizational, and financial topics to produce evidence reports and technology assessments (AHRQ, 2004a,b). Such reviews can form the foundation of evidence-based guidelines. Professional organizations (e.g., those representing oncology, primary care, nursing) also have a role to play in developing interdisciplinary guidelines. Achieving consensus on CPGs across medical specialties and provider groups is essential in promoting conformance to CPGs. The guideline development process is a costly one, and public and private support is needed to improve and expedite the development process. The development of guidelines is currently impeded by the lack of good evidence to support most surveillance strategies.

A model for guideline development can be found in the efforts of the Children's Oncology Group (COG). COG has developed systematic guidelines for long-term follow-up of survivors of childhood, adolescent, and young adult cancers and has made them widely available through the internet (Children's Oncology Group, 2005; Landier et al., 2004). A complementary set of patient educational materials has also been developed to broaden the application of the guidelines.

Rigorously developed evidence-based guidelines can minimize the potential harms of surveillance (e.g., morbidity and mortality associated with the follow-up of false-positive screening tests) (Woolf et al., 1999; Woolf, 2000). They are, however, only one option for improving the quality of care. On a practical level, it is difficult for providers to obtain reimbursement from insurance companies for needed surveillance (e.g., cardiac and pulmonary function testing) without evidence-based CPGs. Balancing this is the likelihood that some testing strategies will be found to be excessively intensive; savings are likely to result from discontinuing ineffective tests and procedures.

Cancer treatments are constantly evolving and consequently, what is known about today's cohort of cancer survivors may not be relevant to those benefiting from new therapies. Newer therapies hold the promise of limiting the late effects of cancer, but mechanisms to monitor long-term effects need to put in place. The science on which clinical decisions must be based is far from perfect. Compared to the number of studies on the effectiveness of cancer therapies, relatively few have addressed late effects and the value of cancer follow-up policies. A greater investment in research is needed to learn more about late effects and their management. Mechanisms are also needed to communicate new research findings of relevance to cancer survivors and their providers.

APPENDIX 3A
EXAMPLES OF END-OF-TREATMENT CONSULTATION NOTES

Example of an End-of-Treatment Consultation Note: Breast Cancer

Date of note: April 12, 2005
Name: Jane Doe Age: 39
Date of tissue diagnosis of cancer: August 4, 2004

Diagnosis: Breast cancer
Stage of cancer: T1N1M0 Stage II
Pathologic findings: 1.5 cm. infiltrating ductal cancer in the left breast, moderately differentiated, ER positive, PR negative, Her2Neu negative; 3 of 10 nodes positive for metastatic cancer

Initial treatment plan:

- Surgery: Lumpectomy and axillary dissection
- Radiation therapy: 6 weeks of radiation therapy to the left breast
- Chemotherapy: 4 cycles of AC followed by Taxol; dose-dense regimen

Treatment received (specify dates, location, and providers):
Surgery performed as planned by Dr. David Smith at Happy Valley Hospital on 8/23/04.
Chemotherapy administered by Dr. Mary Scott at Westside Oncology Center from 9/15/04 to 2/1/05. Patient received full dose as specified in published protocol Citron et al., JCO, 2003, CALGB 9751 trial, doxorubicin 60 mg/m^2 and cyclophosphamide 600 mg/m^2 q 2 weeks × 4 cycles followed by paclitaxel 175 mg/m^2 q 2 weeks × 4 cycles. Total dose of doxorubicin was 240 mg/m^2.
Radiation therapy was given to the left breast by Dr. Mark Schwartz at Happy Valley Hospital from 2/15/05 to 4/6/05.
Dr. Scott initiated therapy with tamoxifen on 4/12/05.

Unusual or unexpected toxicities during treatment:
There were some treatment delays due to neutropenia and patient required blood transfusions on two occasions.

Expected short- and long-term effects of treatment:
Patient has some fatigue and alopecia at this time, but these are likely to recover over the next 3–6 months. The patient became amenorrheic after the first two cycles of chemotherapy and has severe hot flashes at this time

that may worsen on tamoxifen. She may well have resumption of menses and should use some form of barrier contraception at this time as she may still ovulate. If hot flashes persist, then she may want to consider one of several non-estrogen therapies, as described in the March 21, 2005, NIH State of the Science conference on management of menopausal symptoms. This patient also requires a baseline bone density with follow-up every 2 years to assess for premature osteoporosis.

Late toxicity monitoring needed:
The dose of radiation received is unlikely to cause much risk for hypothyroidism, but periodic evaluation should be considered.
Patient needs to be reminded of lymphedema precautions re: trauma and infection.
She will need regular pelvic examinations to monitor for tamoxifen effects and second malignancies.

Surveillance needed for potential recurrence of cancer:
Needs annual mammograms and breast examinations every 6 months forever. No recommendations for radiological studies or blood tests except to monitor for potential tamoxifen toxicity with annual CBC and chemistry panel.

Surveillance needed for second malignancies:
This patient has a strong family history of breast and ovarian cancer. Given her young age, she may benefit from consideration of genetic testing for BRCA1/2, as well as preventive oophorectomy.

Physicians responsible for monitoring of toxicity, recurrence, second malignancies:
Dr. Scott will see patient every 3–4 months for the next 2 years, and then every 6 months to monitor for tamoxifen therapy and local recurrence of breast cancer.
Dr. Ian Chen, the patient's family physician, will monitor patient with pelvic examination and bone density as well as routine health maintenance issues (contraception, hot flashes); he will arrange for referral for genetic counseling.

Identified psychosocial issues or concerns:
The patient is very concerned about her potential loss of fertility and possible risk for permanent menopause. She is attending the support group at Happy Valley Hospital, but may need individual counseling, depending on whether or not her menses resume. Her husband is very supportive, but he is also concerned about this lost opportunity in their lives.

Recommended preventive behaviors, interventions, or genetic testing:
This patient already has a very health lifestyle and habits, but she is encouraged to avoid weight gain and to remain physically active. Genetic testing has been advised as noted earlier. Patient given NCI booklet, *Life After Cancer Treatment*, and the NCCS "Cancer Survival Toolbox: An Audio Resource Program" that address medical and psychosocial issues, including those related to health insurance and employment.

NOTE: All individual and hospital names are fictitious.
SOURCE: Patricia Ganz, committee member, 2005.

Example of an End-of-Treatment Consultation Note: Prostate Cancer

Date of note: April 20, 2005
Name: John Doe Age: 65
Date of tissue diagnosis of cancer: October 21, 2001

Diagnosis: Prostate cancer
Stage of cancer: Clinical T1c
Pathologic findings: pT2cN0M0, Gleason 4+4, 2.3 cm

Initial treatment plan:

- Surgery: Yes
- Radiation therapy: None
- Chemotherapy: None

Treatment received (specify dates, location, and providers):
Radical prostatectomy with nerve sparing on December 1, 2001, Eastside Medical Center, Dr. Roger Smith

Unusual or unexpected toxicities during treatment:
None

Expected short- and long-term effects of treatment:
Mild urinary leakage for 3 weeks, now dry
Sexual dysfunction for 3 months, now potent with occasional sildenafil

Late toxicity monitoring needed:
None

Surveillance needed for potential recurrence of cancer:
Semi-annual PSA until 5 years post-op, then annual PSA; annual digital rectal exam

Surveillance needed for second malignancies:
None

Physicians responsible for monitoring of toxicity, recurrence, second malignancies:
Dr. Smith will be following Mr. Doe for recurrence and will also assess treatment side effects.

Identified psychosocial issues or concerns:
Short-term depression following surgery, resolved with counseling and support group. Assess psychosocial distress during follow-up visits.

Recommended preventive behaviors, interventions, or genetic testing:
Patient counseled regarding diet/exercise (avoidance of obesity). At follow-up visits assess sexual function and depression. Patient given NCI booklet, *Life After Cancer Treatment*, and the NCCS "Cancer Survival Toolbox: An Audio Resource Program" that address medical and psychosocial issues, including those related to health insurance and employment.

NOTE: All individual and hospital names are fictitious.
SOURCE: Mark Litwin, committee member, 2005.

Example of an End-of-Treatment Consultation Note: Colorectal Cancer

Date of note: April 18, 2005
Name: John Smith Age: 70
Date of tissue diagnosis of cancer: September 15, 2004

Diagnosis: Colon cancer
Stage of cancer: T3N2M0 (IIIB)

Pathologic findings: Moderately differentiated adenocarcinoma penetrating through the muscularis propria. No lymphovascular or perineural invasion. 5/13 regional lymph nodes positive for cancer.

Initial treatment plan:

- Surgery: Left hemicolectomy 9/28/04
- Radiation therapy: None
- Chemotherapy: FOLFOX (5-FU 400 mg/m^2 bolus followed by

1,200 mg/m^2/d for 2 days, leucovorin 400 mg/m^2, oxaliplatin 85 mg/m^2) × 12 cycles

Treatment received (specify dates, location, and providers):
Received FOLFOX from 11/10/04 to 04/13/05 at Northside Cancer Institute under the supervision of Dr. Jane Marks.

Unusual or unexpected toxicities during treatment:
None

Expected short- and long-term effects of treatment:
Sixth cycle held 1 week for thrombocytopenia, requiring a dose reduction in oxaliplatin to 65 mg/m^2. Experienced cold-induced paresthesias in the hands and feet, but no residual neuropathy.

Late toxicity monitoring needed:
None

Surveillance needed for potential recurrence of cancer:
Clinical assessments and bloodwork including CEA every 3 months for 2 years, every 4 months for 1 year, then every 6 months for 2 years. After 5 years, either follow up on an as-needed basis or every 1–2 years, depending on patient choice.

Surveillance needed for second malignancies:
Colonoscopy 1 year after hemicolectomy. Subsequent schedule to depend on the findings. If not polyps or other disease, repeat every 3 to 5 years.

Physicians responsible for monitoring of toxicity, recurrence, second malignancies:
Dr. Jane Marks

Identified psychosocial issues or concerns:
Normal anxiety. Has contact with social worker, David Jones, as needed.

Recommended preventive behaviors, interventions, or genetic testing:
None specific for this cancer. Routine medical care recommended. Patient counseled regarding diet/nutrition. Patient given NCI booklet, *Life After Cancer Treatment*, and the NCCS "Cancer Survival Toolbox: An Audio Resource Program" that address medical and psychosocial issues, including those related to health insurance and employment.

NOTE: All individual and hospital names are fictitious.
SOURCE: Craig Earle, committee member, 2005.

Example of an End-of-Treatment Consultation Note: Hodgkin's Disease

Date of note: April 15, 2005
Name: Jane Smith Age: 28
Date of tissue diagnosis of cancer: November 15, 2004

Diagnosis: Hodgkin's disease
Stage of cancer: Clinical stage IIA
Pathologic findings: Classical Hodgkin's disease

Initial treatment plan:

- Surgery: Biopsy, left supraclavicular lymph note
- Radiation therapy: 30 Gy radiation, to modified mantle field (i.e., bilateral supraclavicular and mediastinal), as consolidation after chemotherapy
- Chemotherapy: Stanford V chemotherapy for 12 weeks

Treatment received (specify dates, location, and providers):
Stanford V chemotherapy 12/1/04–3/2/05; full doses, on schedule; Dr. Kay, Eastern University Medical Center
Radiation therapy 3/15/05–4/15/05; Dr. Smith, Eastern University Medical Center

Unusual or unexpected toxicities during treatment:
None

Expected short- and long-term effects of treatment:
Short term—partial alopecia, hospitalization for fever with neutropenia, 2/15/05 to 2/17/05—given granulocyte colony-stimulating factor and red blood cell transfusion.

Late toxicity monitoring needed:
Thyroid function tests, annually—thyroid-stimulating hormone (TSH) and free T4.
Pulmonary function tests and echocardiograms are not customary or recommended to perform routinely. In particular, it is established that pulmonary function tests within 12 months of thoracic radiation may show mild abnormalities which improve over time.
Careful auscultation of the heart is recommended during follow-up, particularly for patients receiving chest irradiation and anthracycline chemotherapy.
Assessment of fertility—birth control pills for at least 2 years. Monitoring of menstrual functioning. Referral to GYN if requested.

Surveillance needed for potential recurrence of cancer:
History and physical examination every 3 months × 1 year; every 4 months × 1 year; every 6 months × 1 year;: annually thereafter. Appropriate laboratory and imaging studies if symptomatic.

Surveillance needed for second malignancies:
Annual mammograms, beginning 2010; breast self-exam, monthly; breast exam by all follow-up physicians (primary care provider, medical oncologist, radiation oncologist).
Skin assessment annually.
Thyroid exam annually.
Laboratory and imaging studies according to National Comprehensive Cancer Network guidelines for the follow-up of Hodgkin's disease.

Physicians responsible for monitoring of toxicity, recurrence, second malignancies:
Primary care provider: Assess for general medical issues, weight, exercise, diet, annual influenza vaccination.
Medical oncologist: Assess for fertility, infections, cardiopulmonary function, surveillance imaging exams. Visits alternated with radiation oncologist.
Radiation oncologist: Assess for thyroid function, second malignancy, surveillance imaging exams. Visits alternated with medical oncologist.

Identified psychosocial issues or concerns:
None identified, but needs evaluation and consultation as appropriate if specific issues arise. Patient has no children and desires them in the future. Although her therapy is not known to cause fertility problems, counseling was provided on fertility and reproduction.

Recommended preventive behaviors, interventions, or genetic testing:
Patient was counseled regarding diet and exercise for cardiovascular health, and avoidance of sun exposure to minimize risk of skin cancer. Annual flu vaccination is recommended. Recommend psychosocial assessment at follow-up. Patient given NCI booklet, *Life After Cancer Treatment*, and the NCCS "Cancer Survival Toolbox: An Audio Resource Program" that address medical and psychosocial issues, including those related to health insurance and employment.

NOTE: All individual and hospital names are fictitious.
SOURCE: Sarah Donaldson, committee member, 2005.

REFERENCES

AACE (American Association of Clinical Endocrinologists). 1999. AACE medical guidelines for clinical practice for management of menopause. *Endocrine Practice* 5(6):354–366.

ACS (American Cancer Society). 2000. *Guide to Complementary and Alternative Cancer Methods.* Atlanta, GA: ACS.

ACS. 2004a. *Eating Well, Staying Well During and After Cancer.* Atlanta, GA: ACS.

ACS. 2004b. *Sexuality for Women and Their Partners.* [Online]. Available: http://www.cancer.org/docroot/MIT/MIT_7_1x_SexualityforWomenandTheirPartners.asp [accessed September 30, 2004].

Ahles TA, Saykin AJ. 2002. Breast cancer chemotherapy-related cognitive dysfunction. *Clin Breast Cancer* 3(Suppl 3):S84–S90.

Ahles TA, Saykin AJ, Noll WW, Furstenberg CT, Guerin S, Cole B, Mott LA. 2003. The relationship of APOE genotype to neuropsychological performance in long-term cancer survivors treated with standard dose chemotherapy. *Psychooncology* 12(6):612–619.

Ahles TA, Saykin AJ, Furstenberg CT, Cole B, Mott LA, Titus-Ernstoff L, Skalla K, Bakitas M, Silberfarb PM. 2005. Quality of life of long-term survivors of breast cancer and lymphoma treated with standard-dose chemotherapy or local therapy. *J Clin Oncol* 23(19):4399-4405.

AHRQ (Agency for Healthcare Research and Quality). 1998. *Invitation to Submit Guidelines to the National Guideline Clearinghouse.* [Online]. Available: http://www.ahrq.gov/fund/ngcguidl.htm [accessed April 19, 2005].

AHRQ. 2002. *Management of Cancer Symptoms: Pain, Depression, and Fatigue. Summary, Evidence Report/Technology Assessment: Number 61.* AHRQ Publication No. 02-E031. [Online]. Available: http://www.ahrq.gov/clinic/epcsums/csympsum.htm [accessed December 21, 2004].

AHRQ. 2004a. *Evidence-based Practice Centers.* [Online]. Available: http://www.ahrq.gov/clinic/epc/ [accessed October 18, 2004].

AHRQ. 2004b. *National Guideline Clearinghouse.* [Online]. Available: http://www.guideline.gov [accessed December 6, 2004].

AICR (American Institute for Cancer Research). 2004. *Nutrition Guidelines for Cancer Survivors After Treatment.* [Online]. Available: http://www.aicr.org/information/survivor/guidelines.lasso [accessed December 8, 2004].

Aisner J, Wiernik PH, Pearl P. 1993. Pregnancy outcome in patients treated for Hodgkin's disease. *J Clin Oncol* 11(3):507–512.

Amato P, Christophe S, Mellon PL. 2002. Estrogenic activity of herbs commonly used as remedies for menopausal symptoms. *Menopause* 9(2):145–150.

American Psychiatric Association. 1994. *Diagnostic and Statistical Manual of Mental Disorders.* 4th ed. Washington, DC: American Psychiatric Association.

Amling CL, Riffenburgh RH, Sun L, Moul JW, Lance RS, Kusuda L, Sexton WJ, Soderdahl DW, Donahue TF, Foley JP, Chung AK, McLeod DG. 2004. Pathologic variables and recurrence rates as related to obesity and race in men with prostate cancer undergoing radical prostatectomy. *J Clin Oncol* 22(3):439–445.

Andersen BL, Farrar WB, Golden-Kreutz DM, Glaser R, Emery CF, Crespin TR, Shapiro CL, Carson WE III. 2004. Psychological, behavioral, and immune changes after a psychological intervention: A clinical trial. *J Clin Oncol* 22(17):3570–3580.

Anthony T, Simmang C, Hyman N, Buie D, Kim D, Cataldo P, Orsay C, Church J, Otchy D, Cohen J, Perry WB, Dunn G, Rafferty J, Ellis CN, Rakinic J, Fleshner P, Stahl T, Gregorcyk S, Ternent C, Kilkenny JW III, Whiteford M. 2004. Practice parameters for the surveillance and follow-up of patients with colon and rectal cancer. *Dis Colon Rectum* 47(6):807–817.

Antman K, Benson MC, Chabot J, Cobrinik D, Grann VR, Jacobson JS, Joe AK, Katz AE, Kelly K, Neugut AI, Russo D, Tiersten A, Weinstein IB. 2001. Complementary and alternative medicine: The role of the cancer center. *J Clin Oncol* 19(18 Suppl):55S–60S.

Antoniou A, Pharoah PD, Narod S, Risch HA, Eyfjord JE, Hopper JL, Loman N, Olsson H, Johannsson O, Borg A, Pasini B, Radice P, Manoukian S, Eccles DM, Tang N, Olah E, Anton-Culver H, Warner E, Lubinski J, Gronwald J, Gorski B, Tulinius H, Thorlacius S, Eerola H, Nevanlinna H, Syrjakoski K, Kallioniemi OP, Thompson D, Evans C, Peto J, Lalloo F, Evans DG, Easton DF. 2003. Average risks of breast and ovarian cancer associated with BRCA1 or BRCA2 mutations detected in case series unselected for family history: A combined analysis of 22 studies. *Am J Hum Genet* 72(5):1117–1130.

Arterbery VE, Frazier A, Dalmia P, Siefer J, Lutz M, Porter A. 1997. Quality of life after permanent prostate implant. *Semin Surg Oncol* 13(6):461–464.

ASCO (American Society of Clinical Oncology). 2003. American Society of Clinical Oncology policy statement update: Genetic testing for cancer susceptibility. *J Clin Oncol* 21(12):2397–2406.

Ashing-Giwa K, Ganz PA, Petersen L. 1999. Quality of life of African-American and white long term breast carcinoma survivors. *Cancer* 85(2):418–426.

Avis N, Crawford S, Manuel J. 2005. Quality of life among younger women with breast cancer. *J Clin Oncol* 23(15):3322-3330.

Aziz NM, Rowland JH. 2003. Trends and advances in cancer survivorship research: Challenge and opportunity. *Semin Radiat Oncol* 13(3):248–266.

Bacon CG, Giovannucci E, Testa M, Glass TA, Kawachi I. 2002. The association of treatment-related symptoms with quality-of-life outcomes for localized prostate carcinoma patients. *Cancer* 94(3):862–871.

Badger C, Preston N, Seers K, Mortimer P. 2004a. Benzo-pyrones for reducing and controlling lymphoedema of the limbs. *Cochrane Database Syst Rev* (2):CD003140.

Badger C, Preston N, Seers K, Mortimer P. 2004b. Physical therapies for reducing and controlling lymphoedema of the limbs. *Cochrane Database Syst Rev* (4):CD003141.

Badger C, Seers K, Preston N, Mortimer P. 2004c. Antibiotics/anti-inflammatories for reducing acute inflammatory episodes in lymphoedema of the limbs. *Cochrane Database Syst Rev* (2):CD003143.

Baniel J, Israilov S, Segenreich E, Livne PM. 2001. Comparative evaluation of treatments for erectile dysfunction in patients with prostate cancer after radical retropubic prostatectomy. *BJU Int* 88(1):58–62.

Barnes PM, Powell-Griner E, McFann K, Nahin RL. 2004. Complementary and alternative medicine use among adults: United States, 2002. *Adv Data* (343):1–19.

Bast RC Jr, Ravdin P, Hayes DF, Bates S, Fritsche H Jr, Jessup JM, Kemeny N, Locker GY, Mennel RG, Somerfield MR. 2001. 2000 update of recommendations for the use of tumor markers in breast and colorectal cancer: Clinical practice guidelines of the American Society of Clinical Oncology. *J Clin Oncol* 19(6):1865–1878.

Baxter NN, Tepper JE, Durham SB, Rothenberger DA, Virnig BA. 2005. Increased risk of rectal cancer after prostate radiation: A population-based study. *Gastroenterology* 128(4):819–824.

Benson AB III, Desch CE, Flynn PJ, Krause C, Loprinzi CL, Minsky BD, Petrelli NJ, Pfister DG, Smith TJ, Somerfield MR. 2000. 2000 update of American Society of Clinical Oncology colorectal cancer surveillance guidelines. *J Clin Oncol* 18(20):3586–3588.

Bethge W, Guggenberger D, Bamberg M, Kanz L, Bokemeyer C. 2000. Thyroid toxicity of treatment for Hodgkin's disease. *Ann Hematol* 79(3):114–118.

Blamey RW. 2002. Guidelines on endocrine therapy of breast cancer EUSOMA. *Eur J Cancer* 38(5):615–634.

Blanchard CM, Denniston MM, Baker F, Ainsworth SR, Courneya KS, Hann DM, Gesme DH, Reding D, Flynn T, Kennedy JS. 2003a. Do adults change their lifestyle behaviors after a cancer diagnosis? *Am J Health Behav* 27(3):246–256.

Blanchard DK, Donohue JH, Reynolds C, Grant CS. 2003b. Relapse and morbidity in patients undergoing sentinel lymph node biopsy alone or with axillary dissection for breast cancer. *Arch Surg* 138(5):482–487; discussion 487–488.

Blank TO. 2005. Gay men and prostate cancer: Invisible diversity. *J Clin Oncol* 23(12):2593–2596.

Bloom JR, Fobair P, Gritz E, Wellisch D, Spiegel D, Varghese A, Hoppe R. 1993. Psychosocial outcomes of cancer: A comparative analysis of Hodgkin's disease and testicular cancer. *J Clin Oncol* 11(5):979–988.

Bloom JR, Stewart SL, Chang S, Banks PJ. 2004. Then and now: Quality of life of young breast cancer survivors. *Psychooncology* 13(3):147–160.

Bower JE, Ganz PA, Desmond KA, Rowland JH, Meyerowitz BE, Belin TR. 2000. Fatigue in breast cancer survivors: Occurrence, correlates, and impact on quality of life. *J Clin Oncol* 18(4):743–753.

Bradbury BD, Lash TL, Kaye JA, Jick SS. 2004. Tamoxifen and cataracts: A null association. *Breast Cancer Res Treat* 87(2):189–196.

Bradbury BD, Lash TL, Kaye JA, Jick SS. 2005. Tamoxifen-treated breast carcinoma patients and the risk of acute myocardial infarction and newly-diagnosed angina. *Cancer* 103(6):1114–1121.

Brennan J. 2001. Adjustment to cancer—coping or personal transition? *Psychooncology* 10(1):1–18.

Brezden CB, Phillips KA, Abdolell M, Bunston T, Tannock IF. 2000. Cognitive function in breast cancer patients receiving adjuvant chemotherapy. *J Clin Oncol* 18(14):2695–2701.

British Columbia Cancer Agency. 2002a. *Gastrointestinal—05 Colon*. [Online]. Available: http://www.bccancer.bc.ca/HPI/CancerManagementGuidelines/Gastrointestinal/05.Colon/default.htm [accessed March 16, 2004].

British Columbia Cancer Agency. 2002b. *Hodgkin's Lymphoma*. [Online]. Available: http://www.bccancer.bc.ca/HPI/CancerManagementGuidelines/Lymphoma/HodgkinsDisease.htm [accessed March 16, 2004].

British Columbia Cancer Agency. 2004a. *Breast*. [Online]. Available: http://www. bccancer.bc.ca/HPI/CancerManagementGuidelines/Breast/Followup/default.htm [accessed March 16, 2004].

British Columbia Cancer Agency. 2004b. *Genitourinary—Prostate*. [Online]. Available: http://www.bccancer.bc.ca/HPI/CancerManagementGuidelines/Genitourinary/Prostate/default.htm [accessed March 16, 2004].

British Columbia Guidelines and Protocols Advisory Committee. 2004. *Follow-up of Patients after Curative Resection of Colorectal Cancer*. [Online]. Available: http://www.healthservices.gov.bc.ca/msp/protoguides/gps/colorectal.pdf [accessed December 6, 2004].

Brown JK, Byers T, Doyle C, Courneya KS, Demark-Wahnefried W, Kushi LH, McTiernan A, Rock CL, Aziz N, Bloch AS, Eldridge B, Hamilton K, Katzin C, Koonce A, Main J, Mobley C, Morra ME, Pierce MS, Sawyer KA. 2003. Nutrition and physical activity during and after cancer treatment: An American Cancer Society guide for informed choices. *CA Cancer J Clin* 53(5):268–291.

Burstein HJ. 2000. Discussing complementary therapies with cancer patients: What should we be talking about? *J Clin Oncol* 18(13):2501–2504.

Burstein HJ, Winer EP. 2000. Primary care for survivors of breast cancer. *N Engl J Med* 343(15):1086–1094.

Burstein HJ, Gelber S, Guadagnoli E, Weeks JC. 1999. Use of alternative medicine by women with early-stage breast cancer. *N Engl J Med* 340(22):1733–1739.

Bushnell CD, Goldstein LB. 2004. Risk of ischemic stroke with tamoxifen treatment for breast cancer: A meta-analysis. *Neurology* 63(7):1230–1233.

Calvert PM, Frucht H. 2002. The genetics of colorectal cancer. *Ann Intern Med* 137(7):603–612.

Campos SM. 2004. Aromatase inhibitors for breast cancer in postmenopausal women. *Oncologist* 9(2):126–136.

Canales MK, Geller BM. 2003. Surviving breast cancer: The role of complementary therapies. *Fam Community Health* 26(1):11–24.

Cancer Care Ontario. 2005. *Supportive Care Practice Guidelines.* [Online]. Available: http://www.cancercare.on.ca/index_supportiveCareguidelines.htm [accessed May 9, 2005].

Carmichael AR, Bates T. 2004. Obesity and breast cancer: A review of the literature. *Breast* 13(2):85–92.

Carter CL, Key J, Marsh L, Graves K. 2001. Contemporary perspectives in tobacco cessation: What oncologists need to know. *Oncologist* 6(6):496–505.

Casso D, Buist DS, Taplin S. 2004. Quality of life of 5–10 year breast cancer survivors diagnosed between age 40 and 49. *Health Qual Life Outcomes* 2(1):25.

Cella DF. 1995. Methods and problems in measuring quality of life. *Support Care Cancer* 3(1):11–22.

Cella DF, Tross S. 1986. Psychological adjustment to survival from Hodgkin's disease. *J Consult Clin Psychol* 54(5):616–622.

Chen Z, Maricic M, Bassford TL, Pettinger M, Ritenbaugh C, Lopez AM, Barad DH, Gass M, Leboff MS. 2005. Fracture risk among breast cancer survivors: Results from the Women's Health Initiative Observational Study. *Arch Intern Med* 165(5):552–558.

Children's Oncology Group. 2005. *Long-Term Follow-Up Guidelines for Survivors of Childhood, Adolescent, and Young Adult Cancers.* [Online] Available: http://www.survivorshipguidelines.org/ [accessed July 15, 2005).

Chlebowski RT. 2005a. Obesity and early-stage breast cancer. *J Clin Oncol* 23(7):1345–1347.

Chlebowski RT. 2005b. Bone health in women with early-stage breast cancer. *Clin Breast Cancer* 5(Suppl 2):S35–S40.

Chlebowski RT, Aiello E, McTiernan A. 2002a. Weight loss in breast cancer patient management. *J Clin Oncol* 20(4):1128–1143.

Chlebowski RT, Blackburn GL, Elashoff RE, Thomson C, Goodman MT, Shapiro A, Giuliano AE, Karanja N, Hoy MK, Nixon DW. 2005 (May 13–17). *Dietary fat reduction in postmenopausal women with primary breast cancer: Phase III Women's Intervention Nutrition Study (WINS). Presentation at the ASCO Annual Meeting, Orlando, FL.* [Online]. Available: http://www.asco.org/ac/1,1003,_12-002643-00_18-0034-00_19-0031414,00.asp [accessed May 20, 2005].

Chlebowski RT, Col N, Winer EP, Collyar DE, Cummings SR, Vogel VG III, Burstein HJ, Eisen A, Lipkus I, Pfister DG. 2002b. American Society of Clinical Oncology technology assessment of pharmacologic interventions for breast cancer risk reduction including tamoxifen, raloxifene, and aromatase inhibition. *J Clin Oncol* 20(15):3328–3343.

Chlebowski RT, Kim JA, Col NF. 2003. Estrogen deficiency symptom management in breast cancer survivors in the changing context of menopausal hormone therapy. *Semin Oncol* 30(6):776–788.

Chun TY. 1997. Coincidence of bladder and prostate cancer. *J Urol* 157(1):65–67.

Church J, Simmang C. 2003. Practice parameters for the treatment of patients with dominantly inherited colorectal cancer (familial adenomatous polyposis and hereditary nonpolyposis colorectal cancer). *Dis Colon Rectum* 46(8):1001–1012.

Citron ML, Berry DA, Cirrincione C, Hudis C, Winer EP, Gradishar WJ, Davidson NE, Martino S, Livingston R, Ingle JN, Perez EA, Carpenter J, Hurd D, Holland JF, Smith BL, Sartor CI, Leung EH, Abrams J, Schilsky RL, Muss HB, Norton L. 2003. Randomized trial of dose-dense versus conventionally scheduled and sequential versus concurrent combination chemotherapy as postoperative adjuvant treatment of node-positive primary breast cancer: First report of Intergroup Trial C9741/Cancer and Leukemia Group B Trial 9741. *J Clin Oncol* 21(8):1431–1439.

City of Hope Beckman Research Institute. 2004. *Quality of Life*. [Online]. Available: http://www.cityofhope.org/prc/pdf/cancer_survivor_QOL.pdf [accessed September 7, 2004].

Clark JA, Inui TS, Silliman RA, Bokhour BG, Krasnow SH, Robinson RA, Spaulding M, Talcott JA. 2003. Patients' perceptions of quality of life after treatment for early prostate cancer. *J Clin Oncol* 21(20):3777–3784.

CMS (Centers for Medicare and Medicaid Services). 2005. *Medicare Adds Coverage of Smoking and Other Tobacco Use Cessation Services*. [Online]. Available: http://www.cms.hhs.gov/media/press/release.asp?Counter=1395 [accessed March 29, 2005].

Cooperberg MR, Broering JM, Litwin MS, Lubeck DP, Mehta SS, Henning JM, Carroll PR. 2004. The contemporary management of prostate cancer in the United States: Lessons from the Cancer of the Prostate Strategic Urologic Research Endeavor (CaPSURE), a national disease registry. *J Urol* 171(4):1393–1401.

Cordova MJ, Cunningham LL, Carlson CR, Andrykowski MA. 2001. Post-traumatic growth following breast cancer: A controlled comparison study. *Health Psychol* 20(3):176–185.

Courneya KS, Friedenreich CM. 2001. Framework PEACE: An organizational model for examining physical exercise across the cancer experience. *Ann Behav Med* 23(4):263–272.

Courneya KS, Friedenreich CM, Quinney HA, Fields AL, Jones LW, Fairey AS. 2003a. A randomized trial of exercise and quality of life in colorectal cancer survivors. *Eur J Cancer Care (Engl)* 12(4):347–357.

Courneya KS, Mackey JR, Bell GJ, Jones LW, Field CJ, Fairey AS. 2003b. Randomized controlled trial of exercise training in postmenopausal breast cancer survivors: Cardiopulmonary and quality of life outcomes. *J Clin Oncol* 21(9):1660–1668.

Cox LS, Africano NL, Tercyak KP, Taylor KL. 2003. Nicotine dependence treatment for patients with cancer. *Cancer* 98(3):632–644.

Crandall C, Petersen L, Ganz PA, Greendale GA. 2004. Association of breast cancer and its therapy with menopause-related symptoms. *Menopause* 11(5):519–530.

Cuzick J. 2005. Radiotherapy for breast cancer. *J Natl Cancer Inst* 97(6):406–407.

Day R, Ganz PA, Costantino JP. 2001. Tamoxifen and depression: More evidence from the National Surgical Adjuvant Breast and Bowel Project's Breast Cancer Prevention (P-1) Randomized Study. *J Natl Cancer Inst* 93(21):1615–1623.

Day R, Ganz PA, Costantino JP, Cronin WM, Wickerham DL, Fisher B. 1999. Health-related quality of life and tamoxifen in breast cancer prevention: A report from the National Surgical Adjuvant Breast and Bowel Project P-1 Study. *J Clin Oncol* 17(9):2659–2669.

de Jong, N, Courtens AM, Abu-Saad HH, and Schouten HC. 2002. Fatigue in patients with breast cancer receiving adjuvant chemotherapy: A review of the literature. *Cancer Nurs.* 25(4):283–297; quiz 298–299.

Demark-Wahnefried W, Rock CL. 2003. Nutrition-related issues for the breast cancer survivor. *Semin Oncol* 30(6):789–798.

Demark-Wahnefried W, Aziz NM, Rowland JH, and Pinto BM. 2005. Riding the crest of the teachable moment: Promoting long-term health after the diagnosis of cancer. *J Clin Oncol* 23(24):1–17.

Demark-Wahnefried W, Peterson B, McBride C, Lipkus I, Clipp E. 2000. Current health behaviors and readiness to pursue life-style changes among men and women diagnosed with early stage prostate and breast carcinomas. *Cancer* 88(3):674–684.

DiGianni LM, Garber JE, Winer EP. 2002. Complementary and alternative medicine use among women with breast cancer. *J Clin Oncol* 20(18 Suppl):34S–38S.

Dignam JJ, Mamounas EP. 2004. Obesity and breast cancer prognosis: An expanding body of evidence. *Ann Oncol* 15(6):850–851.

Djuric Z, DiLaura NM, Jenkins I, Darga L, Jen CK, Mood D, Bradley E, Hryniuk WM. 2002. Combining weight-loss counseling with the Weight Watchers plan for obese breast cancer survivors. *Obes Res* 10(7):657–665.

Donaldson SS, Hancock SL, Hoppe RT. 1999. The Janeway Lecture. Hodgkin's disease—finding the balance between cure and late effects. *Cancer J Sci Am* 5(6):325–333.

Donnez J, Dolmans MM, Demylle D, Jadoul P, Pirard C, Squifflet J, Martinez-Madrid B, Van Langendonckt A. 2004. Live birth after orthotopic transplantation of cryopreserved ovarian tissue. *Lancet* 364(9443):1405–1410.

Dores GM, Metayer C, Curtis RE, Lynch CF, Clarke EA, Glimelius B, Storm H, Pukkala E, van Leeuwen FE, Holowaty EJ, Andersson M, Wiklund T, Joensuu T, van't Veer MB, Stovall M, Gospodarowicz M, Travis LB. 2002. Second malignant neoplasms among long-term survivors of Hodgkin's disease: A population-based evaluation over 25 years. *J Clin Oncol* 20(16):3484–3494.

Dorval M, Guay S, Mondor M, Mâsse B, Falardeau M, Robidoux A, Deschênes L, Maunsell E. 2005. Couples who get closer after breast cancer: Frequency and predictors in a prospective investigation. *J Clin Oncol* 23(15):3588-3596.

Dorval M, Maunsell E, Deschenes L, Brisson J. 1998. Type of mastectomy and quality of life for long-term breast carcinoma survivors. *Cancer* 83(10):2130–2138.

Dow KH, Ferrell BR, Leigh S, Ly J, Gulasekaram P. 1996. An evaluation of the quality of life among long-term survivors of breast cancer. *Breast Cancer Res Treat* 39(3):261–273.

Dresler CM. 2003. Is it more important to quit smoking than which chemotherapy is used? *Lung Cancer* 39(2):119–124.

Dunlop MG. 2002. Guidance on gastrointestinal surveillance for hereditary non-polyposis colorectal cancer, familial adenomatous polyposis, juvenile polyposis, and Peutz-Jeghers syndrome. *Gut* 51(Suppl 5):V21–V27.

Early Breast Cancer Trialists' Collaborative Group. 2004a. Multi-agent chemotherapy for early breast cancer (Cochrane Review). In: *The Cochrane Library.* Issue 3. Chichester, UK: John Wiley & Sons, Ltd.

Early Breast Cancer Trialists' Collaborative Group. 2004b. Tamoxifen for early breast cancer (Cochrane Review). In: *The Cochrane Library.* Issue 3. Chichester, UK: John Wiley & Sons, Ltd.

Easton DF, Hopper JL, Thomas DC, Antoniou A, Pharoah PD, Whittemore AS, Haile RW. 2004. Breast cancer risks for BRCA1/2 carriers. *Science* 306(5705):2187–2191; author reply 2187–2191.

Elston Lafata J, Simpkins J, Schultz L, Chase GA, Johnson CC, Yood MU, Lamerato L, Nathanson D, Cooper G. 2005. Routine surveillance care after cancer treatment with curative intent. *Med Care* 43(6):592-599.

Emens LA, Davidson NE. 2003. The follow-up of breast cancer. *Semin Oncol* 30(3):338–348.

Erickson VS, Pearson ML, Ganz PA, Adams J, Kahn KL. 2001. Arm edema in breast cancer patients. *J Natl Cancer Inst* 93(2):96–111.

ESMO (European Society of Medical Oncology). 2003. *Minimum Clinical Recommendations for Diagnosis, Adjuvant Treatment and Follow-up of Primary Breast Cancer.* [Online]. Available: http://www.esmo.org/reference/referenceGuidelines/pdf/new_pdf/ESMO_01_primary_breast.pdf [accessed December 13, 2004].

Eton DT, Lepore SJ. 2002. Prostate cancer and health-related quality of life: A review of the literature. *Psychooncology* 11(4):307–326.

Eton DT, Lepore SJ, Helgeson VS. 2001. Early quality of life in patients with localized prostate carcinoma: An examination of treatment-related, demographic, and psychosocial factors. *Cancer* 92(6):1451–1459.

Evans HS, Moller H, Robinson D, Lewis CM, Bell CM, Hodgson SV. 2002. The risk of subsequent primary cancers after colorectal cancer in southeast England. *Gut* 50(5):647–652.

Ewer MS, Lippman SM. 2005. Type II chemotherapy-related cardiac dysfunction: Time to recognize a new entity. *J Clin Oncol* 23(13):2900–2902.

FACS. 2005. *FACS Trial.* [Online]. Available: http://www.facs.soton.ac.uk/ [accessed April 19, 2005].

Fallowfield L, Fleissig A, Edwards R, West A, Powles TJ, Howell A, Cuzick J. 2001. Tamoxifen for the prevention of breast cancer: Psychosocial impact on women participating in two randomized controlled trials. *J Clin Oncol* 19(7):1885–1892.

Ferrans CE. 2005. Definitions and conceptual models of quality of life. In: *Outcomes Assessment in Cancer: Measures, Methods, and Applications.* Cambridge, UK: Cambridge University Press. Pp. 14–30.

Ferrell BR. 2004 (October 27–29). *Quality of Life Issues: Cancer Patients' Perspectives.* Presentation at the meeting of the IOM Committee on Cancer Survivorship Meeting, Irvine, CA.

Ferrell BR, Grant M, Funk B, Otis-Green S, Garcia N. 1997a. Quality of life in breast cancer. Part I: Physical and social well-being. *Cancer Nurs* 20(6):398–408.

Ferrell BR, Grant MM, Funk B, Otis-Green S, Garcia N. 1997b. Quality of life in breast cancer survivors as identified by focus groups. *Psychooncology* 6(1):13–23.

Ferrell BR, Grant M, Funk B, Otis-Green S, Garcia N. 1998. Quality of life in breast cancer. Part II: Psychological and spiritual well-being. *Cancer Nurs* 21(1):1–9.

Figueredo A, Rumble RB, Maroun J, Earle CC, Cummings B, McLeod R, Zuraw L, Zwaal C. 2003. Follow-up of patients with curatively resected colorectal cancer: A practice guideline. *BMC Cancer* 3(1):26.

Finnish Medical Society Duodecim. 2001. *Postoperative Follow-up of Colorectal Cancer.* [Online]. Available: http://195.236.0.10/ltk-root/eng/htm/ebm/ebm00199.htm [accessed June 2, 2004].

Finnish Medical Society Duodecim. 2002. *Carcinoma of the Prostate.* [Online]. Available: http://195.236.0.10/ltk-root/eng/htm/ebm/ebm00247.htm [accessed June 2, 2004].

Fiorica J. 2004. Association of breast cancer and its therapy with menopause-related symptoms. *Menopause* 11(5):502–504.

Fisher B, Anderson S, Bryant J, Margolese RG, Deutsch M, Fisher ER, Jeong JH, Wolmark N. 2002. Twenty-year follow-up of a randomized trial comparing total mastectomy, lumpectomy, and lumpectomy plus irradiation for the treatment of invasive breast cancer. *N Engl J Med* 347(16):1233–1241.

Fisher B, Anderson S, DeCillis A, Dimitrov N, Atkins JN, Fehrenbacher L, Henry PH, Romond EH, Lanier KS, Davila E, Kardinal CG, Laufman L, Pierce HI, Abramson N, Keller AM, Hamm JT, Wickerham DL, Begovic M, Tan-Chiu E, Tian W, Wolmark N. 1999. Further evaluation of intensified and increased total dose of cyclophosphamide for the treatment of primary breast cancer: Findings from National Surgical Adjuvant Breast and Bowel Project B-25. *J Clin Oncol* 17(11):3374–3388.

Flechtner H, Bottomley A. 2003. Fatigue and quality of life: Lessons from the real world. *Oncologist* 8(Suppl 1):5–9.

Fobair P, Hoppe RT, Bloom J, Cox R, Varghese A, Spiegel D. 1986. Psychosocial problems among survivors of Hodgkin's disease. *J Clin Oncol* 4(5):805–814.

Ford D, Easton DF, Stratton M, Narod S, Goldgar D, Devilee P, Bishop DT, Weber B, Lenoir G, Chang-Claude J, Sobol H, Teare MD, Struewing J, Arason A, Scherneck S, Peto J, Rebbeck TR, Tonin P, Neuhausen S, Barkardottir R, Eyfjord J, Lynch H, Ponder BA, Gayther SA, Zelada-Hedman M, et al. 1998. Genetic heterogeneity and penetrance analysis of the BRCA1 and BRCA2 genes in breast cancer families. The Breast Cancer Linkage Consortium. *Am J Hum Genet* 62(3):676–689.

Fransson P, Widmark A. 1999. Late side effects unchanged 4–8 years after radiotherapy for prostate carcinoma: A comparison with age-matched controls. *Cancer* 85(3):678–688.

Freedland SJ, Aronson WJ, Kane CJ, Presti JC Jr, Amling CL, Elashoff D, Terris MK. 2004. Impact of obesity on biochemical control after radical prostatectomy for clinically localized prostate cancer: A report by the Shared Equal Access Regional Cancer Hospital database study group. *J Clin Oncol* 22(3):446–453.

Friedlander M, Thewes B. 2003. Counting the costs of treatment: The reproductive and gynaecological consequences of adjuvant therapy in young women with breast cancer. *Intern Med J* 33(8):372–379.

Gallo-Silver L. 2000. The sexual rehabilitation of persons with cancer. *Cancer Pract* 8(1): 10–15.

Galvao DA, Newton RU. 2005. Review of exercise intervention studies in cancer patients. *J Clin Oncol* 23(4):899–909.

Ganz PA. 1998. Cognitive dysfunction following adjuvant treatment of breast cancer: A new dose-limiting toxic effect? *J Natl Cancer Inst* 90(3):182–183.

Ganz PA. 2000. Quality of life across the continuum of breast cancer care. *Breast J* 6(5):324–330.

Ganz PA. 2001a. Impact of tamoxifen adjuvant therapy on symptoms, functioning, and quality of life. *J Natl Cancer Inst Monogr* 30:130–134.

Ganz PA. 2001b. Menopause and breast cancer: Symptoms, late effects, and their management. *Semin Oncol* 28(3):274–283.

Ganz PA. 2002a. What outcomes matter to patients: A physician-researcher point of view. *Med Care* 40(6 Suppl):III11–19.

Ganz PA. 2002b. The price of anticancer intervention. Treatment-induced malignancy. *Lancet Oncol* 3(9):575–576.

Ganz PA. 2002c. *Adult Cancer Survivors: Understanding the Late Effects of Cancer and Its Treatment.* Paper commissioned for the National Cancer Policy Board. Unpublished.

Ganz PA. 2004 (July 27). *Understanding the Late Effects of Cancer Treatment: Making the Case for Systematic Follow-up.* Presentation at the meeting of the IOM Committee on Cancer Survivorship, Woods Hole, MA.

Ganz PA. 2005. A teachable moment for oncologists: Cancer survivors, 10 million strong and growing! *J Clin Oncol* 23(24):1–3.

Ganz PA, Coscarelli A, Fred C, Kahn B, Polinsky ML, Petersen L. 1996. Breast cancer survivors: Psychosocial concerns and quality of life. *Breast Cancer Res Treat* 38(2):183–199.

Ganz PA, Desmond KA, Belin TR, Meyerowitz BE, Rowland JH. 1999. Predictors of sexual health in women after a breast cancer diagnosis. *J Clin Oncol* 17(8):2371–2380.

Ganz PA, Desmond KA, Leedham B, Rowland JH, Meyerowitz BE, Belin TR. 2002. Quality of life in long-term, disease-free survivors of breast cancer: A follow-up study. *J Natl Cancer Inst* 94(1):39–49.

Ganz PA, Greendale GA, Petersen L, Kahn B, Bower JE. 2003a. Breast cancer in younger women: Reproductive and late health effects of treatment. *J Clin Oncol* 21(22):4184–4193.

Ganz PA, Greendale GA, Petersen L, Zibecchi L, Kahn B, Belin TR. 2000. Managing menopausal symptoms in breast cancer survivors: Results of a randomized controlled trial. *J Natl Cancer Inst* 92(13):1054–1064.

Ganz PA, Guadagnoli E, Landrum MB, Lash TL, Rakowski W, Silliman RA. 2003b. Breast cancer in older women: Quality of life and psychosocial adjustment in the 15 months after diagnosis. *J Clin Oncol* 21(21):4027–4033.

Ganz PA, Hirji K, Sim MS, Schag CA, Fred C, Polinsky ML. 1993. Predicting psychosocial risk in patients with breast cancer. *Med Care* 31(5):419–431.

Ganz PA, Kwan L, Stanton AL, Krupnick JL, Rowland JH, Meyerowitz BE, Bower JE, Belin TR. 2004a. Quality of life at the end of primary treatment of breast cancer: First results from the moving beyond cancer randomized trial. *J Natl Cancer Inst* 96(5):376–387.

Ganz PA, Lee JJ, Sim MS, Polinsky ML, Schag CA. 1992. Exploring the influence of multiple variables on the relationship of age to quality of life in women with breast cancer. *J Clin Epidemiol* 45(5):473–485.

Ganz PA, Moinpour CM, McCoy S, Pauler DK, Press OW, Fisher RI. 2004b. Predictors of vitality (energy/fatigue) in early stage Hodgkin's disease (HD): Results from Southwest Oncology Group (SWOG) Study 9133. *J Clin Oncol* 22(14S):569S.

Ganz PA, Moinpour CM, Pauler DK, Kornblith AB, Gaynor ER, Balcerzak SP, Gatti GS, Erba HP, McCoy S, Press OW, Fisher RI. 2003c. Health status and quality of life in patients with early-stage Hodgkin's disease treated on Southwest Oncology Group Study 9133. *J Clin Oncol* 21(18):3512–3519.

Ganz PA, Rowland JH, Desmond K, Meyerowitz BE, Wyatt GE. 1998a. Life after breast cancer: Understanding women's health-related quality of life and sexual functioning. *J Clin Oncol* 16(2):501–514.

Ganz PA, Rowland JH, Meyerowitz BE, Desmond KA. 1998b. Impact of different adjuvant therapy strategies on quality of life in breast cancer survivors. *Recent Results Cancer Res* 152:396–411.

Garces YI, Hays JT. 2003. Tobacco dependence: Why should an oncologist care? *J Clin Oncol* 21(9):1884–1886.

Giedzinska AS, Meyerowitz BE, Ganz PA, Rowland JH. 2004. Health-related quality of life in a multiethnic sample of breast cancer survivors. *Ann Behav Med* 28(1):39–51.

Giordano SH, Kuo YF, Freeman JL, Buchholz TA, Hortobagyi GN, Goodwin JS. 2005. Risk of cardiac death after adjuvant radiotherapy for breast cancer. *J Natl Cancer Inst* 97(6):419–424.

GIVIO. 1994. Impact of follow-up testing on survival and health-related quality of life in breast cancer patients. A multicenter randomized controlled trial. The GIVIO Investigators. *JAMA* 271(20):1587–1592.

Goodwin P, Esplen MJ, Butler K, Winocur J, Pritchard K, Brazel S, Gao J, Miller A. 1998. Multidisciplinary weight management in locoregional breast cancer: Results of a Phase II study. *Breast Cancer Res Treat* 48(1):53–64.

Goodwin PJ, Ennis M, Pritchard KI, McCready D, Koo J, Sidlofsky S, Trudeau M, Hood N, Redwood S. 1999a. Adjuvant treatment and onset of menopause predict weight gain after breast cancer diagnosis. *J Clin Oncol* 17(1):120–129.

Goodwin PJ, Ennis M, Pritchard KI, Trudeau M, Hood N. 1999b. Risk of menopause during the first year after breast cancer diagnosis. *J Clin Oncol* 17(8):2365–2370.

Gore JL, Krupski T, Kwan L, Maliski S, Litwin MS. 2005. Partnership status influences quality of life in low-income, uninsured men with prostate cancer. *Cancer* 104 (1): 191–198.

Grady WM, Russell K. 2005. Ionizing radiation and rectal cancer: Victims of our own success. *Gastroenterology* 128(4):1114–1117.

Green HJ, Pakenham KI, Headley BC, Yaxley J, Nicol DL, Mactaggart PN, Swanson C, Watson RB, Gardiner RA. 2002a. Altered cognitive function in men treated for prostate cancer with luteinizing hormone-releasing hormone analogues and cyproterone acetate: A randomized controlled trial. *BJU Int* 90(4):427–432.

Green RJ, Metlay JP, Propert K, Catalano PJ, Macdonald JS, Mayer RJ, Haller DG. 2002b. Surveillance for second primary colorectal cancer after adjuvant chemotherapy: An analysis of Intergroup 0089. *Ann Intern Med* 136(4):261–269.

Grise P, Thurman S. 2001. Urinary incontinence following treatment of localized prostate cancer. *Cancer Control* 8(6):532–539.

Grossfeld GD, Stier DM, Flanders SC, Henning JM, Schonfeld W, Warolin K, Carroll PR. 1998. Use of second treatment following definitive local therapy for prostate cancer: Data from the CaPSURE database. *J Urol* 160(4):1398–1404.

Grunfeld E, Dhesy-Thind S, Levine M. 2005. Clinical practice guidelines for the care and treatment of breast cancer: 9. Follow-up after treatment for breast cancer (2005 update). [Online]. Available: http://www.cmaj.ca/cgi/data/172/10/1319/DC1/2 [accessed July 14, 2005].

Guay AT, Spark RF, Bansal S, Cunningham GR, Goodman NF, Nankin HR, Petak SM, Perez JB, Law B Jr, Garber JR, Levy P, Jovanovic LG, Hamilton CR Jr, Rodbard HW, Palumbo PJ, Service FJ, Stoffer SS, Rettinger HI, Shankar TP, and Mechanick JI. 2003. American Association of Clinical Endocrinologists medical guidelines for clinical practice for the evaluation and treatment of male sexual dysfunction: A couple's problem—2003 update. *Endocr Pract* 9(1):77–95.

Gulliford T, Opomu M, Wilson E, Hanham I, Epstein R. 1997. Popularity of less frequent follow up for breast cancer in randomised study: Initial findings from the hotline study. *BMJ* 314(7075):174–177.

Hammerlid E, Taft C. 2001. Health-related quality of life in long-term head and neck cancer survivors: A comparison with general population norms. *Br J Cancer* 84(2):149–156.

Hancock SL. 1999. *Cardiovascular Late Effects After Treatment of Hodgkin's Disease.* New York, NY: Lippincott Williams & Wilkins.

Hancock SL, Tucker MA, Hoppe RT. 1993. Breast cancer after treatment of Hodgkin's disease. *J Natl Cancer Inst* 85(1):25–31.

Hanson Frost M, Suman VJ, Rummans TA, Dose AM, Taylor M, Novotny P, Johnson R, Evans RE. 2000. Physical, psychological and social well-being of women with breast cancer: The influence of disease phase. *Psychooncology* 9(3):221–231.

Harris JR, Lippman ME, Morrow M, Osborne CK. 2004. *Diseases of the Breast.* 3rd ed. New York, NY: Lippincott Williams & Wilkins.

Harris SR, Hugi MR, Olivotto IA, Levine M. 2001. Clinical practice guidelines for the care and treatment of breast cancer: Lymphedema. *CMAJ* 164(2):191–199.

Helewa M, Levesque P, Provencher D, Lea RH, Rosolowich V, Shapiro HM. 2002. Breast cancer, pregnancy, and breastfeeding. *J Obstet Gynaecol Can* 24(2):164–180; quiz 181–184.

Henderson IC, Berry DA, Demetri GD, Cirrincione CT, Goldstein LJ, Martino S, Ingle JN, Cooper MR, Hayes DF, Tkaczuk KH, Fleming G, Holland JF, Duggan DB, Carpenter JT, Frei E III, Schilsky RL, Wood WC, Muss HB, Norton L. 2003. Improved outcomes from adding sequential paclitaxel but not from escalating doxorubicin dose in an adjuvant chemotherapy regimen for patients with node-positive primary breast cancer. *J Clin Oncol* 21(6):976–983.

Herman DR, Ganz PA, Petersen L, Greendale GA. In press. Obesity and cardiovascular risk factors in younger breast cancer survivors: The Cancer and Menopause Study (CAMS). *Breast Cancer Res Treat.*

Herold AH, Roetzheim RG. 1992. Cancer survivors. *Prim Care* 19(4):779–791.

Hewitt M, Rowland JH, and Yancik R. 2003. Cancer survivors in the United States: Age, health, and disability. *J Gerontol A Biol Sci Med Sci* 58(1):82–91.

Hillner BE, Ingle JN, Chlebowski RT, Gralow J, Yee GC, Janjan NA, Cauley JA, Blumenstein BA, Albain KS, Lipton A, Brown S. 2003. American Society of Clinical Oncology 2003 update on the role of bisphosphonates and bone health issues in women with breast cancer. *J Clin Oncol* 21(21):4042–4057.

Hoda D, Perez DG, Loprinzi CL. 2003. Hot flashes in breast cancer survivors. *Breast J* 9(5):431–438.

Hoffman RD, Saltzman CL, Buckwalter JA. 2002. Outcome of lower extremity malignancy survivors treated with transfemoral amputation. *Arch Phys Med Rehabil* 83(2):177–182.

Holmes MD, Chen WY, Feskanich D, Kroenke CH, Colditz GA. 2005. Physical activity and survival after breast cancer diagnosis. *JAMA* 293(20): 479–2486.

Holmes MD, Kroenke CH. 2004. Beyond treatment: Lifestyle choices after breast cancer to enhance quality of life and survival. *Women's Health Issues* 14(1):11–13.

Holtzman J, Schmitz K, Babes G, Kane RL, Duval S, Wilt TJ, MacDonald RM, Rutks I (Minnesota Evidence-based Practice Center, under Contract No. 290-02-009). 2004. *Effectiveness of Behavioral Interventions to Modify Physical Activity Behaviors in General Populations and Cancer Patients and Survivors.* Evidence Report/Technology Assessment No. 102. Rockville, MD: Agency for Healthcare Research and Quality.

Hu JC, Kwan L, Saigal CS, Litwin MS. 2003. Regret in men treated for localized prostate cancer. *J Urol* 169(6):2279–2283.

Hurria A, Hudis C. 2003. Follow-up care of breast cancer survivors. *Crit Rev Oncol Hematol* 48(1):89–99.

ICSI (Institute for Clinical Systems Improvement). 2003. *Health Care Guideline: Breast Cancer Treatment.* Bloomington, MN: ICSI.

IOM (Institute of Medicine). 1990. *Clinical Practice Guidelines: Directions for a New Program.* Field MJ, Lohr KN, eds. Washington, DC: National Academy Press.

IOM. 2003. *Fulfilling the Potential of Cancer Prevention and Early Detection.* Curry SJ, Byers T, Hewitt M, eds. Washington, DC: The National Academies Press.

IOM. 2004. *Meeting the Psychosocial Needs of Women with Breast Cancer.* Hewitt M, Herdman R, Holland J, eds. Washington, DC: The National Academies Press.

Irwin ML, Crumley D, McTiernan A, Bernstein L, Baumgartner R, Gilliland FD, Kriska A, Ballard-Barbash R. 2003. Physical activity levels before and after a diagnosis of breast carcinoma: The Health, Eating, Activity, and Lifestyle (HEAL) study. *Cancer* 97(7):1746–1757.

Isaacs C, Peshkin BN, Schwartz M. 2004. Evaluation and management of women with a strong family history. In: Harris JR, Lippman ME, Morrow M, Osborne CK, eds. *Diseases of the Breast.* 3rd ed. New York, NY: Lippincott Williams & Wilkins. Pp. 315–345.

Jacobson JS, Troxel AB, Evans J, Klaus L, Vahdat L, Kinne D, Lo KM, Moore A, Rosenman PJ, Kaufman EL, Neugut AI, Grann VR. 2001. Randomized trial of black cohosh for the treatment of hot flashes among women with a history of breast cancer. *J Clin Oncol* 19(10):2739–2745.

Jen KL, Djuric Z, DiLaura NM, Buison A, Redd JN, Maranci V, Hryniuk WM. 2004. Improvement of metabolism among obese breast cancer survivors in differing weight loss regimens. *Obes Res* 12(2):306–312.

Jenkins I, Djuric Z, Darga L, DiLaura NM, Magnan M, Hryniuk WM. 2003. Relationship of psychiatric diagnosis and weight loss maintenance in obese breast cancer survivors. *Obes Res* 11(11):1369–1375.

Johansson K, Ohlsson K, Ingvar C, Albertsson M, Ekdahl C. 2002. Factors associated with the development of arm lymphedema following breast cancer treatment: A match pair case-control study. *Lymphology* 35(2):59–71.

Johnson FE, Virgo KS. 1997. *Cancer Patient Follow-Up*. St. Louis, MO: Mosby.

Johnson FE, Virgo KS, Fossati R. 2004. Follow-up for patients with colorectal cancer after curative-intent primary treatment. *J Clin Oncol* 22(8):1363–1365.

Joly F, Henry-Amar M, Arveux P, Reman O, Tanguy A, Peny AM, Lebailly P, Mace-Lesec'h J, Vie B, Genot JY, Busson A, Troussard X, Leporrier M. 1996. Late psychosocial sequelae in Hodgkin's disease survivors: A French population-based case-control study. *J Clin Oncol* 14(9):2444–2453.

Jones LW, Courneya KS. 2002. Exercise discussions during cancer treatment consultations. *Cancer Pract* 10(2):66–74.

Jones LW, Courneya KS, Fairey AS, Mackey JR. 2004. Effects of an oncologist's recommendation to exercise on self-reported exercise behavior in newly diagnosed breast cancer survivors: A single-blind, randomized controlled trial. *Ann Behav Med* 28(2):105–113.

Justice B. 1999. Why do women treated for breast cancer report good health despite disease or disability? A pilot study. *Psychol Rep* 84(2):392–394.

Kattlove H, Winn RJ. 2003. Ongoing care of patients after primary treatment for their cancer. *CA Cancer J Clin* 53(3):172–196.

King MC, Marks JH, Mandell JB. 2003. Breast and ovarian cancer risks due to inherited mutations in BRCA1 and BRCA2. *Science* 302(5645):643–646.

Kligman L, Wong RK, Johnston M, Laetsch NS. 2004. The treatment of lymphedema related to breast cancer: A systematic review and evidence summary. *Support Care Cancer* 12(6):421–431.

Knobel H, Havard Loge J, Brit Lund M, Forfang K, Nome O, Kaasa S. 2001. Late medical complications and fatigue in Hodgkin's disease survivors. *J Clin Oncol* 19(13):3226–3233.

Knols R, Aaronson NK, Uebelhart D, Fransen J, Aufdemkampe G. 2005. Physical exercise in cancer patients during and after medical treatment: A systematic review of randomized and controlled clinical trials. *J Clin Oncol* 23(16):3830–3842.

Kornblith AB. 1998. Psychosocial adaptation of cancer survivors. In: Holland JC, ed. *Psycho-Oncology*. New York: Oxford University Press.

Kornblith AB, Ligibel J. 2003. Psychosocial and sexual functioning of survivors of breast cancer. *Semin Oncol* 30(6):799–813.

Kornblith AB, Anderson J, Cella DF, Tross S, Zuckerman E, Cherin E, Henderson E, Weiss RB, Cooper MR, Silver RT, et al. 1992. Hodgkin's disease survivors at increased risk for problems in psychosocial adaptation. The Cancer and Leukemia Group B. *Cancer* 70(8):2214–2224.

Kornblith AB, Herndon JE II, Weiss RB, Zhang C, Zuckerman EL, Rosenberg S, Mertz M, Payne D, Massie MJ, Holland JF, Wingate P, Norton L, Holland JC. 2003. Long-term adjustment of survivors of early-stage breast carcinoma, 20 years after adjuvant chemotherapy. *Cancer* 98(4):679–689.

Kornblith AB, Herndon JE II, Zuckerman E, Cella DF, Cherin E, Wolchok S, Weiss RB, Diehl LF, Henderson E, Cooper MR, Schiffer C, Canellos GP, Mayer RJ, Silver RT, Schilling A, Peterson BA, Greenberg D, Holland JC. 1998. Comparison of psychosocial adaptation of advanced stage Hodgkin's disease and acute leukemia survivors. Cancer and Leukemia Group B. *Ann Oncol* 9(3):297–306.

Koupparis A, Ramsden A, Persad R. 2004. Cognitive effects of hormonal treatment for prostate cancer. *BJU Int* 93(7):915–916.

Krag DN, Julian TB, Harlow SP, Weaver DL, Ashikaga T, Bryant J, Single RM, Wolmark N. 2004. NSABP-32: Phase III, randomized trial comparing axillary resection with sentinal lymph node dissection: A description of the trial. *Ann Surg Oncol* 11(3 Suppl):208S–210S.

Kroenke CH, Chen WY, Rosner B, Holmes MD. 2005. Weight, weight gain, and survival after breast cancer diagnosis. *J Clin Oncol* 23(7):1370–1380.

Kroenke CH, Rosner B, Chen WY, Kawachi I, Colditz GA, Holmes MD. 2004. Functional impact of breast cancer by age at diagnosis. *J Clin Oncol* 22(10):1849–1856.

Krupski T, Petroni GR, Bissonette EA, Theodorescu D. 2000. Quality-of-life comparison of radical prostatectomy and interstitial brachytherapy in the treatment of clinically localized prostate cancer. *Urology* 55(5):736–742.

Krupski TL, Smith MR, Lee WC, Pashos CL, Brandman J, Wang Q, Botteman M, Litwin MS. 2004. Natural history of bone complications in men with prostate carcinoma initiating androgen deprivation therapy. *Cancer* 101(3):541–549.

Landier W, Bhatia S, Eshelman DA, Forte KJ, Sweeny T, Hester AL, Darling J, Armstrong FD, Blatt J, Constine LS, Freeman CR, Friedman DL, Green DM, Marina N, Meadows AT, Neglia JP, Oeffinger KC, Robison LL, Ruccione KS, Sklar CA, Hudson MM. 2004. Development of risk-based guidelines for pediatric cancer survivors: The Children's Oncology Group Long-Term Follow-Up Guidelines from the Children's Oncology Group Late Effects Committee and Nursing Discipline. *J Clin Oncol* 22(24):4979–4990.

Lamont EB, Christakis NA, Lauderdale DS. 2003. Favorable cardiac risk among elderly breast carcinoma survivors. *Cancer* 98(1):2–10.

Lamont EB, Lauderdale DS. 2003. Low risk of hip fracture among elderly breast cancer survivors. *Ann Epidemiol* 13(10):698–703.

Langer AS. 2001. Side effects, quality-of-life issues, and trade-offs: The patient perspective. *J Natl Cancer Inst Monogr* 30:125–129.

Lea R, Bannister E, Case A, Levesque P, Miller D, Provencher D, Rosolovich V. 2004. Use of hormonal replacement therapy after treatment of breast cancer. *J Obstet Gynaecol Can* 26(1):49–60; quiz 62–64.

Lee MM, Lin SS, Wrensch MR, Adler SR, Eisenberg D. 2000. Alternative therapies used by women with breast cancer in four ethnic populations. *J Natl Cancer Inst* 92(1):42–47.

Lee-Jones C, Humphris G, Dixon R, Hatcher MB. 1997. Fear of cancer recurrence—a literature review and proposed cognitive formulation to explain exacerbation of recurrence fears. *Psychooncology* 6(2):95–105.

Leedham B, Ganz PA. 1999. Psychosocial concerns and quality of life in breast cancer survivors. *Cancer Invest* 17(5):342–348.

Lepore SJ, Helgeson VS, Eton DT, Schulz R. 2003. Improving quality of life in men with prostate cancer: A randomized controlled trial of group education interventions. *Health Psychol* 22(5):443–452.

Levi F, Te VC, Randimbison L, La Vecchia C. 2003. Cancer risk in women with previous breast cancer. *Ann Oncol* 14(1):71–73.

Liberati A. 1995. The GIVIO trial on the impact of follow-up care on survival and quality of life in breast cancer patients. Interdisciplinary Group for Cancer Care Evaluation. *Ann Oncol* 6(Suppl 2):41–46.

Litwin MS. 2003. Quality of life following definitive therapy for localized prostate cancer: Potential impact of multiple therapies. *Curr Opin Urol* 13(2):153–156.

Litwin MS, Ron DH, Fink A, Ganz PA, Leake B, Brook RH. 2004. *UCLA Prostate Cancer Index, including the RAND 36-Item Health Survey v2 (SF-36 v2).* [Online]. Available: http://www.proqolid.org/public/UCLA-PCI.html [accessed February 15, 2005].

Loge JH, Abrahamsen AF, Ekeberg O, Kaasa S. 1999. Hodgkin's disease survivors more fatigued than the general population. *J Clin Oncol* 17(1):253–261.

Loge JH, Abrahamsen AF, Ekeberg O, Kaasa S. 2000. Fatigue and psychiatric morbidity among Hodgkin's disease survivors. *J Pain Symptom Manage* 19(2):91–99.

Loprinzi CL, Kugler JW, Sloan JA, Rooke TW, Quella SK, Novotny P, Mowat RB, Michalak JC, Stella PJ, Levitt R, Tschetter LK, Windschitl H. 1999. Lack of effect of coumarin in women with lymphedema after treatment for breast cancer. *N Engl J Med* 340(5):346–350.

Loprinzi CL, Sloan JA, Perez EA, Quella SK, Stella PJ, Mailliard JA, Halyard MY, Pruthi S, Novotny PJ, Rummans TA. 2002. Phase III evaluation of fluoxetine for treatment of hot flashes. *J Clin Oncol* 20(6):1578–1583.

Lu-Yao GL, Potosky AL, Albertsen PC, Wasson JH, Barry MJ, Wennberg JE. 1996. Follow-up prostate cancer treatments after radical prostatectomy: A population-based study. *J Natl Cancer Inst* 88(3–4):166–173.

Mackey JR, Joy AA. 2005. Skeletal health in postmenopausal survivors of early breast cancer. *Int J Cancer* 114(6):1010–1015.

Mandelblatt JS, Eisenberg JM. 1995. Historical and methodological perspectives on cancer outcomes research. *Oncology (Huntingt)* 9(11 Suppl):23–32.

Mandelblatt J, Figueiredo M, Cullen J. 2003. Outcomes and quality of life following breast cancer treatment in older women: When, why, how much, and what do women want? *Health Qual Life Outcomes* 1(1):45.

Manne SL. 2002. Prostate cancer support and advocacy groups: Their role for patients and family members. *Semin Urol Oncol* 20(1):45–54.

Marcus AD. 2004, September 8. A wife's struggle with cancer takes an unexpected toll. *The Wall Street Journal*. P. A1.

Massie MJ. 2004. Prevalence of depression in patients with cancer. *J Natl Cancer Inst Monogr* 32:57–71.

Massie MJ, Holland JC. 1991. Psychological reactions to breast cancer in the pre- and post-surgical treatment period. *Semin Surg Oncol* 7(5):320–325.

Matesich SM, Shapiro CL. 2003. Second cancers after breast cancer treatment. *Semin Oncol* 30(6):740–748.

Mauch PM, Armitage JO, Diehl V, Hoppe RT, Weiss LM, eds. 1999. *Hodgkin's Disease*. New York, NY: Lippincott, Williams & Wilkins.

Maunsell E, Brisson J, Deschenes L. 1989. Psychological distress after initial treatment for breast cancer: A comparison of partial and total mastectomy. *J Clin Epidemiol* 42(8):765–71.

Maunsell E, Brisson J, Deschenes L. 1992. Psychological distress after initial treatment of breast cancer. Assessment of potential risk factors. *Cancer* 70(1):120–125.

Maunsell E, Brisson J, Deschenes L. 1995. Social support and survival among women with breast cancer. *Cancer* 76(4):631–637.

McBride CM, Ostroff JS. 2003. Teachable moments for promoting smoking cessation: The context of cancer care and survivorship. *Cancer Control* 10(4):325–333.

McEvoy MD, McCorkle R. 1990. Quality of life issues in patients with disseminated breast cancer. *Cancer* 66(6 Suppl):1416–1421.

McKinley ED. 2000. Under Toad days: Surviving the uncertainty of cancer recurrence. *Ann Intern Med* 133(6):479–480.

McTiernan A. 2004. Physical activity after cancer: Physiologic outcomes. *Cancer Invest* 22(1):68–81.

McTiernan A, Rajan KB, Tworoger SS, Irwin M, Bernstein L, Baumgartner R, Gilliland F, Stanczyk FZ, Yasui Y, Ballard-Barbash R. 2003. Adiposity and sex hormones in post-menopausal breast cancer survivors. *J Clin Oncol* 21(10):1961–1966.

Mehta SS, Lubeck DP, Pasta DJ, Litwin MS. 2003. Fear of cancer recurrence in patients undergoing definitive treatment for prostate cancer: Results from CaPSURE. *J Urol* 170(5):1931–1933.

Meyerhardt JA, Mayer RJ. 2003. Follow-up strategies after curative resection of colorectal cancer. *Semin Oncol* 30(3):349–360.

Meyerowitz BE, Desmond KA, Rowland JH, Wyatt GE, Ganz PA. 1999. Sexuality following breast cancer. *J Sex Marital Ther* 25(3):237–250.

Meyers CA. 2000. Neurocognitive dysfunction in cancer patients. *Oncology (Huntingt)* 14(1):75–79; discussion 79, 81–82, 85.

Michael YL, Berkman LF, Colditz GA, Holmes MD, Kawachi I. 2002. Social networks and health-related quality of life in breast cancer survivors: A prospective study. *J Psychosom Res* 52(5):285–293.

Michael YL, Kawachi I, Berkman LF, Holmes MD, Colditz GA. 2000. The persistent impact of breast carcinoma on functional health status: Prospective evidence from the Nurses' Health Study. *Cancer* 89(11):2176–2186.

Miller DC, Sanda MG, Dunn RL, Montie JE, Pimentel H, Sandler HM, McLaughlin WP, Wei JT. 2005. Long-term outcomes among localized prostate cancer survivors: Health-related quality-of-life changes after radical prostatectomy, external radiation, and brachytherapy. *J Clin Oncol* 23(12):2772–2780.

Moertel CG, Fleming TR, Macdonald JS, Haller DG, Laurie JA, Tangen C. 1993. An evaluation of the carcinoembryonic antigen (CEA) test for monitoring patients with resected colon cancer. *JAMA* 270(8):943–947.

Montazeri A, Gillis CR, McEwen J. 1996. Measuring quality of life in oncology: Is it worthwhile? Meaning, purposes and controversies. *Eur J Cancer Care (Engl)* 5(3):159–167.

Mor V, Malin M, Allen S. 1994. Age differences in the psychosocial problems encountered by breast cancer patients. *J Natl Cancer Inst Monogr* (16):191–197.

Morrow M, Strom EA, Bassett LW, Dershaw DD, Fowble B, Giuliano A, Harris JR, O'Malley F, Schnitt SJ, Singletary SE, Winchester DP. 2002a. Standard for breast conservation therapy in the management of invasive breast carcinoma. *CA Cancer J Clin* 52(5):277–300.

Morrow M, Strom EA, Bassett LW, Dershaw DD, Fowble B, Harris JR, O'Malley F, Schnitt SJ, Singletary SE, Winchester DP. 2002b. Standard for the management of ductal carcinoma in situ of the breast (DCIS). *CA Cancer J Clin* 52(5):256–276.

Mortimer P, Bates D, Brassington H, Stanton A, Strachan D, Levick J. 1996. The prevalence of arm oedema following treatment for breast cancer. *QJM* 89(5):337–380.

Mrozek E, Shapiro CL. 2005. Survivorship and complications of treatment in breast cancer. *Clinical Advances in Hematology & Oncology* 3(3):211–222.

Mukand JA, Blackinton DD, Crincoli MG, Lee JJ, Santos BB. 2001. Incidence of neurologic deficits and rehabilitation of patients with brain tumors. *Am J Phys Med Rehabil* 80(5):346–350.

Muzzin LJ, Anderson NJ, Figueredo AT, Gudelis SO. 1994. The experience of cancer. *Soc Sci Med* 38(9):1201–1208.

National Surgical Adjuvant Breast and Bowel Project. 2004. *NSABP Clinical Trials Overview: Protocol B-32*. [Online]. Available: http://www.nsabp.pitt.edu/b-32.htm [accessed August 30, 2004].

Navo MA, Phan J, Vaughan C, Palmer JL, Michaud L, Jones KL, Bodurka DC, Basen-Engquist K, Hortobagyi GN, Kavanagh JJ, Smith JA. 2004. An assessment of the utilization of complementary and alternative medication in women with gynecologic or breast malignancies. *J Clin Oncol* 22(4):671–677.

NBCC (National Breast Cancer Centre). 2001. *Clinical Practice Guidelines for the Management of Early Breast Cancer*. Canberra, Australia: National Health and Medical Research Council.

NBCC and NCCI (National Breast Cancer Center and National Cancer Control Initiative). 2004. *Clinical Practice Guidelines for the Management and Support of Younger Women With Breast Cancer*. Camperdown, NSW, Australia: National Breast Cancer Center.

NCCAM (National Center for Complementary and Alternative Medicine). 2002. *What Is Complementary and Alternative Medicine (CAM)?* [Online]. Available: http://nccam.nih.gov/health/whatiscam/ [accessed February 26, 2005].

NCCN (National Comprehensive Cancer Network). 1999. NCCN practice guidelines for the management of psychosocial distress. *Oncology (Huntingt)* 13(5A):113–147.

NCCN. 2004a. *Breast Cancer Treatment Guidelines for Patients, Version VI. Breast Cancer Treatment.* [Online]. Available: http://www.nccn.org/patients/patient_gls/_english/_breast/5_treatment.asp#consider [accessed May 9, 2005].

NCCN. 2004b. *Clinical Practice Guidelines in Oncology-v.1.2004. Breast Cancer.* [Online]. Available: http://www.nccn.org/professionals/physician_gls/PDF/breast.pdf [accessed December 6, 2004].

NCCN. 2004c. *Clinical Practice Guidelines in Oncology-v.1.2004. Colorectal Screening.* [Online]. Available: http://www.nccn.org/professionals/physician_gls/PDF/colorectal_screening.pdf [accessed December 6, 2004].

NCCN. 2004d. *Clinical Practice Guidelines in Oncology-v.1.2004. Distress Management.* [Online]. Available: http://www.nccn.org/physician_gls/f_guidelines.html [accessed December 6, 2004].

NCCN. 2004e. *Clinical Practice Guidelines in Oncology-v.1.2004. Genetic/Familial High-Risk Assessment: Breast and Ovarian.* [Online]. Available: http://www.nccn.org/professionals/physician_gls/PDF/genetics_screening.pdf [accessed December 6, 2004].

NCCN. 2004f. *Clinical Practice Guidelines in Oncology-v.1.2004. Hodgkin's Disease.* [Online]. Available: http://www.nccn.org/professionals/physician_gls/PDF/hodgkins.pdf [accessed December 6, 2004].

NCCN. 2004g. *Clinical Practice Guidelines in Oncology-v.1.2004. Prostate Cancer.* [Online]. Available: http://www.nccn.org/professionals/physician_gls/PDF/prostate.pdf [accessed December 6, 2004].

NCCN. 2004h. *Clinical Practice Guidelines in Oncology-v.2.2004. Colon Cancer.* [Online]. Available: http://www.nccn.org/professionals/physician_gls/PDF/colon.pdf [accessed December 6, 2004].

NCCN. 2004i. *NCCN Treatment Guidelines for Patients.* [Online]. Available: http://www.nccn.org/patients/patient_gls.asp [accessed September 11, 2004].

NCCN. 2005. *Clinical Practice Guidelines in Oncology-v.2.2005. Cancer-Related Fatigue.* [Online]. Available: http://www.nccn.org/professionals/physician_gls/PDF/fatigue.pdf [accessed July 22, 2005].

NCI (National Cancer Institute). 2004a. *Breast Cancer (PDQ): Treatment.* [Online]. Available: http://www.cancer.gov/cancertopics/pdq/treatment/breast/healthprofessional/allpages [accessed September 2004].

NCI. 2004b. *Genetics of Breast and Ovarian Cancer (PDQ) Health Professional Version.* [Online]. Available: http://www.cancer.gov/cancertopics/pdq/genetics/breast-and-ovarian/healthprofessional [accessed October 6, 2004].

NCI. 2005a. *Adult Hodgkin's Lymphoma (PDQ®): Treatment.* [Online]. Available: http://www.nci.nih.gov/cancertopics/pdq/treatment/adulthodgkins/Patient/page4 [accessed February 10, 2005].

NCI. 2005b. *Colon Cancer PDQ: Treatment.* [Online]. Available: http://www.cancer.gov/cancertopics/pdq/treatment/colon/healthprofessional [accessed February 7, 2005].

NCI and NCCAM (National Cancer Institute and National Center for Complementary and Alternative Medicine). 2004. *Cancer Facts: Complementary and Alternative Medicine.* [Online]. Available: http://cis.nci.nih.gov/fact/9_14.htm [accessed December 8, 2004].

Ng AK, Mauch PM. 2004. Late complications of therapy of Hodgkin's disease: Prevention and management. *Curr Hematol Rep* 3(1):27–33.

NIH (National Institutes of Health). 2000. Adjuvant therapy for breast cancer. *NIH Consensus Statement* 17(4):1–35.

Northover J. 2003. Follow-up after curative surgery for colorectal cancer. *Scand J Surg* 92(1):84–89.

Oktay K. 2001. Ovarian tissue cryopreservation and transplantation: Preliminary findings and implications for cancer patients. *Hum Reprod Update* 7(6):526–534.

Oktay K, Sonmezer M. 2004. Ovarian tissue banking for cancer patients: Fertility preservation, not just ovarian cryopreservation. *Hum Reprod* 19(3):477–480.

Oktay K, Buyuk E, Davis O, Yermakova I, Veeck L, Rosenwaks Z. 2003. Fertility preservation in breast cancer patients: IVF and embryo cryopreservation after ovarian stimulation with tamoxifen. *Hum Reprod* 18(1):90–95.

Oktay K, Buyuk E, Libertella N, Akar M, Rosenwaks Z. 2005. Fertility preservation in breast cancer patients: A prospective controlled comparison of ovarian stimulation with tamoxifen and letrozole for embryo cryopreservation. *J Clin Oncol* 23(19):4347–4353.

Omne-Ponten M, Holmberg L, Sjoden PO. 1994. Psychosocial adjustment among women with breast cancer Stages I and II: Six-year follow-up of consecutive patients. *J Clin Oncol* 12(9):1778–1782.

Paik S, Shak S, Tang G, Kim C, Baker J, Cronin M, Baehner FL, Walker MG, Watson D, Park T, Hiller W, Fisher ER, Wickerham DL, Bryant J, Wolmark N. 2004. A multigene assay to predict recurrence of tamoxifen-treated, node-negative breast cancer. *N Engl J Med* 351(27):2817–2826.

Palli D, Russo A, Saieva C, Ciatto S, Rosselli Del Turco M, Distante V, Pacini P. 1999. Intensive vs clinical follow-up after treatment of primary breast cancer: 10-year update of a randomized trial. National Research Council Project on Breast Cancer Follow-up. *JAMA* 281(17):1586.

Park RE, Fink A, Brook RH, Chassin MR, Kahn KL, Merrick NJ, Kosecoff J, Solomon DH. 1986. Physician ratings of appropriate indications for six medical and surgical procedures. *Am J Public Health* 76(7):766–772.

Parker-Pope T. 2004 (June 1). Efforts mount to combat lymphedema, a devastating side effect of cancer care. *The Wall Street Journal.* P. D1.

Partridge AH, Winer EP. 2005. Fertility after breast cancer: Questions abound. *J Clin Oncol* 23(19):4259-4261.

Partridge AH, Burstein HJ, Winer EP. 2001. Side effects of chemotherapy and combined chemohormonal therapy in women with early-stage breast cancer. *J Natl Cancer Inst Monogr* 30:135–142.

Partridge AH, Winer EP, Burstein HJ. 2003. Follow-up care of breast cancer survivors. *Semin Oncol* 30(6):817–825.

Paskett ED. 2003. Empowering women with breast cancer: One survivor's story. *Semin Oncol* 30(6):814–816.

Penson DF, Litwin MS. 2003a. The physical burden of prostate cancer. *Urol Clin North Am* 30(2):305–313.

Penson DF, Litwin MS. 2003b. Quality of life after treatment for prostate cancer. *Curr Urol Rep* 4(3):185–195.

Penson DF, Sokoloff MH. 2004. Management of side effects of prostate cancer therapy. In: Carroll P, Nelson WG, eds. *Report to the Nation on Prostate Cancer.* Santa Monica, CA: Prostate Cancer Foundation.

Petrie KJ, Buick DL, Weinman J, Booth RJ. 1999. Positive effects of illness reported by myocardial infarction and breast cancer patients. *J Psychosom Res* 47(6):537–543.

Phillips KA, Bernhard J. 2003. Adjuvant breast cancer treatment and cognitive function: Current knowledge and research directions. *J Natl Cancer Inst* 95(3):190–197.

Pierce R, Chadiha LA, Vargas A, Mosley M. 2003. Prostate cancer and psychosocial concerns in African American men: Literature synthesis and recommendations. *Health Soc Work* 28(4):302–311.

Pinto BM, Maruyama NC. 1999. Exercise in the rehabilitation of breast cancer survivors. *Psychooncology* 8(3):191–206.

Pinto BM, Eakin E, Maruyama NC. 2000. Health behavior changes after a cancer diagnosis: What do we know and where do we go from here? *Ann Behav Med* 22(1):38–52.

Pinto BM, Frierson GM, Rabin C, Trunzo JJ, Marcus BH. 2005. Home-based physical activity intervention for breast cancer patients. *J Clin Oncol* 23(15):3577–3587.

Pinto BM, Maruyama NC, Clark MM, Cruess DG, Park E, Roberts M. 2002. Motivation to modify lifestyle risk behaviors in women treated for breast cancer. *Mayo Clin Proc* 77(2):122–129.

Posther KE, Wilke LG, Giuliano AE. 2004. Sentinel lymph node dissection and the current status of American trials on breast lymphatic mapping. *Semin Oncol* 31(3):426–436.

Pound CR, Partin AW, Eisenberger MA, Chan DW, Pearson JD, Walsh PC. 1999. Natural history of progression after PSA elevation following radical prostatectomy. *JAMA* 281(17):1591–1597.

President's Cancer Panel. 2004. *Living Beyond Cancer: Finding a New Balance*. Bethesda, MD: National Cancer Institute.

Pritchard KI, Khan H, Levine M. 2002. Clinical practice guidelines for the care and treatment of breast cancer: The role of hormone replacement therapy in women with a previous diagnosis of breast cancer. *CMAJ* 166(8):1017–1022.

Quigley KM. 1989. The adult cancer survivor: Psychosocial consequences of cure. *Semin Oncol Nurs* 5(1):63–69.

Ramaswamy B, Shapiro CL. 2003. Osteopenia and osteoporosis in women with breast cancer. *Semin Oncol* 30(6):763–775.

Ramsey SD, Berry K, Moinpour C, Giedzinska A, Andersen MR. 2002. Quality of life in long term survivors of colorectal cancer. *Am J Gastroenterol* 97(5):1228–1234.

Rao A, Cohen HJ. 2004. Symptom management in the elderly cancer patient: Fatigue, pain, and depression. *J Natl Cancer Inst Monogr* 32:150–157.

Rauch P, Miny J, Conroy T, Neyton L, Guillemin F. 2004. Quality of life among disease-free survivors of rectal cancer. *J Clin Oncol* 22(2):354–360.

Recht A, Edge SB, Solin LJ, Robinson DS, Estabrook A, Fine RE, Fleming GF, Formenti S, Hudis C, Kirshner JJ, Krause DA, Kuske RR, Langer AS, Sledge GW Jr, Whelan TJ, Pfister DG. 2001. Postmastectomy radiotherapy: Clinical practice guidelines of the American Society of Clinical Oncology. *J Clin Oncol* 19(5):1539–1569.

Richardson MA, Sanders T, Palmer JL, Greisinger A, Singletary SE. 2000. Complementary/alternative medicine use in a comprehensive cancer center and the implications for oncology. *J Clin Oncol* 18(13):2505–2514.

Ries LAG, Eisner MP, Kosary CL, Hankey BF, Miller BA, Clegg L, Mariotto A, Feuer EJ, Edwards BK, eds. 2004. *SEER Cancer Statistics Review, 1975–2001*. Bethesda, MD: National Cancer Institute.

Robinson JW, Moritz S, Fung T. 2002. Meta-analysis of rates of erectile function after treatment of localized prostate carcinoma. *Int J Radiat Oncol Biol Phys* 54(4):1063–1068.

Rock CL, Demark-Wahnefried W. 2002. Nutrition and survival after the diagnosis of breast cancer: A review of the evidence. *J Clin Oncol* 20(15):3302–3316.

Rojas M, Telaro E, Russo A, Moschetti I, Coe L, Fossati R, Palli D, Roselli TM, Liberati A. 2005. Follow-up strategies for women treated for early breast cancer. *Cochrane Database Syst Rev* (1):CD001768.

Rosselli Del Turco M, Palli D, Cariddi A, Ciatto S, Pacini P, Distante V. 1994. Intensive diagnostic follow-up after treatment of primary breast cancer. A randomized trial. National Research Council Project on Breast Cancer follow-up. *JAMA* 271(20):1593–1597.

Rowland JH, Desmond KA, Meyerowitz BE, Belin TR, Wyatt GE, Ganz PA. 2000. Role of breast reconstructive surgery in physical and emotional outcomes among breast cancer survivors. *J Natl Cancer Inst* 92(17):1422–1429.

Rugo HS, Ahles T. 2003. The impact of adjuvant therapy for breast cancer on cognitive function: Current evidence and directions for research. *Semin Oncol* 30(6):749–762.

Sadler IJ, Jacobsen PB. 2001. Progress in understanding fatigue associated with breast cancer treatment. *Cancer Invest* 19(7):723–731.

Salminen EK, Portin RI, Koskinen AI, Helenius HY, Nurmi MJ. 2005. Estradiol and cognition during androgen deprivation in men with prostate carcinoma. *Cancer* 103(7):1381–1387.

Sapp AL, Trentham-Dietz A, Newcomb PA, Hampton JM, Moinpour CM, Remington PL (University of Wisconsin Comprehensive Cancer Center). 2003. Social networks and quality of life among female long-term colorectal cancer survivors. *Cancer* 98(8):1749–1758.

Satia JA, Campbell MK, Galanko JA, James A, Carr C, Sandler RS. 2004. Longitudinal changes in lifestyle behaviors and health status in colon cancer survivors. *Cancer Epidemiol Biomarkers Prev* 13(6):1022–1031.

Saykin AJ, Ahles TA, McDonald BC. 2003. Mechanisms of chemotherapy-induced cognitive disorders: Neuropsychological, pathophysiological, and neuroimaging perspectives. *Semin Clin Neuropsychiatry* 8(4):201–216.

Schag CA, Ganz PA, Polinsky ML, Fred C, Hirji K, Petersen L. 1993. Characteristics of women at risk for psychosocial distress in the year after breast cancer. *J Clin Oncol* 11(4):783–793.

Schnoll RA, Zhang B, Rue M, Krook JE, Spears WT, Marcus AC, Engstrom PF. 2003. Brief physician-initiated quit-smoking strategies for clinical oncology settings: A trial coordinated by the Eastern Cooperative Oncology Group. *J Clin Oncol* 21(2):355–365.

Scholefield JH, Steele RJ. 2002. Guidelines for follow up after resection of colorectal cancer. *Gut* 51(Suppl 5):V3–V5.

Schover LR. 1994. Sexuality and body image in younger women with breast cancer. *J Natl Cancer Inst Monogr* 16:177–182.

Schover LR. 2004. Myth-busters: Telling the true story of breast cancer survivorship. *J Natl Cancer Inst* 96(24):1800–1801.

Schover LR. 2005. Motivation for parenthood after cancer: A review. *J Natl Cancer Inst Monogr* 34:2–5.

Schover LR, Fouladi RT, Warneke CL, Neese L, Klein EA, Zippe C, Kupelian PA. 2002. The use of treatments for erectile dysfunction among survivors of prostate carcinoma. *Cancer* 95(11):2397–2407.

Schover LR, Fouladi RT, Warneke CL, Neese L, Klein EA, Zippe C, Kupelian PA. 2004. Seeking help for erectile dysfunction after treatment for prostate cancer. *Arch Sex Behav* 33(5):443–454.

Schover LR, Yetman RJ, Tuason LJ, Meisler E, Esselstyn CB, Hermann RE, Grundfest-Broniatowski S, Dowden RV. 1995. Partial mastectomy and breast reconstruction. A comparison of their effects on psychosocial adjustment, body image, and sexuality. *Cancer* 75(1):54–64.

Schwartz D, Billingsley K, Wallner K. 2000. Follow-up care for cancer: Making the benefits equal the cost. *Oncology (Huntingt)* 14(10):1493–1498, 1501; discussion 1502–1505.

Schwartz GF. 2004. Clinical practice guidelines for the use of axillary sentinel lymph node biopsy in carcinoma of the breast: Current update. *Breast J* 10(2):85–88.

Shapiro CL, Recht A. 2001. Side effects of adjuvant treatment of breast cancer. *N Engl J Med* 344(26):1997–2008.

Shapiro CL, Manola J, Leboff M. 2001. Ovarian failure after adjuvant chemotherapy is associated with rapid bone loss in women with early-stage breast cancer. *J Clin Oncol* 19(14):3306–3311.

Shekelle PG, Ortiz E, Rhodes S, Morton SC, Eccles MP, Grimshaw JM, Woolf SH. 2001. Validity of the Agency for Healthcare Research and Quality clinical practice guidelines: How quickly do guidelines become outdated? *JAMA* 286(12):1461–1467.

Shimozuma K, Ganz PA, Petersen L, Hirji K. 1999. Quality of life in the first year after breast cancer surgery: Rehabilitation needs and patterns of recovery. *Breast Cancer Res Treat* 56(1):45–57.

Short PF, Mallonee EL. In press. Income disparities in the quality of life of cancer survivors. *Med Care.*

SIGN (Scottish Intercollegiate Guidelines Network). 1998. *Breast Cancer in Women: A National Clinical Guideline.* Edinburgh, Scotland: SIGN.

SIGN. 2003. *Management of Colorectal Cancer.* Edinburgh, Scotland: SIGN.

Simmang CL, Senatore P, Lowry A, Hicks T, Burnstein M, Dentsman F, Fazio V, Glennon E, Hyman N, Kerner B, Kilkenny J, Moore R, Peters W, Ross T, Savoca P, Vernava A, Wong WD. 1999. Practice parameters for detection of colorectal neoplasms. The Standards Committee, The American Society of Colon and Rectal Surgeons. *Dis Colon Rectum* 42(9):1123–1129.

Singh GK, Miller BA, Hankey BF, Edwards BK. 2003. *Area Socioeconomic Variations in U.S. Cancer Incidence, Mortality, Stage, Treatment, and Survival, 1975–1999.* NCI Cancer Surveillance Monograph Series, No. 4. Bethesda, MD: National Cancer Institute.

Smith K, Lesko LM. 1988. Psychosocial problems in cancer survivors. *Oncology (Huntingt)* 2(1):33–44.

Smith MR. 2003. Bisphosphonates to prevent osteoporosis in men receiving androgen deprivation therapy for prostate cancer. *Drugs Aging* 20(3):175–183.

Smith TJ, Hillner BE. 2001. Ensuring quality cancer care by the use of clinical practice guidelines and critical pathways. *J Clin Oncol* 19(11):2886–2897.

Smith TJ, Davidson NE, Schapira DV, Grunfeld E, Muss HB, Vogel VG III, Somerfield MR. 1999. American Society of Clinical Oncology 1998 update of recommended breast cancer surveillance guidelines. *J Clin Oncol* 17(3):1080–1082.

Soloway CT, Soloway MS, Kim SS, Kava BR. 2005. Sexual, psychological and dyadic qualities of the prostate cancer "couple". *BJU International* 95:780-785.

Sparaco A, Fentiman IS. 2002. Arm lymphoedema following breast cancer treatment. *Int J Clin Pract* 56(2):107–110.

Sparreboom A, Cox MC, Acharya MR, Figg WD. 2004. Herbal remedies in the United States: Potential adverse interactions with anticancer agents. *J Clin Oncol* 22(12):2489–2503.

Sprangers MA, Taal BG, Aaronson NK, te Velde A. 1995. Quality of life in colorectal cancer. Stoma vs. nonstoma patients. *Dis Colon Rectum* 38(4):361–369.

Stanford JL, Feng Z, Hamilton AS, Gilliland FD, Stephenson RA, Eley JW, Albertsen PC, Harlan LC, Potosky AL. 2000. Urinary and sexual function after radical prostatectomy for clinically localized prostate cancer: The Prostate Cancer Outcomes Study. *JAMA* 283(3):354–360.

Stanton AL, Ganz PA, Bower JE, Kwan L, Meyerowitz BE, Rowland JH, Krupnick JL. 2004. The Moving Beyond Cancer Trial: A psycho-educational intervention for women with breast cancer. *J Clin Oncol, 2004 ASCO Annual Meeting Proceedings (Post-Meeting Edition)* 22(14S):8011.

Stearns V, Davidson NE. 2004. Adjuvant chemotherapy and chemoendocrine therapy. In: Harris JR, Lippman ME, Morrow M, Osborne CK, eds. *Diseases of the Breast.* 3rd ed. New York: Lippincott Williams & Wilkins. Pp. 893–919.

Tannock IF, Ahles TA, Ganz PA, Van Dam FS. 2004. Cognitive impairment associated with chemotherapy for cancer: Report of a workshop. *J Clin Oncol* 22(11):2233–2239.

Taxel P, Stevens MC, Trahiotis M, Zimmerman J, Kaplan RF. 2004. The effect of short-term estradiol therapy on cognitive function in older men receiving hormonal suppression therapy for prostate cancer. *J Am Geriatr Soc* 52(2):269–273.

Teloken C. 2001. Management of erectile dysfunction secondary to treatment for localized prostate cancer. *Cancer Control* 8(6):540–545.

Temple LK, Wang EE, McLeod RS. 1999. Preventive health care, 1999 update: Follow-up after breast cancer. Canadian Task Force on Preventive Health Care. *CMAJ* 161(8):1001–1008.

Thellenberg C, Malmer B, Tavelin B, Gronberg H. 2003. Second primary cancers in men with prostate cancer: An increased risk of male breast cancer. *J Urol* 169(4):1345–1348.

Theodoulou M, Seidman AD. 2003. Cardiac effects of adjuvant therapy for early breast cancer. *Semin Oncol* 30(6):730–739.

Thors CL, Broeckel JA, Jacobsen PB. 2001. Sexual functioning in breast cancer survivors. *Cancer Control* 8(5):442–448.

Thorsen L, Skovlund E, Stromme SB, Hornslien K, Dahl AA, Fossa SD. 2005. Effectiveness of physical activity on cardiorespiratory fitness and health-related quality of life in young and middle-aged cancer patients shortly after chemotherapy. *J Clin Oncol* 23(10):2378–2388.

Tice JA, Ettinger B, Ensrud K, Wallace R, Blackwell T, Cummings SR. 2003. Phytoestrogen supplements for the treatment of hot flashes: The Isoflavone Clover Extract (ICE) Study: A randomized controlled trial. *JAMA* 290(2):207–214.

Tomich PL, Helgeson VS. 2002. Five years later: A cross-sectional comparison of breast cancer survivors with healthy women. *Psychooncology* 11(2):154–169.

Torrey MJ, Poen JC, Hoppe RT. 1997. Detection of relapse in early-stage Hodgkin's disease: Role of routine follow-up studies. *J Clin Oncol* 15(3):1123–1130.

Trask PC. 2004. Assessment of depression in cancer patients. *J Natl Cancer Inst Monogr* 32:80–92.

Travis LB, Gospodarowicz M, Curtis RE, Clarke EA, Andersson M, Glimelius B, Joensuu T, Lynch CF, van Leeuwen FE, Holowaty E, Storm H, Glimelius I, Pukkala E, Stovall M, Fraumeni JF Jr, Boice JD Jr, Gilbert E. 2002. Lung cancer following chemotherapy and radiotherapy for Hodgkin's disease. *J Natl Cancer Inst* 94(3):182–192.

Travis LB, Hill DA, Dores GM, Gospodarowicz M, van Leeuwen FE, Holowaty E, Glimelius B, Andersson M, Wiklund T, Lynch CF, Van't Veer MB, Glimelius I, Storm H, Pukkala E, Stovall M, Curtis R, Boice JD Jr, Gilbert E. 2003. Breast cancer following radiotherapy and chemotherapy among young women with Hodgkin's disease. *JAMA* 290(4):465–475.

Trentham-Dietz A, Remington PL, Moinpour CM, Hampton JM, Sapp AL, Newcomb PA (University of Wisconsin Comprehensive Cancer Center). 2003. Health-related quality of life in female long-term colorectal cancer survivors. *Oncologist* 8(4):342–349.

USPSTF (U.S. Preventive Services Task Force). 2003. *Counseling to Prevent Tobacco Use and Tobacco-Related Diseases: Recommendation Statement*. [Online]. Available: http://www.ahrq.gov/clinic/3rduspstf/tobacccoun/tobcounrs.htm [accessed December 8, 2004].

Vachon ML. 2001. The meaning of illness to a long-term survivor. *Semin Oncol Nurs* 17(4):279–283.

Van Patten CL, Olivotto IA, Chambers GK, Gelmon KA, Hislop TG, Templeton E, Wattie A, Prior JC. 2002. Effect of soy phytoestrogens on hot flashes in postmenopausal women with breast cancer: A randomized, controlled clinical trial. *J Clin Oncol* 20(6):1449–1455.

Villers A, Pommier P, Bataillard A, Fervers B, Bachaud JM, Berger N, Bertrand AF, Bouvier R, Brune D, Daver A, Fontaine E, Haillot O, Lagrange JL, Molinie V, Muratet JP, Pabot du Chatelard P, Peneau M, Prapotnich D, Ravery V, Richaud P, Rossi D, Soulie M. 2003. Summary of the Standards, Options and Recommendations for the management of patients with nonmetastatic prostate cancer (2001). *Br J Cancer* 89(Suppl 1):S50–S58.

Visser A, van Andel G. 2003. Psychosocial and educational aspects in prostate cancer patients. *Patient Educ Couns* 49(3):203–206.

Warner E, Plewes DB, Hill KA, Causer PA, Zubovits JT, Jong RA, Cutrara MR, DeBoer G, Yaffe MJ, Messner SJ, Meschino WS, Piron CA, Narod SA. 2004. Surveillance of BRCA1 and BRCA2 mutation carriers with magnetic resonance imaging, ultrasound, mammography, and clinical breast examination. *JAMA* 292(11):1317–1325.

Wassertheil-Smoller S, Hendrix SL, Limacher M, Heiss G, Kooperberg C, Baird A, Kotchen T, Curb JD, Black H, Rossouw JE, Aragaki A, Safford M, Stein E, Laowattana S, Mysiw WJ. 2003. Effect of estrogen plus progestin on stroke in postmenopausal women: The Women's Health Initiative: A randomized trial. *JAMA* 289(20):2673–2684.

Wefel JS, Lenzi R, Theriault R, Buzdar AU, Cruickshank S, Meyers CA. 2004a. 'Chemobrain' in breast carcinoma?: A prologue. *Cancer* 101(3):466–475.

Wefel JS, Lenzi R, Theriault RL, Davis RN, Meyers CA. 2004b. The cognitive sequelae of standard-dose adjuvant chemotherapy in women with breast carcinoma: Results of a prospective, randomized, longitudinal trial. *Cancer* 100(11):2292–2299.

Weiger WA, Smith M, Boon H, Richardson MA, Kaptchuk TJ, Eisenberg DM. 2002. Advising patients who seek complementary and alternative medical therapies for cancer. *Ann Intern Med* 137(11):889–903.

Wenzel L, Dogan-Ates A, Habbal R, Berkowitz R, Goldstein DP, Bernstein M, Kluhsman BC, Osann K, Newlands E, Seckl MJ, Hancock B, Cella D. 2005. Defining and measuring reproductive concerns of female cancer survivors. *J Natl Cancer Inst Monogr* 34:94–98.

Wenzel LB, Fairclough DL, Brady MJ, Cella D, Garrett KM, Kluhsman BC, Crane LA, Marcus AC. 1999. Age-related differences in the quality of life of breast carcinoma patients after treatment. *Cancer* 86(9):1768–1774.

White RL Jr, Wilke LG. 2004. Update on the NSABP and ACOSOG breast cancer sentinel node trials. *Am Surg* 70(5):420–424.

Winawer S, Fletcher R, Rex D, Bond J, Burt R, Ferrucci J, Ganiats T, Levin T, Woolf S, Johnson D, Kirk L, Litin S, Simmang C. 2003. Colorectal cancer screening and surveillance: Clinical guidelines and rationale—Update based on new evidence. *Gastroenterology* 124(2):544–560.

Winer EP, Hudis C, Burstein HJ, Wolff AC, Pritchard KI, Ingle JN, Chlebowski RT, Gelber R, Edge SB, Gralow J, Cobleigh MA, Mamounas EP, Goldstein LJ, Whelan TJ, Powles TJ, Bryant J, Perkins C, Perotti J, Braun S, Langer AS, Browman GP, Somerfield MR. 2005. American Society of Clinical Oncology technology assessment on the use of aromatase inhibitors as adjuvant therapy for postmenopausal women with hormone receptor-positive breast cancer: Status report 2004. *J Clin Oncol* 23(3):619–629.

Winn RJ. 2002. *Clinical Practice Guidelines and Survivorship*. Paper commissioned for the National Cancer Policy Board. Unpublished.

Winn RJ, Botnick WZ. 1997. The NCCN Guideline Program: A conceptual framework. *Oncology (Huntingt)* 11(11A):25–32.

Wooldridge JE, Link BK. 2003. Post-treatment surveillance of patients with lymphoma treated with curative intent. *Semin Oncol* 30(3):375–381.

Woolf SH. 1992. Practice guidelines, a new reality in medicine. Methods of developing guidelines. *Arch Intern Med* 152(5):946–952.

Woolf SH. 2000. Evidence-based medicine and practice guidelines: An overview. *Cancer Control* 7(4):362–367.

Woolf SH, Grol R, Hutchinson A, Eccles M, Grimshaw J. 1999. Clinical guidelines: Potential benefits, limitations, and harms of clinical guidelines. *BMJ* 318(7182):527–530.

Wyatt GE, Desmond KA, Ganz PA, Rowland JH, Ashing-Giwa K, Meyerowitz BE. 1998. Sexual functioning and intimacy in African American and white breast cancer survivors: A descriptive study. *Women's Health* 4(4):385–405.

Yao SL, Dipaola RS. 2003. An evidence-based approach to prostate cancer follow-up. *Semin Oncol* 30(3):390–400.

Yeh ET, Tong AT, Lenihan DJ, Yusuf SW, Swafford J, Champion C, Durand JB, Gibbs H, Zafarmand AA, Ewer MS. 2004. Cardiovascular complications of cancer therapy: Diagnosis, pathogenesis, and management. *Circulation* 109(25):3122–3131.

Zebrack BJ, Ganz PA, Bernaards CA, Peterson L, Abraham L. 2003. Impact of cancer instrument: A new assessment tool for long-term cancer survivors. *Proceedings of ASCO* 22:531.

Zibecchi L, Greendale GA, Ganz PA. 2003. Continuing education: Comprehensive menopausal assessment: An approach to managing vasomotor and urogenital symptoms in breast cancer survivors. *Oncol Nurs Forum* 30(3):393–407.

4

Delivering Cancer Survivorship Care

Cancer survivorship is a distinct phase of the cancer trajectory, with many opportunities to intervene to improve care. The current system for delivering care to the growing number of cancer survivors is inadequate. This chapter begins with a description of the attributes of an ideal follow-up system that would meet the needs of individuals surviving their cancer. Next, the gap between this ideal system and the current health care delivery system is illustrated in terms of problems faced by survivors in obtaining care and by providers in delivering care. Barriers that patients face in receiving appropriate care include a fragmented and poorly coordinated health care system, an absence of a locus of responsibility for follow-up care, and a lack of guidance on how cancer survivors can maximize their own health outcomes. Barriers that health care providers face in delivering care include not having necessary tools to provide consistent quality care, such as evidence-based clinical practice guidelines. Providers also lack delivery system supports such as information technology that would allow them to overcome some of the obstacles posed by the fragmented nature of cancer care in the United States. The chapter next reviews alternative models for delivering survivorship care. Survivorship clinics are being developed at a few cancer centers to meet the long-term needs of cancer survivors, but other promising models for delivering survivorship care are emerging and are examined. A description of the U.S. cancer care infrastructure is then described, highlighting existing programs to meet the needs of cancer survivors. Finally, the chapter puts forward steps that could be taken to implement the envisioned cancer survivorship system of care. Issues related to provider education and training are covered in Chapter 5. Overriding problems in accessing care due to a lack of health insurance coverage and inadequate insurance coverage are described in Chapter 6.

OPTIMAL CANCER SURVIVORSHIP CARE

For years cancer survivors have voiced concerns about access to appropriate services following their primary treatment. A decade ago, the National Coalition for Cancer Survivorship promulgated 12 principles that it believed were imperatives for quality cancer care (NCCS, 1996). Two of the principles relate to the delivery of care to cancer survivors:

- "People with histories of cancer have the right to continued medical follow-up with basic standards of care that include the specific needs of long-term survivors." (Principle 6)
- "Long-term survivors should have access to specialized follow-up clinics that focus on health promotion, disease prevention, rehabilitation, and identification of physiologic and psychological problems. Communication with the primary care physician must be maintained." (Principle 7)

The committee agreed with the underlying premise of these principles—that an organized system of care is needed to ensure the provision of survivorship care. In its deliberations, the committee sought a clear definition of the essential components of survivorship care and examples of delivery models that could be adopted throughout the nation in communities with varying characteristics and needs. The committee, following its review of the post-treatment clinical and psychosocial needs of cancer survivors, concluded that survivorship care represents a distinct phase of the cancer care trajectory. In its effort to better define this phase of care, the committee addressed key questions concerning the content of survivorship care, its recipients, and attributes of a system of care for this population.

What Are the Essential Components of Survivorship Care?

Survivorship care includes four components: (1) prevention and detection of new cancers and recurrent cancer; (2) surveillance for cancer spread, recurrence, or second cancers; (3) intervention for consequences of cancer and its treatment (e.g., medical problems such as lymphedema and sexual dysfunction; symptoms, including pain and fatigue; psychological distress experienced by cancer survivors and their caregivers; and concerns related to employment and insurance); and (4) coordination between specialists and primary care providers to ensure that all of the survivor's health needs are met (e.g., health promotion, immunizations, screening for both cancer and noncancerous conditions, and the care of concurrent conditions).

Essential to survivorship care is a patient-centered approach, including responsiveness to patients' needs, effective communication and information sharing, encouragement of the adoption of healthy lifestyles, and assistance in accessing community support services. Survivorship care has a focus on prevention—identifying treatable cancer recurrences, second cancers, and late effects; ensuring access to effective interventions; and helping patients to improve their quality of life.

Who Should Receive Survivorship Care?

Every individual should receive survivorship care following their treatment. The need for specific services will vary from survivor to survivor because of the heterogeneity of cancer and late effects. Survivors of early-stage cancer whose treatment was limited to surgery may require minimal follow-up care. In contrast, survivors with more advanced disease treated with combinations of surgery, chemotherapy, radiation, and hormone therapies may need long-term rehabilitative and supportive care. Some individuals treated for a predisposition to cancer (e.g., those who have genetic mutations, such as BRCA mutations) may also benefit from survivorship care.

When Does Survivorship Care Start and End?

An organized plan for survivorship care should be developed by the time primary treatment ends.[1] Discussions of long-term effects of cancer and its treatment often begin at the time when treatment decisions are made. Later in the course of care, discussion of a survivorship care plan can provide hope and practical guidance. The transition from primary treatment into survivorship care is not always clear cut because some individuals require ongoing treatment such as adjuvant therapy. The committee viewed this period of adjuvant therapy as within the spectrum of survivorship care. Survivorship care lasts until recurrence, a second cancer, or death. Individuals who experience a recurrence or second cancer may reenter the acute phase of care for a time and then resume survivorship care. Individuals with chronic or intermittent disease may receive ongoing treatment for their disease, but benefit from survivorship care as they live with their disease (Figure 4-1). These individuals are generally under the long-term care of an oncology provider who can help ensure that survivorship needs are met. Some individuals who cease treatment prematurely may not benefit from a care plan if they are not formally discharged from care.

---

[1]Primary treatment is the first course of therapy provided with the intention to cure cancer.

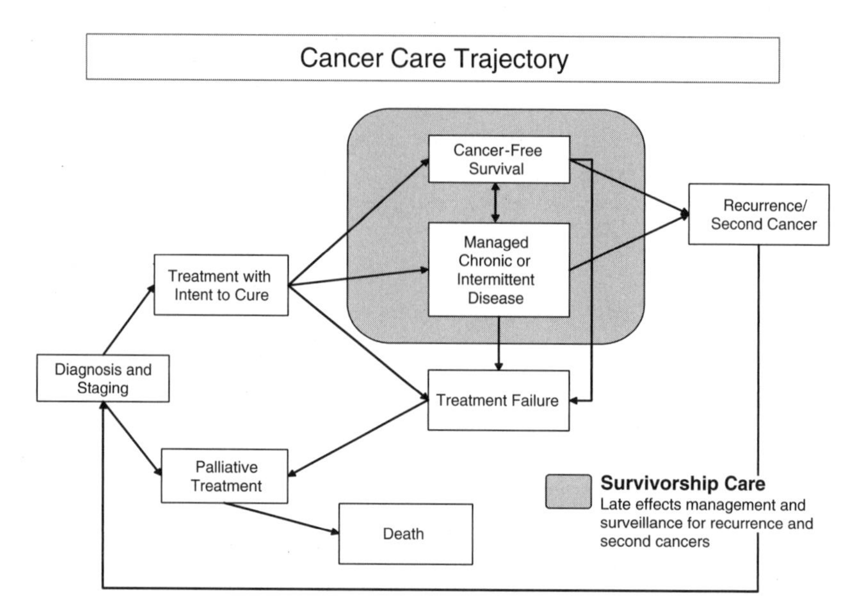

FIGURE 4-1 Cancer care trajectory.
NOTE: Palliative care is provided throughout the cancer care trajectory.

Who Should Provide Survivorship Care?

Survivorship care can be provided by either specialists or primary care providers. These providers can come from various care backgrounds—physicians, nurses, psychologists, and social workers—but optimally a designated individual is responsible for coordinating survivorship care, and care is viewed as a shared responsibility. Cancer survivors should be informed care partners, but providers within the health care system must take primary responsibility for coordinating care.

How Should Survivorship Care Be Provided?

Different models can be used to deliver optimal cancer survivorship care (see discussion below). Information technology, electronic medical records, and other health care delivery support systems can facilitate the delivery of integrated, coordinated, and multidisciplinary survivorship care. Survivorship care should embody rules set forth by the Institute of Medicine's (IOM's) Committee on Health Care Quality in America in its report *Crossing the Quality Chasm* (Box 4-1).

Receipt of optimal survivorship care depends on a patient-centered

BOX 4-1
Recommendation from the Institute of Medicine Committee on Health Care Quality in America

Recommendation: Private and public purchasers, health care organizations, clinicians, and patients should work together to redesign health care processes in accordance with the following rules:

1. **Care based on continuous healing relationships.** Patients should receive care whenever they need it and in many forms, not just face-to-face visits. This rule implies that the health care system should be responsive at all times (24 hours a day, every day) and that access to care should be provided over the Internet, by telephone, and by other means in addition to face-to-face visits.

2. **Customization based on patient needs and values.** The system of care should be designed to meet the most common types of needs, but have the capability to respond to individual patient choices and preferences.

3. **The patient as the source of control.** Patients should be given the necessary information and the opportunity to exercise the degree of control they choose over health care decisions that affect them. The health system should be able to accommodate differences in patient preferences and encourage shared decision making.

4. **Shared knowledge and the free flow of information.** Patients should have unfettered access to their own medical information and to clinical knowledge. Clinicians and patients should communicate effectively and share information.

5. **Evidence-based decision making.** Patients should receive care based on the best available scientific knowledge. Care should not vary illogically from clinician to clinician or from place to place.

6. **Safety as a system property.** Patients should be safe from injury caused by the care system. Reducing risk and ensuring safety require greater attention to systems that help prevent and mitigate errors.

7. **The need for transparency.** The health care system should make information available to patients and their families that allows them to make informed decisions when selecting a health plan, hospital, or clinical practice, or when choosing among alternative treatments. This should include information describing the system's performance on safety, evidence-based practice, and patient satisfaction.

8. **Anticipation of needs.** The health system should anticipate patient needs, rather than simply reacting to events.

9. **Continuous decrease in waste.** The health system should not waste resources or patient time.

10. **Cooperation among clinicians**. Clinicians and institutions should actively collaborate and communicate to ensure an appropriate exchange of information and coordination of care.

SOURCE: IOM (2001).

approach in which care is structured around the needs and preferences of patients themselves (Berry et al., 2003). A call for such an approach has been made by physician-researchers William Tierney and Elizabeth McKinley in their description of their cancer experience from the patient's perspective (Tierney and McKinley, 2002):

> Providers must try to understand the impact of cancer on their patients' lives and the lives of their patients' caregivers. They should focus on both the negative and positive effects of cancer and its treatment, and be as energetic and considerate in treating the cancer patient (and hopefully, survivor) as they are in treating the cancer itself.

BARRIERS TO OPTIMAL CANCER SURVIVORSHIP CARE

Cancer survivors now generally receive some kind of follow-up, either from their cancer care specialist or primary care physician, but the focus of care has usually been on surveillance for recurrence and second cancers, not on the other key elements of care identified above. What barriers impede the delivery of optimal survivorship care? As this phase of care has only recently gained wide public attention, there is relatively little experience and research on how to deliver comprehensive and multidisciplinary survivorship care. This section of the chapter reviews significant barriers that both cancer survivors and their caregivers face in achieving satisfactory survivorship care.

Barriers Facing Cancer Survivors

Fragmented Delivery System

Individuals with chronic conditions face many obstacles in obtaining medical care that meets their needs for effective clinical management, psychological support, and information (Wagner et al., 2001). Cancer survivors, like other individuals with chronic conditions, face a common set of challenges—dealing with symptoms, disability, emotional upheaval, complex medication regimens, difficult lifestyle adjustments, and the need to obtain helpful medical care. While in treatment, cancer patients often see multiple specialists—surgeons, medical oncologists, and radiation oncologists—in addition to their primary care provider. Assuring coordinated, multidisciplinary care for primary treatment can be difficult and may affect access to subsequent survivorship care. It is generally the primary treatment specialist who informs survivors of their need for long-term follow-up, but continuity of that care is not always assured. A focus on continuity of care is central to quality of care throughout the cancer care trajectory, including survivorship. The concept of continuity of care in oncology has been defined as:

> The systematic assurance of uninterrupted, integrated medical and psychosocial care of the patient, in accord with the patient's wishes, from assessment of symptoms in the prediagnostic period, throughout the phase of active treatment, and for the duration of posttreatment monitoring and/or palliative care. (Lauria, 1991)

When the systems responsible for coordinating individuals' cancer care have been evaluated, they have often come up short. A qualitative study of mechanisms present within several New York hospitals to coordinate care for women with early breast cancer found that no site had the ability to systematically track care provided by multiple specialists (Bickell and Young, 2001). Mechanisms that hospitals relied on included tracking of referrals, patient support such as education and navigator programs, regularly scheduled multidisciplinary meetings, feedback of performance data, use of protocols, computerized systems, and a single physical location for care.

One consequence of poorly coordinated care is poor-quality care. Cancer survivors may not receive necessary noncancer care if their cancer diagnosis shifts attention away from care that is routine but necessary. Colorectal cancer survivors in one study were less likely than controls to receive appropriate follow-up for heart failure, necessary diabetic care, and recommended preventive services (Earle and Neville, 2004). Having both primary care physicians and oncologists involved in follow-up appeared to ameliorate this effect significantly, suggesting that a collaborative approach to follow-up is needed. This study focused on the care experience of Medicare beneficiaries who had survived 5 years past their diagnosis of colorectal cancer. In contrast to the findings in this study, breast cancer survivors received more preventive services (i.e., influenza vaccination, blood lipid testing, cervical and colon cancer screening, bone densitometry for osteoporosis) than controls in a similar study of Medicare beneficiaries (Earle et al., 2003). Breast cancer survivors who were followed by oncology specialists were more likely to receive mammograms; those who were followed by primary care physicians were more likely to receive all other noncancer-related preventive services; and those who saw both types of practitioners received more of both types of services. Both studies point to the importance of care that is coordinated and involves both primary and specialty providers.

Evidence from studies of surveillance practices in the United States suggests that follow-up care is not being provided as guidelines recommend (Johnson and Virgo, 1997) (see Appendix 4A for a summary of relevant studies). Rates of follow-up are not uniformly high for patients with a history of breast cancer with annual mammography (Hillner et al., 1997; Andersen and Urban, 1998; Schapira et al., 2000; Lash and Silliman, 2001; Geller et al., 2003), for patients with a history of colorectal cancer with colorectal examinations (Cooper et al., 1999, 2000; Elston Lafata et al., 2001, 2005; Knopf et al., 2001; Ellison et al., 2003; Rulyak et al., 2004), and for patients with a history of bladder cancer with cystoscopy (Schrag et al., 2003). When examined, racial/ethnic and income differences usually account for significant variation in surveillance practices. The use of testing for metastatic disease that is not recommneded in guidelines has been found to be commonplace among cancer survivors (Elston Lafata et al., 2005). Adherence to adjuvant tamoxifen therapy among women with breast cancer is not uniformly high, with some studies finding nearly one-fourth of patients at risk for inadequate clinical response because of poor adherence (Demissie et al., 2001; Partridge et al., 2003; Fink et al., 2004). Evidence also suggests that the psychosocial needs of cancer patients are not being addressed. For example, oncologists often underdiagnose depression and fail to refer patients to mental health services (Passik et al., 1998; Fallowfield et al., 2001; Eakin and Strycker, 2001; Ell et al., 2005). Reports of unmet mental health needs because of cost have been reported to be significantly higher among cancer survivors relative to those without such a history (Hewitt and Rowland, 2002).

Optimal survivorship care is characterized by an organized plan for follow-up that is shared with patients so they can take responsibility for their care. There has been little research in the United States on the extent to which such plans are developed or communicated to patients. One Canadian study found that more than a third of cancer survivors surveyed after completion of treatment were not sure which physician was in charge of their cancer follow-up care (Miedema et al., 2003). This study relied on an unrepresentative sample of cancer survivors and so may not be generalizable to the broader population.

Relatively little is known of cancer survivors' desires and perspectives regarding follow-up. Interviews conducted in England with breast cancer survivors on their views of routine follow-up indicated that women wanted, but were not receiving, continuity of care and an unrushed consultation (Adewuyi-Dalton et al., 1998).

A management model has emerged to guide the redesign of delivery systems and to improve care for individuals with chronic conditions. Six elements of the model are relevant to cancer survivorship care (Improving Chronic Illness Care, 2004):

1. Mobilize community resources to meet needs of patients.
2. Create a culture, organization, and mechanisms that promote safe, high-quality care.

3. Empower and prepare patients to manage their health and health care.
4. Assure the delivery of effective, efficient clinical care and self-management support.
5. Promote clinical care that is consistent with scientific evidence and patient preferences.
6. Organize patient and population data to facilitate efficient and effective care.

The chronic disease model has been implemented in primary care practices to improve care for individuals with diabetes, asthma, and congestive heart failure and has had some success in terms of improved outcome measures and reduced health care costs (Bodenheimer et al., 2002a,b). The Centers for Medicare and Medicaid Services (CMS) has supported several demonstration programs to improve care coordination and disease management in Medicare (MedPAC, 2004b). The Medicare Coordinated Care Demonstration, for example, is testing models of coordinated care to improve quality of services and manage Medicare expenditures at 15 sites, with 1 site focused on cancer care (CMS, 2004). The cancer care coordination project provides Medicare beneficiaries in South Florida with an oncology nurse advocate to help them understand their disease and better manage the side effects and symptoms of cancer and its treatment (Quality Oncology Inc., 2003).

Improvements in cancer care coordination could also come from initiatives aimed at improving care for the chronically ill. For example, the Academic Chronic Care Collaborative, an initiative of the American Association of Medical Colleges Institute for Improving Clinical Care, has been launched in partnership with the Robert Wood Johnson Foundation's national chronic illness care program. The collaborative involves 22 academic medical centers that will undergo extensive redesign of their chronic care strategies (AAMC, 2005).

The complexities of the health care system can be particularly daunting for those whose language is not English, who are uninsured, who reside in a rural area, or who have other difficulties in accessing care. One mechanism that is being evaluated to reduce cancer health disparities is "Patient Navigation" (Freeman and Clanton, 2004). A patient navigator is a trained patient advocate and guide who helps individuals and their families navigate their way through the maze of doctors' offices, clinics, hospitals, outpatient centers, insurance and payment systems, patient support organizations, and other components of the health care system (NCI, 2004). Navigation services include: facilitating communication and information exchange for patients; coordinating care among medical service providers; and arranging for financial support, transportation, or child care services.

Lack of Awareness of the Late Effects of Cancer and Its Treatment

A prerequisite to obtaining appropriate cancer follow-up care is an awareness of one's increased risk and knowledge of what should be done to reduce risk or ameliorate adverse outcomes. Late effects that are known to be associated with cancer treatments may be discussed in the context of making treatment decisions and obtaining informed consent. Given the stressful nature of this phase of care, cancer patients may have difficulty retaining the information. Patients do not routinely receive a summary of their treatments or possible late effects. Cancer survivors are beginning to be informed about what to expect after treatment through the efforts of patient advocacy organizations. For example, the American Cancer Society (ACS) has provided information on "What Happens After Treatment" for most cancer types (ACS, 2005a) and the Lance Armstrong Foundation has provided a guide to help survivors summarize their medical treatment and plan for follow-up care (LAF, 2004a). A few studies have assessed adult cancer survivors' awareness of their increased risk and need for follow-up:

- Female adult survivors of Hodgkin's disease treated at a young age with mantle irradiation are at high risk for subsequent cancer, but only 47 percent reported having had a mammogram in the past 2 years (Diller et al., 2002). As many as 40 percent of women were unaware of their increased risk.
- Breast cancer survivors report knowing little about lymphedema before developing it, and physicians report not routinely counseling women or providing written information on lymphedema prevention to their patients with breast cancer (Paskett and Stark, 2000).
- Only about half of men and women with cancer who are of child-bearing age receive timely information from their health care providers about their risk of infertility and options to preserve or restore fertility (Canada and Schover, 2005).
- Breast cancer survivors often do not recall discussing the reproductive health impact of their treatment, and many report that their concerns are not adequately addressed (Partridge et al., 2004; Duffy et al., 2005).
- Relatively few (22 percent) survivors of colorectal cancer could identify risk indicators for recurrence, but most (64 percent) agreed that they would like to be told what to look for (Papagrigoriadis and Heyman, 2003).

More is known about the awareness of late effects among survivors of childhood cancer. As part of the Childhood Cancer Survivorship Study (CCSS), members of a large cohort of 5-year childhood cancer survivors have been surveyed to learn more about their health status, health care behavior, attitudes, and perceptions. When 635 members of this cohort were asked if past therapies could cause a serious health problem with the passage of time, 35 percent responded affirmatively, 46 percent responded negatively, and 19 percent did not know (Kadan-Lottick et al., 2002). Only 15 percent reported that they had ever received a written statement of their diagnoses and treatments to keep as a reference in the future. To learn more about the experiences of survivors of adult cancer, a large cohort study, similar in design to the CCSS, could be initiated (see details of its design in Chapter 7).

Barriers to Communication

Some research suggests there is a disjuncture between patients' expectations and physicians' perceptions of cancer follow-up. Most women being followed after breast cancer treatment want to be asked about nutrition, pain, and emotional/family problems, but relatively few want to be asked about sexual problems, according to an American study of patients' expectations of follow-up visits and perceptions of the value of follow-up tests and examinations. Women in this study overestimated the value of laboratory and imaging studies and underestimated the value of the medical history and physical examination (Muss et al., 1991). Studies conducted among European cancer survivors indicate that information on long-term effects of treatment and prognosis, prevention of cancer, and hereditary factors was desired, as was access to cancer expertise, diagnostic tests, and specialist facilities (Adewuyi-Dalton et al., 1998; de Bock et al., 2004).

Anticipation of a follow-up visit can engender anxiety, and providers must balance providing realistic information with remaining hopeful and reassuring. In one British study of asymptomatic and disease-free survivors' views on follow-up of colorectal cancer, anticipation of the follow-up appointment caused anxiety (35 percent), sleep problems (27 percent), and decreased appetite (8 percent) (Papagrigoriadis and Heyman, 2003). Most patients (78 percent), however, felt reassured and optimistic for the future after receiving results of tests performed at their visit. This finding that follow-up clinic visits are generally perceived as reassuring has been found in other research (Kiebert et al., 1993; GIVIO, 1994; Stiggelbout et al., 1997).

When cancer survivors seek follow-up care, all components of survivorship care may not be addressed. In a study of follow-up care for women with breast cancer in England, for example, visits were focused on detection of recurrent disease by clinical examination, but little attention was paid to patient education and psychosocial needs (Beaver and Luker, 2004). There is anecdotal evidence for this same pattern of care in the United States. One recent unscientific poll of cancer survivors found that nearly half (49 percent) felt their psychosocial needs were not being met by the health care system (LAF, 2004b). Cancer survivors expressed dissatisfaction with their oncologist's provision of support in dealing with the secondary aspects of cancer, such as depression, fear of recurrence, chronic pain, ongoing health challenges, infertility, sexual dysfunction, difficulty with relationships, and financial or job insecurity.

As part of a major effort to gauge cancer patients' experience with cancer within the British National Health System, a nationwide survey was conducted in 2000 (Airey et al., 2002).[2] Dissatisfaction with some aspects of post-treatment care mirror those identified in the United States. Nearly one in five (19 percent) survivors reported that doctors and nurses did not spend enough time, or spent no time at all, telling them what would happen when they left the hospital after their first treatment; 26 percent reported not being given written or printed information about what they should or shouldn't do following their discharge; and 36 percent reported not being told about a support or self-help group. Results of surveys were made available to each group of cancer care providers so they could compare their results with other providers and make efforts to improve care.

Relatively little is known about the content of follow-up care provided in the United States. According to national surveys of ambulatory care, relatively little counseling takes place during cancer-related visits.[3] Among cancer-related visits made by individuals who use tobacco, for example, physicians report smoking cessation counseling or referral during only 18 percent of visits (Table 4-1). Guidelines for smoking cessation recommend routinely counseling individuals who smoke (USPSTF, 2003). These estimates are for all cancer-related visits and would include visits for both primary treatment and survivorship care.[4]

Barriers to communication are compounded for the 90 million American adults who lack the needed literacy skills to effectively use the U.S. health system (IOM, 2004a). The problem of limited health literacy is often greater among older adults, people with limited education, and those with limited English proficiency. For individuals whose native language is not

---

[2]Nearly three-quarters (74 percent) of patients identified through hospital records responded to the survey. See Appendix 4C for more information on the survey and how it has been used to redesign cancer care systems.

[3]See Appendix 4B for details of the ambulatory care surveys and their analysis.

[4]A limitation of these estimates is the underreporting by physicians on the delivery of health behavior counseling. There was only fair to moderate agreement among physician reports on the provision of counseling on smoking, exercise, and diet and directly observed physician behaviors during clinical visits. Reporting by physicians of procedures and tests is more accurate (Gilchrist et al., 2004).

TABLE 4-1 The Provision of Counseling During Adult Cancer-Related Ambulatory Care Visits, United States, 2001–2002[a]

Characteristic	Total
Annual number of visits (in 1,000s)	20,574
Services ordered or provided (% yes)	
Mental health or psychotherapy	4
Diet counseling/education	11
Exercise counseling/education	6
Smoking cessation	2
Smoking cessation for visits made by patients who used tobacco (9% of visits made by tobacco users)	18

[a]Adults were categorized as being aged 25 and older. Visits for non-melanoma skin cancer were excluded. Radiologists were excluded from the sample of office-based physicians. Clinics providing chemotherapy, radiotherapy, physical medicine, and rehabilitation were excluded from the sample of hospital out-patient departments.
SOURCE: Committee staff analyses of the 2001 and 2002 National Ambulatory Medical Care Survey and the National Hospital Ambulatory Medical Care Survey. See Appendix 4B for details of analyses.

English, issues of health literacy are compounded by issues of basic communication and the specialized vocabulary used to convey health information. In addition, communication barriers may arise that relate to sociocultural differences between survivors and their health care providers (IOM, 2002). These differences may relate to commonly held attitudes, norms, beliefs, and practices for those with certain life experiences (e.g., poverty, membership in a racial or ethnic minority group) or environments (e.g., communities with poor access to health care services).

In summary, there is a limited amount of research regarding cancer survivors' expectations and experience with their care following primary treatment. Available evidence points to systemic problems in health care delivery that in some cases lead to poor-quality care, such as underuse of post-treatment screening for cancer. When evaluated, problems in survivorship care appear to stem from a lack of coordination between primary care providers and cancer care providers. There is anecdotal evidence of general dissatisfaction with post-treatment care, with cancer survivors reporting too little attention being paid to their many psychosocial concerns, such as depression, fear of recurrence, sexual dysfunction, and financial issues. Why the expectations of cancer survivors are not being met is not clear, but factors that could be at play include a lack of recognition of the value of these aspects of care, the presence of communication barriers, and a lack of delineation of responsibility on the part of providers to address these concerns. There is little information regarding the difficulties survivors may have in communication that are related to low literacy levels and to sociocultural factors.

Barriers Facing Providers

Health care providers face many of the same problems as cancer survivors in dealing with a fragmented system of care. Providers are also hampered in their provision of survivorship care by a lack of training on survivorship and an absence of agreed-upon standards of survivorship care. Such standards are essential to ensuring the delivery of the full complement of services that cancer survivors may need (see discussion of guidelines in Chapter 3). Furthermore, without agreed-upon practice guidelines for care, reimbursement for care can be problematic. Communication issues are also a major challenge to those providing and coordinating survivorship care because individuals with cancer often have multiple providers at different sites of care. Compounding these problems are concerns about the capacity of the primary care and oncology care systems to accommodate the follow-up needs of the large and growing population of cancer survivors.

Fragmented Delivery System Hampers Delivery of Coordinated Care

The fragmented nature of the U.S. health care system hampers the delivery of coordinated survivorship care. Providing such care is a challenge because cancer care is delivered by multiple providers over extended periods of time and through multiple phases of illness. These providers often wish to provide coordinated care, but usually do not work within systems of care that facilitate its delivery. The goal of care coordination is to establish and support a continuous healing relationship, enabled by an integrated clinical environment and characterized by the proactive delivery of evidence-based care and follow-up (IOM, 2001). Clinical integration is further defined as the extent to which patient care services are coordinated across people, functions, activities, and sites over time so as to maximize the value of services delivered to patients. Coordination encompasses a set of practitioner behaviors and information systems intended to bring together health services, patient needs, and streams of information to facilitate the delivery of quality care. Such coordination can be facilitated by procedures for engaging community resources, including social and public health services.

Key strategies that enhance care coordination are often lacking. These include: providing educational supports; instituting patient-centered health records supported by modern information technology; ensuring accountability and defining roles for providers of care; and aligning financial incentives to ensure the delivery of coordinated care (IOM, 2001). The extent to which these strategies operate for providers of survivorship care are described in the following sections.

Lack of Education and Training

Often physicians, nurses, and other providers of cancer survivorship care have not had optimal relevant formal education, training, and continuing medical education. The status of education and training for physicians, nurses, social workers, and other providers of survivorship care is detailed in Chapter 5. The recognition of cancer survivorship as a phase of care associated with an extensive set of management issues is relatively new. Educational and training opportunities are likely to increase as a consensus is reached regarding the content of such care and its delivery, but for now the notion of cancer survivorship as a distinct clinical entity is not prevalent in the provider community. In addition to their lack to education and training regarding cancer survivorship, health care providers report being ill-equipped and -trained to manage the care of patients with chronic conditions. According to one survey conducted in 2000 and 2001, practicing physicians reported that their training did not adequately prepare them to coordinate in-home and community services (66 percent), educate patients with chronic conditions (66 percent), or manage the psychological and social aspects of chronic care (64 percent) (Partnership for Solutions, 2002).

Lack of Survivorship Standards of Care

Health care providers, before being held accountable for providing quality care, need to have clear evidence-based guidance. As described in Chapter 3, such guidance for survivorship care exists for some aspects of care, but it is not readily available to clinicians.[5] There are practice guidelines for the follow-up of breast and colorectal cancer, but the focus of the guidelines is generally limited to detecting recurrences and second cancers. There are also guidelines for the management of certain late effects (e.g., lymphedema, osteoporosis, depression), but these have not been widely disseminated to the primary care clinicians most likely to encounter patients presenting with these symptoms. For many aspects of survivorship care—for example, health promotion (exercise and healthy diet)—clear

[5] As described in Chapter 3, a comprehensive set of guidelines has been developed by the Children's Oncology Group for survivors of childhood, adolescent, and young adult cancers (Landier et al., 2004).

guidance is not available. For most types of cancer, the research needed to support such guidelines has not been conducted, but assembling that information is critical to informing clinicians and patients on appropriate post-treatment care. Clinical guidelines can also help avoid unnecessary and expensive care, and without them physicians may be under considerable pressure from patients to provide follow-up tests (Loprinzi et al., 2000). Without established guidelines, follow-up practices and expenditures have been shown to vary widely (Virgo et al., 1995; Johnson and Virgo, 1997).

Although guidelines for most aspects of survivorship care are lacking, providers are not following the guidelines that are available. This general phenomenon in medicine (Mendelson and Carino, 2005; Timmermans and Mauck, 2005) is apparent in survivorship care as well. For example, adherence to post-treatment surveillance guidelines is not uniformly high; depression is not routinely assessed; patients complete their primary treatment without knowing about their risks of late effects such as lymphedema; and individuals are not apprised of the implications of their cancer history to employment and health insurance (see Appendix 4A for a summary of studies of U.S. surveillance practice patterns).

Ultimately, health care quality measures will be developed to monitor quality problems in survivorship care. There are three types of quality problems in health care: too little care; too much care; and the wrong care (IOM, 1998). Too little care (underuse) is when patients do not receive evidence-based care. Too much care (overuse) is when patients receive unnecessary health care services that may cause side effects or pose other health risks. The wrong care (misuse) is when diagnoses are missed or delayed, ineffective treatments are used, effective procedures are done poorly, or errors are made. A framework has been created for identifying measures of quality for cancer care (McGlynn, 2002; McGlynn and Malin, 2002). Some quality measures have already been developed (Schachter et al., 2004; AHRQ, 2004a; Greenberg et al., 2005; IOM, 2005) or are under review (NQF, 2005). Few of the measures identified thus far are directly related to survivorship care. Some potential quality of care measures relevant to cancer survivorship are shown in Box 4-2. Such measures, if found to be clinically important, evidence based, practical to measure, and meaningful to providers and patients, could facilitate improvements in care.

The use of quality of care measures has a dual purpose: evaluating progress and motivating change (IOM, 2005). Monitoring systems may help to assess progress according to a particular set of indicators, but may also motivate change though a new focus on processes of care and outcomes. Quality of care measures for other chronic conditions such as diabetes have been developed through public/private partnerships and adopted by health systems to improve care (National Diabetes Quality Improvement Alliance, 2005).

BOX 4-2
Potential Survivorship Quality of Care Measures

Processes of care

- Provision of a survivorship care plan, a written post-treatment summary outlining the proposed follow-up plan
- Assessment of psychosocial distress, referral to mental health providers
- Assessment of employment, insurance, and financial issues, referral to rehabilitation and social work providers
- Provision of written information on available community support services

Screening guidelines

- Adherence to evidence-based follow-up and surveillance guidelines, where available (e.g., annual mammography for breast cancer survivors; nonroutine use of inappropriate follow-up scans and tests for breast cancer; follow-up colonoscopy for colorectal cancer survivors)

Survivorship interventions

- Adherence to adjuvant therapy (e.g., hormonal therapy for breast cancer)
- Assessment and management of pain
- When appropriate, referral to enterostomal care
- When appropriate, referral for lymphedema management
- When appropriate, assessment of sexual function and referral to sexuality counseling
- When appropriate, referral to genetic counseling
- Recommendation of exercise for fatigue
- Smoking cessation counseling, if necessary

Survivor assessments of care

- Ratings by survivors of their satisfaction with care, coordination of care, and quality of care

When quality measures for survivorship care are developed and then adopted by health systems, office supports such as computerized reminder systems, the involvement of nonphysician providers in care, and standing orders for screening tests that have been shown to be effective in promoting preventive health services will likely also prove useful in prompting the delivery of appropriate survivorship care (IOM, 2003b).

Difficulties in Communication

Communication issues are a major challenge to those providing and coordinating survivorship care because individuals with cancer often have multiple providers at different sites of care. Discharge plans that are clear to the oncologist may not be clear to the primary care provider. The migration of patients across health plans and the geographic movement that characterizes contemporary mobile society create a turnover in health providers. Large separations of time are characteristic of survivorship care, which can extend over a period of decades. Clinicians unfamiliar with the patient's medical history may have difficulty in determining the names of the original doctors or health care institutions or in obtaining documentation of the cancer diagnosis and treatment regimen.

Relatively few health care providers have access to information systems and electronic medical records that would facilitate communication regarding survivorship care (Burt and Hing, 2005; Berner et al., 2005; Ash and Bates, 2005). According to a survey of U.S. physicians in 2003, only 7 percent said they routinely use e-mail to communicate with other doctors, and only 27 percent used electronic medical records (Audet et al., 2004). Perceived barriers to the adoption of information technology included the costs of system start-up and maintenance, lack of standards, and lack of time to consider acquiring, implementing, and using a new system. The investigators concluded that widespread adoption of information technology in health care would require federal leadership, potentially in the form of federal grants, increased physician reimbursement, and loans. A 2004 health information technology initiative, if fully implemented, would further the adoption of these communication tools (Thompson and Brailer, 2004). As part of this effort, a strategic framework for action has been developed to inform clinical practice, interconnect clinicians, personalize care, and improve population health. Although these developments are encouraging, improvements in information technology and adoption of electronic medical records must be viewed as enabling technologies. Improvements in the quality and coordination of care will require investments in medical practice support systems, financial rewards for quality improvement, and improved information technology infrastructure (Miller and Sim, 2004).

There are a few examples of technological innovation to improve communication between primary care providers and cancer specialists. An interactive Internet resource, Passport for Care, is being developed for survivors of childhood cancer. Elements of the website include: a guidelines generator that dynamically assembles recommendations for care individualized to each survivor according to his or her treatment history;[6] an end-of-treatment summary, completed by the treating institution and available

[6]Comprehensive guidelines for survivors of childhood cancer are available through the Children's Oncology Group (Children's Oncology Group, 2005).

to the survivor, that can be securely shared with providers at the direction of the survivors; individualized survivor education resources that are customized to the needs of each patient based on his/her disease and its treatment (and accessible to the survivor's health care provider); an online survivor forum; and a section for survivor news and stories (Personal communication, M. Horowitz, Baylor College of Medicine, February 23, 2005). Once completed and evaluated, it is planned to encompass adult cancer survivors as well. Another initiative is the Cancer Survivor Virtual Information Center, a website with information for cancer survivors and their physicians. It is undergoing a pilot feasibility study targeting survivors of childhood Hodgkin's lymphoma (Personal communication, K. Oeffinger, University of Texas–Southwestern, June 24, 2004). The website contains information about survivorship, but does not provide specific information about individual patients. As part of a Patient Gateway initiative at Partners HealthCare, a web-based information system is being piloted in oncology to enhance care coordination across multiple practices, including medical oncology, radiation oncology, and primary care (Personal communication, J. Wald, Partners HealthCare, March 22, 2005).

The Improving Cancer Care in Massachusetts (CAMA) project, sponsored by the Dana-Farber/Harvard Cancer Center, aims to improve cancer treatment in Massachusetts through the use of more efficient and timely data on cancer care quality (Ayanian, 2004). The CAMA investigators plan to assess the feasibility of a personal health record that integrates care information from multiple care sites. The plan is to give patients web-based access to relevant information from their medical records, and enable them to share information with their clinicians. The CAMA system would give clinicians more complete and timely medical information on their patients, including information from other care sites.

In Europe, a few systems are already in place. One hospital in Italy has, with cancer patients' consent, made information about cancer care available to each patient's primary care physician through a protected website (Personal communication, F. Testore, Head of Oncology Division, Ospedale Civile di Asti, Asti, Italy, November 22, 2004). Community-based physicians can also send e-mail requests to specialists through this system to get information about their patients. In a similar fashion, a secure ONCONET system has been established in the German federal state of Saxony-Anhalt to facilitate the shared care of cancer patients (Blobel, 2000). The system aids communication among 57 clinics and more than 160 general practitioners involved in oncology. The system includes an electronic health care record, scheduling functions, and the creation of doctor's reports. It also supports research activities and quality assurance efforts for cancer care. Many other systems are being developed to improve communication between patients and physicians, such as Internet-based tools. Such systems can be used to send e-mail, view the medical chart, provide health information, and send personalized reminders about care.

Until information technology advances and standard systems are in place to facilitate communications, cancer care providers need to rely on mechanisms at hand, such as a letter from a specialist to a primary care provider detailing the nature of a patient's cancer, a summary of primary treatment, risks of late effects, and a survivorship care plan (see Chapter 3 for more information on individual survivorship care plans). Such a summary and cancer survivorship care plan should also be provided to survivors so they can be alerted to possible late effects, engage in recommended health promotion activities, and actively seek necessary care.

The Capacity for Delivering Survivorship Care

Both oncologists and primary care providers want to provide follow-up care to cancer patients after their treatment (Bope, 1987; Williams, 1994). However, when survivorship care is delivered, there is often no clear plan or designated responsibility. Some models of care that foster shared care with designated responsibilities are emerging, but these have not been extensively tested (see discussion of alternative models below). The creation of alternative models of delivery is needed to accommodate the growing numbers of cancer survivors.

Primary care clinicians, who manage general health and survivorship needs, must have systems in place to coordinate ongoing care with the work of oncologists and other specialists to provide streamlined attention to cancer-related issues. The primary care system is under tremendous stress, and only innovative models of coordination will serve to accommodate the expanded workload that will come from a growing survivor population.

Handling the cancer-related issues of the survivor population may also become more difficult for oncologists. While surveillance for recurrence, cancer spread, and second cancers is usually the responsibility of oncologists, many of the late effects of cancer are most appropriately managed by other providers such as physiatrists, cardiologists, fertility specialists, and psychologists. Oncologists will need the help of other clinicians to steer patients to the most appropriate specialists and to coordinate the delivery of care. The increasing volume of cancer survivors may also hamper their ability to see new patients. Gauging resource use according to the National Comprehensive Cancer Network (NCCN) guidelines provides one indicator of the magnitude of the problem. If NCCN guidelines are adhered to for breast cancer, a breast cancer survivor would make 10 to 15 visits over the course of 5 years. For colorectal cancer, the recommended number of visits is 14. The NCCN site-specific guidelines only cover issues related to the detection of recurrence and second cancer, not the full complement of survivorship care that the committee recommends. The workload generated for specialists by cancer survivors can be significant. In one study, 210 patients who had achieved a complete or partial remission following treatment for Hodgkin's disease between 1984 and 1990 generated 2,512 outpatient follow-up visits during the follow-up period (Radford et al., 1997). In another study of resource use, 535 women with breast cancer (all stages) made 8,206 follow-up visits during the first 5 years of follow-up (Kaija et al., 1996). With demographic trends predicting a surge in new cancer patients in need of follow-up care, there is an imperative to assess alternative models that will deliver needed services to cancer survivors.

In summary, physicians share some of the same frustrations as cancer survivors in terms of fragmentation of care, poor mechanisms for communication, and a lack of agreement on what constitutes survivorship care and how it should be provided. Of note is the apparent universality of fragmented chronic care, irrespective of delivery system. Such fragmentation in survivorship care is evident in studies carried out in European countries with national health plans (see Appendix 4C). Overcoming fragmentation rests on building an integrated systems approach—getting primary care providers, oncologists, and other care providers to work together as a team, to agree on how to communicate with each other, and to work out streamlined transitions in care.

Facilitating such an integrated system of care are improvements in communication technology. Efforts underway to improve the health care information technology infrastructure will likely help in overcoming problems of fragmentation and enhance chronic care delivery. Innovative applications of the Internet to promote shared care for cancer patients have been implemented in Europe and hold promise in furthering coordination of care. Until such innovations are more widely available, however, the burden of overcoming problems related to fragmentation largely rests with combined efforts of primary care and oncology providers. Office supports such as reminder systems, standing orders for certain screening tests, and standardized letters to primary care providers are among the tools available now. Providers of survivorship care should welcome consideration of new models for delivering this post-treatment care in light of the enormous resource use posed by the expansion of the survivorship population and a more comprehensive definition of what constitutes good survivorship care.

MODELS FOR DELIVERING SURVIVORSHIP CARE

How different follow-up delivery strategies affect health outcomes and costs, perceptions of quality of life, and satisfaction with care is relatively unexplored. Most research in the area has been conducted in the context of breast cancer care. A recent systematic review on the effectiveness of follow-up services concluded that there is insufficient primary empirical evidence on which to draw broad conclusions regarding best practice for breast cancer follow-up in terms of patient involvement in care, reductions in morbidity, and cost-effectiveness of service provision (Collins et al., 2004).

Some promising models of follow-up care have emerged, including a shared-care model that integrates oncology with primary care follow-up, a nurse-led model of care, and specialized multidisciplinary survivorship follow-up clinics. Relatively little is known regarding cancer survivors' preferences for care, but there is a growing recognition of the need for flexible options for survivors who may have different needs and circumstances (Koinberg et al., 2002).

Shared-Care Model of Follow-up Care

Shared care has been defined as "care which applies when the responsibility for the health care of the patient is shared between individuals or teams who are part of separate organizations, or where substantial organizational boundaries exist" (Pritchard and Hughes, 1995). Such a model implies personal communication and organized transfer of knowledge from specialists to primary care practitioners as well as patient involvement (Nielsen et al., 2003). Cancer patients may face several care transitions, for example, from their active treatment phase, to survivorship care, to care for a recurrence, and finally to palliative and end-of-life care. With such transitions, the focus of care can shift toward specialty care or toward primary care. When the shift is toward primary care, a smooth transition is more likely when the primary care physician receives relevant and timely information from cancer specialists (Braun et al., 2003).

Primary care physicians are actively providing cancer-related care according to ambulatory care surveys of U.S. office-based and hospital-based physicians. Of all the cancer-related visits that were made to physicians' offices in 2001 and 2002, nearly one-third (32 percent) were made to primary care physicians (Table 4-2). Relatively fewer such visits were made to oncologists (18 percent). Cancer-related primary care visits were somewhat more common when they were for prostate cancer and lung cancer, which may indicate primary care providers' active role in symptom management, palliative care, and end-of-life care.

The role of the primary care clinician in the shared-care model is to ensure that all of the physical and emotional health needs of the patient are addressed, to assume responsibility for aspects of care of the chronic disease that are feasible in the primary care setting, to refer the patient to specialists for periodic reevaluations and to address issues that require focused expertise, and to consult with specialists on areas of uncertainty. The role of the

TABLE 4-2 Distribution of Adult Ambulatory Cancer Care Visits, by Site of Visit, Physician Specialty, and Clinic Type, United States, 2001–2002[a]

Visit Characteristic	Number/Percentage
Annual number of visits (in 1,000s)	20,574
Site of visits (%)	
Physician's office	89
Hospital outpatient department	11
Physician office visits[b] (%)	
Oncology	18
Primary care	32
General surgery	10
Specialty surgery	3
Dermatology	7
Urology	14
Other medical specialty	15
Hospital outpatient department[c] (%)	
General medicine	78
Surgery	14
Other	8

[a]Adults were categorized as being aged 25 and older. Visits for non-melanoma skin cancer were excluded.

[b]Radiologists were excluded from the sample of office-based physicians.

[c]Clinics providing chemotherapy, radiotherapy, physical medicine, and rehabilitation were excluded from the sample of hospital outpatient departments.

SOURCE: Committee staff analyses of the 2001 and 2002 National Ambulatory Medical Care Survey and the National Hospital Ambulatory Medical Care Survey. See Appendix 4B for details on analyses.

specialist who participates in shared care is to provide guidance and treatment in the area of expertise, to keep the primary care clinician informed of the treatment plan, and to return the patient to the primary care provider for implementation of the treatment plan and for care of other health needs. This model is applicable for many conditions, including when primary care providers share care for the management of chronic heart failure (working with cardiologists), multiple sclerosis (working with neurologists), bipolar disorder (working with psychiatrists), and chronic renal failure (working with nephrologists).

The shared care model depends on the specialist and generalist having a common understanding of expected components of care and respective roles, and works best when providers communicate clearly with each other. Shared care may not be fully understood or practiced. Specialists may

TABLE 4-3 Proportion of Adult Cancer-Related Ambulatory Care Visits for Which Care Was Shared by Other Physicians, by Site of Care, United States, 2001–2002[a]

Characteristic	Total	Physician Office-Based Visits	Hospital Outpatient Department Visits
Annual number of visits (in 1,000s)	20,574	18,311	2,263
Other physicians share care for problem (%)			
Yes	47	46	55
No	41	43	24
Unknown	12	11	20

[a]Adults were categorized as being aged 25 and older. Visits for non-melanoma skin cancer were excluded. Radiologists were excluded from the sample of office-based physicians. Clinics providing chemotherapy, radiotherapy, physical medicine, and rehabilitation were excluded from the sample of hospital outpatient departments.

SOURCE: Committee staff analyses of the 2001 and 2002 National Ambulatory Medical Care Survey and the National Hospital Ambulatory Medical Care Survey. See Appendix 4B for details of analyses.

believe that it is their obligation to follow up on their patients and that patients prefer to see them for their cancer-related care, even when that care could be provided by a primary care physician. They may also question the ability of primary care physicians to handle all components of follow-up care (e.g., detection of recurrence) (Steinberg and Rose, 1996). For their part, primary care physicians may not have been informed by care specialists of the important role they have to play in the ongoing care of cancer survivors. A balance between primary care and specialty care is clearly needed, as evidenced by the research of Earle and colleagues cited above (Earle et al., 2003; Earle and Neville, 2004).

Studies of shared cancer follow-up care in the United States are limited. According to national surveys, U.S. physicians report that care is shared by other physicians for nearly half (47 percent) of cancer-related visits (Table 4-3).[7] Shared care is reported more often by physicians in hospital outpa-

[7]Information is not available on the nature of the shared care described. For example, physicians reporting that other physicians share care for the problem may be referring to sharing care within their own group practice or sharing care with other physicians outside of their practice.

tient departments than by physicians in office-based practices (for 55 versus 46 percent of visits, respectively).

In Europe, Canada, and Australia, several research initiatives have been undertaken to promote shared care (see Appendix 4C). Findings from this research suggest that cancer-related follow-up care can be provided by primary care providers and at lower cost without sacrificing patient satisfaction, but that a minority of patients wish to continue to see specialists for their follow-up care (Grunfeld et al., 1996, 1999a,b). The timely transfer of information from one care sector to another is critical to the concept of shared care. Addressing patient anxiety is also key to a successful transfer from specialty to primary care, and simple strategies, such as discussing plans for follow-up with patients and designing a standardized discharge letter, can ease the transition (Glynne-Jones et al., 1997; Braun et al., 2003). Successful shared-care models depend on professional training; general practitioners viewing their role in cancer care as enhancing patient care and improving their job satisfaction; and appropriate remuneration (Nielsen et al., 2003; Maher and Millar, 2003).

In summary, the shared-care delivery model appears to be especially relevant for the transition from active cancer treatment to survivorship care. U.S. primary care physicians are playing a significant role in cancer care, and nearly half of cancer-related ambulatory visits are characterized as shared care, but with available information it is not clear what the relative roles of specialists and primary care providers are in these settings. Research points to the importance of setting expectations and planning for follow-up early in the care process. Demonstrations and evaluations of shared survivorship care are needed, as are assessments of the shared-care model's effects on resource use and costs.

Nurse-Led Model of Cancer Follow-up Care

Nurses have successfully led comprehensive, long-term follow-up clinics for survivors of childhood cancer throughout the United States (Hobbie and Hollen, 1993; Hollen and Hobbie, 1995; IOM, 2003a). Clinical nurse specialists have also delivered post-treatment oncology care in rural areas (White et al., 1996; Desch et al., 1999), successfully managed cancer symptoms (Given et al., 2002), promoted continuity of care (Smith et al., 1998), played a key role in cancer disease management programs (Lee, 2004), provided survivorship care in research settings (Ganz et al., 2000), and conducted survivorship research (Ferrell et al., 1992, 1995, 1997, 1998, 2003a,b; Dow et al., 1999; Ritz et al., 2000). Nurse-led follow-up services are acceptable, appropriate, and effective, according to a comprehensive review of the literature evaluating the impact of nurse-led follow-up in cancer care. Although the evidence base for the review was far from complete, the review concluded that nurse follow-up can be an efficient means of maintaining contact with a large client group, providing vital support to vulnerable patients during their move into aftercare and beyond (Cox and Wilson, 2003). A nurse-led case management program also appears promising in improving cancer care for individuals with low incomes (Maliski et al., 2004).

Nurses would appear to be very well suited to providing survivorship care, given the emphasis in nursing education and training on patient assessment, symptom management, psychosocial care, and care planning. Nurses have assumed important roles in survivorship care in Europe and Australia. Research related to their integration into care systems is described in Appendix 4C. Most of these studies have found that cancer survivors are satisfied with follow-up care from nurses, but some cancer survivors prefer to remain with a specialist physician for their post-treatment long-term care (Earnshaw and Stephenson, 1997; Pennery and Mallet, 2000; Renton et al., 2002; Brown et al., 2002; Papagrigoriadis and Heyman, 2003; Koinberg et al., 2004). Creative strategies for harnessing the talents of American nurses in cancer survivorship have been proposed (Leigh, 1998; Pelusi, 2001). Despite the obvious appeal of a nurse-led model of cancer follow-up care, such a model has not been widely implemented or evaluated in the United States.

A factor limiting the feasibility of having nurses provide survivorship care is the short supply of nurses (see Chapter 5). In addition, nurses are more likely to work in hospitals than in outpatient or community-based settings, where cancer follow-up care is most likely to be delivered (see Chapter 5).

According to national surveys of ambulatory care, registered nurses or physician assistants are involved in 27 percent of cancer-related ambulatory care visits. Nurses are much more likely to be involved in care during visits to hospital outpatient departments than physician office-based practices (67 versus 22 percent, respectively) (Table 4-4). The focus of the surveys represented in Table 4-4 is on ambulatory care settings where individual encounters with physicians take place. Nurses are often involved in the administration of chemotherapy and in the provision of supportive care, but the estimates provided in Table 4-4 excluded patient visits to freestanding ambulatory care centers and hospital outpatient chemotherapy, radiotherapy, physical medicine, and rehabilitation clinics.

In summary, although a nurse-led model of cancer follow-up appears to be promising, there is relatively little research available to judge its effectiveness and acceptance in the United States. Nurses are central to any interdisciplinary effort in survivorship care and in some instances, nurses may be the best survivorship care providers. Barriers to adopting nurse-led models of survivorship care include a shortage of trained oncology nurses,

TABLE 4-4 Percentage of Adult Cancer-Related Ambulatory Care Visits During Which Patients Saw an RN, PA, or NP, by Site of Care, United States, 2001–2002[a]

Characteristic	Total	Physician Office-Based Visits	Hospital Outpatient Department Visits
Annual number of visits (in 1,000s)	20,574	18,311	2,263
Saw RN, PA, NP during visit (%)			
Yes	27	22	67
No	73	78	33

[a]Adults were categorized as being aged 25 and older. Visits for non-melanoma skin cancer were excluded. Radiologists were excluded from the sample of office-based physicians. Clinics providing chemotherapy, radiotherapy, physical medicine, and rehabilitation were excluded from the sample of hospital outpatient departments.
NOTE: RN = registered nurse; PA = physician assistant; NP = nurse practitioner.
SOURCE: Committee staff analyses of the 2001 and 2002 National Ambulatory Medical Care Survey and the National Hospital Ambulatory Medical Care Survey. See Appendix 4B for details of analyses.

especially in outpatient settings (see Chapter 5), and the potential preference on the part of some cancer patients to receiving follow-up care from physicians.

Survivorship Follow-up Clinics

A few academic centers have developed cancer survivorship clinics that concentrate needed expertise to provide follow-up care in one location. Such programs can facilitate the application of a holistic and coordinated approach to medical and psychosocial problems. One potential disadvantage of such clinics is the separation of survivorship care from other routine care and the attendant difficulties of communication and coordination. Selected attributes of the few clinics for survivors of adult cancers are described in Table 4-5.

According to representatives of these clinics, they are labor intensive and the respective roles of physicians and other personnel are not well established. Many of the services available in the clinics are provided by expert oncology nurses and nurse practitioners. A barrier to the dissemination of such clinics is the uncertainty regarding adequate reimbursement for

TABLE 4-5 Adult Cancer Survivorship Clinics

Clinic Name and Location	Clinic Characteristics
University of Texas M.D. Anderson Cancer Center: Life After Cancer Care No external support http://www.mdanderson.org/departments/lacc	• **Year founded:** 2001. • **Patient population:** Accepts survivors with all cancer diagnoses, although most are breast cancer survivors who are cancer free and are no longer seen by their oncologist. • **Staff:** Endocrinologist and nurse practitioner. • **Clinical focus:** General evaluation and check-ups of survivors with recommendations for follow-up and screening provided to primary care physicians. Late effects identification and management, especially premature menopause and endocrine dysfunction. • **Research:** An online survey has been completed by nearly 11,000 survivors and is used for studies of survivor needs and late effects. • **Barriers:** Fewer patients from outside M.D. Anderson than expected, possibly because patients do not expect or look for survivorship care.
University of Michigan: Breast Cancer Survivor Clinic No external support http://www.cancer.med.umich.edu/clinic/breastwellclinic.htm	• **Year founded:** 2000. • **Patient population:** Breast cancer survivors who have been followed at the cancer center and are 5 years post-diagnosis. • **Staff:** Medical oncologist and five nurse practitioners. • **Clinical focus:** Management of menopause, osteoporosis, lymphedema, and cancer screening and prevention. Screening exams and mammography are performed. Referrals to support groups and genetic counseling are available. The clinic does not serve as a primary care clinic, but rather refers survivors back to primary care physicians with appropriate recommendations for follow-up care. • **Research:** Clinical trials conducted in the past, but no currently active clinical trials. • **Barriers:** Some insurance companies will not reimburse for nurse practitioner visits.
University of Pennsylvania: Living Well After Cancer Program Supported by the Lance Armstrong Foundation http://www.penncancer.org/cancerprograms_detail.cfm?id=32	• **Year founded:** 2001. • **Patient population:** Survivors of testicular cancer and lymphoma, and adult survivors of childhood cancers who have completed primary treatment and are at least 2 years post-diagnosis. Also provides a consultative service for breast cancer survivors, but does not actually see them in the clinic.

TABLE 4-5 Continued

Clinic Name and Location	Clinic Characteristics
	• **Staff:** Senior oncology nurse practitioner, two medical oncologists, a cardiologist, two primary care physicians, social workers, a nutrition specialist, and a psychologist. Referrals are made for genetic and psychosocial counseling. • **Clinical focus:** Clinical surveillance and follow-up for testicular cancer patients and adult survivors of childhood cancers. Also provides a consultative and research service for breast cancer survivors, which involves surveying breast cancer survivors by mail to identify issues affecting quality of life, and then communicating surveillance and treatment suggestions to their oncologist. • **Research:** Active research program. • **Barriers:** Visibility of the program to patients and oncologists. Obtaining funding for survivorship research.
Dana-Farber Cancer Institute: Lance Armstrong Foundation Adult Survivorship Clinic Supported by the Lance Armstrong Foundation http://www.dana-farber.org/survivor	• **Year founded:** 2004. • **Patient population:** All cancer survivors after completion of primary therapy. • **Staff:** Medical oncologist, nurse practitioner, cardiologist, medical educator, and mental health provider. • **Clinical focus:** General survivorship, especially late effects of disease and treatment. • **Research:** Active research program. • **Barriers:** Part of the research focus will be to characterize barriers to providing survivorship services.

the range of services provided, especially because nonphysician personnel deliver much of the care. In addition, referrals to the clinics are limited because many cancer survivors and oncologists are not aware of the clinics, probably because they were established only in the past few years. Also, some patients prefer to continue seeing their oncologists, and some oncologists would rather follow patients themselves.

Although relatively few survivors of adult cancer are cared for in specialized survivorship clinics, specialized follow-up clinics for survivors of childhood cancer have emerged as an acceptable model in the past decade. There are 35 comprehensive follow-up programs for survivors of pediatric cancer, according to the website of the Association of Cancer Online Resources (Pediatric Oncology Resource Center, 2003).[8] According to a 2000 survey, 44 percent of childhood cancer survivors reported that they had attended a clinic expressly for follow-up of their cancer (Kadan-Lottick et al., 2002). Information collected on health behaviors during an earlier period indicated that 42 percent of young adult survivors reported having had a cancer-related visit and 19 percent a visit at a cancer center (Oeffinger et al., 2004). The clinics diagnose and manage treatment-related sequelae; provide education and counseling; develop surveillance recommendations; address issues related to insurance, education, and employment; and conduct research on late effects (IOM, 2003a).

Pediatric nurse practitioners trained in oncology generally manage the clinics in collaboration with one or more pediatric oncologists. Additional personnel involved, usually on a referral basis, include social workers, psychologists, and other specialists (e.g., cardiologists, fertility specialists, genetic counselors). Well-established programs typically assess 300 to 400 survivors annually, while newer programs or those serving smaller patient populations report seeing only 50 or 60 patients each year. Most programs picked up patients after they had completed their care from their treating oncologist, generally when they were 2 years removed from the completion of therapy and/or 3 to 5 years from diagnosis, and disease free.

Although these comprehensive follow-up programs are addressing the concerns of cancer survivors and their families, there have been no evaluations of their effectiveness or value. As a consequence, a referral to a long-term follow-up program is often initially met by denial from health insurers who contend that such care is not medically necessary. Efforts to overturn these denials usually succeed in securing authorization for follow-up care, but insurers often stipulate that all laboratory and diagnostic tests be performed within network. This can present logistical problems to patients who must travel extended distances to access follow-up care. In addition, reimbursement for services provided in long-term follow-up clinics typically falls far short of compensation for the time and effort required to evaluate and manage these patients. In fact, many services garner no reimbursement for surveillance programs, including those provided by social workers, education specialists, genetic counselors, nutritionists, or dentists. Consequently, hospitals often rely on grant support or philanthropic dona-

[8]Comprehensive programs are those that have a dedicated time and place for the clinic, meet at least twice a month, are staffed by a doctor with experience in the late effects after treatment for childhood cancer, have a nurse coordinator, provide state-of-the-art screening for individual's risks of late effects, provide referrals to appropriate specialists, and provide wellness education.

tions to partially subsidize the costs of providing long-term follow-up care. Similar issues will likely arise for clinics serving survivors of adult cancer.

Although some cancer centers have focused on survivorship care by creating specialized survivor clinics, Memorial-Sloan Kettering Cancer Center is integrating survivorship care into disease-site-specific clinics. After completing primary therapy, survivors continue to be seen in the same medical clinic where they received treatment, but receive follow-up care from a provider with expertise in survivorship, usually a nurse practitioner. This model is currently being pilot-tested in lung, head and neck, prostate cancer, and lymphoma clinics (Personal communication, M. McCabe, Memorial Sloan-Kettering Cancer Center, March 23, 2005). Core evaluation criteria for survivors are being developed and will be used institutionwide, with specialized items added for each disease site. In addition to medical evaluation, Memorial Sloan-Kettering is also piloting a psychosocial screening effort. A screening questionnaire to evaluate emotional functioning and facilitate immediate referrals is currently being pilot-tested and, if successful, will be put into general use (Personal communication, J. Ford, Memorial Sloan-Kettering Cancer Center, March 23, 2005). A sexual health clinic, smoking cessation services, and fertility preservation services are being established or expanded to supplement the survivorship services that are provided in each site-specific clinic. These efforts expand on Memorial Sloan-Kettering's existing survivorship infrastructure, which includes the Post-Treatment Resource Program, an education and support center that has served more than 50,000 people since it was established in the 1980s. This program is open to all survivors, regardless of where they received primary treatment, and provides seminars and workshops on late effects and other survivorship issues, consultation on insurance and employment issues, and professionally led educational support groups (MSKCC, 2004).

At cancer centers that do not have a dedicated survivorship clinic, support services and educational programs are still often available to survivors. For example, a program similar to the Sloan-Kettering Post-Treatment Resource Program is being developed at the Nevada Cancer Institute with the support of the Lance Armstrong Foundation (LAF, 2005a; NVCI, 2005). The Lance Armstrong Foundation Cancer Survivorship Center, which will be located in the patient library at the Nevada Cancer Institute, will provide educational programs, translation and interpretation services, navigation services, and general support to survivors and their families. The program, which is currently in development, will be tailored to the needs of survivors in Nevada as identified by a survey being conducted of cancer survivors in the state.

In addition to the general cancer survivorship clinics described in Table 4-5, there are a number of more narrowly focused referral clinics that provide some aspects of survivorship care. For example, The University of

Texas M.D. Anderson Cancer Center has a clinic for the diagnosis and management of fatigue (M.D. Anderson Cancer Center, 2004); Beth Israel Hospital in New York has a sexuality clinic to address post-treatment sexual late effects (Continuum Health Partners, 2005); and the Fox Chase Cancer Center has a family risk assessment program to provide screening, genetic counseling and testing, and follow-up services (Fox Chase Cancer Center, 2004). Psychosocial interventions, lymphedema care, and menopausal symptom management are other types of care that could be handled by such specialized referral clinics.

In summary, a handful of dedicated clinics have been established to meet the needs of survivors of adult cancer, but they see relatively few patients and have not been formally evaluated. Other clinics are available to manage particular late effects, for example, fatigue, sexual dysfunction, genetic risk, and symptoms of menopause. These specialized clinics are available to individuals with and without cancer and so may be more economically viable. There is virtually no information on the cost-effectiveness and acceptability to patients and providers of either generalized cancer survivorship clinics or the more specialized cancer-related ancillary clinics. There is more experience with clinics that have been established to meet the needs of childhood cancer survivors, but here too, there has been no research to evaluate their cost-effectiveness. Difficulties in obtaining reimbursement for services through these clinics will persist until evidence of their effectiveness has been demonstrated.

THE INFRASTRUCTURE FOR DELIVERING SURVIVORSHIP CARE

Much of the research on the organization of cancer survivorship care has been conducted in Europe and Canada (findings from international studies are summarized in Appendix 4C). While much can be learned from the experience in other countries, the U.S. health care system is somewhat unique. First, adequacy of insurance coverage varies greatly, from no coverage at all for an estimated 11 percent of individuals ages 25 to 64 with a history of cancer, to somewhat generous coverage for elderly cancer survivors enrolled in Medicare who, in addition, have private supplemental coverage (see Chapter 6 for a review of insurance issues). In addition to the confusing array of health insurance products that are available, health care consumers in the United States face a heterogeneous delivery system that includes, at one extreme, managed care, with its focus on controlling costs and coordinating care, and, at the other extreme, fee-for-service care that optimizes choice of health care providers, but leaves care coordination to the patient and doctor. Although the United States lacks a comprehensive national system of care, there is an organized federally supported infrastructure for cancer-related clinical research and care.

This section of the chapter reviews the limited information on where cancer-related care is delivered and what survivorship services are available within the U.S. cancer care system. Although most cancer care is provided in outpatient settings, little information is available on survivorship care or service availability in these settings. More information is available on survivorship-related services that are provided in hospitals with well-developed cancer programs. Examples of the delivery of certain cancer survivorship services are described in Appendix 4D (genetic counseling, rehabilitation, and psychosocial services).

Cancer-Related Hospital and Ambulatory Care

Until the early 1980s most cancer care was delivered in hospitals. The dramatic shift from hospital to ambulatory care began in 1983 when Medicare's inpatient Diagnostic Related Group payment system went into effect. With the added cost-constraining influence of managed care, cancer care has shifted largely to outpatient settings. Mastectomy and other breast surgical procedures, for example, have been increasingly performed in outpatient day-hospital settings (Case et al., 2001). The implication of this shift in site of care is that people cared for in outpatient settings may no longer have access to the many supportive care personnel that are hospital based, such as social workers, nurse educators, psychologists, and clergy. According to national health care surveys, there were an estimated 1.2 million cancer-related hospitalizations and 20.6 million ambulatory care visits in 2002 (Tables 4-6 and 4-2).

When a person with cancer is hospitalized, the availability of ancillary services that might be needed long term (oncology social workers, rehabilitation specialists) often vary by care setting. A rich array of hospital-based specialists and services may, for example, be available in larger hospitals, but absent in smaller hospitals. Fifteen percent of cancer-related hospital discharges are from hospitals with fewer than 100 beds where ancillary and supportive care resources may not be widely available. An equal share of cancer-related hospital discharges are from bigger hospitals (500 or more beds) that likely have more supportive care resources.

In terms of ambulatory care among adults, most cancer-related visits are to physicians' offices, with only 11 percent of visits made to hospital-based outpatient departments where supportive care specialists tend to be available. For example, a registered nurse, nurse practitioner, or physician's assistant is three times more likely (67 versus 22 percent) to be involved in a cancer-related visit to a hospital outpatient department than a physician's office (Table 4-4).

Efforts to improve services to members of minority racial/ethnic groups or to the uninsured could focus on hospital outpatient departments because

TABLE 4-6 Characteristics of Cancer-Related Hospital Discharges, United States, 2002[a]

Characteristic	Cancer-Related Hospital Discharges (in 1,000s)	Percent Distribution
Type of cancer[b]		
All types	1,175.1	100.0
Lung, other respiratory	146.5	12.5
Female breast	85.1	7.2
Prostate	92.0	7.8
Colon, rectum	155.4	13.2
Lymphatic and hematopoietic	128.6	10.9
Gynecologic	73.3	6.2
Bladder	32.6	2.8
All others	461.5	39.3
Hospital size (no. of beds)	1,175.1	100.0
6-99	171.4	14.6
100-199	240.6	20.5
200-299	258.1	22.0
300-499	324.7	27.6
≥500	180.3	15.3

[a]Based on a sample of 11,033 hospital discharges from nonfederal, short-stay hospitals with a primary diagnosis of cancer. Numbers and percentages are adjusted using sampling weights to produce national estimates. Numbers and percentages may not add to total because of rounding.

[b]According to the Ninth Revision of the International Classification of Diseases, Clinical Modification (ICD-9-CM): Lung, other respiratory = 161, 162; female breast = 174; prostate = 185; colon, rectum = 153, 154; lymphatic and hematopoietic = 200-208; gynecologic = 179-184; bladder = 188; other = all other malignancies (ICD-9-CM 140 to 208 and V10).

SOURCE: Committee Staff analyses of the 2002 National Hospital Discharge Survey (NCHS, 2004).

disproportionately more cancer-related care is provided to these groups at these sites of ambulatory care than in physician offices (Table 4-7).

Changes in the organization of cancer care can facilitate the shared-care model. Comprehensive breast care programs have been developed over the past decade to put under one roof the many providers and services that an individual with breast cancer might need to make breast care simpler and to provide "one-stop" care. Typically, these programs employ physician specialists, clinical nurse specialists, social workers, psychologists, and other providers to meet the range of breast cancer needs throughout diagnosis, treatment, and follow-up. While care in such settings is likely more

TABLE 4-7 Patient's Race/Ethnicity and Payment Source for Adult Cancer-Related Ambulatory Care Visits, by Site of Care, United States, 2001–2002[a]

Characteristic	Total	Physician Office-Based Visits	Hospital Outpatient Department Visits
Annual number of visits (in 1,000s)	20,574	18,311	2,263
Race/ethnicity (%)			
White, non-Hispanic	85	87	73
White, Hispanic	3	2	9
Black	9	9	15
Other	2	2	3
Main payment source (%)			
Private insurance	41	42	37
Medicare	46	47	37
Medicaid	4	3	12
Uninsured (self-pay/no charge)	2	2	4
Other, unknown source	6	6	10

NOTE: Percentages may not add to 100 because of rounding.

[a]Adults were categorized as being aged 25 and older. Visits for non-melanoma skin cancer were excluded. Radiologists were excluded from the sample of office-based physicians. Clinics providing chemotherapy, radiotherapy, physical medicine, and rehabilitation were excluded from the sample of hospital outpatient departments.

SOURCE: Committee staff analyses of the 2001 and 2002 National Ambulatory Medical Care Survey and the National Hospital Ambulatory Medical Care Survey. See Appendix 4B for details of analyses.

integrated, some evidence suggests that surveillance tests for breast cancer are overused in breast cancer centers (Lash and Silliman, 2001). There are no data on how many individuals with breast cancer are seen in such programs, but it is likely to be a small fraction of the total number of breast cancer patients (Frost et al., 1999; Rabinowitz, 2002). Analyses of care provided to Medicare beneficiaries during 1994–1995 suggest that surgical treatment for older women with breast cancer is decentralized and being provided primarily by surgeons in low-volume settings (Neuner et al., 2004). Most (55 percent) surgeons providing breast cancer surgery worked in solo or two-physician practices. Only 12 percent of surgeons worked in hospital-based practices.

Cancer survivorship is a distinct phase of care, but it is difficult to know where the 10 million cancer survivors are along the cancer care trajectory. One study of Medicare beneficiaries diagnosed with colorectal cancer between 1975 and 1996 assessed the type of care survivors were receiving in 1996. Investigators classified care into four categories:

1. Initial diagnosis treated with curative intent
2. Post-diagnostic monitoring
3. Treatment for recurrent/metastatic disease or second primaries
4. Terminal care

More than one-third (38 percent) of beneficiaries were determined to have received post-diagnostic monitoring care (Mariotto et al., 2003). The prevalence of type of care in 1996 is shown in Figure 4-2 by years since diagnosis. Those diagnosed within the past 2 years were usually in the initial phase of care. After 2 years, however, the monitoring phase of care predominates. This first study of "care prevalence" relied on analysis of the linked Surveillance, Epidemiology, and End Results (SEER)-Medicare database,[9] which allows investigators to examine the health care claims of individuals following their diagnosis of cancer.

Survivorship Services Within Cancer Centers

With the limited number of dedicated cancer survivorship programs and large and growing population of cancer survivors, the committee attempted to assess the availability and scope of survivor-oriented services within cancer centers. Information was sought for the following sites of care:

- National Cancer Institute-designated Comprehensive Cancer Centers
- Cancer programs approved by the American College of Surgeons' Commission on Cancer
- Community cancer centers that are members of the Association of Community Cancer Centers

NCI-Designated Comprehensive Cancer Centers

The National Cancer Institute (NCI) supports 60 major academic and research institutions throughout the United States to sustain interdisciplinary programs in cancer research (NCI, 2005a). A relatively small proportion of individuals with cancer are cared for within these institutions, but

[9]The SEER-Medicare database is described in Chapter 7.

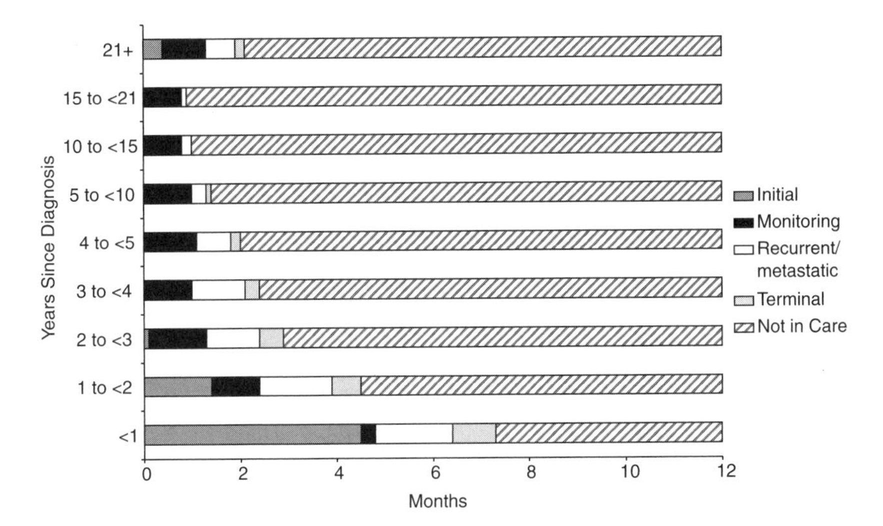

FIGURE 4-2 Average number of months of phase of care in 1996 among patients diagnosed with colorectal cancer from 1975 to 1996, by years since diagnosis. SOURCE: Mariotto et al. (2003).

they provide important opportunities for participation in clinical trials and other research. Cancer Center Support Grants fund the scientific infrastructure of the cancer centers, and recipients of these grants are recognized as NCI-designated cancer centers. Two types of cancer centers are designated based on the degree of specialization of their research activities (Figure 4-3): (1) comprehensive cancer centers integrate research activities across laboratory, clinical, and population-based research (there were 38 such centers in 2005); and (2) cancer centers not designated as "comprehensive" have a scientific agenda that is primarily focused on basic sciences, population sciences, or clinical research, or any two of the three components (there were 22 such cancer centers in 2005).

Although NCI grants are used solely to support the research infrastructure at cancer centers, all designated cancer centers also provide clinical care and service for cancer patients. In addition, comprehensive cancer centers have extensive ancillary cancer-related activities such as outreach, education, and information dissemination. The NCI-designated cancer centers are viewed as playing "an important role in their communities and regions and serve to influence standards of cancer prevention and treatment" (NCI, 2005a).

A telephone survey conducted in 2001 of representatives of all NCI-designated comprehensive cancer centers (there were 37 such centers at the time) found varying degrees of availability of medical and psychosocial

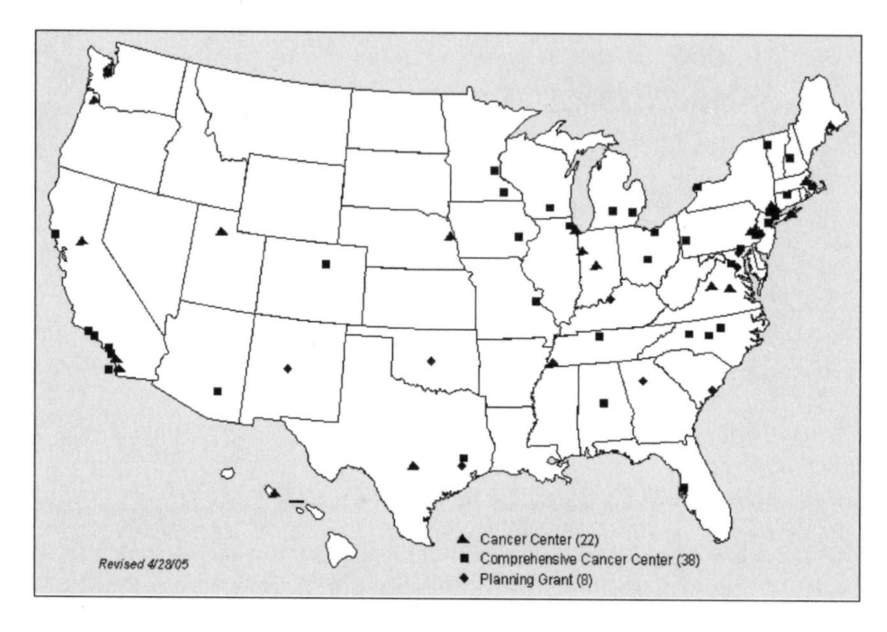

FIGURE 4-3 NCI-designated cancer centers.
SOURCE: NCI (2005a).

services for cancer survivors (Table 4-8) (Tesauro et al., 2002). Although most (70 percent) centers had a lymphedema management program in place, fewer than half had professionally led support groups (49 percent) and long-term medical care programs (38 percent). Relatively few (14 percent) had programs to provide counseling regarding nutrition, fertility, and sexual concerns. Surveys of NCI clinical and comprehensive cancer centers conducted in the early 1990s indicate that virtually all of the responding cancer

TABLE 4-8 Survivorship Services in NCI-Designated Comprehensive Cancer Centers

Service	Availability (percentage)
Lymphedema management	70
Professionally led support groups	49
Long-term medical care	38
Nutrition counseling	14
Fertility and sexual counseling	14

SOURCE: Tesauro et al. (2002).

centers offered group support programs (Presberg and Levenson, 1993; Coluzzi et al., 1995; Gruman and Convissor, 1995). A recent survey on genetics services at NCI clinical and comprehensive cancer centers indicates that that most centers provide such services for evaluation of familial cancer (82 percent) (Epplein et al., 2005).

Cancer Programs Approved by the American College of Surgeons' Commission on Cancer

Most people with cancer are treated in community hospitals close to their homes. In an effort to assure the quality of cancer care throughout the nation, the American College of Surgeons in 1922 established a Commission on Cancer (CoC) that sets standards for quality multidisciplinary cancer care, surveys hospitals to assess compliance with those standards, collects data from approved hospitals to measure treatment patterns and outcomes, and uses the data to improve cancer care outcomes at the national and local levels (Personal communication, K. Phair, Cancer Liaison Program Administrator, CoC, November 9, 2004).[10] As of 2003, there were more than 1,400 CoC-approved cancer programs in the United States and Puerto Rico, representing nearly 25 percent of all hospitals (CoC, 2003). More than 70 percent of all newly diagnosed cancer patients are treated in CoC-approved cancer programs, either as an inpatient or when visiting an outpatient hospital-based practice or clinic. Some of the CoC standards pertain to services of potential benefit to cancer survivors (Box 4-3).

CoC staff provided information to the committee on the supportive care services offered at CoC-approved facilities in the previous year. The information provided is self-reported by the institutions on a web-based application, which is updated twice a year (Personal communication, K. Phair, Cancer Liaison Program Administrator, CoC, November 9, 2004). Cancer centers submit detailed information on their programs in advance of their onsite survey. A service was considered to be present if it was provided at the facility, in a staff physician's office, or by referral. At least some level of supportive care was available through the reporting sites, for example, psychology and mental health providers were available in 88 percent of programs, a pain management service was available in 92 percent of programs, and lymphedema rehabilitation services were available in 77 percent of programs (Table 4-9).

---

[10]Findings of the CoC survey are used as part of the Joint Commission for the Accreditation of Healthcare Organizations (JCAHO) accreditation process for JCAHO-accredited organizations that house a cancer center.

BOX 4-3
Selected Survivorship-Related Standards of the American College of Surgeons' Commission on Cancer

Rehabilitation services are provided onsite or by referral (Standard 4.7). Rehabilitation services include, but are not limited to:

- Career counseling
- Physical therapy
- Speech therapy
- Stomal therapy

Supportive services are provided onsite or coordinated with local agencies and facilities (Standard 6.1). Supportive services include, but are not limited to:

- Genetic testing and counseling
- Grief counseling
- Home care and/or hospice
- Nutritional counseling
- Pastoral services
- Reference library
- Support groups

The cancer committee monitors the community outreach activities on an annual basis. The findings are documented (Standard 6.3). Supportive services, prevention, and early detection programs are monitored to ensure that appropriate services are provided to patients and the community.

SOURCE: Commission on Cancer (2003).

Although the level of survivorship services appears relatively high in CoC-approved cancer programs, it is difficult to know precisely how accessible services are to cancer survivors. Many of the positive responses may represent services provided hospitalwide. If there were only one psychologist available within an institution, for example, the availability of psychological services may be stretched thin. Unclear also is the level of training of staff regarding issues related to cancer survivorship. Some services may be limited to patients on active treatment, leaving a void for long-term survivors. Because referral sources were included as positive responses, the logistics of accessing care at a distance may have a major impact on the true availability of services. Although many important areas are included in the CoC survey, information on significant areas of survivorship care such as genetic counseling or sexuality counseling is not available.[11] Although these data have some shortcomings, they provide important information on the

[11]Information on the availability of genetic counseling services will be available in subsequent years. See Appendix 4D for a description of the delivery of cancer-related genetic counseling services.

TABLE 4-9 Number (and Percentage) of Programs Approved by the American College of Surgeons' Commission on Cancer That Provide Support Services, 2004

	Programs Offering Service[b]	
Service[a]	Number	Percent
Support services:		
Home care	1,224	89
Hospice	1,263	92
Nutrition	1,008	73
Pain management	1,272	92
Lymphedema rehabilitation	1,068	77
Family services	1,143	83
Reference library	1,272	92
Providers:		
Oncology Nursing Society-certified nurse	1,329	96
Physical therapist	1,290	94
Pastoral care	1,290	94
Psychiatric	1,243	90
Psychology/mental health	1,220	88
Social services	940	68
Enterostomal care	1,044	76
Speech therapy	1,267	92
Support activities:		
Breast cancer specific:		
Reach to Recovery[c]	1,198	87
Prostate cancer specific:		
Man to Man[d]	844	61
Us TOO[e]	573	42
Any cancer type:		
CanSurmount[f]	490	36
I Can Cope[g]	935	68
Other support groups	951	69

[a]Services may be available directly from the institution or by referral to appropriate resource.

[b]Pediatric hospitals were excluded from these estimates.

[c]A support group sponsored by the American Cancer Society for individuals with breast cancer.

[d]A support group sponsored by the American Cancer Society for men who are prostate cancer survivors.

[e]Us TOO provides information, local support groups, counseling, and educational meetings to assist men with prostate cancer as they make decisions about their treatment and continued quality of life.

[f]A program that puts a patient in touch with a person who has experienced the same kind of cancer.

[g]A 7-week educational series for cancer patients and their families sponsored by the American Cancer Society.

availability of supportive services, at some level, within the CoC-approved cancer program. Unknown entirely is how available support services are for the approximately 30 percent of patients treated in non-CoC-approved hospitals.

Association of Community Cancer Centers

The Association of Community Cancer Centers (ACCC) is a membership organization that includes 650 medical centers, hospitals, oncology practices, and cancer programs that are generally recognized to have structured cancer programs. The organization estimates that its members provide services to 40 percent of all new cancer patients in the United States (ACCC, 2004a). ACCC has issued voluntary guidelines for cancer programs to encourage the development of comprehensive and interdisciplinary programs. Several guidelines relate to care for cancer survivors. Shown in Box 4-4 are guidelines for rehabilitation and patient advocacy and cancer survivorship. Other guidelines are available for pain management, nutritional support services, and genetic risk assessment, counseling, and testing (ACCC, 2004b).

To learn more about survivorship services available within ACCC cancer centers, an informal survey was conducted in 2002 of cancer center program coordinators.[12] Program coordinators were asked about the availability of several survivorship-related services.[13] The service did not have to be housed in the center: referrals to external organizations or facilities at other centers, including local academic institutions, were considered to serve the center's needs. As stated above, many of the clinics/organizations served both survivors and patients in active treatment, and it was not possible to identify services that were dedicated only to survivors. Table 4-10 shows the availability of these services across responding centers. The availability of lymphedema services and support groups appears to be somewhat lower in these ACCC-member cancer centers than in the NCI-designated comprehensive cancer centers (Table 4-8).[14]

With the information at hand, it is difficult to gauge the availability of cancer survivorship clinical and supportive services in cancer centers. In

---

[12]A convenience sample of 83 centers was selected from the roster of institutions who are ACCC members. Two members were selected from each state with three or more members, one member was selected if there were only one or two members. Community centers were selected from different cities in a state, and larger city or larger institutional centers were preferentially selected. Telephone calls were placed to the designated program coordinator of each of the 83 centers. No follow-up calls were made. Responses were obtained from 56 institutions (67 percent).

[13]The questions about survivorship services were asked in an open-ended format. Respondents were not asked whether they were provided a given set of survivorship services.

[14]See Appendix 4D for a description of the delivery of cancer rehabilitation services.

part, the difficulty in ascertainment may be due to the lack of clear definitions relating to survivorship care. The availability of certain specialized services among cancer centers appears to vary substantially. Lymphedema services were, for example, reported in 77 percent of CoC-approved cancer programs according to 2004 CoC survey data, 70 percent of comprehensive cancer centers according to a 2001 NCI-sponsored telephone survey, and 38 percent of ACCC-member cancer centers according to a 2002 informal survey. Likewise, the availability of general or disease-specific support groups seems to vary widely. Sexuality counseling and dedicated fatigue management appear to be rarely available.

To better understand the adequacy of cancer survivorship clinical and support services, an in-depth survey from the perspectives of both survivors and providers of oncology and primary care is needed. This survey would allow conclusions to be drawn about such issues as the spectrum of services that are needed, levels of unmet need, the respective roles of specialty and primary care providers, and the role of specialized clinics versus integration of survivorship care into routine oncology and primary care practice. Such a survey would also assist in the development of standardized survivor instruments to facilitate needs assessments and remedial interventions. Ultimately, a set of quality indicators and benchmarks is needed so that survivorship care can be evaluated, regardless of the setting in which it is provided or the particular type of practitioner involved in care.

Community-Based Support Services

An important element of the chronic disease model is mobilizing community resources to meet needs of patients. There is a wealth of cancer-related community support services available through voluntary organizations, many of them at no cost. Many supportive services are offered through call centers, web-based information and discussion boards, and direct service delivery. Table 4-11 describes some of the programs that are available nationally. Among the services these programs offer are information, peer support, individual support by telephone, information on nutrition and exercise, and assistance with appearance, for example, wigs and breast prostheses.

Cancer patients make frequent inquiries about supportive services. Health providers are often asked about support groups, counseling, nutrition, financial aid, health insurance, and employment, according to a survey of physicians, nurses, and social workers providing cancer care (Matthews et al., 2004). Although community-based support services are of great interest, some evidence suggests that health care providers are not providing their patients with information or referral to support groups and other resources in their communities (Guidry et al., 1997; Matthews et al., 2002). Furthermore, a recent review of the role of community-based and

BOX 4-4
Guidelines for Rehabilitation and for Patient Advocacy and Survivorship: Association of Community Cancer Centers Standards for Cancer Programs

Rehabilitation Guidelines: Comprehensive rehabilitation services are available to cancer patients and their families.

Cancer is a chronic disease that may require adjustment in the physical, social, financial, and emotional aspects of life in order to maximize independence and quality of life. Professionals experienced in rehabilitation are best suited to meet the needs of cancer patients.

The rehabilitation team includes, but is not limited to:

- Oncology nursing services
- Psychosocial services
- Nutritional support services
- Pharmacy services
- Pastoral care services
- Physical, occupational, and recreational therapy services
- Speech pathology services
- Comprehensive, multidisciplinary lymphedema services
- Enterostomal therapy services
- A discharge planner to address home care and community and/or extended care facility services and needs
- Qualified volunteers to provide support and advocacy for cancer patients and their families
- Other complementary services, such as music/art therapy, relaxation, massage, and others, may be used in conjunction with rehabilitation disciplines

Each health care discipline is available on staff or by consult to facilitate continuity of care for rehabilitation services. All outsourced services should be provided by properly credentialed individuals whose performance is reviewed annually.

Rehabilitation services are a part of the organizational structure of the program and follow proper policies and procedures.

philanthropic organizations in meeting the needs of cancer patients and caregivers found gaps in service provision for assistance with practical needs such as transportation, home care, child care, financial assistance, and psychosocial support (Shelby et al., 2002). The authors note that with increasing use of outpatient care for cancer patients, a greater demand for practical assistance can be expected in the future.

Ongoing educational opportunities are available to members of rehabilitation services.

A mechanism is in place to inform patients and family members of the services available.

Patient Advocacy and Survivorship Guidelines: Information and programs specific to patient advocacy and survivorship issues are available to cancer patients and their families.

Programs and educational resources for survivors and their families should include but are not limited to the following:

1. Access to information about cancer prevention, early detection, genetics, disease treatment, symptom management, and psychosocial, spiritual, and financial concerns through written materials and/or referrals to same via the Internet, other experts, or support organizations.
2. Information about local, regional, and national resources on any aspect of cancer, cancer care, research, advocacy, and survivorship.
3. Access to support groups onsite or through referrals to local or web-based support groups and other support mechanisms, such as telephone connection programs linking survivors together.
4. Information about specific survivorship issues, such as employment rights, insurance coverage, late and long-term effects of disease and treatment, advance directives, living will and durable power of attorney, estate planning, options for recurrent disease management, and end-of-life care planning.
5. Programmatic opportunities to participate with the care team to develop community outreach education and support programs for quality cancer care in the community and to educate professional staff about the cancer experience.

Resources are allocated to provide a robust advocacy and survivorship program.

National standards for advocacy and survivorship will be incorporated into program planning, implementation, and evaluation.

SOURCE: ACCC (2004c,d).

This section of the chapter highlights selected programs that provide services nationally, those offered by the American Cancer Society and the Wellness Community, selected programs that focus on the needs of Hispanic and African-American cancer survivors, and support available by telephone or online. Appendix 4D includes a description of the delivery of psychosocial services for women with breast cancer to illustrate some of the barriers to access to care.

TABLE 4-10 Survivorship Services in Selected ACCC Cancer Centers

Survivorship Service	Number (n = 56)	Percentage
At least one survivorship service	47	84
No survivorship services	9	16
Lymphedema services	21	38
Genetic counseling	19	34
Support groups, professionally run		
All cancer	19	34
Breast	13	23
Prostate	8	14
Gynecologic	4	7
Brain	2	4
Lymphoma/leukemia	2	4
Support groups, peer led	13	23
Sexuality counseling	4	7
Yoga/relaxation	2	4
Symptom management	2	4
Prevention	2	4
Prosthesis lending	1	2

SOURCE: Winn (2002).

American Cancer Society Programs

The American Cancer Society provides extensive information on cancer patient support and special topics in survivorship issues and sponsors several programs for cancer survivors (see Table 4-11; Box 4-5). Detailed guides on what to expect after treatment for the most common cancers, including surveillance practices, are available at the ACS website. Also available is information on adopting healthy lifestyles after cancer treatment. The ACS's Cancer Survivors Network is a web-based program supporting online interaction among cancer survivors. Participants can create a personal website; post pictures, poems, and other expressions; listen to or read prerecorded stories of other survivors; and engage in online discussions in English, Spanish, and Chinese.

The I Can Cope program started as a series of classes for individuals with cancer, but has been adapted for use as multiple standalone modules on a variety of topics ranging from financial management to coping with side effects. A health care navigator program is under development by ACS that will direct individuals to resources within their community.

The Reach to Recovery program, offered since 1960, provides peer support to women with breast cancer. Initially designed for women in the hospital after mastectomy, the program is now offered largely in the community. Attempts are made to match volunteer mentors with women with breast cancer by age, type of procedure, and cancer stage. Trained volunteers made nearly 65,000 visits in 2003 (Teschendorf, 2005). Road to Recovery is a community-based program that provides rides to individuals with cancer who need transportation to treatment. Although the program is already offered in various forms in many states, it continues to expand nationwide. An estimated 66,000 people were served nationally by this program in 2003 (Teschendorf, 2005).

Since 1989, the Look Good...Feel Better (LGFB) program has provided assistance with makeup, skin care, and other aspects of appearance (e.g., information on wigs, turbans). The program is co-sponsored by the Cosmetic, Toiletry, and Fragrance Association Foundation, the National Cosmetology Association, and ACS. In 2003 the LGFB program reached about 31,000 women (Teschendorf, 2005). A magazine and catalogue called *tlc*, or Tender Loving Care, combines articles, information, and products for women coping with cancer treatment (e.g., wigs, mastectomy forms and products, hats and head coverings, bathing suits, and lingerie) (ACS, 2004).

The ACS's Man to Man program helps men cope with prostate cancer by providing community-based education and support to patients and their family members. A major part of the program is the self-help and/or support group. Volunteers organize free monthly meetings where speakers and participants learn about and discuss information about prostate cancer, treatment, side effects, and how to cope with the disease and its treatment. Approximately 27,000 men participated in Man to Man in 2003 (Teschendorf, 2005).

The Wellness Community

The Wellness Community, founded in 1982, is an international nonprofit organization that provides free education and support services to individuals with cancer and their families (see Table 4-11) (The Wellness Community, 2004b). The founding principle of The Wellness Community is the "Patient Active Concept," which states that patients who participate in recovery improve the quality of their lives and may enhance the possibility of recovery. In 2004, The Wellness Community reached more than 150,000 people affected by cancer. The free programs are led by licensed health care professionals, including social workers, psychotherapists, nurses, and psychologists, and all programs and training curricula are uniform throughout the country. Its online resources include webcasts, relaxation exercises, cancer-specific educational materials, continuing education for oncology nurses, and online support groups hosted through "The Virtual Wellness Community" (The Wellness Community, 2004a). Many of the online programs are also available in Spanish.

TABLE 4-11 Selected National Community-Based Psychosocial Resources

Program Name, Sponsor	Services and Availability
Generic Cancer Programs	
Cancer Care http://www.cancercare.org	• One-on-one counseling • Group therapy • Information and education Available nationwide by telephone and via the Internet
I Can Cope ACS http://www.cancer.org	• Series of classes taught by doctors, nurses, social workers, and others • Information, peer support, and practical coping skills Available nationwide
The Wellness Community http://www.thewellnesscommunity.org	• Nutrition • Support groups • Online support groups • Nutrition/exercise, mind/body programs • Physician lectures • Stress reduction workshops Available in 22 locations throughout the United States, and nationwide via the Internet
Cancer Hope Network http://www.cancerhopenetwork.org	• One-on-one peer support (in-person or by telephone) Available nationwide by telephone, or in person at some locations
ACOR (Association of Cancer Online Resources) http://www.acor.org	• Group discussion and peer support • Information and education Available nationwide via the Internet
Gilda's Club http://www.gildasclub.org	• Support groups • Education Available in 18 centers nationwide, with 7 centers in development
Cancer Survivors Project http://www.cancersurvivorsproject.org	• Online education Available nationwide via the Internet

Content of Services	Eligibility
• Emotional support and encouragement • Psychological counseling from social worker • Teleconferences for cancer information • Group peer support via telephone or Internet • Financial advice and assistance	Survivors, family, and loved ones
• Diagnosis, treatment, side effects of treatment • Emotions and self-esteem, cancer and intimacy • Communication skills • Community resources, financial concerns • Pain management	Survivors and family
• Psychosocial interventions: emotional support, coping strategies, relaxation/visualization training • Information and education • Exercise techniques and nutritional guidance	Survivors and family
• Emotional support and encouragement from cancer survivor	Survivors
• E-mail listservs, networks, and chat rooms monitored by health care professionals; survivorship-related networks include long-term survivorship, fertility, sexuality, fatigue, osteoporosis, and financial issues • Cancer information	Survivors and family
• Emotional support for survivors and families • Support program specifically for post-treatment survivors • Education: topics include stress reduction, nutrition, managing pain, meditation, exercise, yoga, etc.	Survivors, family, and friends
• Information on physiological and psychosocial late effects, preventive care, and long-term follow-up • Survivor stories	Survivors, family, and friends

Continued

TABLE 4-11 Continued

Program Name, Sponsor	Services and Availability
LIVESTRONG, Lance Armstrong Foundation and Centers for Disease Control and Prevention http://www.livestrong.org	• Information and education Available nationwide via the Internet and by telephone
Breast Cancer	
Reach to Recovery ACS http://www.cancer.org	• One-on-one peer support and education (in-person or by telephone) Available nationwide
Look Good...Feel Better, ACS; Cosmetic, Toiletry, and Fragrance Association Foundation; and the National Cosmetology Association http://www.lookgoodfeelbetter.org	• Information and hands-on instruction on makeup and skin care and suggestions for using wigs, turbans, and scarves Available nationwide
Other groups (Y-Me, Bosom Buddies, Sisters Network, YWCA, Circle of Life, TOUCH)	• Group therapy Available in regions nationwide
Prostate Cancer	
Man to Man ACS http://www.cancer.org	• Group or one-on-one peer support and education Services and activities vary depending on location
Us TOO http://www.ustoo.org	• Support groups • Online information and mailing lists Support groups available nationwide, with more than 330 chapters worldwide
Colon Cancer	
Colon Cancer Alliance http://www.ccalliance.org	• Online support groups • One-on-one peer support • Information and education Available nationwide through the Internet

Content of Services	Eligibility
• Survivor stories • Health management and organization tools, such as the "Survivorship Notebook" • Partnership with CancerCare and Patient Advocate Foundation for emotional, legal, and financial needs.	Survivors, family, and friends
• Emotional support from cancer survivors • Information and education • Assistance obtaining prostheses	Breast cancer survivors
• Teaching women how to cope with the appearance-related side effects of cancer • Enhancing appearance and makeovers • Learning to use wigs, hair pieces, turbans, etc.	Breast cancer survivors
• Emotional support, coping strategies • Group psychotherapy	Breast cancer survivors and family
• Emotional support from cancer survivors • Information and education	Prostate cancer survivors
• Support groups for patients and survivors • Us TOO Partners support groups for women whose partners or family members have prostate cancer • Prostate Pointers website with 13 focused listservs on topics such as intimacy and sexuality, treatment modalities, and spirituality	Prostate cancer survivors and partners
• Emotional support • Educational materials on quality of life • Survivor stories	Colorectal cancer survivors and family

Continued

TABLE 4-11 Continued

Program Name, Sponsor	Services and Availability
Blood Cancers	
The Leukemia and Lymphoma Society http://www.leukemia-lymphoma.org	• Group support • One-on-one peer telephone support • Educational programs and physician lectures • Call center staffed with social workers, nurses, and health educators 59 local chapters, and information available nationwide by telephone
Thyroid Cancer	
ThyCa: Thyroid Cancer Survivors Association, Inc. http://www.thyca.org	• Group support • One-on-one peer support • Email support groups Available nationwide during the internet, and in person in some locations

Community-based educational programs are offered at all The Wellness Community locations and at some independent cancer clinics. A variety of topics are covered, and programs are designed to help people with cancer and their caregivers feel a greater sense of hope, control over their situation, and community. National education programs are focused on coping with cancer as a chronic condition, with strategies for managing the disease, its side effects, and a host of lifestyle and emotional concerns that arise over time. The *Frankly Speaking about New Discoveries in Cancer* program, developed in 2004, covers information about the most current medical and psychosocial advances, and addresses topics such as complementary and alternative medicine and psychological concerns (The Wellness Community, 2005).

Evaluations of The Wellness Community programs are underway and include a comparison of face-to-face and online support services, an examination of provider best practices, and analyses of outcomes associated with interventions (Lieberman et al., 2003). Research partners include Stanford University, University of California–San Francisco, M.D. Anderson Cancer Center, Catholic University, and the National Coalition for Cancer Survivorship.

Content of Services	Eligibility
• Emotional support • "Keys to Survivorship" educational programs on fatigue, insurance, employment, and self-care • Caregiver information	Leukemia and lymphoma survivors, family, and caregivers
• Emotional support • Group focusing specifically on mental challenges • Thyroid cancer information	Thyroid cancer survivors and caregivers

Community-Based Support Targeted to Racial and Ethnic Minority Groups

A number of psychosocial support programs are targeted to members of racial and ethnic minority groups. Nueva Vida, a program to meet the needs of Hispanic women in the District of Columbia, was established in 1996 and offers support groups, crisis intervention, and peer support to breast cancer survivors (Nueva Vida, 2005a). Because many women served are poor, uninsured, and speak Spanish, Nueva Vida provides "patient navigation" services to help women make appointments and get appropriate follow-up care, assistance with health insurance applications and claim translation, and social supports (assistance with transportation, babysitting). Support groups focus on stress reduction, education (e.g., nutrition), and the implications of cancer for families. Nueva Vida maintains a national psychosocial support resource directory for Hispanic women with breast cancer; the directory includes programs in 20 states (Nueva Vida, 2005b). The most pressing needs of Hispanic women identified by programs surveyed thus far are related to poor access to health care, information, and psychosocial support, and difficulties navigating the health care system.

Sisters Network, Inc., was founded in 1993 to address the needs of African-American women with breast cancer (Sisters Network, Inc., 2005). The only national African-American breast cancer survivors' organization

BOX 4-5
American Cancer Society Survivorship-Related Books

- *Eating Well, Staying Well During and After Cancer*
- *Guide to Complementary and Alternative Cancer Methods*
- *Couples Confronting Cancer: Keeping Your Relationship Strong*
- *Crossing Divides: A Couple's Story of Cancer, Hope, and Hiking Montana's Continental Divide*
- *Cancer in the Family: Helping Children Cope with a Parent's Illness*
- *Our Mom Has Cancer (Book for Children)*
- *Coming to Terms with Cancer*
- *Caregiving: A Step-By-Step Resource for Caring for the Person with Cancer at Home*
- *Guide to Pain Control: Powerful Methods to Overcome Cancer Pain*
- *When the Focus Is on Care: Palliative Care and Cancer*
- *A Breast Cancer Journey: Your Personal Guidebook*
- *Social Work in Oncology: Supporting Survivors, Families, and Caregivers*

SOURCE: ACS (2004).

in the United States, Sisters Network has 39 affiliate chapters across the country. More than 3,000 members are involved in providing breast health training, attending conferences, and serving on various national boards and review committees. Chapters offer individual and group support, community education, advocacy, and research-related activities (e.g., promoting access to clinical trials). The 2005 national Sisters Network Conference "The New Spirit of Survivorship" focused on disparities, risk factors, and survivorship (CDC, 2005a).

The Prostate Health Education Network (PHEN) was founded by a prostate cancer survivor to raise awareness of prostate cancer among those at high risk, especially African-American men (PHEN, 2005). PHEN is establishing "brotherhoods" of prostate cancer survivors across the country that will focus on educating men about prostate cancer and mentoring and counseling those newly diagnosed with the disease, but will also provide support to each other as survivors. The Dana-Farber Cancer Institute and PHEN recently partnered to establish the first prostate cancer support group for African-American men in the Boston area (Dana-Farber Cancer Institute, 2005).

Support Available by Telephone and Online

Many psychosocial support services are available by phone to residents of rural areas and those living far from cancer centers, and increasingly online through the World Wide Web. This section of the report describes three such programs: Cancer Care, the Association of Cancer Online Resources (ACOR), and CHESS (Comprehensive Health Enhancement Support System). In addition, a referral resource is available online to help locate psychosocial and mental health services through the American Psychosocial Oncology Society (APOS, 2004). There are other organized online lay information and support groups, including Fertile Hope (FertileHope.org), Living Beyond Breast Cancer (lbbc.org), and Cancer and Careers: Living and Working with Cancer (cancerandcareers.org), and many Internet chat rooms. There are also radio resources, for example, the Group Room weekly cancer talk radio show (and Internet simulcast) provided by Vital Options® International, which can reach rural areas. Chapter 6 reviews some online resources related to employment and insurance programs. The potential for these resources to help survivors, provide psychosocial care, and engage in research is not clear but merits investigation.

CancerCare Since 1944, CancerCare has provided emotional support, information, and practical help to people with cancer and their families. With a staff of more than 40 professional oncology social workers, this nonprofit social service agency provides individual and family counseling, group counseling (in-person, online, or by telephone), referrals to other resources, direct financial assistance, and teleconference programs that allow people to listen via telephone to experts in oncology or related fields (CancerCare, 2005a). Previous teleconference programs have covered coping strategies for side effects, communicating with one's health care team, and how best to maintain quality of life while living with cancer. CancerCare has recently teamed with the Lance Armstrong Foundation to create a counseling program specifically for cancer survivors that includes an online forum for survivors and individualized counseling (CancerCare, 2005b). In addition, CancerCare also hosts an annual teleconference series on survivorship; the 2005 workshop covered care after treatment, fatigue and memory long-term effects, and health-promoting behaviors. In 2004, CancerCare provided services to more than 90,000 people, and all services are provided free of charge. According to an analysis of requests for assistance made to CancerCare from 1983 to 1997, the most commonly reported problems relate to personal adjustment to illness and financial, home care, and transportation needs (Shelby et al., 2002).

CancerCare is also involved in professional education and training, offering seminars, workshops, and teleconferences in all fields of oncology care. Distance learning programs are conducted entirely on the website. (Chapter 6 includes a description of services related to employment and insurance issues.)

Association of Cancer Online Resources ACOR provides opportunities for individuals with cancer to interact with other cancer patients, therapists, or doctors through chat rooms, e-mail, or listservs. Psychosocial support is available through listservs dedicated to breast cancer, cancer-related depression, and caregivers. Another feature of ACOR is the provision of information about cancer from sources deemed to be credible (ACOR, 2004a).

CHESS (Comprehensive Health Enhancement Support System) CHESS provides information, social support, and decision-making assistance via personal computers placed in a patient's home. Women of all ages and varied socioeconomic backgrounds have successfully used the program to become active participants in their care following a diagnosis of breast cancer. CHESS allows participants to talk anonymously with peers, question experts, learn where to obtain help and how to use it, read stories about people who have survived similar crises, read relevant articles, monitor their health status, consider decision options, and plan how to implement decisions (Gustafson et al., 1993; Shaw et al., 2000). Support group use is the most popular aspect of CHESS. CHESS support groups are monitored by a facilitator. CHESS is undergoing further development as part of NCI's Centers of Excellence in Cancer Communications Research Initiative (NCI, 2005c).

In addition to these support services, many sources of information are available on survivorship issues (Box 4-6).

Statewide Comprehensive Cancer Control

Opportunities in the United States to develop regional approaches to care for cancer survivors could be facilitated by the Centers for Disease Control and Prevention's (CDC's) efforts to build the capacities of states—and, in turn, their local partners—to both develop and implement comprehensive cancer control plans (Brady, 2004). As part of CDC's National Comprehensive Cancer Control Program, such plans have been defined as those with an integrated and coordinated approach to reducing the incidence and rates of morbidity and mortality from cancer through prevention, early detection, treatment, rehabilitation, and palliation (CDC, 2004a).

CDC has identified a useful framework for the establishment of a state cancer control program and has provided various models for comprehensive planning and evaluation. Essential elements of a comprehensive plan include (Abed et al., 2000a,b) the following:

- Strategies and mechanisms for developing and maintaining partnerships,

BOX 4-6
Examples of Information on Survivorship Available to Cancer Survivors and Their Families

Cancer advocacy

- Cancer Survival Toolbox: An audio resource program, National Coalition for Cancer Survivorship (NCCS), Oncology Nursing Society, Association of Oncology Social Work, National Association of Social Workers (also available online and in Spanish and Chinese) (NCCS, 2004)
- Facing Forward—Ways You Can Make a Difference in Cancer, National Cancer Institute (NCI, 2002b).
- Life Beyond Cancer, women's retreat and conference on advocacy, US Oncology (US Oncology, 2005)
- People Living Through Cancer, Inc., trains volunteer cancer survivors as group facilitators in New Mexico, including American Indians (PLTC, 2005)

Print

- Cure magazine, Heal magazine
- Facing Forward—Life After Cancer Treatment, National Cancer Institute (also in Spanish) (NCI, 2002)
- A Cancer Survivor's Almanac, NCCS (Hoffman, 2004)

Web

- Cancer: After Treatment, from the American Academy of Family Practice "familydoctor.org" website (AAFP, 2002)
- CancerCare (CancerCare, 2005a)
- Cancer: Keys to Survivorship, webcasts of live teleconferences, NCCS and The Leukemia & Lymphoma Society (NCCS, 2005)
  - Strategies for Self Improvement and Communicating with Healthcare Providers
  - Working It Out: Your Employment Rights as a Cancer Survivor
  - What Cancer Survivors Need to Know About Health Insurance
- CancerSymptoms.org website, Oncology Nursing Society (ONS, 2005)
- Cancer Survivors Network, American Cancer Society (ACS, 2005b)
- Life After Cancer Care, M.D. Anderson Cancer Center (M.D. Anderson, 2005)
- LIVESTRONG, Lance Armstrong Foundation (LAF, 2005b).
- Long-term survivors discussion group through the Association of Cancer Online Resources (ACOR, 2004b)
- People Living With Cancer (American Society of Clinical Oncology) (ASCO, 2005)

Radio

- The Group Room, syndicated live cancer talk radio show, produced by Vital Options® International (Vital Options, 2005)

Telephone

- American Cancer Society National Cancer Information Center, 800-ACS-2345
- Cancer Information Service, National Cancer Institute, 800-4-CANCER
- CancerCare, 800-813-HOPE

- Assessments and surveillance,
- Infrastructure development,
- Public education,
- Professional education,
- Policy and legislative activities, and
- Evaluation and monitoring.

An online resource called Cancer Control Planet helps states to assess program priorities, identify potential partners, determine the effectiveness of different intervention approaches, find research-tested programs and products, and plan and evaluate their program (Cancer Control Planet, 2004). A locus at the site on survivorship issues is under development (Rowland, 2005). All but 1 state (Idaho) receive support from CDC for their comprehensive cancer control program; 28 states are implementing their plans; and 21 states and the District of Columbia are developing their plans (Figure 4-4) (CDC, 2004b).

With an understanding that cancer survivors could benefit tremendously from a coordinated public health effort, CDC in collaboration with the Lance Armstrong Foundation developed *A National Action Plan for Cancer Survivorship: Advancing Public Health Strategies* (CDC and LAF, 2004). The plan includes four goals:

1. Preventing secondary cancers and recurrence of cancer whenever possible.
2. Promoting appropriate disease management following diagnosis and treatment to ensure the maximum number of years of healthy life for cancer survivors.
3. Minimizing preventable pain, disability, and psychosocial distress for those living with, through, and beyond cancer.
4. Assisting cancer survivors in accessing family, peer, and community support and other resources they need for coping with their disease.

This action plan and the strategies outlined within the plan shown in Box 4-7 will serve as a guide to states as they expand their comprehensive cancer control plans to include survivorship. As part of a pilot project, CDC is analyzing four organizations' survivorship-related activities that are national in scope (i.e., those of the American Cancer Society, CancerCare, the Lance Armstrong Foundation, and the National Coalition for Cancer Survivorship). The results of this pilot project will help CDC determine how it can most effectively address gaps in cancer survivorship within the realm of public health (Personal communication, P. Thompson, CDC, April 26, 2005).

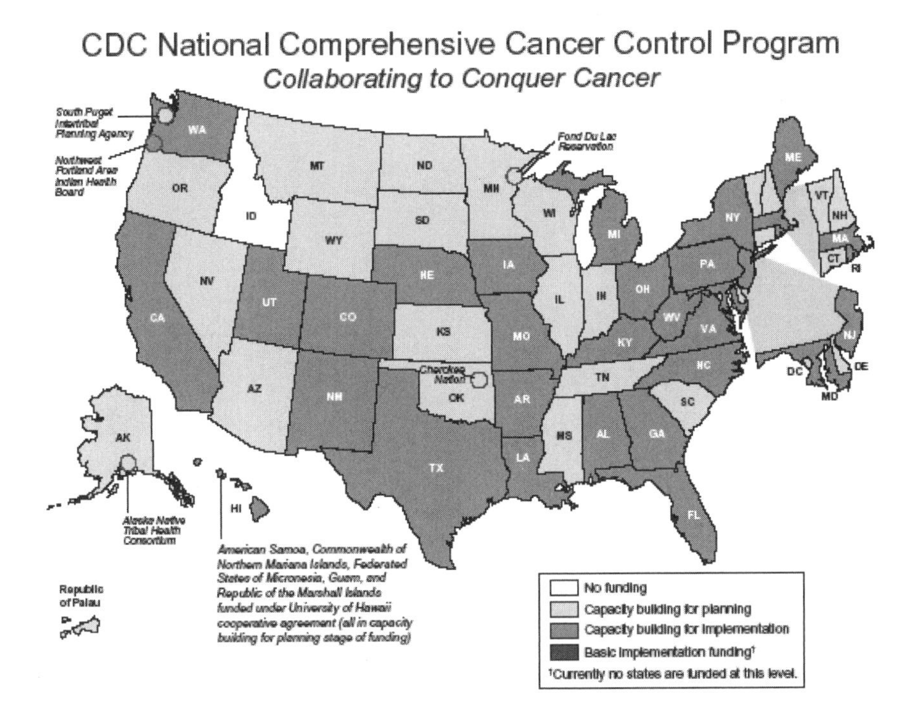

FIGURE 4-4 Status of CDC State Comprehensive Cancer Control Plans.
SOURCE: CDC (2004a).

The CDC-funded comprehensive cancer control activities vary by state depending on local needs and preferences. Comprehensive cancer control plans have been oriented to primary and secondary prevention activities such as tobacco control and cancer screening; however, states have recently been adding some survivorship elements to their plans (True, 2004; Texas Cancer Council, 2005). In the area of data collection, some plans describe expanding current cancer registry activities to obtain information on survival, rehabilitation, and palliative care. In the area of consumer education, some plans address the need for better information regarding side effects of treatment and quality of life issues. Ensuring appropriate and continuous psychosocial support is addressed in some plans. There is little consistency across plans on how survivorship is defined and addressed, but when implemented, these plans provide an opportunity to approach survivorship with a public health focus. The Maryland Comprehensive Control Plan is a good example of how survivorship can be integrated into a cancer control plan.

BOX 4-7
A National Action Plan for Cancer Survivorship: Advancing Public Health Strategies

The *National Action Plan* identifies and prioritizes cancer survivorship needs and proposes strategies for addressing those needs within four core public health components:

- Surveillance and applied research
  1. Enhance the existing surveillance and applied research infrastructure.
  2. Identify factors associated with ongoing health concerns of cancer survivors.
  3. Determine programs and services that best address the needs of cancer survivors.
  4. Conduct research on preventive interventions to evaluate their impact on issues related to cancer survivorship.
  5. Translate applied research into practice.

- Communication, education, and training
  1. Develop strategies to educate the public that cancer can be a chronic disease that people can and do survive.
  2. Educate policy and decision makers about the role and value of long-term follow-up care, addressing quality of life issues and legal needs, and ensuring access to clinical trials and ancillary services for cancer survivors.
  3. Empower survivors with advocacy skills.
  4. Develop, test, maintain, and promote patient navigation systems for people living with cancer.
  5. Teach survivors how to access and evaluate available information.
  6. Educate health care providers about cancer survivorship issues from diagnosis through long-term treatment effects and end-of-life care.

However, the state has limited resources with which to implement its plan (Box 4-8) (Family Health Administration, 2005). The comprehensive cancer control plans have not yet been evaluated and evidence is needed of their effects on statewide access to cancer-related services, the quality and comprehensiveness of those services, and the extent to which the needs of cancer patients and survivors are being met. The National Conference of State Legislators (NCSL) is working with the Lance Armstrong Foundation to develop state-level policy indicators for survivorship (Personal communication, S. Wasserman, NCSL, March 21, 2005). This effort will include a survey of state best practices. An opportunity for state and tribal representatives to meet and discuss issues related to their comprehensive cancer control efforts is provided by the Comprehensive Cancer Control Leader-

- Programs, policies, and infrastructure
  1. Develop, test, maintain, and promote patient navigation or case management programs that facilitate optimum care.
  2. Develop and disseminate public education programs that empower survivors to make informed decisions.
  3. Identify and implement programs proven to be effective (i.e., best practices).
  4. Implement evidence-based cancer plans that include all stages of cancer survivorship.
  5. Establish clinical practice guidelines for each stage of cancer survivorship.
  6. Promote policy changes that support addressing cancer as a long-term, chronic disease.
  7. Develop infrastructure to obtain quality data on all cancer management activities to support programmatic action.

- Access to quality care and services
  1. Develop, test, maintain, and promote a patient navigation system for cancer survivors.
  2. Educate decision makers about economic and insurance barriers related to health care for cancer survivors.
  3. Establish and/or disseminate guidelines that support quality and timely service provision to cancer survivors.
  4. Assess and enhance provision of palliative services to cancer survivors.
  5. Establish integrated multidisciplinary teams of health care providers.

SOURCE: CDC and LAF (2004).

ship Institutes.[15] These 2- to 3-day regional meetings bring together up to 15 people from each state to participate in lectures, discussions, and exercises to assist them in their cancer control efforts (Personal communication, P. Thompson, CDC, May 2, 2005). Survivorship will be among the topics addressed at the Institutes in 2006 (Personal communication, P. Thompson, CDC, April 26, 2005).

[15]The Comprehensive Cancer Control Leadership Institutes are a collaborative effort convened by the American Cancer Society, the American College of Surgeons, the Association of State and Territorial Health Officers, C-Change, the Centers for Disease Control and Prevention, the Chronic Disease Directors, the Intercultural Cancer Council, the National Cancer Institute, and the North American Association of Central Cancer Registries (CDC, 2005b).

BOX 4-8
Comprehensive Cancer Control and Survivorship in Maryland

The Maryland Comprehensive Cancer Control plan, released in 2004, includes a chapter entitled "Patient Issues and Cancer Survivorship" that recognizes many of the problems faced by cancer survivors, and presents public health strategies for overcoming them, with the overall goal of enhancing quality of life for all cancer survivors in Maryland. The Maryland plan identifies four objectives relating to survivorship:

1. To enhance access to information and resources for Maryland cancer survivors, their friends, and families;
2. To reduce the financial burden on cancer survivors and their families;
3. To ensure that all cancer survivors have access to psychosocial support services throughout all phases of their cancer experience; and
4. To address the needs of long-term cancer survivors.

Selected strategies to reach these goals include (see state plan for a list of all strategies):

- Establish and market a comprehensive cancer information clearinghouse in the form of a website plus a staffed, toll-free telephone number.
- Encourage oncologists to distribute copies of the National Cancer Institute publications *Facing Forward* and *Life After Cancer Treatment* to all patients.
- Examine the cost of cancer services and develop a statewide financial aid system to help offset the expense of cancer diagnosis and treatment services.
- Initiate a review of the Maryland Medicaid system with attention to cancer costs.
- Educate health care practitioners to be aware of, and sensitive to, the psychosocial needs of their patients. Educate providers about existing mental health services and other psychosocial support services for cancer survivors and the urgent need for increased numbers of timely referrals for mental health services.
- Establish an annual conference sponsored by the Maryland Department of Health & Mental Hygiene, academic health centers, and Maryland professional organizations to address psychosocial issues of cancer survivors.
- Establish new and expand existing long-term survivorship clinics in Maryland for both childhood and adult cancer survivors. These clinics should be designed to follow survivors after treatment and to provide them with comprehensive care to address the unique needs of cancer survivors.
- Educate oncologists and other health care providers about long-term survivorship issues. Providers should be encouraged to explain the long-term effects of the different treatment options available and help their patients make treatment decisions with regard to these long-term effects.
- Educate oncologists about the need to refer their patients to neurologists, cardiologists, physical therapists, or other specialists as necessary for the management of long-term side effects.
- Identify or create new programs to address occupational issues of cancer survivors such as job retraining and workplace reintegration.

SOURCES: Family Health Administration (2005); Maryland Comprehensive Cancer Control Plan; Personal communication, R. Villanueva, Maryland State Council on Cancer Control, February 16, 2005.

FINDINGS AND RECOMMENDATIONS

Survivorship care represents a unique phase of the cancer care trajectory following primary treatment and lasting until recurrence, a second cancer, or death. An ideal system of survivorship care would provide all cancer survivors with preventive services, surveillance, necessary interventions, and coordination with primary care to ensure that all of the survivor's care needs are met. Many cancer survivors do not receive comprehensive survivorship care. They are, in effect, lost to follow-up. Some survivors may receive aspects of post-treatment care from their cancer care or primary care providers, but such care is rarely comprehensive or coordinated. Many survivors are not aware of their increased risk for late effects and do not seek the care they need. Primary care physicians are often willing to assume follow-up responsibilities, but do not receive explicit guidance from oncology specialists on what they should do. Improvements in information systems and electronic health records hold promise to improve communications between providers involved in cancer care, but such systems are not yet widely available. Education and training opportunities on survivorship care are limited and comprehensive evidence-based clinical practice guidelines have not been developed. Promising models of delivering survivorship care have been tested in Europe, but have not been formally evaluated in the United States. The chronic disease model of care is emerging in the United States, but has not been applied in the context of cancer survivorship.

Defining Quality Health Care for Cancer Survivors

The National Cancer Policy Board, in its 1999 report, *Ensuring Quality Cancer Care*, recommended that systems of care "measure and monitor the quality of care using a core set of quality measures" and specified some of the attributes and applications of such measures (Box 4-9) (IOM, 1999). Since the IOM report was published, the American Society of Clinical Oncology, the Susan G. Komen Foundation, the National Cancer Insitute, and others have supported research and activities to further the development of quality measures for cancer care.

For certain types of cancer, some evidence-based measures of quality survivorship care exist. Survivors of breast cancer, for example, need to receive annual mammograms, survivors of prostate cancer need periodic testing with the prostate-specific antigen (PSA) test, and survivors of colon cancer require periodic colon examinations. Other measures could likely be developed with available evidence, for example, the need to monitor some individuals treated with certain chemotherapeutic agents for heart conditions and to monitor certain individuals treated by radiotherapy for thyroid

BOX 4-9
Recommendation from *Ensuring Quality Cancer Care*

Cancer care is optimally delivered in systems of care that "measure and monitor the quality of care using a core set of quality measures."

Cancer care quality measures should:

- Span the continuum of cancer care and be developed through a coordinated public–private effort.
- Be used to hold providers, including health care systems, health plans, and physicians, accountable for demonstrating that they provide and improve quality of care.
- Be applied to care provided through the Medicare and Medicaid programs as a requirement for participation in these programs.
- Be disseminated widely and communicated to purchasers, providers, consumer organizations, individuals with cancer, policy makers, and health services researchers, in a form that is relevant and useful for health care decision making.

SOURCE: IOM (1999).

conditions. In contrast to these disease-specific or treatment-specific measures, some evidence-based measures of quality apply broadly across all types of cancer. For example, routinely assessing cancer survivors for psychosocial distress is warranted because it often exists and effective treatments are available. Given the frequency of other common and treatable symptoms such as fatigue and sexual dysfunction, other measures of survivorship care quality could likely be formulated with available evidence that would be broadly applicable to cancer survivors.

Recommendation 4: Quality of survivorship care measures should be developed through public/private partnerships and quality assurance programs implemented by health systems to monitor and improve the care that all survivors receive.

Overcoming Delivery System Challenges

The problems that cancer survivors face in getting comprehensive and coordinated care are common to those faced by others with chronic health conditions. Because cancer is a complex disease and its management involves the expertise of many specialists, often practicing in different settings, cancer illustrates well the "quality chasm" that exists within the U.S.

health care system and the need for health insurance reforms and innovations in health care delivery.

The Survivorship Committee recognizes that underlying flaws in the organization of health care delivery hamper appropriate survivorship care. The committee endorses the conclusions and recommendations in the IOM report, *Crossing the Quality Chasm* (IOM, 2001). That report provided the rationale and a strategic direction for redesigning the health care delivery system. It concluded that fundamental reform of health care is needed to ensure that all Americans receive care that is safe, effective, patient centered, timely, efficient, and equitable. To that end, health care organizations need to design and implement more effective organizational support processes to make change in the delivery of care possible. Purchasers, regulators, health professionals, educational institutions, and the Department of Health and Human Services need to create an environment that fosters and rewards improvement by (1) creating an infrastructure to support evidence-based practice, (2) facilitating the use of information technology, (3) aligning payment incentives, and (4) preparing the workforce to better serve patients in a world of expanding knowledge and rapid change.[16]

Barriers facing cancer survivors and their providers in achieving quality survivorship care include: a fragmented and poorly coordinated cancer care system; the absence of a locus of responsibility for follow-up care; poor mechanisms for communication; a lack of guidance on the specific tests, examinations, and advice that make up survivorship care; inadequate reimbursement from insurers for some aspects of care; and limited experience on how best to deliver care.

Recommendation 5: The Centers for Medicare and Medicaid Services (CMS), National Cancer Institute (NCI), Agency for Healthcare Research and Quality (AHRQ), Department of Veterans Affairs (VA), and other qualified organizations should support demonstration programs to test models of coordinated, interdisciplinary survivorship care in diverse communities and across systems of care.

Several promising models for delivering survivorship care are emerging, including:

1. A shared-care model in which specialists work collaboratively with primary care providers,

[16]The IOM will be publishing a series of reports starting in late 2005 on performance measures, payment systems, and performance improvement programs.

2. A nurse-led model in which nurses take responsibility for cancer-related follow-up care with oversight from physicians, and
3. Specialized survivorship clinics in which multidisciplinary care is offered at one site.

There is limited evidence on which of these, or other, delivery strategies is feasible, cost-effective, or acceptable to survivors and clinicians. It is likely that different care models will be preferred and appropriate for different survivor groups and communities. Models for delivering survivorship care should address the fact that oncology specialists, facing an expanding population of cancer survivors, will become overburdened with follow-up care at the expense of being able to evaluate and treat new patients. The proposed demonstration program could include the development of an infrastructure for integrated care to enable primary care clinicians to coordinate with specialists as a team to ensure that cancer survivors receive timely and complete care for cancer-related and other health needs. Such an infrastructure could include advanced information systems, such as electronic health records, virtual consultations, smart cards, and web-based approaches. Less technology-dependent interventions could also yield results. Having a community's cancer specialists and primary care providers agree to a plan on how to coordinate care for survivors—including clarifying roles, specifying referral procedures, agreeing on consultation letters, and providing feedback to primary care—could all enhance coordinated care. More than 60 percent of cancer survivors are aged 65 and older, so the Medicare program should have a strong interest in identifying cost-effective models of care.

Survivorship as a Public Health Concern

CDC and the Lance Armstrong Foundation have developed a public health approach to survivorship care that may assist communities in identifying and addressing the survivorship needs of individuals, their families, and their health care providers (CDC and LAF, 2004; CDC, 2004a). Among the public health capacities that could be addressed include:

- Population-based surveillance systems for survivorship care and quality of life;
- Areawide community-based resource guides for survivors and health care providers;
- Service needs assessments;
- A clearinghouse for health care provider education and training opportunities;

- Provision of primary and secondary prevention services (e.g., smoking cessation, cancer screening);
- Program evaluation and identification of best practices.

Health departments have had a long tradition of managing cancer registries, offering health education, and providing community-based health promotion and disease prevention activities. Interventions for common chronic public health problems such as heart disease and diabetes could well be germane to cancer survivors and their families. These public health approaches are early in their development and resources are needed to evaluate the effectiveness of community-based services and comprehensive cancer control plans in improving the care and quality of life of cancer survivors.

Recommendation 6: Congress should support the Centers for Disease Control and Prevention (CDC), other collaborating institutions, and the states in developing comprehensive cancer control plans that include consideration of survivorship care, and promoting the implementation, evaluation, and refinement of existing state cancer control plans.

APPENDIX 4A
SUMMARY OF ARTICLES DESCRIBING U.S. SURVEILLANCE PRACTICE PATTERNS, BY CANCER SITE (LIMITED TO ARTICLES PUBLISHED FROM 1994 TO 2005)

Breast Cancer

Reference/ Study Question	Methods
Mammography surveillance following breast cancer (Geller et al., 2003) ________ When do women diagnosed with breast cancer return for their first mammogram? What factors predict women's return for surveillance?	*Method:* Linkage of data from seven mammography registries (NCI's Breast Cancer Surveillance Consortium (BCSC)) to population-based cancer and pathology registries. *Sample:* 2,503 women diagnosed with breast cancer (DCIS or invasive) within 1 year of a 1996 BCSC mammogram were followed to see if they returned for surveillance mammography. *Statistical methods:* Kaplan-Meier curves were used to depict time from diagnosis to first surveillance mammogram during the defined follow-up period. *Explanatory variables:* Age, race, education, stage, detection by screening, family history, treatment.
Quality of non-breast cancer health maintenance among elderly breast cancer survivors (Earle et al., 2003) ________ What is the quality of preventive health care for breast cancer survivors? What patient and provider characteristics are associated with high-quality care?	*Method:* Retrospective cohort study using SEER-Medicare data. *Sample:* 5,965 elderly women who were diagnosed with nonmetastatic breast cancer in 1991 or 1992 while living in a SEER tumor registry area and who survived to the end of 1998 without evidence of cancer recurrence. *Statistical methods:* Multivariate analyses were used to develop explanatory models. *Explanatory variables:* Preventive service use among cancer survivors was compared to controls matched for age, race, and geographic location.
Medical surveillance after breast cancer diagnosis (Lash and Silliman, 2001)	*Method:* Study of surveillance practices in five Boston hospitals.

Results
78% of women with breast cancer returned for mammography between 7 and 30 months following the diagnosis. Women most likely to undergo surveillance mammography were 60–69 (OR 1.9 relative to women 40–49) with Stage 0, I, or II breast cancer (relative to Stage III) and had received radiation therapy in addition to surgery. 74% of women who returned had two or more mammograms. ASCO guidelines do not recommend biannual surveillance mammography, but many providers are following women after treatment with breast-conserving surgery with mammography every 6 months for the first 2–3 years.
Breast cancer survivors received more preventive services (influenza vaccination, lipid testing, cervical and colon screening, and bone densitometry) in 1997–1998 than matched controls. Survivors who continued to see oncology specialists were more likely to receive appropriate follow-up mammography for their cancer, but those who were monitored by primary care physicians were more likely to receive all other noncancer-related preventive services. Those who saw both types of practitioners received more of both types of services. Among both groups, those who were younger, non-African American, of higher socioeconomic status, living in urban areas, and receiving care in a teaching center were most likely to receive high-quality health maintenance. Mammography use in 1997–1998 was 74% among survivors.
92% of women had some surveillance testing. 47% of women received less than guideline surveillance.

Continued

Breast Cancer (continued)

Reference/ Study Question	Methods
________ What tests are ordered for surveillance of breast cancer recurrence in the 4 years after breast cancer diagnosis by surgeons, medical oncologists, and radiation oncologists? To what extent are guidelines for follow-up adhered to? Adherence measured according to ASCO guideline of annual physical examination and mammography.	*Sample:* 303 Stage I or II breast cancer patients aged 55 years or older and diagnosed at one of five Boston hospitals and followed for at least 4 years were interviewed and their medical records abstracted. Year of completion of primary therapy ranged from 1992 to 1994. 78% of women eligible to participate did so. Nonparticipants were on average 3 years older than participants. Medical records were examined for the following nine surveillance tests: 1. Patient history and physical examination 2. Mammography 3. Liver function studies 4. Complete blood count 5. Carcinoembryonic antigen (CEA) 6. Chest X ray 7. Skeletal survey 8. Bone scan 9. Liver scan Tests ordered because of suspected recurrence were excluded. Surveillance information from primary care physicians was not examined. *Statistical methods:* Stepwise proportional hazards regression used to determine predictive model of failure to receive 4 consecutive years of surveillance. *Explanatory variables:* Physician specialty, patient age, education, marital status, household composition, employment status, cancer stage, treatment, comorbidity.
Underutilization of mammography in older breast cancer survivors (Schapira et al., 2000) ________ How frequently do older breast cancer survivors obtain annual mammography? What determines mammography use?	*Method:* Retrospective cohort study using SEER-Medicare data. *Sample:* 3,885 breast cancer survivors aged 65 and older diagnosed with early-stage breast cancer in 1991. Examined mammography use in 2-year period following initial breast cancer treatment. *Statistical methods:* Multivariate analyses (logistic regression).

Results

Women ages 75 to 90 years were at higher risk for failure to complete 4 consecutive years of surveillance and for receipt of less than recommended guideline surveillance.

Women treated at a breast center and women treated with radiation therapy were more likely to get mammograms.

In the 4 years of follow-up, a mean of 22 tests were ordered for 279 women getting any type of surveillance. Most tests were ordered by medical oncologists. The most common test was a mammogram (mean = 3.9), which was most often ordered by a surgeon.

Liver function studies were ordered on average 2.5 times over the 4-year follow-up period for 279 women, CEA tests 2 times, and chest X rays 0.4 times.

62% of women underwent annual mammography, an additional 23% underwent mammography in 1 of 2 years, and 15% had no mammography claim in the 2 years evaluated.

Women treated with breast-conserving surgery without radiotherapy, those with higher stage of disease or greater comorbidity were less likely to have had annual mammography.

When use of mammography in the 2-year period was examined, black women were less likely than white women to have any mammography (OR 0.54).

Continued

Breast Cancer (continued)

Reference/ Study Question	Methods
	Explanatory variables: Age, race, cancer stage, type of treatment, comorbidity, census tract income, education, population density.
The use of mammography by survivors of breast cancer (Andersen and Urban, 1998) ——— To what extent are rural breast cancer survivors getting annual mammograms?	*Method:* Reinterview of women identified with breast cancer by survey (cancer diagnoses were not confirmed with medical records or registry). *Sample:* 248 women who had reported a history of breast cancer in a 1994 survey of women ages 50 to 80 living in 40 communities in predominantly rural areas of Washington state were reinterviewed in 1996 regarding mammography use. 83% (351/423) of eligible women recontacted in 1996 for the survey agreed to participate. Of these 71% (248/351) were included in the study. Excluded women were being treated for cancer, diagnosed recently, or had had a double mastectomy. *Statistical analysis:* Multiple logistic regression analysis. *Explanatory variables:* Age, insurance status, years since diagnosis, detection of cancer by mammogram, treatment, recent recommendation of mammography.
Measuring standards of care for early breast cancer in an insured population (Hillner et al., 1997) ——— Can available information be used to develop measurements regarding standards of quality and efficiency of oncologic care? What surveillance occurs following breast cancer treatment for privately insured women under age 64?	*Method:* Private insurance claims linked to state cancer registry data. Procedural and hospital claims from Blue Cross/Blue Shield of Virginia were linked with clinical stage data from the Virginia Cancer Registry from 1989 to 1991. *Sample:* 918 women <64 with local or regional breast cancer. *Statistical method:* Univariate descriptive statistics used to develop a quality-of-care "report card." *Explanatory variables:* Age, node status.

Results

70% of breast cancer survivors reported having received a mammogram within the past year. 72% reported having had a mammogram in the past 2 years.

Women who had a recent physician recommendation for mammography and those whose breast cancer had been originally detected by mammography were more likely to have had a recent mammogram.

Mammography
81% of women had at least one mammogram within 3 years of diagnosis. 76% had a mammogram by 18 months and 66% between 18 and 36 months.

Diagnostic imaging
Within 36 months, 34% of women had a bone scan and 21% had a CT scan. For each of the 18-month periods, approximately 24% of women had one or more bone scans and 14% had a CT scan of some type.

Continued

Prostate Cancer

Reference/ Study Question	Methods
Breast cancer evaluation and follow-up: A survey of the Ohio Chapter of the American College of Surgeons (Stark and Crowe, 1996) ________ What are the practice philosophies of Ohio general surgeon fellows regarding evaluation and follow-up?	*Method:* 1994 survey of 764 general surgeons, fellows in the Ohio chapter of the American College of Surgeons. *Sample:* 261 responses to the survey were evaluable (RR = 34%). *Statistical method:* Descriptive statistics. *Explanatory variables:* None.
Geographic variation in patient surveillance after radical prostatectomy (Powell et al., 2000) How tumor stage affects American urologists' surveillance strategies after prostate cancer surgery (Johnson et al., 2000) Current follow-up strategies after radical prostatectomy: A survey of American Urological Association urologists (Oh et al., 1999) The age of the urologist affects the postoperative care of prostate carcinoma patients (Tsai et al., 1999) ________ How does tumor stage and urologist geographic location and age influence variability of surveillance after radical prostatectomy (Stage TNM I-II, III)?	*Method:* 1997 physician survey. Examined three frequently used modalities: 1. Digital rectal exam 2. Urinalysis 3. Serum PSA And eight infrequently used modalities: 1. Chest X ray 2. Computed tomography of abdomen and pelvis 3. Magnetic resonance imaging (MRI) 4. Radionuclide bone scan 5. Multichannel blood chemistry 6. Complete blood count (CBC) 7. Serum prostatic acid phosphatase 8. Monoclonal antibody scan Attitudes toward follow-up were also assessed. *Sample:* 4,467 members of the American Urological Association (randomly selected from total of 12,500 members) mailed survey in 1997. RR = 32% (1,416/4,467); 1,050/1,416 responses were usable; 28% of usable responses (290/1,050) were from urologists practicing outside of United States. *Statistical methods:* Repeated measures analysis of variance. *Explanatory variables:* Location in 24 MSAs, U.S. census region, HMO penetration.

Results

Essentially all surgeons indicated that physical exam and mammograms are important for post-treatment follow-up. Complete blood cell count, liver function studies, and chest X rays are used by more than half of the surgeons. 39% used bone scans. 44% had had difficulty with third-party payors covering the costs of surveillance studies. 88% of surgeons wanted the state chapter of the ACS to establish clinical guidelines or practice parameters.

Geographic variation
Surveillance practices were not affected by MSA, census region, or area HMO penetration rate.

Urologists reported an average of 4.02 office visits, 3.43 PSA tests, and 2.99 urinalyses by patients in the postoperative year after radical prostatectomy (TNM stages I–II).

With the exception of CBC and blood chemistry, other modalities were used very infrequently (0.20 or fewer tests).

Very large standard deviations for the total population estimates indicate wide variation in practices.

72% indicated that the literature does not document significant survival benefits of follow-up testing. Nevertheless, 59% of urologists thought that failure to perform follow-up testing at least once yearly constitutes malpractice.

Stage
The analysis of the effect of stage on follow-up practice by Johnson et al. was limited to 760 U.S. urologists.

Intensity of follow-up differed only slightly by TNM stage (data on Gleason score was not collected).

Urologist age
There was a small but significant influence of urologist age on surveillance practice. Older urologists ordered more PSA levels and CT scans, whereas younger urologists ordered more bone scans. Optimism and belief in the survival benefits of routine surveillance increase with age, but this did not translate into substantially more frequent usage of follow-up modalities.

Continued

Colorectal Cancer

Reference/ Study Question	Methods
Clinical and sociodemographic factors associated with colon surveillance among patients with a history of colorectal cancer (Rulyak et al., 2004)	*Method:* Analysis of HMO automated clinical records for evidence of colonoscopy or flexible sigmoidoscopy, together with barium contrast radiography. *Sample:* 1,002 patients diagnosed with local or regional colon or rectal cancer between January 1993 and December 1999. *Statistical methods:* Survival analysis. *Explanatory variables:* Cancer site, age, SES, marital status, race/ethnicity.
Racial differences in the receipt of bowel surveillance following potentially curative colorectal cancer surgery (Ellison et al., 2003) _________ How does race/ethnicity affect patient surveillance following colorectal surgery?	*Method:* Retrospective cohort study using SEER-Medicare data. *Sample:* 44,768 non-Hispanic white, 2,921 black, and 4,416 patients from other racial/ethnic groups aged 65 and older at diagnosis, with a diagnosis of local or regional colorectal cancer between 1986 and 1996, and followed through December 31, 1998. Surveillance procedures examined included colonoscopy, sigmoidoscopy, endoscopy, and barium enema. *Statistical methods:* Cox proportional hazards models. *Explanatory variables:* Race, gender, age at diagnosis, geographic region, census tract education, comorbidity, hospital ownership, size, teaching status.

Results
61% of patients had colon examinations within 18 months of diagnosis and 80% of patients within 5 years of diagnosis. Less likely to undergo surveillance were patients over 80 years of age, with rectal cancer, and African Americans. More likely to undergo surveillance were patients with higher SES, married, and those of "other" race/ethnicity.
The chance of surveillance within 18 months of surgery was 57 percent, 48 percent, and 45 percent for non-Hispanic whites, blacks, and other, respectively. After adjusting for sociodemographic, hospital, and clinical characteristics, blacks were 25% less likely than whites to receive surveillance if diagnosed between 1991 and 1996 (RR = 0.75). This result was not explained by measured racial differences in sociodemographic, hospital, and clinical characteristics. More than 70% of the bowel surveillance procedures received were colonoscopy. Blacks were nearly 40% more likely than non-Hispanic whites to receive post-treatment bowel surveillance with barium enema.

Continued

Colorectal Cancer (continued)

Reference/ Study Question	Methods
Bowel surveillance patterns after a diagnosis of colorectal cancer in Medicare beneficiaries (Knopf et al., 2001) ——— To what extent are recommendations for postoperative colon surveillance followed for patients with local/regional colorectal cancer? Have practices improved over time?	*Method:* Retrospective cohort study using SEER-Medicare data. *Sample:* 52,283 patients aged ≥65 with colorectal cancer treated between 1986 and 1996. Surveillance patterns through 1998 were examined. Proportion of surviving patients' use of procedures at four time periods after treatment were assessed: 2 to 14 months, 15 to 50 months, 51 to 86 months, and more than 97 months. Surveillance procedures examined included colonoscopy, sigmoidoscopy, endoscopy, and barium enema. *Statistical methods:* Kaplan-Meier method survival analysis. *Explanatory variables:* Age, stage at diagnosis, year of diagnosis.
Sociodemographic differences in the receipt of colorectal cancer surveillance care following treatment with curative intent (Elston Lafata et al., 2001) ——— Are there differences in surveillance care within an HMO population that are explained by race and/or income?	*Method:* Retrospective cohort study based on HMO claims. *Sample:* 251 patients aged ≥40 with colorectal cancer diagnosis from 1990 to 1995 and treated with curative intent. *Statistical methods:* Cumulative incidences of service receipt were estimated using Kaplan-Meier survival analyses. Cox proportional hazard models were used to evaluate the relationship between patient sociodemographic and clinical characteristics and service receipt. Patients were followed through the first of either recurrence, death, health plan disenrollment, or December 1997. Average 8-year medical care expenditures were calculated, adjusted for inflation. *Explanatory variables:* Age, sex, race, census tract income, comorbidity.

Results

Low use of post-diagnosis colon surveillance was observed. No surveillance occurred for 17% of the cohort. The proportions of the cohort that underwent no surveillance during each of the four time periods were 54%, 52%, 60%, and 69%. The proportions of the cohort that underwent surveillance at a greater-than-annual frequency for each of the four periods were 10%, 8%, 5%, and 4%.

Median times to first through fifth surveillance events were 20, 14, 15, 15, and 15 months, respectively.

Surveillance improved with time (1994–1998 versus 1986–1993). Younger patients were more likely to undergo surveillance. Surveillance was not related to stage.

Within 18 months of treatment, 55% of the cohort received a colon examination (colonoscopy, barium enema, sigmoidoscopy), 71% received CEA testing, and 59% received metastatic disease testing (CT scans, ultrasounds, MRI, chest X ray, serum liver transaminases testing). Whites were more likely than minorities to receive CEA testing (RR = 1.47). As the median household income of a patient's zip code of residence increased, so too did the likelihood of colon examination and metastatic disease testing receipt (RR = 1.09, RR = 1.12, respectively). Average 8-year medical care expenditures among the cohort were $30,247.

Continued

Colorectal Cancer (continued)

Reference/ Study Question	Methods
Patterns of endoscopic follow-up after surgery for nonmetastatic colorectal cancer (Cooper et al., 2000) ________ How frequently are colorectal patients followed up? How do surveillance practices vary by patient characteristics and geography?	*Method:* Retrospective cohort study using SEER-Medicare data. *Sample:* 5,716 patients aged ≥65 with local or regional stage colorectal cancer diagnosed in 1991. Medicare claims from 6 months after diagnosis through the end of 1994 were examined to determine use of endoscopic procedures. *Statistical methods:* Chi-square testing. Study did not account for censoring in the data. *Explanatory variables:* Age, gender, race, SEER site, cancer site, stage.
Geographic and patient variation among Medicare beneficiaries in the use of follow-up testing after surgery for nonmetastatic colorectal carcinoma (Cooper et al., 1999) ________ How frequently are colorectal patients followed up? How do surveillance practices vary by patient characteristics and geography?	Same sample and study design as above.
Colorectal cancer screening and surveillance practices by primary care physicians: Results of a national survey (Sharma et al., 2000) ________ To what extent are primary care providers providing screening and surveillance tests for colorectal cancer?	*Method:* 1997 mailed questionnaire to 2,310 primary care physicians (family practice, internal medicine). Stratified sampling from a national database (TAP Pharmaceutical Inc.) to obtain 40–50 physicians per state. *Sample:* Used 417 responses from 2,135 questionnaires that could be delivered (RR 20%). *Statistical methods:* Descriptive statistics. *Explanatory variables:* None.

Results

One or more colonoscopies were performed in 51%, with an average of 2.9 procedures performed among those tested; sigmoidoscopy was performed in 17%. The rate of colonoscopy was highest during the initial 18 months. Polypectomy was performed in 21% of all patients, and subsequent primary colorectal tumors were diagnosed in 1.3%. Factors associated with colonoscopy and sigmoidoscopy use included younger age, survival through follow-up, and geographic region; sigmoidoscopy was also more common in relation to rectal cancers.

The most commonly performed tests among the 5,716 patients identified were liver enzymes, chest X rays, colonoscopy, and CT scans. Lower rates of testing generally were observed with older age groups, patients with fewer comorbidities, and patients who did not survive through the follow-up period. Among all procedures studies, there was also significant variation in the rates of testing across the nine SEER areas, varying from 1.5-fold to 3.6-fold. The geographic variation persisted in multivariate models adjusting for potentially confounding factors.

On the question related to follow-up of a patient with an adenomatous colon polyp diagnosed 10 years previously, 83% of physicians recommended colonoscopy, 10% recommended flexible sigmoidoscopy (FS), 4% recommended FS and barium enema, and 3% recommended FOBT.

Continued

Colorectal Cancer (continued)

Reference/ Study Question	Methods
Geographic variation in patient surveillance after colon cancer surgery (Johnson et al., 1996a) How practice patterns in colon cancer patient follow-up are affected by surgeon age (Johnson et al., 1996c) How tumor stage affects surgeons' surveillance strategies after colon cancer surgery (Johnson et al., 1995) Surveillance after curative colon cancer resection: Practice patterns of surgical subspecialists (Virgo et al., 1995) Current follow-up strategies after resection of colon cancer: Results of a survey of members of the American Society of Colon and Rectal Surgeons (Vernava et al., 1994)	*Method*: These five articles describe variation in patient surveillance after colon cancer surgery as reported in two provider surveys. *Sample:* 1,663 members of the American Society of Colon and Rectal Surgeons (ASCRS) were asked in 1992 by mailed questionnaire how often they request these nine follow-up evaluations for their patients treated for cure with TNM Stage I, II, or III colon cancer over the first 5 post-treatment years: 1. Clinic visits 2. Complete blood count 3. Liver function tests 4. Serum carcinoembryonic antigen (CEA) level 5. Chest X ray 6. Bone scan 7. CT scan 8. Colonoscopy 9. Sigmoidoscopy 46% (757/1,663) of ASCRS members completed the survey and 39% (646/1,663) provided evaluable data. The same questionnaire was administered to 1,070 members of the Society of Surgical Oncology (SSO) in 1993. 33% (349/1,070) of SSO members provided evaluable responses. *Statistical methods:* Repeat measures of analysis of variance. *Explanatory variables:* Tumor stage and year post-surgery, MSA/city and MSA size, surgeon age, training period, and country of practice (United States versus foreign).

Results

According to ASCRS members, routine clinic visits and CEA levels were the most frequently performed items for each of the 5 years. More than three-quarters of surgeons see their patients every 3 to 6 months for years 1 and 2, and then every 6 to 12 months for years 3, 4, and 5. Approximately 80% of respondents obtain CEA levels every 3 to 6 months for years 1, 2, and 3, and every 6 to 12 months for years 4 and 5. Colonoscopy is performed annually by 46% to 70% of respondents, depending on the year. A chest X ray is obtained yearly by 46% to 56%, depending on the year. The majority of ASCRS members do not routinely request CT scans or bone scans. There was great variation in the pattern of use of CBC and liver function tests.

Office visits and CEA tests were performed most frequently. SSO members generally see patients every 3 months in years 1–2, every 6 months in years 3–4, and annually thereafter. There was wide variability in test ordering patterns and moderate variation between SSO and ASCRS members.

With responses from ASCRS and SSO combined, seven of the nine surveillance modalities were performed, significantly more frequently with increasing TNM stage. This effect persisted through 5 years of follow-up. Bone/CT scans were performed too infrequently for analysis.

Surgeon age was not predictive of post-treatment surveillance practice patterns, suggesting that post-graduate physician education homogenizes practitioner behavior.

MSA population size and geographic location generally did not explain variation in surveillance practices.

Continued

Hodgkin's Disease

Reference/ Study Question	Methods
Breast cancer screening in women previously treated for Hodgkin's disease: A prospective cohort study (Diller et al., 2002)	*Method:* Prospective cohort study. *Sample:* 90 female long-term survivors of Hodgkin's disease treated 8 or more years previously with mantle irradiation (ages 24 to 51 years, diagnosed under age 30). 75% of contacted patients were enrolled in the study.
How aware are long-term female survivors of Hodgkin's disease of their risk for breast cancer? What are their breast cancer screening practices?	Participants completed surveys of their perceptions of risk and screening behaviors and received written recommendations for breast examinations and mammography. Annual follow-up was conducted through medical records, telephone, and/or mailed questionnaires. *Statistical methods:* Descriptive statistics and multivariate logistic regression modeling. *Explanatory variables:* Age, age at diagnosis, year of diagnosis, stage, treatment, radiation dose.

Results

At baseline, 40% of women were unaware of their increased risk of breast cancer. Only 47% reported having had a mammogram in the previous 24 months. 10 women developed 12 breast cancers during the study, all evident on mammogram (2 detected at baseline; median time of follow-up 3.1 years).

Six women in the cohort refused mammography because they thought they were "too young" (n = 3), "breasts are too dense according to primary physician" (n = 1), and no reason given (n = 2).

Four patients withdrew from the study because of "no time" (n = 1), "too upsetting to deal with" (n = 1), and no reason (n = 2).

Women who perceived themselves to be at high risk were not more likely to have had a mammogram in the previous 2 years.

Older patients were more likely to have had a mammogram.

Nine patients in the cohort developed other primary tumors during the follow-up period (thyroid, pancreas, stomach, lung, sarcoma, non-Hodgkin's lymphoma).

Continued

Bladder Cancer

Reference/ Study Question	Methods
Adherence to surveillance among patients with superficial bladder cancer (Schrag et al., 2003) ——— How frequently do patients with superficial bladder cancer undergo recommended surveillance procedures? What patient and primary care provider characteristics are associated with nonadherence?	*Method:* Retrospective cohort study using SEER-Medicare data. *Sample:* 6,717 patients aged ≥65 years diagnosed with superficial bladder cancer from 1992 through 1996 and who survived for at least 3 years after diagnosis, but did not have a total cystectomy. Surveillance examination of the bladder during each of five contiguous 6-month intervals from month 7 to month 36 were examined. *Statistical methods:* Logistic regression. *Explanatory variables:* Patient race, sex, age at diagnosis, year of diagnosis, registry location, census tract income, MSA residence, comorbidity; physician Medicare case volume, characteristics from AMA masterfile (e.g., board certification, year of medical school graduation). (AUA and NCCN guidelines recommend that patients with superficial bladder cancer receive cystoscopic surveillance at least every 3–6 months for the first 3 years after diagnosis and at least annually thereafter.)

Results

Only 40% of the entire cohort had an examination during all five intervals; 18% had low-intensity surveillance (bladder exam during fewer than two of the five contiguous 6-month intervals). Patient characteristics that were associated with low-intensity surveillance were being aged 75 years or older (OR = 1.54), being nonwhite (OR = 1.94), having favorable tumor histology (OR = 0.59 for poorly differentiated versus referent well-differentiated tumor grade), and having high comorbidity (OR = 1.72). Residence in an urban area or in a census tract with low median income was also associated with low-intensity surveillance.

Physician characteristics associated with low adherence include solo practice, lower case volume, and year of medical school graduation before 1980.

Continued

Lung Cancer

Reference/ Study Question	Methods
Geographic variation in the conduct of patient surveillance after lung cancer surgery (Johnson et al., 1996b) Clinical surveillance testing after lung cancer operations (Naunheim et al., 1995) ——— What are the surveillance practices of thoracic surgeons for their patients with lung cancer?	*Method:* Physician mail survey. *Sample:* 3,700 active members (U.S. and foreign) of the Society of Thoracic Surgeons (STS) surveyed in 1994. 54% responded (2,009/3,700), and of these, 768 were found to both operate on and provide long-term follow-up for lung cancer patients. Profiles of hypothetical patients suitable for post-operative surveillance and a detailed questionnaire based on the profiles were mailed to STS members. *Statistical methods:* One-way analysis of variance. *Explanatory variables:* None.
Lung cancer patient follow-up: Motivation of thoracic surgeons (Virgo et al., 1998) ——— Do physician characteristics and beliefs explain follow-up intensity?	*Method:* Same as above. *Sample:* Same as above. *Statistical methods:* Logistic regression to examine test use by stage and ordinary least squares regression to examine intensity of use. *Explanatory variables:* Age, professional society memberships, practice type, percentage of practice that was noncardiac, practice location.

Results

The follow-up methods most frequently used during a 5-year follow-up period include clinic visit, chest X ray, CBC, liver function testing, and chest CT scan. Sputum cytology, head CT scan, bone scanning, chest MRI, and bronchoscopy are used infrequently. Although there is wide variation in the frequency of use of the follow-up methods, there is a decrease in the frequency of testing over time since primary therapy.

Fewer than half of respondents believe surveillance testing would yield a survival benefit for either Stage I (44%) or advanced-stage patients (17%) after lung cancer resection. Only one of four respondents believed that the current literature documents any survival benefit. Other reasons for follow-up include maintenance of rapport with colleagues (42%) or patients (69%) and medicolegal liability concerns (49%).

TNM stage and year post-surgery affect follow-up practice. Geographic setting has rather little effect on surveillance strategies.

Physician characteristics and beliefs predicted a less than expected amount of the variation in self-reported follow-up intensity by TNM stage.

Continued

Melanoma

Reference/ Study Question	Methods
Current practice of patient follow-up after potentially curative resection of cutaneous melanoma (Virgo et al., 2000) How surgeon age affects post-treatment surveillance strategies for melanoma patients (Margenthaler et al., 2001) Effect of initial tumor stage on patient follow-up after potentially curative surgery for cutaneous melanoma (Johnson et al., 2001) Geographic variation in post-treatment surveillance intensity for patients with cutaneous melanoma (Margenthaler et al., 2003)	*Method:* Physician mail survey. *Sample:* 3,032 members of the American Society of Plastic and Reconstructive Surgeons (ASPRS; randomly chosen from the 4,320 members) surveyed in 1998 on use of 14 follow-up modalities during years 1–5 and 10 following primary treatment for patients with cutaneous melanoma. 1. Office visit 2. CBC 3. Liver function tests 4. CEA 5. Alpha-fetoprotein 6. Chest X ray 7. 5S-cysteinyl dopa 8. Abdominal ultrasound 9. CT brain 10. CT chest/abdomen 11. MRI brain 12. MRI chest/abdomen 13. PET scan 14. Bone scan RR = 38% (1,142/3,032); 35% (395/1,142) were evaluable because practice included follow-up in addition to treatment. *Statistical methods:* Repeated-measures analysis of variance. *Explanatory variables:* TNM stage, year post-surgery, and physician age.

Results

Plastic surgeons often do not provide post-operative follow-up themselves. When they do, surveillance relies most heavily on office visits, chest X ray, CBC, and liver function tests. All other modalities are used infrequently. Surgeons use the most common modalities similarly by TNM stage.

The intensity of post-treatment surveillance practice patterns of ASPRS members caring for patients with cutaneous melanoma varies markedly. Factors accounting for this variation include geography, MCO penetration rate (chest X ray highest in areas with low MCO penetration rate; 5S-cysteinyl dopa testing highest in areas with high MCO penetration rate).

Surveillance varies only marginally with physician age.

Continued

Melanoma (continued)

Reference/ Study Question	Methods
Geographic and patient variation in receipt of surveillance procedures after local excision of cutaneous melanoma (Barzilai et al., 2004) What are the surveillance practices for Medicare beneficiaries with invasive melanoma?	*Method:* Retrospective cohort study using SEER-Medicare data. *Sample:* 3,389 patients aged ≥65 years diagnosed with invasive melanoma from 1992 through 1996 and who survived for at least 2 years after diagnosis. Surveillance examination and tests were examined (CBC, liver enzymes or lactic dehydrogenase, chest X ray, CT scans, and MRI). *Statistical methods:* Kaplan-Meier analysis and log-rank test. *Explanatory variables:* Gender and age, tumor stage and thickness, geographic area. (The American Academy of Dermatology does not recommend a specific follow-up interval schedule, but recommended follow-up in some situations, including patient education, examination of the skin, and laboratory/radiologic examination between one and four times per year for the first 2 years after diagnosis and one to two times per year thereafter. Routine laboratory tests and imaging tests are not required in asymptomatic patients with melanoma ≤4 mm in depth for initial staging or routine follow-up.)

Results
Surveillance testing was relatively common, ranging from 13% for abdominal ultrasound to 80% for laboratory testing. Follow-up skin examinations were performed in 70% to 90% of patients. The use of most surveillance procedures was associated with younger age, male gender, regional stage tumors, and geographic area.

Continued

Upper Aerodigestive Tract Cancer (UADT)

Reference/ Study Question	Methods
How tumor stage affects surgeons' surveillance strategies after surgery for carcinoma of the upper aerodigestive tract (Johnson et al., 1998) How surgeon age affects post-treatment surveillance strategies for upper aerodigestive tract cancer patients (Clark et al., 1999) Surgical decision making in upper aerodigestive tract cancer patient follow-up (Virgo et al., 2002) ________ Does tumor stage and surgeon age affect surveillance practices? Do clinical beliefs explain follow-up practices?	*Method:* Mail survey of head and neck surgeons. *Sample:* 824 members of the Society of Head and Neck Surgeons (SHNS) and 522 members of the American Society for Head and Neck Surgery (ASHNS) who were not members of the SHNS were surveyed by mail in 1996 on use of 14 follow-up modalities for patients with resectable UADT cancer during years 1 to 5 after potentially curative primary treatment. 1. Office visit 2. CBC 3. Serum electrolytes (calcium level) 4. Serum liver function tests 5. Serum tumor marker measurement 6. Thyroid function tests 7. Chest X ray 8. Bone scan 9. Chest CT 10. Head and neck CT 11. Head and neck MRI 12. Sonogram of the head and neck 13. Flexible esophagoscopy 14. Flexible bronchoscopy RR = 24% (199/824) for SHNS and 42% (221/522) for ASHNS. *Statistical methods:* Repeated-measures analysis of variance. The relationship between clinical beliefs and test ordering practices was examined using Poisson and negative binomial regression analysis. *Explanatory variables:* TNM stage, year post-surgery, and surgeon age clinical beliefs.

Results
Ten of the 14 most commonly used surveillance modalities were ordered significantly more frequently with increasing TNM stage. The effect persisted through 5 years of follow-up. Surveillance practice patterns of surgeons do not vary substantially with practitioner age. Intensity of follow-up decreases with time post-surgery. Two clinical beliefs with the greatest impact on surgical decision making are that surveillance: (1) permits palliative treatment and improves quality of life, and (2) provides no survival benefit for patients with TNM Stage I cancer.

Continued

Head and Neck Cancers

Reference/ Study Question	Methods
Practice patterns and clinical guidelines for post-treatment follow-up of head and neck cancers (Paniello et al., 1999) _________ How does current clinical practice compare to recommendations in published clinical practice guidelines?	*Method:* 1996 mail survey of head and neck surgeons. *Sample:* 640 members of the ASHNS and 824 members of the Society of Head and Neck Surgeons (SHNS) (1,322 were members of one society or the other) were asked about the following surveillance tests: Imaging: • Chest radiography • CT of head and neck, chest • MRI of head and neck • Sonogram of head and neck • Bone scan Blood tests • Complete blood count, electrolytes (with or without calcium) • Liver function tests, thyroid function tests • Specific tumor markers Other • Bronchoscopy • Esophagoscopy RR = 610 were returned (46%); 420 evaluable (32%). *Statistical methods:* Analysis of variance. *Explanatory variables:* Stage, group membership, post-operative year.

Results
Most surgeons relied on directed history, physical examination, and routine chest radiograph at varying intervals for detection of recurrences and second primary tumors. Other tests were used sporadically. The proportion of surgeons who followed published guidelines varied from 97% in post-operative year 1 to 62% in post-operative year 5.

Continued

Extremity Soft-Tissue Sarcoma

Reference/ Study Question	Methods
Current follow-up strategies after potentially curative resection of extremity soft-tissue sarcomas: Results of a survey of members of the Society of Surgical Oncology (Beitler et al., 2000) How surgeon age affects surveillance strategies for extremity soft-tissue sarcoma patients after potentially curative treatment (Sakata et al., 2002) Extremity soft-tissue sarcoma patient follow-up: Tumor grade and size affect surveillance strategies after potentially curative surgery (Sakata et al., 2003) ________ What surveillance modalities are used? Does tumor stage, grade, and size and surgeon age affect surveillance practices?	*Method:* Physician mail survey. *Sample:* 1,592 members of the SSO surveyed in 1997 regarding their follow-up practices for extremity sarcoma patients treated for cure. Respondents reported on 12 surveillance modalities performed annually during the first 5 years and the 10th year after surgery. 1. Office visit 2. CBC 3. Liver function test 4. Serum electrolytes 5. Urinalysis 6. Erythrocyte sedimentation rate 7. Chest X ray 8. Chest CT 9. Extremity X ray 10. Extremity CT 11. Extremity MRI 12. Bone scan 45% (716/1,592) surgeons completed the survey. Of the 343 respondents who performed sarcoma surgery, 318 (93%) also provided long-term post-operative follow-up. *Statistical methods:* Repeated measures analysis of variance. *Explanatory variables:* Physician age and years since completion of training, tumor grade and size, and year post-surgery.

Results

Routine office visits and chest X ray were the most frequently performed items for each of the years. The frequency of office visits and chest X ray increased with tumor size and grade and decreased with post-operative year. CBC and liver function tests were the most commonly ordered blood tests, but many respondents did not order any blood tests routinely. Imaging studies of the extremities were performed on the majority of patients with large (> 5 cm) low-grade lesions and on both large and small high-grade lesions during the first post-operative year.

The post-treatment surveillance practice patterns of the members of the SSO vary only marginally with the length of time since completion of training.

Tumor grade and size significantly impacted physician practice patterns in post-treatment follow-up, although the degree of variation attributable to these variables was modest. Office visit, complete blood count, liver function tests, chest X ray, chest CT, extremity CT, and extremity MRI were ordered more frequently with increasing tumor grade and size.

Continued

Multiple Sites

Reference/ Study Question	Methods
Heterogeneity of cancer surveillance practices among medical oncologists in Washington and Oregon (Richert-Boe, 1995) What are the surveillance practices for breast, prostate, and colorectal cancer in Washington and Oregon?	*Method:* Physician mail survey. Clinical scenarios were presented with options for testing for each cancer site. *Sample:* 113 medical oncologists, members of the American Society of Clinical Oncology (ASCO) residing in Washington or Oregon. 105 members were determined to be eligible; RR = 70% (73/105). *Statistical methods:* Descriptive statistics. *Explanatory variables:* Physician age, year of graduation, practice type, state of residence.
Screening for second cancers and osteoporosis in long-term survivors (Mahon et al., 2000) What do nurses know about follow-up of cancer survivors?	*Method:* Nurse mail survey. *Sample:* 321 nurses, members of the Oncology Nursing Society. 321 of 668 outpatient nurses surveyed responded (RR = 48%). *Statistical methods:* Descriptive statistics. *Explanatory variables:* None.
Routine surveillance care after cancer treatment with curative intent (Elston Lafata et al., 2005) To what extent do post-treatment surveillance practices vary and conform to available guidelines?	*Method*: Medical record abstraction *Sample*: Cohorts of patients aged 30 years or older diagnosed with breast, colorectal, endometrial, lung, or prostate cancer between 1990 and 1995 and treated with curative intent (100 cases for each site). Eligible patients were receiving care from physicians practicing with a 900-member multispecialty, salaried group practice in the Midwest. *Statistical methods*: Kaplan-Meier estimation *Explanatory variables*: None.

NOTE: AMA = American Medical Association; ASCO = American Society of Clinical Oncology; AUA = American Urologic Association; CBC = complete blood cell count; CT = computed tomography; DCIS = ductal carcinoma *in situ*; FOBT = fecal occult blood test; MCO = managed care organization; MRI = magnetic resonance imaging; MSA = Metropolitan Statis-

Results

All respondents reported an intention to provide some level of follow-up testing of their cancer patients. There was considerable variation in testing practices that was not explained by physician age, year of graduation, practice type, or state of residence.

The most consistently performed screenings reported by nurses were mammogram, professional breast examination, and Pap test and pelvic examination. The least frequently performed screenings were flexible sigmoidoscopy/colonoscopy, and bone mineral density testing. Less than one-third of survivors are offered counseling on strategies to promote bone health.

Most cancer patients received the recommended minimum number of physical examinations after treatment. A sizable number received physical examinations at a frequency in excess of what is currently recommended. Most survivors received recommended testing for local recurrence, however, less than two-thirds of colorectal cancer patients received recommended colon examinations in the initial year after treatment. Evidence of overtesting for local recurrent cancer was found. Testing for metastatic disease was commonplace despite its not being recommended in guidelines.

tical Area; NCCN = National Comprehensive Cancer Network; PET = positron emission tomography; RR = response rate; SEER = Surveillance, Epidemiology, and End Results Program (a cancer registry maintained by NCI); SES = socioeconomic status; TNM = tumor, node, metastasis stage.

APPENDIX 4B
INFORMATION ON AMBULATORY CARE SURVEY DATA

The information on ambulatory care in Tables 4-1 to 4-4, 4-6, and 4-7 comes from two large population-based surveys conducted by the National Centers for Health Statistics, the National Ambulatory Medical Care Survey (NAMCS) and the National Hospital Ambulatory Care Survey (NHAMCS). Two years (2001 and 2002) of data from both surveys were combined to yield sufficient sample sizes for cancer site-specific estimates. Information on 3,773 cancer-related ambulatory care visits was available from the 2001 and 2002 NAMCS and NHAMCS. Cancer-related visits are those for which cancer was recorded as the first, second, or third diagnosis associated with the visit according to the International Classification of Diseases (Clinical Modification), Ninth Edition (ICD-9-CM). Cancer-related visits were those where the reason for the visit was coded for history of cancer (V10) and malignant neoplasms (ICD-9 code 140 to 208, but excluding skin, nonmelanoma [173]). All numbers and percentages presented in tables are adjusted using sampling weights to produce national estimates.

NAMCS

NAMCS is a national probability sample survey of visits to office-based physicians. In 2001, information on 24,281 patient visits was received from the 1,230 physicians who participated in NAMCS (64 percent response rate). In 2002, information on 28,738 patient visits was received from 1,474 physicians (70 percent response rate). For each participating physician, a random sample of visits was obtained during a 1-week period. In the tables describing type of physician, "oncology" includes medical oncology and hematology/oncology; "primary care" includes family practice, internal medicine, and general practice; "specialty surgery" includes the following surgical specialties: orthopedic, plastic, vascular, neurological, thoracic, colorectal, and head and neck. "Other medical specialty" includes obstetrics and gynecology, ophthalmology, cardiovascular diseases, psychiatry, gastroenterology, otolaryngology, hematology, pulmonary disease, and others. Estimates of cancer-related ambulatory care are somewhat hampered by the exclusion of radiologists from the sampling frame of office-based providers.

NHAMCS

NHAMCS provides information on ambulatory care provided in hospital outpatient departments. In 2001, information on 33,567 patient visits was provided by 1,036 clinics in 224 hospitals (overall response rate, 74 percent). In 2002, information on 35,586 patient visits was provided by 1,041 clinics in 224 hospitals (overall response rate, 75 percent). For each participating outpatient department clinic, a random sample of visits was obtained during a 4-week period. Excluded from the sampling frame of the hospital outpatient departments are clinics providing chemotherapy, radiation therapy, infusion therapy, physical medicine, and rehabilitation because, in these settings, much of the care is provided by nonphysician providers (e.g., oncology nurses, radiation technicians, physical therapists). The purpose of the surveys is to capture physician-patient encounters.

APPENDIX 4C
WHAT HAS BEEN LEARNED ABOUT MODELS OF SURVIVORSHIP CARE IN OTHER COUNTRIES?

Investigators in Europe, Canada, and Australia have evaluated delivery system issues, often in an effort to improve national health programs. Much of the work of relevance to the delivery of cancer survivorship care comes from the United Kingdom, where cancer care is being reorganized and the results of restructuring efforts are being evaluated through clinical audits (Tattersall and Thomas, 1999). Here, traditional disciplinary divisions of medicine, surgery, obstetrics, and gynecology are being replaced by disease- and organ-based multidisciplinary groupings. The goals of the reorganization are to facilitate improvements in quality, reduce geographic disparities in outcomes of treatment, and provide better coordinated care.

As part of a major effort to gauge cancer patients' experience with cancer within the British National Health System, a nationwide survey was conducted in 2000 (Airey et al., 2002). The survey covered access to care, diagnosis, first treatment, hospital care, and outpatient care.[17] Some aspects of follow-up care were assessed as part of this survey:

- 19 percent of cancer patients reported that doctors and nurses did not spend enough time, or spent no time at all, telling them what would happen when they left the hospital after their first treatment.
- 26 percent of patients were not given written or printed information about what they should or shouldn't do following their discharge.
- 36 percent of cancer patients were not told about a support or self-help group.

[17]Nearly three-quarters (74 percent) of patients identified through hospital records responded to the survey.

The cancer care survey involved more than 65,000 patients who had been treated in 1999 and 2000. Cancer care in England has recently been organized into 172 networks or "Trusts." Data from the survey were made available to each Trust so they could compare their results with other care providers. The position of "Primary Care Cancer Lead Clinician" has been created as part of this reorganization to improve communication between primary and specialty care providers, raise awareness of cancer in primary care, and improve palliative care (Leese et al., 2004).

Several clinical trials have been conducted in Europe to assess alternative models of survivorship care. A shared cancer care program implemented and tested as part of a clinical trial had a positive effect on patients' evaluation of cooperation between the primary care providers and specialists (Nielsen et al., 2003).

The trial involved patients with several types of cancer seen in a Danish university hospital-based practice. The intervention involved knowledge transfer, communication channels, and active patient involvement (Box 4C-1). The shared care program increased contacts with the general practitioner and did not adversely effect quality of life.

A commentary that accompanied the publication of this trial emphasized the importance of the involvement of both patients and providers in formal shared-care arrangements in cancer (Maher and Millar, 2003). In

BOX 4C-1
Components of Shared-Care Program Tested in a Clinical Trial

Knowledge transfer

- Discharge summary letters following predefined guidelines
- Specific information on the disease and its treatment
- General information about chemotherapy and radiotherapy
- General information about pain treatment
- Information about treatment of induced nausea and sickness
- Information about some acute oncologic conditions

Communication channels

- Names and phone numbers of doctors and nurses responsible for the patient were attached to the discharge summary letter to the general practitioner (GP)

Active patient involvement

- In the intervention group the patients received oral as well as written information about the information package to their GP
- The patients were encouraged to contact their GP when facing problems they assumed could be solved in this setting

SOURCE: Nielsen et al. (2003).

addition, shared-care models depend on (1) professional training, (2) general practitioners viewing their role in cancer care as enhancing patient care and improving their job satisfaction, and (3) appropriate remuneration.

Long-term cancer survivors who have been followed for many years by specialists are sometimes reluctant to return to their primary care physician for follow-up, even when reassured that they are at low risk of recurrence. One group of British clinicians noted that a feeling often expressed by patients seen for many years in their specialty clinics was "As long as I keep coming here I feel I'll be alright" (Glynne-Jones et al., 1997). These clinicians concluded that reassurance rather than the detection of recurrence was the most important function of follow-up and so developed a formal system of discharge from their hospital-based oncology clinic to primary care providers for follow-up. As part of the planned discharge, patients were counseled and given a written contract reassuring them of their good prognosis and commitment to continued care from the specialist if necessary. Primary care physicians were informed of the discharge plan. Of the long-term cancer survivors invited to participate, 63 percent agreed to be discharged to primary care. Of the patients who agreed to the contract, 85 percent remained with their primary care provider at 13 months. The planned discharge was viewed as successful, and investigators noted the need to address patients' expectations regarding follow-up and the duration of specialty follow-up early in the treatment process. Investigators highlighted the need to address anxiety among patients as this is a deterrent to acceptance of a transfer to primary care.

A trial conducted at a breast clinic in London showed that reducing the number of hospital-based follow-up visits was not associated with increased visits to local practitioners or to higher use of a telephone hotline (Gulliford et al., 1997). Women diagnosed within the past 5 years were seen every 3 to 6 months in the conventional arm of the trial, but annually during the visit for mammography in the reduced visit arm (for women treated with lumpectomy). Nearly all (93 percent) women were willing to participate in the trial. Twice as many patients in both groups preferred reducing rather than increasing follow-up visits.[18]

Evidence that generalists are as effective as specialists in providing follow-up care for women with breast cancer is available from clinical trials. General practitioner follow-up did not increase length of time to diagnosis of a recurrent cancer (as measured at 18 months) or adversely effect quality of life (Grunfeld et al., 1996). Women who had follow-up

[18]This study was not designed to assess differences in survival or length of time to diagnose recurrent cancer.

care provided by their general practitioner reported greater satisfaction with care than did those followed up in the hospital by specialty providers (Grunfeld et al., 1999a). Costs associated with follow-up were lower when provided by general practitioners (even though they ordered more tests) (Grunfeld et al., 1995, 1996, 1999b).[19] This trial was conducted at two district hospitals in England where one-third of women declined to participate in the trial, indicating that this model of care is not acceptable to all patients. As part of the intervention, general practitioners were sent a letter with recommended follow-up protocols that varied according to initial treatment and patient age. Specialists and general practitioners, when surveyed, indicated that their specialty group should provide follow-up care. These findings have prompted some British hospitals to limit specialty follow-up after treatment for breast cancer to 2 years, after which time oncology providers coordinate with local general practitioners and arrange for patients to be seen by their general practitioners with immediate access to specialist review in the breast care unit if needed (Donnelly et al., 2001).

A Canadian trial also examined the question of specialist versus primary care follow-up for women with early breast cancer (Grunfeld et al., 2004). Women randomized to follow-up by cancer center specialists or family physicians had similar rates of death, recurrence, serious clinical events (e.g., poor functional status), and quality of life. Median period of follow-up was 3.5 years. The results of this trial appear to have affected follow-up care in other parts of the country. A survey conducted in Manitoba of cancer patients regarding their care 6 to 12 months after diagnosis found that relatively few (10 percent) were getting mainly specialist care; roughly 40 percent were getting "parallel care" in which cancer specialists looked after everything to do with cancer and the family doctor looked after most other health problems; about 40 percent were getting "shared care" in which the family doctor and cancer specialists both had been involved in taking care of cancer and the family doctor looked after most other health problems; and 10 percent described other health care situations (Sisler et al., 2004). The most commonly cited kinds of help that women reported needing from family practitioners were:

- Helps with medical problems unrelated to my cancer
- Gets me an appointment with a surgeon or other cancer specialist fairly quickly

[19]Earlier descriptive, nonrandomized research suggested that women preferred specialty follow-up as compared to follow-up by a general practitioner (Morris et al., 1992). This research, however, was limited to women questioned about their preferences while being seen at a hospital breast cancer clinic.

- Takes extra time with me during a visit
- Sees me quickly in the office if I think it's necessary
- Answers my questions about cancer and cancer treatments
- Discusses how I am feeling about having cancer
- Helps with common cancer-related problems, like pain, nausea, depression, and bowel problems

Focus groups held with family physicians throughout Canada to discuss communication between family physicians and oncologists suggest that family physicians would like to have more contact with oncologists, preferably by phone or in person, to negotiate their respective roles, and to discuss the patient's prognosis and the effectiveness of proposed treatments (Dworkind et al., 1999). According to qualitative interviews with oncologists in a Canadian regional cancer center, collaboration with family physicians in the remission phase was identified as desirable, but inhibited by variable and unpredictable interest, poor communication with family physicians, and patients' own preferences for follow-up. Oncologists perceived the cancer system structure as a "black box" within which multidisciplinary teams worked well but seldom included family physicians. Oncologists expressed a need to see healthy patients and to have more understanding and support from family physicians, preferably through sharing follow-up care. Developing dialogue and a more collaborative approach were suggested (Wood and McWilliam, 1996).

A few studies have been carried out to evaluate how to improve communication among cancer specialists, primary care providers, and cancer patients. To encourage breast cancer patients to seek information about cancer from their general practitioners, one group of investigators in England tested giving women cards with specific information about their treatment to take to their general practitioner (Luker et al., 2000). Results of the small clinical trial suggested that the cards did not encourage women to seek information from their primary care physician. Women's information-seeking behavior was more determined by their longstanding relationship with their general practitioner, their perception that their general practitioner lacked specialist knowledge, and the perception that information seeking was not a reason to seek primary care.

A standardized discharge letter improved communication from oncologists to family physicians with respect to the relevance, timeliness, format, and amount of information conveyed (Braun et al., 2003). In this Canadian study, the letter was intended to communicate information about the palliative care needs of patients with lung cancer and included information about diagnosis, stage of disease, current problem(s), treatment plan, potential problems, prognosis, discussion with family, follow-up, and home-care arrangements.

Several European and Australian studies have assessed nurse-led follow-up care. Nurse-led follow-up of patients with lung cancer was found to be acceptable and led to positive outcomes when compared to conventional medical follow-up in an English randomized trial (Moore et al., 2002). Other assessments in the United Kingdom also suggest that breast cancer survivors are accepting of a specialist nurse-led system of follow-up care (Earnshaw and Stephenson, 1997; Pennery and Mallet, 2000; Renton et al., 2002). One British study of patients' views on follow-up of colorectal cancer, however, indicated that fewer than half (47 percent) would accept follow-up care from a specialist nurse, and even fewer (27 percent) were willing to be followed by their general practitioner (Papagrigoriadis and Heyman, 2003). A Swedish randomized trial compared routine physician follow-up and "on-demand" care by a specialist nurse for women with early-stage breast cancer and found no differences between groups in terms of survivors' satisfaction, perceptions regarding accessibility of care, anxiety, and depression when measured over a 5-year period (Koinberg et al., 2004). Another smaller clinical trial conducted in the United Kingdom compared standard clinic follow-up with on-demand care through a breast care nurse (Brown et al., 2002). Women in the on-demand care group were given written information on the signs and symptoms of recurrence and were instructed to contact the breast care nurse if they encountered any problems. There were no major differences in quality of life and psychological morbidity between the two groups and no observed adverse effects associated with patient-initiated follow-up. Of note, however, is that half of women approached to participate in the trial refused, indicating that this model for follow-up is not acceptable to many women with early-stage breast cancer. Resistance to this model of follow-up was evident in an earlier study indicating that most women desired specialist, hospital-based follow-up (Brown et al., 2002). In Australia, a comprehensive specialist breast nurse model of care has been developed to improve the delivery of care, especially psychosocial services (Hordern, 2000; Liebert et al., 2001, 2003; Parle et al., 2001).

Some research suggests that nurse-based follow-up can meet the needs of cancer survivors and reduce the medical outpatient workload. A British study of a nurse-led clinic for patients being treated for central nervous system tumors and a nurse "phone clinic" for post-treatment follow-up was acceptable to patients and decreased the medical outpatient workload by 30 percent. This medical audit was conducted in a large neurooncology program in an English hospital (James et al., 1994). At this same hospital, patients were very satisfied with a nurse-led telephone clinic in the follow-up of patients with glioma, a cancer with very poor prognosis. The telephone intervention was believed to be able to replace routine specialist care during the short stable phase of disease following treatment (Sardell et al., 2000).

APPENDIX 4D CHALLENGES IN THE DELIVERY OF SELECTED SURVIVORSHIP SERVICES

This appendix illustrates some of the challenges of delivering three survivorship services:

- Genetic counseling
- Cancer rehabilitation
- Psychosocial services for women with breast cancer

Genetic Counseling

It has long been recognized that cancer can run in families, and that people with close relatives who have had cancer may be at greater risk for a cancer diagnosis. The establishment of concrete links between particular genetic mutations and cancer have opened the possibility of genetic testing for increased cancer risk. The complete sequencing of the human genome will likely lead to additional opportunities for risk assessment. Genetic risk assessment and testing holds great promise in helping survivors and their family members plan appropriate screening regimens, consider preventative measures, and make reproductive decisions (NCCN, 2004a,b). However, the appropriate delivery and management of genetic information creates new challenges for the health care system. Among these challenges is a lack of trained personnel available to provide genetic counseling and testing to cancer survivors and their families. This limitation of capacity, if not addressed, will limit the diffusion of this relatively new and potentially vital technology.

Genetic tests are commercially available and may be of value for certain cancer survivors and their family members. For example, women diagnosed with breast cancer who have a strong family history of breast and/or ovarian cancer are often tested to determine if they are among the estimated 5 to 10 percent of women with breast and ovarian cancer that is caused by mutations in the BRCA1 and BRCA2 genes. Likewise, commercially available genetic tests are available for colon cancer survivors who have a strong family history of the disease. An estimated 5 percent of individuals with colon cancer have either familial adenomatous polyposis (FAP) or hereditary nonpolyposis colorectal cancer (HNPCC) (Sifri et al., 2004). As the availability of genetic testing becomes more widely known, it will be increasingly important for primary care providers, oncologists, nurses, and other health professionals to be familiar with the process of genetic counseling and testing.

A complete assessment of genetic risk involves much more than genetic testing. American Society of Clinical Oncology (ASCO) guidelines recommend that genetic testing only be offered to selected patients with personal or family histories suggestive of a hereditary syndrome, in the context of pre- and post-test counseling to discuss the risks and benefits of genetic testing and cancer early detection and prevention methods, and only when the test results can be adequately interpreted and will aid in diagnosis or care management (ASCO, 2003).

A recent national survey of physicians indicated that most do not consider themselves qualified to provide genetic counseling to their cancer patients (Table 4D-1) (Freedman et al., 2003). Although nearly a third of U.S. physicians have offered genetic tests or referred patients to be tested, only 8 percent took responsibility for providing pre- and post-test counseling by ordering the tests directly (Wideroff et al., 2003a). Oncologists express more confidence than other physicians in recommending genetic testing (85 percent) and providing counseling (50 percent), however, these estimates suggest that additional education and training in this area is needed for all providers who are likely to encounter cancer survivors in their practices (see Chapter 5).

Individuals with strong family histories of cancer (or who are considered high risk) may be referred to a genetic counselor. Genetic counselors are usually master's degree-level trained and are certified by the American Board of Genetic Counseling. There are about 1,800 certified genetic counselors in the United States, but only 42 percent provide counseling to cancer patients and their families, and only 16 percent spend more than half their

TABLE 4D-1 Physicians' Qualifications to Provide Genetic Counseling and Recommend Genetic Testing

Specialty	Percentage Who Feel Qualified to Provide Genetic Counseling	Percentage Who Feel Qualified to Recommend Genetic Testing
Primary care	28.8	40.8
Tertiary care (general surgery, gastroenterology, urology)	30.7	58.2
Oncology	50.0	84.6

SOURCE: Freedman et al. (2003).

time on cancer genetics (Parrott et al., 2002, 2003). Access to genetic counselors with cancer-related experience may be further limited, as more than half of cancer genetic counselors work in university medical centers, and only 27 percent work in private hospitals or medical facilities (Parrott et al., 2003). Another important resource for genetic counseling is oncology nurses trained in genetics, who may play an increasing role in the delivery of cancer genetic services in the future (Bernhardt et al., 2000; Masny et al., 2003).

The demand for genetic counseling and testing is likely to grow as new tests are developed and marketed, and as cancer survivors and their family members become aware of their potential benefits. Approximately 44 percent of the public is already aware of the availability of genetic tests for cancer susceptibility (Wideroff et al., 2003b). One of the greatest predictors of whether a physician has ordered genetic tests or made a referral for genetic counseling is having patients ask for cancer genetic tests (Wideroff et al., 2003a). Unless education and training programs reach more oncology and primary care providers who care for cancer survivors, the public's demand for genetic testing and counseling will likely not be met.

Some patients and providers may be concerned about the possibility of genetic information being used as a basis for employment or insurance discrimination. Bills have been introduced in Congress to prevent discrimination based on genetic information, but no federal protection is currently in place. However, 33 states have laws prohibiting genetic discrimination in employment, and most states restrict employer access to genetic information (NCSL, 2005). Some states extend the protections to inherited characteristics, family history, the test results of family members, and information on receipt of genetic services. In addition, an executive order issued in 2000 protects against discrimination based on genetic information in civilian federal employment. The Health Insurance Portability and Accountability Act (HIPAA) provides some protection against genetic discrimination under group insurance plans, but does not provide any protection for those seeking individual insurance, and does not prevent insurers from accessing genetic information (NIH, 2005).

Cancer Rehabilitation

Rehabilitation services can help cancer survivors regain and improve physical, psychosocial, and vocational functioning within the limitations imposed by the disease and its treatment (Ganz, 1990; Watson, 1992). Although cancer rehabilitation has been recognized as valuable, organized rehabilitation programs for cancer survivors are limited and lag behind those organized for patients with other chronic conditions such as heart disease for which rehabilitation is now considered a part of standard care

(Segal et al., 1999). Some have suggested that rehabilitation programs for cancer patients with physical limitations have been slow to develop because of the nature of cancer and its treatment as compared to other causes of disability (Sliwa and Marciniak, 1999). Physical impairments associated with stroke and brain injury are commonly treated through rehabilitation programs and in these cases, the deficits are fixed, acute care treatment has been completed, and the likelihood of survival following the initial injury or episode is good. In such cases rehabilitation occurs after acute medical treatment and addresses static deficits. In contrast, cancer patients experiencing physical limitation may be in treatment when rehabilitation services are needed and the treatment may not be curative. Complicating cancer rehabilitation further is its heterogeneity. It spans lymphedema management, neurologic and orthopedic rehabilitation, and general conditioning. This breadth of cancer rehabilitation may pose the greatest challenge to service delivery.

The recognition of the need for rehabilitation services for cancer survivors is longstanding, and the U.S. Congress has actively encouraged the development of rehabilitation programs for cancer survivors (Box 4D-1). These congressional actions encouraged the development of cancer rehabilitation programs and centers. One of the earliest cancer rehabilitation programs was established in 1969 by Dietz, a physiatrist who coordinated the resources of an acute care hospital and a cancer center (Dietz, 1974; Grabois, 2001). The expansion of the role of the National Cancer Institute into rehabilitation in 1971 led to the development of related training, demonstration, and research projects. Some observers have noted, however, that cancer rehabilitation was hampered in its development because there was no specific implementation plan, a lack of trained personnel, and a failure to educate referring health care professionals (Grabois, 2001).

Despite these early initiatives, there are now relatively few organized cancer rehabilitation programs. Those that have been developed are usually housed within hospital physical medicine and rehabilitation programs or within large cancer centers. With the shift of cancer care from inpatient settings to outpatient care, some are concerned that cancer survivors' needs are not being met. Oncologists and surgeons report that rehabilitation services are not available, or if available, are not adequately covered by health insurance. While there is anecdotal evidence of problems with access to rehabilitation services for cancer patients, there has been little systematic documentation of such problems among contemporary cancer survivors.

The successful expansion of cancer rehabilitation programs has been hampered by a lack of an evidence base upon which to base decisions regarding: who needs services; what services should be provided; who should deliver services; and where and how services should be delivered. In the absence of evidence, no widely recognized clinical practice guidelines

BOX 4D-1
Congressional Actions Affecting Cancer Rehabilitation

1965—Congress authorized the establishment and maintenance of Regional Medical Programs under the Heart Disease, Cancer and Stroke Amendment (Pub. L. No. 89–239). These programs were to encourage and assist in the establishment of regional cooperative arrangements among medical schools, research institutions, and hospitals for research and training, including continuing education, and for related demonstration of patient care. Fifty-six regions were established across the nation. Rehabilitation units were to be created in association with diagnostic and treatment services. The program was terminated in 1976.

1971—Congress passed the National Cancer Act (Pub. L. No. 92–218) to amend the Public Health Service Act to strengthen the National Cancer Institute. Funds were available for the development of training, demonstration, and research projects in rehabilitation.

1988—Congress passed legislation (Pub. L. No. 100–607) that added rehabilitation research to the mission of the National Cancer Institute as follows:

> The general purpose of the National Cancer Institute is the conduct and support of research, training, health information dissemination and other programs with respect to cause, diagnosis, prevention, and treatment of cancer, rehabilitation from cancer, and the continuing care of cancer patients and the families of cancer patients (42 U.S.C. 285).

1998—Women's Health and Cancer Rights Act (Pub. L. No. 105–277) was enacted to require health insurance policies that cover mastectomy to also provide coverage for reconstructive surgery, prostheses, and physical complications of mastectomy, including lymphedema.

SOURCES: President's Commission on Heart Disease (1964); DeLisa (2001); NLM (2005); NCLAC (2005); NCI (2005b).

have been developed for common cancer-related conditions, and there are few evidence-based mechanisms to ensure appropriate service use. This void has led to the use by Medicare and private insurers of other mechanisms such as caps in benefits or limits on services in order to control rising costs. Such mechanisms can frustrate both providers and patients as they seek care that is viewed as medically necessary.

Evidence Regarding the Risk of Disability and the Need for Services

Relatively few studies adequately document the prevalence of physical and functional limitations among contemporary cancer survivors. Many of the widely cited studies used to document the prevalence of physical impairments imposed by cancer or its treatment are limited because they were conducted many years ago; did not include representative samples of patients; did not use standard evaluation tools to assess functional limitations; and did not include control groups, sometimes making it difficult to distinguish cancer-related limitations from those due to aging. Many studies have been conducted within inpatient units of individual institutions, and virtually none conducted in outpatient settings where most cancer patients now receive their care. Without such studies it is difficult to gauge how many cancer survivors need rehabilitation services and the extent of any access problem that may exist.

Evidence Regarding What Services Should Be Provided

Relatively few clinical trials have been conducted to assess the effectiveness of cancer rehabilitation services, and those that have been conducted have focused on inpatient rehabilitation (especially for patients with cancers of the brain or spinal cord) (Gerber, et al., 2005). A few clinical trials have been conducted to test the role of exercise in cancer rehabilitation (Segal et al., 1999; AHRQ, 2004b). Exercise has been shown to enhance physical performance, reduce fatigue, and improve psychological well-being (see Chapter 3 section on physical activity). A recommendation to exercise is therefore appropriate for most cancer survivors, however, more research is needed to determine what type of exercise regimen is optimal for survivors of different types of cancer and with various levels of physical limitation. Research could also help distinguish those survivors who could safely engage in exercise on their own from those who need the supervision of rehabilitation personnel during exercise.

Much of the literature documenting gains in functioning following cancer rehabilitation is based on observational studies conducted within a single institution (Sabers et al., 1999; Ganz, 1999). The relative lack of evidence on the effectiveness of rehabilitation treatment modalities has serious implications for patients who are facing cancer-related functional limitations. A recent review of the evidence regarding the treatment of lymphedema related to breast cancer found insufficient high-quality evidence on which to base a clinical practice guideline (Kligman et al., 2004). There is also insufficient evidence upon which to counsel women with breast cancer regarding how to prevent lymphedema (Runowicz, 1998). Well-designed controlled clinical trials are needed to reinvigorate cancer rehabilitation, as well as to evaluate the impact of this important clinical care activity on patient outcomes (Ganz, 1999).

BOX 4D-2
Providers of Cancer Rehabilitation Services

- Physiatrists
- Rehabilitation oncology nurses
- Occupational therapists
- Physical therapists
- Prosthetist/orthotists
- Enterostomal therapists
- Nutritionists/dieticians
- Speech-language pathologists
- Vocational rehabilitation counselors
- Recreational therapists

SOURCES: Beck (2003); Ragnarsson and Thomas (2000).

Who Should Deliver Services

Members of the cancer rehabilitation team trained to address the physical, functional, and vocational concerns of cancer survivors are shown in Box 4D-2. Other types of professionals may provide rehabilitative services (e.g., massage therapists, chiropractors), and some referring providers have expressed discomfort over role issues among rehabilitation team members and other medical caregivers (Schmidt, 2001). This discomfort or confusion could lead physicians caring for cancer survivors to fail to refer patients for rehabilitation services. Rehabilitation is underrepresented in medical education and training programs and the role of physical rehabilitation services is not always well understood (Frymark, 1998). This lack of awareness of the specialty may also contribute to underreferral (Schmidt, 2001).

Where and How Services Should Be Delivered

Rehabilitation services are furnished in many different settings, including hospital outpatient departments, outpatient rehabilitation facilities, skilled nursing facilities, home health agencies, and physicians' offices, and by therapists in private practice. Cancer rehabilitation has generally focused on inpatient services, leaving outpatient services not well developed. The exception to this is the many lymphedema clinics that are available. However, there are no estimates of their number, their organization, or their patient populations.

There are few descriptions of existing models for delivering cancer rehabilitation (Harvey et al., 1982; MacLaren, 2003). One U.S. study published in 1982 reviewed 36 cancer rehabilitation programs that were located at cancer centers, university hospitals, or community hospitals. Most programs were organized through oncology departments or departments of rehabilitation medicine (Harvey et al., 1982). Lehmann and colleagues described a model of care that involved systematic assessment and an interdisciplinary team approach to care (Lehmann et al., 1978). A few hospital- or cancer-center-based rehabilitation programs have been described in the literature (Segal et al., 1999; Schmidt, 2001; Grabois, 2001), but there have been no attempts to assess which models of care are more effective or preferred by cancer survivors.

The Consequences of a Lack of Evidence

Without evidence of the effectiveness of services and optimal delivery systems, patients cannot easily make personal health care decisions, health care providers lack the clinical practice guidelines they need to optimize care, and insurers and payors lack the tools they need to ensure that appropriate care is given.

Lacking professionally developed evidence-based guidelines, managed care organizations have attempted to control costs through utilization review mechanisms such as case management programs and authorization for coverage or have set annual limits for coverage. Such programs limit coverage, but without established evidence-based clinical practice guidelines, they cannot distinguish necessary from unnecessary care. Some managed care organizations have attempted to refine their coverage decisions through commercially available therapy guidelines (e.g., InterQual, Milliman & Robertson, Apollo, HealthSouth) and functional assessment and outcome monitoring systems (e.g., LIFEware, Focus on Therapeutic Outcomes or FOTO) (Maxwell and Baseggio, 2000).

Expenditures under Medicare for outpatient therapy services of physical therapists (PTs), occupational therapists (OTs), and speech and language pathologists (SLPs) have increased over time, and Congress has responded by enacting measures to control payment growth (Ciolek and Hwang, 2004). Medicare's coverage policies are fairly broad (Box 4D-3) and, in general, Medicare beneficiaries (with and without cancer) do not report encountering problems in getting special therapy services (which include PT, OT, and SLP services) (MedPAC, 2004a). No limit currently exists on the amount of medically necessary outpatient therapy (PT, OT, or SLP) a beneficiary may receive under Medicare, but this has not always been the case. Payment caps have been imposed intermittently and were suspended at the end of 2003. Without congressional action, payment caps will resume in January 2006 (Ciolek and Hwang, 2004). Most private payors have adopted some kind of controls to limit rehabilitation service

BOX 4D-3
Medicare Coverage of Outpatient Therapy Services

Medicare covers outpatient therapy services as long as the services are furnished by a skilled professional, are appropriate and effective for a patient's condition, and are reasonable in terms of frequency and duration. Furthermore, a physician must refer the patients; review a written plan of care every 30 days; and, for longer term treatment (extending beyond 60 days), reevaluate the patient. In addition, providers must have a physician on call to support emergency medical care. Beneficiaries are expected to improve significantly in a reasonable period of time. Medicare does not cover physical therapy designed to maintain a level of functioning or serve as a general exercise program. Finally, services are not covered when the expected patient gains from therapy are insignificant in relation to the therapy required to reach them or when it has been decided that a patient will not realize treatment goals.

SOURCES: Maxwell and Baseggio (2000); MedPAC, (2004a).

use (e.g., to a predefined number of days or visits per year, such as 60 calendar days from the beginning of an "event" or 30 visits) (Maxwell and Baseggio, 2000).

Some of Medicare's reimbursement policies are not always consistent with the latest evidence on effectiveness. For women with breast cancer, for example, available evidence suggests that nonpharmacologic treatments, especially complex decongestive therapy, is effective for lymphedema. This therapy involves skin care, multilayer low-stretch bandaging, exercise, and massage techniques, followed by long-term fitted elastic compression (Sparaco and Fentiman, 2002; Kligman et al., 2004). Medicare and many private health insurers generally cover the most expensive components of complex lymphedema therapy, including physical therapy, but some aspects of the therapy may not be covered. Medicare, for example, does not cover durable medical equipment, including surgical stockings or hose. Expensive pneumatic compression devices are covered if they are determined to be reasonable and necessary for the treatment of lymphedema and if a trial of conservative therapy (including the use of compression bandages or garments) lasting 4 weeks does not result in improvement. Compression garments are covered only if the patient is also prescribed a pneumatic compression pump.

There are some anecdotal reports that pumps are provided to lymphedema patients with little education or follow-up, and that in some cases, these pumps actually worsen the condition irreversibly, especially if excessive pressures are used. Pumps have not been shown to be effective, are expensive, and because they tether users for a few hours daily, they tend to go unused. Pumps may have a place in patient treatment programs, but it is crucial that other modalities be fully explored first, and to the extent possible, that pumps be combined with other modalities. Although Medicare reimbursement is available for pumps, the scientific evidence supporting their effectiveness is poor compared to that available for most of the other modalities, notably complex decongestive therapy (especially the wrapping component) and compression garments.

Congress has acted to ensure coverage of certain cancer rehabilitation services. The federal Women's Health and Cancer Rights Act of 1998 requires health insurance policies that cover mastectomy to also provide coverage for reconstructive surgery, prostheses, and physical complications of mastectomy, including lymphedema. Certain states have also mandated coverage. Since 2004, Virginia has required health insurers and plans to provide coverage for lymphedema, including equipment, supplies, complex decongestive therapy, and outpatient self-management training and education for the treatment of lymphedema, if prescribed by a health care professional.

Given the complexities of coverage for lymphedema therapy, help in resolving insurance reimbursement problems is frequently requested from the National Lymphedema Network, an advocacy group representing individuals with lymphedema (NLN, 2005).

In summary, evidence of the effectiveness of cancer rehabilitation services, who should deliver such services, and in what manner is critical to guide the decisions of consumers, providers, educators, and payors. Such evidence is needed before the perceived barriers to access to these services can be overcome. Research is critical to better elucidate the post-treatment rehabilitation needs of cancer survivors.

Psychosocial Services for Women with Breast Cancer

Distress in cancer has been defined as an unpleasant emotional experience that may be psychological, social, or spiritual in nature (see Chapter 3). Distress exists on a continuum beginning with the "normal" and expected feelings of fear, worries, sadness, and vulnerability in coping with cancer and its treatment. However, these normal feelings may extend to become more severe, even disabling, symptoms of anxiety or a formal diagnosis of major depression. Severe distress may relate to the illness or its treatment, a severe social problem, or a family problem, or it also may result from a spiritual or existential crisis created by confronting a threat to life or from the complications of treatment (NCCN, 2004c). Logically, psychosocial issues and distress are likely primarily not cancer site-specific, but they have been studied most extensively among women with breast cancer. In particular, women with breast cancer have been examined for the impact on psychological function at each stage of disease and during survivorship. The studies show highest distress at transition points in treatment: at the time of diagnosis, awaiting treatment, during and on completion of treatment, at follow-up visits, at time of recurrence, and at time of treatment failure. Taken overall, approximately 30 percent of women show significant distress at some point during the illness, and the number is greater in women with recurrent disease whose family members are also distressed.

Interventions to address psychosocial problems and distress begin with basic information about the disease and treatment options from the breast cancer care clinician (often a medical oncologist). This clinician, regardless of medical specialty, should express support, encourage patients to voice their fears and concerns, encourage coping, and provide medication when needed to control symptoms like insomnia and anxiety. Psychosocial services should be provided by oncology caregivers as a part of total medical care, but referrals to specialists in psychooncology, social workers, pastoral counselors, and other professionals may be necessary when the level of distress is high. The frequency of visits to a psychooncology professional may vary from a single encounter to several, and the timing and duration may also vary from very brief to extending over months or, at times, even years. Today, there are many community-based services available to women with breast cancer at no charge. Evidence from 31 randomized clinical trials, meta-analyses, and nonrandomized studies of the effectiveness of psychosocial interventions among women with breast cancer supports the inclusion of psychosocial interventions in routine clinical care (IOM, 2004b). This body of research documents that several psychosocial interventions reduce psychosocial problems and distress among women with breast cancer. Psychosocial factors and interventions are also related to other aspects of cancer such as pain and other side effects.

Many women with breast cancer rely solely on family, friends, and clergy for social support. Some may find information and support on the Internet, for example, the American Cancer Society's "Cancer Survivor's Network" or ASCO's "People Living with Cancer." Other women, however, do not have social supports built into their lives. They may also lack access to psychosocial services, either because care providers do not refer them to the available services or because of other barriers (e.g., no health insurance or no reimbursement for services).

Several barriers impede appropriate care. The dramatic shift in the delivery of nearly all cancer care from inpatient hospital to outpatient settings has not included a similar shift in the outpatient psychosocial services to the outpatient clinics and private oncology office practices. Increased complexity of care has limited access even further. Women with breast cancer usually see multiple specialists (e.g., surgeons, radiation oncologists, medical oncologists), and care is often not well coordinated. Fragmentation of care is an added psychological burden; the patient is not given care by a single, trusted physician. In addition, the outpatient offices and clinics are extremely busy; the length of time doctors can spend with patients is often limited; and the opportunity to bring up psychosocial problems may be lost. Receiving adequate information and the ability to ask questions in a comfortable way are basic needs for addressing psychosocial concerns. Breast cancer care occurs primarily in private office-based practices that routinely do not employ psychosocial professionals.

Another barrier is the lack or inadequacy of health insurance coverage. An estimated 5 percent of women ages 25 to 64 with breast cancer are uninsured, or, if patients are insured, there is coverage of mental health services with lower reimbursement levels or placement of mental health services in behavioral health contracts, separate from medical coverage (see Chapter 6). Still other barriers are the reluctance to discuss psychosocial concerns with the busy oncologist provider; the stigma associated with seeking or using mental health services; physicians' failure to ask patients about distressing emotional symptoms; and the lack of simple, rapid instruments for screening for psychosocial distress. All are barriers to the symptoms receiving appropriate recognition, diagnosis, and treatment by supportive and psychosocial services. Also, primary oncology teams in outpatient offices are often not familiar with clinical practice guidelines for managing psychosocial distress; they often work in environments that do not provide psychosocial services onsite; and they often are not aware of the psychosocial resources in their local communities. The situation is complicated additionally by the paucity in many communities of identified professionals with skills in managing psychosocial and mental health issues in patients with cancer. As part of an initiative to help locate appropriate professionals, the American Psychosocial Oncology Society (APOS) now provides a directory online (www.apos-society.org) and a toll-free help line for patients and families (1-866-APOS-4-HELP). Overcoming barriers to appropriate use of psychosocial services will require advocacy, monitoring of psychosocial services through quality assurance programs to ensure compliance with standards of care, physician education, training in communication skills, and research relative to identifying and overcoming barriers.

REFERENCES

AAFP (American Academy of Family Physicians). 2002. *Cancer: After Treatment.* [Online]. Available: http://familydoctor.org/723.xml [accessed April 27, 2005].

AAMC (American Association of Medical Colleges). 2005. *AAMC Launches Chronic Care Initiative.* [Online]. Available: http://www.aamc.org/newsroom/pressrel/2005/050428.htm [accessed May 2, 2005].

Abed J, Reilley B, Butler MO, Kean T, Wong F, Hohman K. 2000a. Comprehensive cancer control initiative of the Centers for Disease Control and Prevention: An example of participatory innovation diffusion. *J Public Health Manag Pract* 6(2):79–92.

Abed J, Reilley B, Butler MO, Kean T, Wong F, Hohman K. 2000b. Developing a framework for comprehensive cancer prevention and control in the United States: An initiative of the Centers for Disease Control and Prevention. *J Public Health Manag Pract* 6(2):67–78.

ACCC (Association of Community Cancer Centers). 2004a. *About ACCC.* [Online]. Available: http://www.accc-cancer.org/about/ [accessed October 21, 2004].

ACCC. 2004b. *Guidelines for Cancer Program.* [Online]. Available: http://www.accc-cancer.org/guidelines.asp [accessed October 21, 2004].

ACCC. 2004c. *Guidelines for Cancer Programs. Chapter 4: Clinical Management and Supportive Care Services.* [Online]. Available: http://www.accc-cancer.org/guidelinesCH4.asp [accessed October 21, 2004].

ACCC. 2004d. *Guidelines for Cancer Programs. Chapter 8: Community Services.* [Online]. Available: http://www.accc-cancer.org/guidelinesCH8.asp [accessed October 21, 2004].

ACOR (Association of Cancer Online Resources). 2004a. *ACOR homepage.* [Online]. Available: http://www.acor.org/ [accessed December 3, 2004].

ACOR. 2004b. *Mailing Lists: Treatments Late Effects.* [Online]. Available: http://www.acor.org/mailing.html?sid=12 [accessed January 31, 2005].

ACS (American Cancer Society). 2004. *tlc Catalog.* [Online]. Available: http://www.tlccatalog.org/ [accessed December 3, 2004].

ACS. 2005a. *All About Cancer (General Information).* [Online]. Available: http://www.cancer.org/docroot/CRI/CRI_2x.asp [accessed March 3, 2005].

ACS. 2005b. *Cancer Survivors' Network.* [Online]. Available: http://www.acscsn.org/ [accessed April 26, 2005].

Adewuyi-Dalton R, Ziebland S, Grunfeld E, Hall A. 1998. Patients' views of routine hospital follow-up: A qualitative study of women with breast cancer in remission. *Psychooncology* 7(5):436–439.

AHRQ (Agency for Healthcare Research and Quality). 2004a. *2004 National Healthcare Quality Report.* Rockville, MD: AHRQ.

AHRQ. 2004b. *Effectiveness of Behavioral Interventions to Modify Physical Activity Behaviors in General Populations and Cancer Patients and Survivors. Evidence Report/Technology Assessment 102.* Rockville, MD: AHRQ.

Airey C, Becher H, Erens B, Fuller E. 2002. *National Surveys of NHS Patients—Cancer: National Overview 1999/2000.* London, England: Department of Health.

Andersen MR, Urban N. 1998. The use of mammography by survivors of breast cancer. *Am J Public Health* 88(11):1713–1714.

APOS (American Psychosocial Oncology Society). 2004. *Referral Information for Cancer Patients and Caregivers.* [Online]. Available: http://www.apos-society.org/patient/default.asp [accessed December 3, 2004].

ASCO (American Society of Clinical Oncology). 2003. American Society of Clinical Oncology policy statement update: Genetic testing for cancer susceptibility. *J Clin Oncol* 21(12):2397–2406.

ASCO. 2005. *People Living with Cancer.* [Online]. Available: http://www.plwc.org [accessed April 15, 2005].

Ash JS, Bates DW. 2005. Factors and forces affecting EHR system adoption: Report of a 2004 ACMI discussion. *J Am Med Inform Assoc* 12(1):8–12.

Audet AM, Doty MM, Peugh J, Shamasdin J, Zapert K, Schoenbaum S. 2004. Information technologies: When will they make it into physician's black bags? *Medscape General Medicine* 6(4) [Online]. Available: http://www.medscape.com/viewarticle/493210 [accessed July 15, 2005].

Ayanian J. 2004. *Improving Cancer Care in Massachusetts (CAMA)*. Dana-Farber/Harvard Cancer Center. Unpublished.

Barzilai DA, Cooper KD, Neuhauser D, Rimm AA, Cooper GS. 2004. Geographic and patient variation in receipt of surveillance procedures after local excision of cutaneous melanoma. *J Invest Dermatol* 122(2):246–255.

Beaver K, Luker KA. 2004. Follow-up in breast cancer clinics: Reassuring for patients rather than detecting recurrence. *Psychooncology* 14(2):94–101.

Beck LA. 2003. Cancer rehabilitation: Does it make a difference? *Rehabil Nurs* 28(2):42–47.

Beitler AL, Virgo KS, Johnson FE, Gibbs JF, Kraybill WG. 2000. Current follow-up strategies after potentially curative resection of extremity sarcomas: Results of a survey of the members of the Society of Surgical Oncology. *Cancer* 88(4):777–785.

Berner ES, Detmer DE, Simborg D. 2005. Will the wave finally break? A brief view of the adoption of electronic medical records in the United States. *J Am Med Inform Assoc* 12(1):3–7.

Bernhardt BA, Geller G, Doksum T, Metz SA. 2000. Evaluation of nurses and genetic counselors as providers of education about breast cancer susceptibility testing. *Oncol Nurs Forum* 27(1):33–39.

Berry LL, Seiders K, Wilder SS. 2003. Innovations in access to care: A patient-centered approach. *Ann Intern Med* 139(7):568–574.

Bickell NA, Young GJ. 2001. Coordination of care for early-stage breast cancer patients. *J Gen Intern Med* 16(11):737–742.

Blobel B. 2000. Onconet: A secure infrastructure to improve cancer patients' care. *Eur J Med Res* 5(8):360–368.

Bodenheimer T, Wagner EH, Grumbach K. 2002a. Improving primary care for patients with chronic illness. *JAMA* 288(14):1775–1779.

Bodenheimer T, Wagner EH, Grumbach K. 2002b. Improving primary care for patients with chronic illness: The chronic care model, Part 2. *JAMA* 288(15):1909–1914.

Bope ET. 1987. Follow-up of the cancer patient: Surveillance for metastases. *Prim Care* 14(2):391–401.

Brady K. 2004 (July 26–27). *Survivorship as a Public Health Issue*. Presentation at the meeting of the IOM Committee on Cancer Survivorship, Woods Hole, MA.

Braun TC, Hagen NA, Smith C, Summers N. 2003. Oncologists and family physicians. Using a standardized letter to improve communication. *Can Fam Physician* 49:882–886.

Brown L, Payne S, Royle G. 2002. Patient initiated follow up of breast cancer. *Psychooncology* 11(4):346–355.

Burt CW, Hing E. 2005. Use of computerized clinical support systems in medical settings: United States, 2001–03. In: *Advance Data From Vital and Health Statistics*. No. 353. Hyattsville, MD: National Center for Health Statistics.

Canada AL, Schover LR. 2005. Research promoting better patient education on reproductive health after cancer. *J Natl Cancer Inst Monogr* 34:98–100.

Cancer Control Planet. 2004. *Cancer Control Planet*. [Online]. Available: http://cancercontrolplanet.cancer.gov/ [accessed November 30, 2004].

CancerCare. 2005a. *CancerCare homepage*. [Online]. Available: http://www.cancercare.org [accessed May 11, 2005].

CancerCare. 2005b. *CancerCare Services for Cancer Survivors*. [Online]. Available: http://www.cancercare.org/CancerCareServices/CancerCareServicesList.cfm?c=878 [accessed May 11, 2005].

Case C, Johantgen M, Steiner C. 2001. Outpatient mastectomy: Clinical, payer, and geographic influences. *Health Serv Res* 36(5):869–884.

CDC (Centers for Disease Control and Prevention). 2004a. *National Comprehensive Cancer Control Program.* [Online]. Available: http://www.cdc.gov/cancer/ncccp/ [accessed November 29, 2004].

CDC. 2004b. *Program Contacts by Funding Status.* [Online]. Available: http://www.cdc.gov/cancer/ncccp/cccstatelist.htm [accessed November 29, 2004].

CDC. 2005a. *The New Spirit of Survivorship.* [Online]. Available: http://www.cdc.gov/cancer/survivorship/newspirit.htm [accessed July 21, 2005].

CDC. 2005b. *Working Together for Comprehensive Cancer Control: Institutes for State Leaders.* [Online]. Available: http://www.cdc.gov/cancer/ncccp/institutes.htm [accessed April 28, 2005].

CDC and LAF (Centers for Disease Control and Prevention and Lance Armstrong Foundation). 2004. *A National Action Plan for Cancer Survivorship: Advancing Public Health Strategies.* Atlanta, GA: CDC.

Children's Oncology Group. 2005. *Cure Search.* [Online]. Available: http://www.childrensoncologygroup.org/ [accessed February 24, 2005].

Ciolek DE, Hwang W. 2004. *Outpatient Rehabilitation Services Payment System Evaluation: Final Project Report.* Columbia, MD: AdvanceMed, prepared for the Centers for Medicare and Medicaid Services.

Clark JG, Virgo KS, Clemente MF, Johnson MH, Paniello RC, Johnson FE. 1999. How surgeon age affects posttreatment surveillance strategies for upper aerodigestive tract cancer patients. *Am J Otolaryngol* 20(4):217–222.

CMS (Centers for Medicare and Medicaid Services). 2004. *Medicare Coordinated Care Demonstration.* [Online]. Available: http://www.cms.hhs.gov/healthplans/research/coorcare.asp [accessed November 22, 2004].

Collins RF, Bekker HL, Dodwell DJ. 2004. Follow-up care of patients treated for breast cancer: A structured review. *Cancer Treat Rev* 30(1):19–35.

Coluzzi PH, Grant M, Doroshow JH, Rhiner M, Ferrell B, Rivera L. 1995. Survey of the provision of supportive care services at National Cancer Institute-designated cancer centers. *J Clin Oncol* 13(3):756–764.

Commission on Cancer. 2003. *Cancer Program Standards, 2004.* Chicago, IL: American College of Surgeons.

Continuum Health Partners. 2005. *Sexual Health and Rehabilitation Program (SHARP).* [Online]. Available: http://www.stoppain.org/services_staff/featuredprogsold.html#sexualhealth [accessed February 23, 2005].

Cooper GS, Yuan Z, Chak A, Rimm AA. 1999. Geographic and patient variation among Medicare beneficiaries in the use of follow-up testing after surgery for nonmetastatic colorectal carcinoma. *Cancer* 85(10):2124–2131.

Cooper GS, Yuan Z, Chak A, Rimm AA. 2000. Patterns of endoscopic follow-up after surgery for nonmetastatic colorectal cancer. *Gastrointest Endosc* 52(1):33–38.

Cox K, Wilson E. 2003. Follow-up for people with cancer: Nurse-led services and telephone interventions. *J Adv Nurs* 43(1):51–61.

Dana-Farber Cancer Institute. 2005. *New Support Group Launched for African-American Men with Prostate Cancer.* [Online]. Available: http://www.dana-farber.org/pat/support/support-2005-03-21.asp [accessed May 11, 2005].

de Bock GH, Bonnema J, Zwaan RE, van de Velde CJ, Kievit J, Stiggelbout AM. 2004. Patient's needs and preferences in routine follow-up after treatment for breast cancer. *Br J Cancer* 90(6):1144–1150.

DeLisa JA. 2001. A history of cancer rehabilitation. *Cancer* 92(4 Suppl):970–974.

Demissie S, Silliman RA, Lash TL. 2001. Adjuvant tamoxifen: Predictors of use, side effects, and discontinuation in older women. *J Clin Oncol* 19(2):322–328.

Desch CE, Grasso MA, McCue MJ, Buonaiuto D, Grasso K, Johantgen MK, Shaw JE, Smith TJ. 1999. A rural cancer outreach program lowers patient care costs and benefits both the rural hospitals and sponsoring academic medical center. *J Rural Health* 15(2):157–167.

Dietz JH. 1974. Rehabilitation of the cancer patient: Its role in the scheme of comprehensive care. *Clin Bull* 4(3):104–107.

Diller L, Medeiros Nancarrow C, Shaffer K, Matulonis U, Mauch P, Neuberg D, Tarbell NJ, Litman H, Garber J. 2002. Breast cancer screening in women previously treated for Hodgkin's disease: A prospective cohort study. *J Clin Oncol* 20(8):2085–2091.

Donnelly J, Mack P, Donaldson LA. 2001. Follow-up of breast cancer: Time for a new approach? *Int J Clin Pract* 55(7):431–433.

Dow KH, Ferrell BR, Haberman MR, Eaton L. 1999. The meaning of quality of life in cancer survivorship. *Oncol Nurs Forum* 26(3):519–528.

Duffy CM, Allen SM, Clark MA. 2005. Discussions regarding reproductive health for young women with breast cancer undergoing chemotherapy. *J Clin Oncol* 23(4):766–773.

Dworkind M, Towers A, Murnaghan D, Guibert R, Iverson D. 1999. Communication between family physicians and oncologists: Qualitative results of an exploratory study. *Cancer Prev Control* 3(2):137–144.

Eakin EG, Strycker LA. 2001. Awareness and barriers to use of cancer support and information resources by HMO patients with breast, prostate, or colon cancer: Patient and provider perspectives. *Psychooncology* 10(2):103–113.

Earle CC, Neville BA. 2004. Under use of necessary care among cancer survivors. *Cancer* 101(8):1712–1719.

Earle CC, Burstein HJ, Winer EP, Weeks JC. 2003. Quality of non-breast cancer health maintenance among elderly breast cancer survivors. *J Clin Oncol* 21(8):1447–1451.

Earnshaw JJ, Stephenson Y. 1997. First two years of a follow-up breast clinic led by a nurse practitioner. *J R Soc Med* 90(5):258–259.

Ell K, Sanchez K, Vourlekis B, Lee PJ, Dwight-Johnson M, Lagomasino I, Muderspach L, Russell C. 2005. Depression, correlates of depression, and receipt of depression care among low-income women with breast or gynecologic cancer. *J Clin Oncol* 23(13):3052–3060.

Ellison GL, Warren JL, Knopf KB, Brown ML. 2003. Racial differences in the receipt of bowel surveillance following potentially curative colorectal cancer surgery. *Health Serv Res* 38(6 Pt 2):1885–1903.

Elston Lafata J, Cole Johnson C, Ben-Menachem T, Morlock RJ. 2001. Sociodemographic differences in the receipt of colorectal cancer surveillance care following treatment with curative intent. *Med Care* 39(4):361–372.

Elston Lafata J, Simpkins J, Schultz L, Chase GA, Johnson CC, Yood MU, Lamerato L, Nathanson D, Cooper G. 2005. Routine surveillance care after cancer treatment with curative intent. *Med Care* 43(6):592-599.

Epplein M, Koon KP, Ramsey SD, Potter JD. 2005. Genetic services for familial cancer patients: A follow-up survey of National Cancer Institute cancer centers. *J Clin Oncol* 23(21):4713–4718.

Fallowfield L, Fleissig A, Edwards R, West A, Powles TJ, Howell A, Cuzick J. 2001. Tamoxifen for the prevention of breast cancer: Psychosocial impact on women participating in two randomized controlled trials. *J Clin Oncol* 19(7):1885–1892.

Family Health Administration. 2005. *The 2004–2008 Maryland Comprehensive Cancer Control Plan: Our Call to Action*. [Online]. Available: http://www.marylandcancerplan.org [accessed February 22, 2005].

Ferrell B, Grant M, Schmidt GM, Rhiner M, Whitehead C, Fonbuena P, Forman SJ. 1992. The meaning of quality of life for bone marrow transplant survivors. Part 1. The impact of bone marrow transplant on quality of life. *Cancer Nurs* 15(3):153–160.

Ferrell B, Smith SL, Cullinane CA, Melancon C. 2003a. Psychological well being and quality of life in ovarian cancer survivors. *Cancer* 98(5):1061–1071.

Ferrell BR. 1996. The quality of lives: 1,525 voices of cancer. *Oncol Nurs Forum* 23(6):909–916.

Ferrell BR, Dow KH, Leigh S, Ly J, Gulasekaram P. 1995. Quality of life in long-term cancer survivors. *Oncol Nurs Forum* 22(6):915–922.

Ferrell BR, Grant MM, Funk B, Otis-Green S, Garcia N. 1997. Quality of life in breast cancer survivors as identified by focus groups. *Psychooncology* 6(1):13–23.

Ferrell BR, Grant MM, Funk BM, Otis-Green SA, Garcia NJ. 1998. Quality of life in breast cancer survivors: Implications for developing support services. *Oncol Nurs Forum* 25(5):887–895.

Ferrell BR, Smith SL, Ervin KS, Itano J, Melancon C. 2003b. A qualitative analysis of social concerns of women with ovarian cancer. *Psychooncology* 12(7):647–663.

Fink AK, Gurwitz J, Rakowski W, Guadagnoli E, Silliman RA. 2004. Patient beliefs and tamoxifen discontinuance in older women with estrogen receptor-positive breast cancer. *J Clin Oncol* 22(16):3309–3315.

Fox Chase Cancer Center. 2004. *The Margaret Dyson Family Risk Assessment Program*. [Online]. Available: http://www.fccc.edu/clinicalresearch/familyriskassessment [accessed December 3, 2004].

Freedman AN, Wideroff L, Olson L, Davis W, Klabunde C, Srinath KP, Reeve BB, Croyle RT, Ballard-Barbash R. 2003. US physicians' attitudes toward genetic testing for cancer susceptibility. *Am J Med Genet A* 120(1):63–71.

Freeman H, Clanton M. 2004. Patient navigator program reduces cancer health disparities. *NCI Cancer Bulletin*. 1(33):1–2.

Frost MH, Arvizu RD, Jayakumar S, Schoonover A, Novotny P, Zahasky K. 1999. A multidisciplinary healthcare delivery model for women with breast cancer: Patient satisfaction and physical and psychosocial adjustment. *Oncol Nurs Forum* 26(10):1673–1680.

Frymark SL. 1998. Taking control. Cancer rehabilitation allows patients to increase the quality of their lives and reclaim independence. *Rehab Manag* 11(3):80, 84–86.

Ganz PA. 1990. Current issues in cancer rehabilitation. *Cancer* 65(3 Suppl):742–751.

Ganz PA. 1999. The status of cancer rehabilitation in the late 1990s. *Mayo Clin Proc* 74(9):939–940.

Ganz PA, Greendale GA, Petersen L, Zibecchi L, Kahn B, Belin TR. 2000. Managing menopausal symptoms in breast cancer survivors: Results of a randomized controlled trial. *J Natl Cancer Inst* 92(13):1054–1064.

Geller BM, Kerlikowske K, Carney PA, Abraham LA, Yankaskas BC, Taplin SH, Ballard-Barbash R, Dignan MB, Rosenberg R, Urban N, Barlow WE. 2003. Mammography surveillance following breast cancer. *Breast Cancer Res Treat* 81(2):107–115.

Gerber LH, Vargo MM, Smith RG. 2005. Chapter 56, Rehabilitation of the Cancer Patient. In: DeVita VT, Hellman S, Rosenberg SA, eds. *Cancer: Principles and Practice of Oncology*. 7th ed. Philadelphia, PA: Lippincott, Wiliams & Wilkins. Pp. 2719–2746.

Gilchrist VJ, Stange KC, Flocke SA, McCord G, Bourguet CC. 2004. A comparison of the National Ambulatory Medical Care Survey (NAMCS) measurement approach with direct observation of outpatient visits. *Med Care* 42(3):276–280.

Given B, Given CW, McCorkle R, Kozachik S, Cimprich B, Rahbar MH, Wojcik C. 2002. Pain and fatigue management: Results of a nursing randomized clinical trial. *Oncol Nurs Forum* 29(6):949–956.

GIVIO. 1994. Impact of follow-up testing on survival and health-related quality of life in breast cancer patients. A multicenter randomized controlled trial. The GIVIO Investigators. *JAMA* 271(20):1587–1592.

Glynne-Jones R, Chait I, Thomas SF. 1997. When and how to discharge cancer survivors in long term remission from follow-up: The effectiveness of a contract. *Clin Oncol (R Coll Radiol)* 9(1):25–29.

Grabois M. 2001. Integrating cancer rehabilitation into medical care at a cancer hospital. *Cancer* 92(4 Suppl):1055–1057.

Greenberg A, Angus H, Sullivan T, Brown AD. 2005. Development of a set of strategy-based system-level cancer care performance indicators in Ontario, Canada. *Int J Qual Health Care* 17(2):107–114.

Gruman J, Convissor R. 1995. *Psychosocial Services in Cancer Care: A Survey of Comprehensive Cancer Centers.* Washington, DC: The Center for the Advancement of Health.

Grunfeld E, Fitzpatrick R, Mant D, Yudkin P, Adewuyi-Dalton R, Stewart J, Cole D, Vessey M. 1999a. Comparison of breast cancer patient satisfaction with follow-up in primary care versus specialist care: Results from a randomized controlled trial. *Br J Gen Pract* 49(446):705–710.

Grunfeld E, Gray A, Mant D, Yudkin P, Adewuyi-Dalton R, Coyle D, Cole D, Stewart J, Fitzpatrick R, Vessey M. 1999b. Follow-up of breast cancer in primary care vs specialist care: Results of an economic evaluation. *Br J Cancer* 79(7–8):1227–1233.

Grunfeld E, Levine M, Julian J, et al. 2004 (June 5–8). *A randomized controlled trial (RCT) of routine follow-up for early stage breast cancer: A comparison of primary care versus specialist care.* Paper presented at the Annual Meeting of the American Society for Clinical Oncology, New Orleans, LA. Abstract No. 665.

Grunfeld E, Mant D, Vessey MP, Yudkin P. 1995. Evaluating primary care follow-up of breast cancer: Methods and preliminary results of three studies. *Ann Oncol* 6(Suppl 2):47–52.

Grunfeld E, Mant D, Yudkin P, Adewuyi-Dalton R, Cole D, Stewart J, Fitzpatrick R, Vessey M. 1996. Routine follow up of breast cancer in primary care: Randomised trial. *BMJ* 313(7058):665–669.

Guidry JJ, Aday LA, Zhang D, Winn RJ. 1997. The role of informal and formal social support networks for patients with cancer. *Cancer Pract* 5(4):241–246.

Gulliford T, Opomu M, Wilson E, Hanham I, Epstein R. 1997. Popularity of less frequent follow up for breast cancer in randomised study: Initial findings from the hotline study. *BMJ* 314(7075):174–177.

Gustafson D, Wise M, McTavish F, Taylor J, Wolberg W, Steward J, Smalley R, Bosworth K. 1993. Development and pilot evaluation of a computer-based support system for women with breast cancer. *Journal of Psychosocial Oncology* 11(4):69–93.

Harvey RF, Jellinek HM, Habeck RV. 1982. Cancer rehabilitation. An analysis of 36 program approaches. *JAMA* 247(15):2127–2131.

Hewitt M, Rowland JH. 2002. Mental health service use among adult cancer survivors: Analyses of the National Health Interview Survey. *J Clin Oncol* 20(23):4581–4590.

Hillner BE, McDonald MK, Penberthy L, Desch CE, Smith TJ, Maddux P, Glasheen WP, Retchin SM. 1997. Measuring standards of care for early breast cancer in an insured population. *J Clin Oncol* 15(4):1401–1408.

Hobbie WL, Hollen PJ. 1993. Pediatric nurse practitioners specializing with survivors of childhood cancer. *J Pediatr Health Care* 7(1):24–30.

Hoffman, B. 2004. *A Cancer Survivor's Almanac: Charting Your Journey.* 3rd ed. Hoboken, NJ: John Wiley & Sons.

Hollen PJ, Hobbie WL. 1995. Establishing comprehensive specialty follow-up clinics for long-term survivors of cancer. Providing systematic physiological and psychosocial support. *Support Care Cancer* 3(1):40–44.

Hordern A. 2000. The emerging role of the breast care nurse in Australia. *Cancer Nurs* 23(2):122–127.

Improving Chronic Illness Care. 2004. *The Community—Resources and Policies.* [Online]. Available: http://www.improvingchroniccare.org/change/model/community.html [accessed November 16, 2004].

IOM (Institute of Medicine). 1998. *Statement on Quality of Care.* National Roundtable on Healthcare Quality. Washington, DC: National Academy Press.

IOM. 1999. *Ensuring Quality Cancer Care.* Hewitt M, Simone JV, eds. Washington, DC: National Academy Press.

IOM. 2001. *Crossing the Quality Chasm: A New Health System for the 21st Century.* Washington, DC: National Academy Press.

IOM. 2002. *Speaking of Health: Assessing Health Communication Strategies for Diverse Populations.* Washington, DC: The National Academies Press.

IOM. 2003a. *Childhood Cancer Survivorship: Improving Care and Quality of Life.* Hewitt M, Weiner SL, Simone JV, eds. Washington, DC: The National Academies Press.

IOM. 2003b. *Fulfilling the Potential of Cancer Prevention and Early Detection.* Curry SJ, Byers T, Hewitt M, eds. Washington, DC: The National Academies Press.

IOM. 2004a. *Health Literacy: A Prescription to End Confusion.* Nielsen-Bohlman L, Panzer AM, Kindig DA, eds. Washington, DC: The National Academies Press.

IOM. 2004b. *Meeting Psychosocial Needs of Women with Breast Cancer.* Hewitt M, Herdman R, Holland J, eds. Washington, DC: The National Academies Press.

IOM. 2005. *Assessing the Quality of Cancer Care: An Approach to Measurement in Georgia.* Eden J, Simone JV, eds. Washington, DC: The National Academies Press.

James ND, Guerrero D, Brada M. 1994. Who should follow up cancer patients? Nurse specialist based outpatient care and the introduction of a phone clinic system. *Clin Oncol (R Coll Radiol)* 6(5):283–287.

Johnson FE, Virgo, KS. 1997. *Cancer Patient Follow-Up.* St. Louis, MO: Mosby.

Johnson FE, Longo WE, Vernava AM, Wade TP, Coplin MA, Virgo KS. 1995. How tumor stage affects surgeons' surveillance strategies after colon cancer surgery. *Cancer* 76(8): 1325–1329.

Johnson FE, McKirgan LW, Coplin MA, Vernava AM, Longo WE, Wade TP, Virgo KS. 1996a. Geographic variation in patient surveillance after colon cancer surgery. *J Clin Oncol* 14(1):183–187.

Johnson FE, Naunheim KS, Coplin MA, Virgo KS. 1996b. Geographic variation in the conduct of patient surveillance after lung cancer surgery. *J Clin Oncol* 14(11):2940–2949.

Johnson FE, Novell LA, Coplin MA, Longo WE, Vernava AM, Wade TP, Virgo KS. 1996c. How practice patterns in colon cancer patient follow-up are affected by surgeon age. *Surg Oncol* 5(3):127–131.

Johnson FE, Virgo KS, Clemente MF, Johnson MH, Paniello RC. 1998. How tumor stage affects surgeons' surveillance strategies after surgery for carcinoma of the upper aerodigestive tract. *Cancer* 82(10):1932–1937.

Johnson FE, Virgo KS, Johnson DY, Chan D, Goshima K, Handler BS. 2001. Effect of initial tumor stage on patient follow-up after potentially curative surgery for cutaneous melanoma. *Int J Oncol* 18(5):973–978.

Johnson FE, Virgo KS, Ornstein DK, Johnson ET, Chan D, Colberg JW. 2000. How tumor stage affects American urologists' surveillance strategies after prostate cancer surgery. *Int J Oncol* 16(6):1221–1225.

Kadan-Lottick NS, Robison LL, Gurney JG, Neglia JP, Yasui Y, Hayashi R, Hudson M, Greenberg M, Mertens AC. 2002. Childhood cancer survivors' knowledge about their past diagnosis and treatment: Childhood Cancer Survivor Study. *JAMA* 287(14):1832–1839.

Kaija H, Matti H, Tapani H. 1996. Use of hospital services by breast cancer patients by stage of the disease: Implications on the costs of cancer control. *Breast Cancer Res Treat* 37(3):237–241.

Kiebert GM, Welvaart K, Kievit J. 1993. Psychological effects of routine follow up on cancer patients after surgery. *Eur J Surg* 159(11–12):601–607.

Kligman L, Wong RK, Johnston M, Laetsch NS. 2004. The treatment of lymphedema related to breast cancer: A systematic review and evidence summary. *Support Care Cancer* 12(6):421–431.

Knopf KB, Warren JL, Feuer EJ, Brown ML. 2001. Bowel surveillance patterns after a diagnosis of colorectal cancer in Medicare beneficiaries. *Gastrointest Endosc* 54(5):563–571.

Koinberg IL, Fridlund B, Engholm GB, Holmberg L. 2004. Nurse-led follow-up on demand or by a physician after breast cancer surgery: A randomised study. *Eur J Oncol Nurs* 8(2):109–117; discussion 118–120.

Koinberg IL, Holmberg L, Fridlund B. 2002. Breast cancer patients' satisfaction with a spontaneous system of check-up visits to a specialist nurse. *Scand J Caring Sci* 16(3):209–215.

LAF (Lance Armstrong Foundation). 2004a. *Cancer Survivor's Medical Treatment Summary*. [Online]. Available: http://www.livestrong.org/portal/needsAssessment/medical_summary.pdf [accessed February 23, 2005].

LAF. 2004b. *LiveStrong Poll Finds Nearly Half of People Living With Cancer Feel Their Non-Medical Needs Are Unmet by the Healthcare System*. Austin, TX: LAF.

LAF. 2005a. *Cancer Survivorship Centers*. [Online]. Available: http://www.laf.org/site/c.beIKLOOrGpF/b.507137/k.8513/Cancer_Survivorship_Centers.htm#5 [accessed May 19, 2005].

LAF. 2005b. *Lance Armstrong Foundation LIVESTRONG*. [Online]. Available: http://www.livestrong.org [accessed July 26, 2005].

Landier W, Bhatia S, Eshelman DA, Forte KJ, Sweeny T, Hester AL, Darling J, Armstrong FD, Blatt J, Constine LS, Freeman CR, Friedman DL, Green DM, Marina N, Meadows AT, Neglia JP, Oeffinger KC, Robison LL, Ruccione KS, Sklar CA, Hudson MM. 2004. Development of risk-based guidelines for pediatric cancer survivors: the Children's Oncology Group Long-Term Follow-Up Guidelines from the Children's Oncology Group Late Effects Committee and Nursing Discipline. *J Clin Oncol* 22(24):4979–4990.

Lash TL, Silliman RA. 2001. Medical surveillance after breast cancer diagnosis. *Med Care* 39(9):945–955.

Lauria MM. 1991. Continuity of cancer care. *Cancer* 67(6 Suppl):1759–1766.

Lee FC. 2004. Employer-based disease management programs in cancer. *Dis Manage Health Outcomes* 12(1):9–17.

Leese B, Din I, Darr A, Walker R, Heywood P, Allgar V. 2004. *'Early Days Yet': The Primary Care Cancer Lead Clinician (PCCL) Initiative Executive Summary*. Leeds, UK: Centre for Research in Primary Care, University of Leeds.

Lehmann JF, DeLisa JA, Warren CG, deLateur BJ, Bryant PL, Nicholson CG. 1978. Cancer rehabilitation: Assessment of need, development, and evaluation of a model of care. *Arch Phys Med Rehabil* 59(9):410–419.

Leigh SA. 1998. The long-term cancer survivor: A challenge for nurse practitioners. *Nurse Pract Forum* 9(3):192–196.

Lieberman MA, Golant M, Giese-Davis J, Winzlenberg A, Benjamin H, Humphreys K, Kronenwetter C, Russo S, Spiegel D. 2003. Electronic support groups for breast carcinoma: A clinical trial of effectiveness. *Cancer* 97(4):920–925.

Liebert B, Parle M, Roberts C, Redman S, Carrick S, Gallagher J, Simpson J, Ng K, Khan MA, White K, Salkeld G, Lewis M, Olver I, Gill G, Marchant M, Coates A, North R, Akers G, Cannon A, Gray C, Liebelt J, Rodger A, Henderson M, Stoney D, Hickey P, Archer S, Metcalf C, Trotter J. 2003. An evidence-based specialist breast nurse role in practice: A multicentre implementation study. *Eur J Cancer Care (Engl)* 12(1):91–97.

Liebert B, Parle M, White K, Rodger A. 2001. Establishing an evidence base for the specialist breast nurse: A model for Australian breast cancer care. *Aust Health Rev* 24(1):192–199.

Loprinzi CL, Hayes D, Smith T. 2000. Doc, shouldn't we be getting some tests? *J Clin Oncol* 18(11):2345–2348.

Luker K, Beaver K, Austin L, Leinster SJ. 2000. An evaluation of information cards as a means of improving communication between hospital and primary care for women with breast cancer. *J Adv Nurs* 31(5):1174–1182.

MacLaren JA. 2003. Models of lymphoedema service provision across Europe: Sharing good practice. *Int J Palliat Nurs* 9(12):538–543.

Maher EJ, Millar D. 2003. Shared care: Step down or step up? *Qual Saf Health Care* 12(4):242.

Mahon SM, Williams MT, Spies MA. 2000. Screening for second cancers and osteoporosis in long-term survivors. *Cancer Pract* 8(6):282–290.

Maliski SL, Clerkin B, Litwin MS. 2004. Describing a nurse case manager intervention to empower low-income men with prostate cancer. *Oncol Nurs Forum* 31(1):57–64.

Margenthaler JA, Meier JD, Virgo KS, Johnson DY, Goshima K, Chan D, Handler BS, Johnson FE. 2003. Geographic variation in post-treatment surveillance intensity for patients with cutaneous melanoma. *Am J Surg* 186(2):194–200.

Margenthaler JA, Virgo KS, Johnson DY, Sugarbaker EM, Handler BS, Johnson FE. 2001. How surgeon age affects post-treatment surveillance strategies for melanoma patients. *Int J Oncol* 19(1):175–180.

Mariotto A, Warren JL, Knopf KB, Feuer EJ. 2003. The prevalence of patients with colorectal carcinoma under care in the U.S. *Cancer* 98(6):1253–1261.

Masny A, Daly M, Ross E, Balshem A, Gillespie D, Weil S. 2003. A training course for oncology nurses in familial cancer risk assessment: Evaluation of knowledge and practice. *J Cancer Educ* 18(1):20–25.

Matthews BA, Baker F, Spillers RL. 2002. Healthcare professionals' awareness of cancer support services. *Cancer Pract* 10(1):36–44.

Matthews BA, Baker F, Spillers RL. 2004. Oncology professionals and patient requests for cancer support services. *Support Care Cancer* 12(10):731–738.

Maxwell S, Baseggio C. 2000. *Outpatient Therapy Services Under Medicare: Background and Policy Issues.* Washington, DC: Urban Institute.

McGlynn EA (RAND). 2002. *Applying the Strategic Framework Board's Model to Selecting National Goals and Core Measures for Stimulating Improved Quality for Cancer Care.* Background Paper No. 1. Bethesda, MD: National Cancer Institute.

McGlynn EA, Malin J (RAND). 2002. *Selecting National Goals and Core Measures of Cancer Care Quality.* Background Paper No. 2. Bethesda, MD: National Cancer Institute.

M.D. Anderson Cancer Center. 2004. *Fatigue & Cancer.* [Online]. Available: http://www.mdanderson.org/topics/fatigue/ [accessed December 3, 2004].

M.D. Anderson Cancer Center. 2005. *Life After Cancer Care.* [Online]. Available: http://www.mdanderson.org/departments/lacc/ [accessed April 25, 2005].

MedPAC (Medicare Payment Advisory Commission). 2004a. *Report to the Congress: Eliminating Physician Referrals to Physical Therapy (December 2004).* [Online]. Available: http://www.medpac.gov/publications/congressional_reports/Dec04_PTaccess.pdf [accessed May 17, 2005].

MedPAC. 2004b. *Report to the Congress: New Approaches in Medicare.* Washington, DC: MEDPAC.

Mendelson D, Carino TV. 2005. Evidence-based medicine in the United States—de rigueur or dream deferred? *Health Aff (Millwood)* 24(1):133–136.

Miedema B, MacDonald I, Tatemichi S. 2003. Cancer follow-up care. Patients' perspectives. *Can Fam Physician* 49:890–895.

Miller RH, Sim I. 2004. Physicians' use of electronic medical records: Barriers and solutions. *Health Aff (Millwood)* 23(2):116–126.

Moore S, Corner J, Haviland J, Wells M, Salmon E, Normand C, Brada M, O'Brien M, Smith I. 2002. Nurse led follow up and conventional medical follow up in management of patients with lung cancer: Randomised trial. *BMJ* 325(7373):1145.

Morris S, Corder AP, Taylor I. 1992. What are the benefits of routine breast cancer follow-up? *Postgrad Med J* 68(805):904–907.

MSKCC (Memorial Sloan-Kettering Cancer Center). 2004. *Post-Treatment Resource Program.* [Online]. Available: http://www.mskcc.org/mskcc/html/19409.cfm [accessed April 27, 2005].

Muss HB, Tell GS, Case LD, Robertson P, Atwell BM. 1991. Perceptions of follow-up care in women with breast cancer. *Am J Clin Oncol* 14(1):55–59.

National Diabetes Quality Improvement Alliance. 2005. *National Diabetes Quality Improvement Alliance homepage.* [Online]. Available: http://www.nationaldiabetesalliance.org [accessed May 10, 2005].

Naunheim KS, Virgo KS, Coplin MA, Johnson FE. 1995. Clinical surveillance testing after lung cancer operations. *Ann Thorac Surg* 60(6):1612–1616.

NCCN (National Comprehensive Cancer Network). 2004a. *Clinical Practice Guidelines in Oncology-v.1.2004. Breast Cancer Screening and Diagnosis Guidelines.* [Online]. Available: http://www.nccn.org/professionals/physician_gls/PDF/breast-screening.pdf [accessed June 3, 2004].

NCCN. 2004b. *Clinical Practice Guidelines in Oncology-v.1.2004. Breast Risk Reduction.* [Online]. Available: http://www.nccn.org/professionals/physician_gls/PDF/breast_risk.pdf [accessed June 3, 2004].

NCCN. 2004c. *Clinical Practice Guidelines in Oncology-v.1.2004. Distress Management.* [Online]. Available: http://www.nccn.org/physician_gls/f_guidelines.html [accessed June 2004].

NCCS (National Coalition for Cancer Survivorship). 1996. *Imperatives for Quality Cancer Care: Access, Advocacy, Action, and Accountability.* Clark EJ, Stovall EL, Leigh S, Siu AL, Austin DK, Rowland JH. Silver Spring, MD: National Coalition for Cancer Survivorship.

NCCS. 2004. *Cancer Survival Toolbox.* Silver Spring, MD: NCCS.

NCCS. 2005. *Cancer: Keys to Survivorship.* [Online]. Available: http://www.canceradvocacy.org/programs/keys.aspx [accessed April 26, 2005].

NCHS (National Center for Health Statistics). 2004. *National Hospital Discharge Survey, 2002: Public Use Data File Documentation.* Hyattsville, MD: NCHS.

NCI (National Cancer Institute). 2002a. *Facing Forward: Life After Cancer Treatment.* Bethesda, MD: NCI.

NCI. 2002b. *Facing Forward Series: Ways You Can Make a Difference in Cancer.* Bethesda, MD: NCI.

NCI. 2004. *Patient Navigator Research Program Introduction & Overview.* [Online]. Available: http://crchd.nci.nih.gov/Navigator/overview.htm [accessed November 8, 2004].

NCI. 2005a. *Description of the Cancer Centers Program.* [Online]. Available: http://www3.cancer.gov/cancercenters/description.html [accessed May 11, 2005].

NCI. 2005b. *National Cancer Act of 1971.* [Online]. Available: http://www3.cancer.gov/legis/1971canc.html [accessed May 12, 2005].

NCI. 2005c. *Centers of Excellence in Cancer Communications Research.* [Online]. Available: http://dccps.nci.nih.gov/ncirb/ceccr [accessed August 29, 2005].

NCLAC (National Cancer Legislation Advisory Committee). 2005. *National Cancer Policy Legislative History.* [Online]. Available: http://www.cancersource.com/nclac/leghistory.htm [accessed May 10, 2005].

NCSL (National Conference of State Legislatures). 2005. *State Genetics Employment Laws.* [Online] http://www.ncls.org/programs/health/genetics/ndiscrim.htm [accessed June 15, 2005].

Neuner JM, Gilligan MA, Sparapani R, Laud PW, Haggstrom D, Nattinger AB. 2004. Decentralization of breast cancer surgery in the United States. *Cancer* 101(6):1323–1329.

Nielsen JD, Palshof T, Mainz J, Jensen AB, Olesen F. 2003. Randomised controlled trial of a shared care programme for newly referred cancer patients: Bridging the gap between general practice and hospital. *Qual Saf Health Care* 12(4):263–272.

NIH. 2005. *Legislative Updates: Genetic Nondiscrimination.* [Online]. Available: http://olpa.od.nih.gov/legislation/109/pendinglegislation/geneticnondiscrimination.asp [accessed June 14, 2005].

NLM (National Library of Medicine). 2005. *Regional Medical Programs.* [Online]. Available: http://rmp.nlm.nih.gov/RM/ [accessed May 12, 2005].

NLN (National Lymphedema Network). 2005. *NLN homepage.* [Online]. Available: http://lymphnet.org/ [accessed May 9, 2005].

NQF (National Quality Forum). 2005. *National Quality Forum Current Activities and Consensus Reports.* [Online]. Available: http://www.qualityforum.org/activities/home.htm [accessed April 15, 2005].

Nueva Vida. 2005a. *Nueva Vida: A Support Network for Latinas with Cancer.* [Online], Available: http://www.nueva-vida.org/index2.htm [accessed May 11, 2005].

Nueva Vida. 2005b. *Nueva Vida: Locate a Local Support Program.* [Online]. Available. http://www.nueva-vida.org/locate.htm [accessed May 11, 2005].

NVCI (Nevada Cancer Institute). 2005. *Survivorship: A Joint Goal of the Nevada Cancer Institute and the Lance Armstrong Foundation.* [Online]. Available: http://www.nevadacancerinstitute.org/communityprograms/survivorship.htm [accessed May 18, 2005].

Oeffinger KC, Mertens AC, Hudson MM, Gurney JG, Casillas J, Chen H, Whitton J, Yeazel M, Yasui Y, Robison LL. 2004. Health care of young adult survivors of childhood cancer: A report from the Childhood Cancer Survivors Study. *Ann Fam Med* 2(1):61–70.

Oh J, Colberg JW, Ornstein DK, Johnson ET, Chan D, Virgo KS, Johnson FE. 1999. Current followup strategies after radical prostatectomy: A survey of American Urological Association urologists. *J Urol* 161(2):520–523.

ONS (Oncology Nursing Society). 2005. *Cancer Symptoms.org.* [Online]. Available: http://cancersymptoms.org [accessed April 26, 2005].

Paniello RC, Virgo KS, Johnson MH, Clemente MF, Johnson FE. 1999. Practice patterns and clinical guidelines for posttreatment follow-up of head and neck cancers: A comparison of 2 professional societies. *Arch Otolaryngol Head Neck Surg* 125(3):309–313.

Papagrigoriadis S, Heyman B. 2003. Patients' views on follow up of colorectal cancer: Implications for risk communication and decision making. *Postgrad Med J* 79(933):403–407.

Parle M, Gallagher J, Gray C, Akers G, Liebert B. 2001. From evidence to practice: Factors affecting the specialist breast nurse's detection of psychological morbidity in women with breast cancer. *Psychooncology* 10(6):503–510.

Parrott S, Clark C, Mahoney Shannon K. 2002. *National Society of Genetic Counselors, Inc. Professional Status Survey 2002.* Waltham, MA: Boston Information Solutions.

Parrott S, Clark C, Mahoney Shannon K. 2003. *National Society of Genetic Counselors, Inc. Professional Status Survey 2002: Cancer Genetics Analysis.* Waltham, MA: Boston Information Solutions.

Partnership for Solutions (Johns Hopkins University). 2002. *Chronic Conditions: Making the Case for Ongoing Care.* Baltimore, MD: Johns Hopkins University.

Partridge AH, Gelber S, Peppercorn J, Sampson E, Knudsen K, Laufer M, Rosenberg R, Przypyszny M, Rein A, Winer EP. 2004. Web-based survey of fertility issues in young women with breast cancer. *J Clin Oncol* 22(20):4174–4183.

Partridge AH, Wang PS, Winer EP, Avorn J. 2003. Nonadherence to adjuvant tamoxifen therapy in women with primary breast cancer. *J Clin Oncol* 21(4):602–606.

Paskett ED, Stark N. 2000. Lymphedema: Knowledge, treatment, and impact among breast cancer survivors. *Breast J* 6(6):373–378.

Passik SD, Dugan W, McDonald MV, Rosenfeld B, Theobald DE, Edgerton S. 1998. Oncologists' recognition of depression in their patients with cancer. *J Clin Oncol* 16(4):1594–1600.

Pediatric Oncology Resource Center. 2003. *Survivors—Follow-up Clinics.* [Online]. Available: http://www.acor.org/ped-onc/treatment/surclinics.html [accessed November 19, 2004].

Pelusi J. 2001. The past sets the stage for the future: Follow-up issues facing long-term cancer survivors. *Semin Oncol Nurs* 17(4):263–267.

Pennery E, Mallet J. 2000. A preliminary study of patients' perceptions of routine follow-up after treatment for breast cancer. *Eur J Oncol Nurs* 4(3):138–145; discussion 146–147.

PHEN (Prostate Health Education Network). 2005. *About PHEN.* [Online]. Available: http://prostatehealthed.org [accessed May 11, 2005].

PLTC (People Living Through Cancer). 2005. *PLTC homepage.* [Online]. Available: http://www.pltc.org/ [accessed April 26, 2005].

Powell TM, Thompsen JP, Virgo KS, Johnson ET, Chan D, Colberg JW, Ornstein DK, Johnson FE. 2000. Geographic variation in patient surveillance after radical prostatectomy. *Ann Surg Oncol* 7(5):339–345.

Presberg BA, Levenson JL. 1993. A survey of cancer support groups provided by National Cancer Institute (NCI) clinical and comprehensive centers. *Psychooncology* 2:215–217.

President's Commission on Heart Disease, Cancer, and Stroke. 1964. *Report to the President: A National Program to Conquer Heart Disease, Cancer, and Stroke.* Washington, DC: U.S. Government Printing Office.

Pritchard P, Hughes J. 1995. *Shared Care the Future Imperative?* London, England: Royal Society of Medicine Press.

Quality Oncology, Inc. 2003. *Quality Oncology, Inc. Announces Progress in Its Federal Pilot Project To Manage Cancer Care for South Florida Medicare Patients.* [Online]. Available: http://www.qualityoncology.com/press/medicare_4_18_03.asp [accessed November 22, 2004].

Rabinowitz B. 2002. Psychosocial issues in breast cancer. *Obstet Gynecol Clin North Am* 29(1):233–247.

Radford JA, Eardley A, Woodman C, Crowther D. 1997. Follow up policy after treatment for Hodgkin's disease: Too many clinic visits and routine tests? A review of hospital records. *BMJ* 314(7077):343–346.

Ragnarsson KT, Thomas DC. 2000. Principles of cancer rehabilitation medicine. In: Bast RC, Kufe DW, Pollock RE, Weichselbaum RR, Holland JF, Frei E, Gansler TS, eds. *Cancer Medicine.* Hamilton, Ontario, Canada: BC Decker. [Online]. Available: http://www.ncbi.nlm.nih.gov/books/bv.fcgi?rid=cmed.section.17163 [accessed July 18, 2005].

Renton JP, Twelves CJ, Yuille FA. 2002. Follow-up in women with breast cancer: The patients' perspective. *Breast* 11(3):257–261.

Richert-Boe KE. 1995. Heterogeneity of cancer surveillance practices among medical oncologists in Washington and Oregon. *Cancer* 75(10):2605–2612.

Ritz LJ, Nissen MJ, Swenson KK, Farrell JB, Sperduto PW, Sladek ML, Lally RM, Schroeder LM. 2000. Effects of advanced nursing care on quality of life and cost outcomes of women diagnosed with breast cancer. *Oncol Nurs Forum* 27(6):923–932.

Rowland J. 2005 (March 24–25). *Update for the IOM Committee on Cancer Survivorship.* Presentation at the meeting of the IOM Committee on Cancer Survivorship, Washington, DC.

Rulyak SJ, Mandelson MT, Brentnall TA, Rutter CM, Wagner EH. 2004. Clinical and sociodemographic factors associated with colon surveillance among patients with a history of colorectal cancer. *Gastrointest Endosc* 59(2):239–247.

Runowicz CD. 1998. Lymphedema: Patient and provider education: Current status and future trends. *Cancer* 83(12 Suppl American):2874–2876.

Sabers SR, Kokal JE, Girardi JC, Philpott CL, Basford JR, Therneau TM, Schmidt KD, Gamble GL. 1999. Evaluation of consultation-based rehabilitation for hospitalized cancer patients with functional impairment. *Mayo Clin Proc* 74(9):855–861.

Sakata K, Beitler AL, Gibbs JF, Kraybill WG, Virgo KS, Johnson FE. 2002. How surgeon age affects surveillance strategies for extremity soft tissue sarcoma patients after potentially curative treatment. *J Surg Res* 108(2):227–234.

Sakata K, Johnson FE, Beitler AL, Kraybill WG, Virgo KS. 2003. Extremity soft tissue sarcoma patient follow-up: Tumor grade and size affect surveillance strategies after potentially curative surgery. *Int J Oncol* 22(6):1335–1343.

Sardell S, Sharpe G, Ashley S, Guerrero D, Brada M. 2000. Evaluation of a nurse-led telephone clinic in the follow-up of patients with malignant glioma. *Clin Oncol (R Coll Radiol)* 12(1):36–41.

Schachter HM, Mamaladze V, Lewin G, Paszat L, Verma S, DeGrasse C, Graham I, Brouwers M, Sampson M, Morrison A, Zhang L, O'Blenis P, Garrity C. 2004. *Measuring the Quality of Breast Cancer Care in Women.* Evidence Report/Technology Assessment No. 105. (Prepared by the University of Ottawa Evidence-based Practice Center under Contract No. 290-02-0021.) AHRQ Publication No. 04-E030-2. Rockville, MD: AHRQ.

Schapira MM, McAuliffe TL, Nattinger AB. 2000. Underutilization of mammography in older breast cancer survivors. *Med Care* 38(3):281–289.

Schmidt KD. 2001. Cancer rehabilitation services in a tertiary care center. *Cancer* 92(4 Suppl):1053–1054.

Schrag D, Hsieh LJ, Rabbani F, Bach PB, Herr H, Begg CB. 2003. Adherence to surveillance among patients with superficial bladder cancer. *J Natl Cancer Inst* 95(8):588–597.

Segal R, Evans W, Johnson D, Smith J, Colletta SP, Corsini L, Reid R. 1999. Oncology Rehabilitation Program at the Ottawa Regional Cancer Centre: Program description. *CMAJ* 161(3):282–285.

Sharma VK, Vasudeva R, Howden CW. 2000. Colorectal cancer screening and surveillance practices by primary care physicians: Results of a national survey. *Am J Gastroenterol* 95(6):1551–1556.

Shaw BR, McTavish F, Hawkins R, Gustafson DH, Pingree S. 2000. Experiences of women with breast cancer: Exchanging social support over the CHESS computer network. *J Health Commun* 5(2):135–159.

Shelby RA, Taylor KL, Kerner JF, Coleman E, Blum D. 2002. The role of community-based and philanthropic organizations in meeting cancer patient and caregiver needs. *CA Cancer J Clin* 52(4):229–246.

Sifri R, Gangadharappa S, Acheson LS. 2004. Identifying and testing for hereditary susceptibility to common cancers. *CA Cancer J Clin* 54(6):309–326.

Sisler JJ, Brown JB, Stewart M. 2004. Family physicians' roles in cancer care. Survey of patients on a provincial cancer registry. *Can Fam Physician* 50:889–896.

Sisters Network, Inc. 2005. *Sisters Network, Inc. Organization Overview*. [Online]. Available: http://www.sistersnetworkinc.org/about-us.asp [accessed May 11, 2005].

Sliwa JA, Marciniak C. 1999. Physical rehabilitation of the cancer patient. *Cancer Treat Res* 100:75–89.

Smith ED, Walsh-Burke K, Crusan C. 1998. Principles of training social workers in oncology. In: Holland JC, ed. *Psycho-Oncology*. New York: Oxford University Press.

Sparaco A, Fentiman IS. 2002. Arm lymphoedema following breast cancer treatment. *Int J Clin Pract* 56(2):107–110.

Stark ME, Crowe JP Jr. 1996. Breast cancer evaluation and follow-up: A survey of The Ohio Chapter of The American College of Surgeons. *Am Surg* 62(6):458–460.

Steinberg ML, Rose CM. 1996. Posttreatment follow-up of radiation oncology patients in a managed care environment. *Int J Radiat Oncol Biol Phys* 35(1):113–116.

Stiggelbout AM, de Haes JC, Vree R, van de Velde CJ, Bruijninckx CM, van Groningen K, Kievit J. 1997. Follow-up of colorectal cancer patients: Quality of life and attitudes towards follow-up. *Br J Cancer* 75(6):914–920.

Tattersall MH, Thomas H. 1999. Recent advances: Oncology. *BMJ* 318(7181):445–448.

Tesauro GM, Rowland JH, Lustig C. 2002. Survivorship resources for post-treatment cancer survivors. *Cancer Pract* 10(6):277–283.

Teschendorf B. 2005 (October 27–28). *ACS Division Survey 2003 Results*. Presentation at the meeting of the IOM Committee on Cancer Survivorship. Irvine, CA.

Texas Cancer Council. 2005. *Texas Cancer Plan: A statewide blueprint for cancer prevention and control in Texas*. 4th ed. Austin, TX: Texas Cancer Council.

The Wellness Community. 2004a. *The Virtual Wellness Community Online Support Groups*. [Online]. Available: http://www.thewellnesscommunity.org/virtual_WC/support.htm [accessed December 3, 2004].

The Wellness Community. 2004b. *The Wellness Community National*. [Online]. Available: http://www.thewellnesscommunity.org/default.asp [accessed October 21, 2004].

The Wellness Community. 2005. *Frankly Speaking About New Discoveries in Cancer*. [Online]. Available: http://www.thewellnesscommunity.org/programs/frankly/newdiscoveries/newdiscoveries_home.htm [accessed March 2, 2005].

Thompson TG, Brailer DJ. 2004. *The Decade of Health Information Technology: Delivering Consumer-Centric and Information-Rich Health Care*. Washington, DC: U.S. Department of Health and Human Services.

Tierney WM, McKinley ED. 2002. When the physician-researcher gets cancer: Understanding cancer, its treatment, and quality of life from the patient's perspective. *Med Care* 40(6 Suppl):III20–III27.

Timmermans S, Mauck A. 2005. The promises and pitfalls of evidence-based medicine. *Health Aff (Millwood)* 24(1):18–28.

True S. 2004 (June 17–18). *Comprehensive Cancer Control and Survivorship*. Presentation at the NCI and ACS Meeting, "Cancer Survivorship: Pathways to Health After Cancer," Washington, DC.

Tsai DY, Virgo KS, Colberg JW, Ornstein DK, Johnson ET, Chan D, Johnson FE. 1999. The age of the urologist affects the postoperative care of prostate carcinoma patients. *Cancer* 86(7):1314–1321.

US Oncology. 2005. *Life Beyond Cancer*. [Online]. Available: http://www.usoncology.com/Resources/LBC.asp [accessed April 25, 2005].

USPSTF (U.S. Preventive Services Task Force). 2003. *Counseling to Prevent Tobacco Use and Tobacco-Related Diseases: Recommendation Statement*. [Online]. Available: http://www.ahrq.gov/clinic/3rduspstf/tobacccoun/tobcounrs.htm [accessed December 8, 2004].

Vernava AM III, Longo WE, Virgo KS, Coplin MA, Wade TP, Johnson FE. 1994. Current follow-up strategies after resection of colon cancer. Results of a survey of members of the American Society of Colon and Rectal Surgeons. *Dis Colon Rectum* 37(6):573–583.

Virgo KS, Chan D, Handler BS, Johnson DY, Goshima K, Johnson FE. 2000. Current practice of patient follow-up after potentially curative resection of cutaneous melanoma. *Plast Reconstr Surg* 106(3):590–597.

Virgo KS, Naunheim KS, Coplin MA, Johnson FE. 1998. Lung cancer patient follow-up: Motivation of thoracic surgeons. *Chest* 114(6):1519–1534.

Virgo KS, Paniello RC, Johnson MH, Clemente MF, Johnson FE. 2002. Surgical decision making in upper aerodigestive tract cancer patient follow-up. *Int J Oncol* 21(5):1101–1109.

Virgo KS, Wade TP, Longo WE, Coplin MA, Vernava AM, Johnson FE. 1995. Surveillance after curative colon cancer resection: Practice patterns of surgical subspecialists. *Ann Surg Oncol* 2(6):472–482.

Vital Options, Inc. 2005. *Cancer Survivorship, Program #466 1/9/2005*. [Online]. Available: http://www.vitaloptions.org/ [accessed April 27, 2005].

Wagner EH, Austin BT, Davis C, Hindmarsh M, Schaefer J, Bonomi A. 2001. Improving chronic illness care: Translating evidence into action. *Health Aff (Millwood)* 20(6):64–78.

Watson PG. 1992. Cancer rehabilitation: An overview. *Semin Oncol Nurs* 8(3):167–173.

White NJ, Given BA, Devoss DN. 1996. The advanced practice nurse: Meeting the information needs of the rural cancer patient. *J Cancer Educ* 11(4):203–209.

Wideroff L, Freedman AN, Olson L, Klabunde CN, Davis W, Srinath KP, Croyle RT, Ballard-Barbash R. 2003a. Physician use of genetic testing for cancer susceptibility: Results of a national survey. *Cancer Epidemiol Biomarkers Prev* 12(4):295–303.

Wideroff L, Vadaparampil ST, Breen N, Croyle RT, Freedman AN. 2003b. Awareness of genetic testing for increased cancer risk in the year 2000 National Health Interview Survey. *Community Genet* 6(3):147–156.

Williams PT. 1994. The role of family physicians in the management of cancer patients. *J Cancer Educ* 9(2):67–72.

Winn R. 2002. *Clinical Practice Guidelines and Survivorship*. Background paper prepared for the National Cancer Policy Board. Unpublished.

Wood ML, McWilliam CL. 1996. Cancer in remission. Challenge in collaboration for family physicians and oncologists. *Can Fam Physician* 42:899–904, 907–910.

5

Providers of Survivorship Care: Their Supply and Education and Training

With the number of cancer survivors in the United States at 10 million and expected to increase, concerns have arisen about the supply of adequately trained health professionals to provide survivorship care. This chapter enumerates providers of survivorship care and then reviews the inclusion of survivorship content in the educational and training programs of selected health professionals involved in survivorship care. Support for professional education and training in survivorship is then described. Finally, the committee puts forth its recommendations to improve the capacity of the survivorship workforce.

SUPPLY OF SURVIVORSHIP CARE PROVIDERS

Survivorship care is by nature multidisciplinary and ideally provided using a team approach. Physicians are the likely coordinators of survivorship care, but as a National Cancer Institute (NCI) Fact Sheet describing the cancer health care team informs consumers, "Your Doctor Is Only the Beginning" (NCI, 2000). Physicians and nurses are often links to many other important care providers, including those in the areas of social work, psychology, rehabilitation, and genetic counseling.

Using the best available data on the supply of health personnel, an attempt is made in Tables 5-1 and 5-2 to assess the availability of selected providers of survivorship care. Table 5-1 shows the numbers of physicians in various disciplines certified by the American Board of Medical Specialties[1] (ABMS) and the membership of related professional societies. For nurses, physical and occupational therapists, social workers, mental health professionals, and other nonphysician providers involved in survivorship care, Table 5-2 shows the number of licensed or certified personnel when applicable and the relevant professional societies.[2] The professional societies of physicians, nurses, and other providers are often the main source of continuing medical education for their specialty and so are key to any effort to raise awareness of survivorship care.

Important disciplines relevant to survivorship care are not represented in these tables. The expertise of cardiologists, neurologists, and endocrinologists, for example, may be needed to diagnose and manage cancer's late effects. Although these estimates are incomplete and imprecise, they point to potential shortages of trained personnel given the size of the survivorship population. Concerns about the future supply of physicians, nurses, and other providers available to care for an older cancer patient population have been voiced since the early 1990s (Kennedy, 1994), but there are few studies of health personnel capacity to gauge the extent of the problem. The Association of American Medical Colleges (AAMC) and the American Society for Clinical Oncology (ASCO) are partnering to study whether the future supply of clinical oncologists will be sufficient to meet future health care needs (ASCO, AAMC to assess clinical oncology workforce, 2005). Better information on all survivorship-related health care personnel is needed to plan for health care delivery and education and training.

STATUS OF PROFESSIONAL EDUCATION AND TRAINING

Cancer survivorship care as a distinct phase of the cancer trajectory is a relatively new construct, and health professional schools' curricula have generally not included much content in this area. This needs to change, but a larger task is providing continuing medical education to professionals who have completed their formal training and are encountering cancer survivors in their practices. The question of who to train is a complicated one because survivorship care encompasses both medical and psychosocial issues and a diverse set of providers can potentially be involved. The content of any survivorship curricula is also not straightforward. Providers need to be apprised of the risks of cancer treatments, the probabilities of cancer recurrence and second cancers, the effectiveness of surveillance and interventions for late effects, the need to address psychosocial concerns, the

[1]By 2003, more than 85 percent of licensed physicians in the United States were certified by at least one ABMS Member Board (ABMS, 2004b).

[2]Membership in a professional association is a very rough marker for supply of specific types of providers because an organization can include members from various professions.

TABLE 5-1 Estimates of the Supply of Selected Physicians Who Provide Survivorship Care

Type of Physician	Number of Physicians	
Physician specialist		
Medical oncology	• Board certified	9,708
	• American Society of Clinical Oncology	12,603
Radiation oncology	• Board certified	4,005
	• American Society for Therapeutic Radiology and Oncology	3,900
Hematology	• Board certified	5,794
	• American Society of Hematology	4,233
Surgery	• Board certified	35,403
	• Society for Surgical Oncology	1,700
Colorectal surgery	• Board certified	1,317
	• American Society of Colon and Rectal Surgeons	1,000
Thoracic surgery	• Board certified	5,693
	• Society of Thoracic Surgeons	4,200[c]
Breast surgery	• American Society of Breast Surgeons	1,900
Ear Nose & Throat (Otolaryngology)	• Board certified	10,165
Urology	• Board certified	10,512
	• American Urological Association	9,738[a]
Gynecologic oncology	• Board certified	718
	• Society of Gynecologic Oncologists	872
Physiatry	• Board certified	6,604
	• American Academy of Physical Medicine and Rehabilitation (AAPM&R)	6,849
	• AAPM&R cancer special interest group	28

benefits to patients of prevention and lifestyle change, and the complexities of integrating survivorship concerns into care for a group of patients of generally advanced age with other chronic conditions.

Education and training must also stress the need for multidisciplinary approaches, integrated and coordinated care, and effective use of community-based resources. Aspects of survivorship that could be considered essential content of survivorship training for health care providers are shown in Box 5-1.

TABLE 5-1 Continued

Type of Physician	Number of Physicians	
Primary care		
Family medicine	• Board certified	64,701
	• American Academy of Family Physicians	94,000
Internal medicine	• Board certified	161,921
	• American College of Physicians: Internal Medicine	118,000[c]
Obstetrics and gynecology	• Board certified	37,057
	• American College of Obstetricians and Gynecologists	46,480[b]
Geriatric medicine	• Board certified	7,287

NOTE: Numbers are estimates based on the number of certifications issued, and may not accurately reflect the number of currently practicing physicians.

[a]Number includes resident members and excludes retired members.

[b]Number includes resident members.

[c]Number includes medical student and resident members.

SOURCES: Number of Board-certified physicians comes from the American Board of Medical Specialties (ABMS, 2004a) and the American Board of Internal Medicine (ABIM, 2005); professional organization membership (limited to physicians of the specified type who may care for adult cancer survivors, in the United States, when possible) comes from: American Society of Clinical Oncology (Personal communication, D. Lopez, ASCO, June 22, 2005); American Society of Breast Surgeons (2005); American Society of Hematology (Personal communication, G. Aklilu, ASH, July 27, 2005); Society of Gynecologic Oncologists (Personal communication, R. Benkert, SGO, January 26, 2005); American Society of Therapeutic Radiation Oncologists (ASTRO, 2002, 2004); Society of Surgical Oncology (Personal communication, R. Slawny, SSO, April 15, 2005); American Urological Association (AUA, 2005); American College of Obstetricians and Gynecologists (Personal communication, C. Flood, ACOG, April 15, 2005); American Society of Colon and Rectal Surgeons (ASCRS, 2005); American College of Physicians (ACP, 2005a); American Society for Therapeutic Radiology and Oncology (Personal communication, S. Smith, ASTRO, June 21, 2005); Society of Thoracic Surgeons (Personal communication, A. Ticoalu, STS, June 23, 2005); American Academy of Family Physicians (AAFP, 2005).

Education and training opportunities for selected physician and nonphysician providers of survivorship care are detailed in the following section. Most of these are oriented to a particular health care discipline, but it is likely that survivorship education and training could be developed for multiple audiences. A few continuing education resources are broadly applicable across professional disciplines. Forthcoming from NCI is a resource for clinicians on cancer survivorship (Personal communication, S. Wilcox, Office of Education and Special Initiatives, NCI, February 2,

TABLE 5-2 Estimates of the Supply of Selected Nonphysician Survivorship-Related Providers

Type of Provider	Number of Providers	
Registered nurses (RNs)	• Licensed	2,201,813[a]
	• Oncology certified nurse	19,132
	• Advanced oncology certified nurse	1,514
	• Oncology Nursing Society	32,000
Physical therapists	• Licensed	120,433
	• American Physical Therapy Association (APTA)	50,035
	• APTA Oncology Section	600
Occupational therapists	• Certified	111,151
	• American Occupational Therapy Association	35,000[b]
Social workers	• Medical and public health social workers	107,000
	• National Association of Social Workers	153,000
Oncology social workers	• Association of Oncology Social Work	1,000
Mental health professionals		
Psychology	• Licensed	85,000
	• American Psychological Assocation (APA)	90,200
	• APA, Health Division	2,947
Psychiatry	• Board certified	34,114
	• Focus on oncology	100
Pastoral counseling	• Certified chaplains	9,100
Genetic counseling	• Board certified	1,811
	• National Society of Genetic Counselors	2,098[c]

[a]Number of RNs employed in nursing, including nurse practitioners.
[b]All members, including occupational therapy assistants and student members.
[c]Includes student members

SOURCES: Number of RNs employed in nursing from the Health Resources and Service Administration (Spratley et al., 2000); number of professional chaplains from a white paper on chaplaincy (VandeCreek and Burton, 2001); number of licensed doctoral level clinically trained psychologists (Personal communication, K. Lewis, APA, July 12, 2005); professional organization membership (limited to U.S. professionals) comes from: Oncology Nursing Society (ONS, 2005); American Physical Therapy Association (Personal communication, K Gardner, APTA, April 27, 2005); American Occupational Therapy Assocation (AOTA, 2005); National Association of Social Workers (NASW, 2005a); National Board for Certification in Occupational Therapy (Personal communication, P. Grace, NBCOT, May 5, 2005); American Board of Genetic Counseling (ABGC, 2003); National Society of Genetic Counselors (Personal communication, L. Brodeur, NSGC, May 17, 2005); Association of Oncology Social Workers (Personal communication, B. Zebrack, AOSW, April 25, 2005); American Psychological Association (Personal communication, K. Cooke, APA, April 25, 2005).

BOX 5-1
Essential Content of Survivorship Training for Health Care Providers

- Prevention of secondary cancers
- General discussion of survivorship
- Long-term complications/sequelae of treatment
- Trends and statistics in health care access
- Health care systems/quality assurance/models of care
- Rehabilitation services
- Quality-of-life issues in survivorship
- Detection of recurrent and secondary cancers
- Pain management
- Palliative care/end-of-life care
- Short-term complications
- Treatment of recurrent cancer

SOURCE: Ferrell et al. (2003).

2005).[3] An educational opportunity available to a cross-section of health professionals is a cancer survivorship biennial conference sponsored by NCI's Office of Cancer Survivorship and the American Cancer Society (ACS) (NCI and ACS, 2002, 2004).

Physicians

The status of undergraduate and graduate medical education is described in this section, followed by some examples of opportunities for continuing medical education on survivorship for practicing physicians.[4] Given their educational potential, the availability of clinical practice guidelines related to cancer survivorship is included in this discussion.

[3]An older, now out-of-date training program for health professionals, *The Cancer Journey: Issues for Survivors*, was developed by NCI in collaboration with the National Coalition for Cancer Survivorship and Ortho Biotech, Inc. It was designed to (1) raise awareness of cancer survivorship; (2) demonstrate how to provide effective support, accurate information, and useful referrals; and (3) promote the empowerment of survivors and their families to work effectively with their health care team, employers, and others concerning issues related to their cancer history (NCI, 1998).

[4]The status of survivorship-related educational opportunities for psychiatrists are described later in the chapter in the section on psychosocial and mental health providers.

Undergraduate Medical Education

Cancer survivorship has not yet been well represented in medical school curricula. Only a few schools were identified as having courses or clerkships pertaining to cancer survivorship when the online database on medical school curriculum maintained by the American Association of Medical Colleges was searched (AAMC, 2005a).[5] Some medical schools have, however, incorporated survivorship issues into the curriculum by including cancer survivors as "standardized patients" in what are referred to as "structured clinical instruction modules" (Plymale et al., 1999). These instruction modules involve medical students interacting with cancer survivors who have been trained to describe their medical history, symptoms, and concerns in a standardized way. Students interview and assess cancer survivors in this simulated, but realistic, clinical setting under the supervision of the faculty. Both the faculty instructor and the cancer survivor provide feedback to the trainees about their performances and, as time allows, the cancer survivor shares additional personal experiences with the trainees. An evaluation of one of these programs found that this method of instruction was considered beneficial for trainees and faculty members alike (Plymale et al., 1999). Emory University has added an educational program, "Survivors Teaching Students: Saving Women's Lives" to the third-year medical students' 6-week gynecology and obstetrics rotation. Survivors from the Georgia Ovarian Cancer Alliance volunteer to discuss their experiences, giving students an opportunity to understand the diagnosis of cancer from the patient's perspective (Emory University, 2004).

A 4-year integrated curriculum in cancer survivorship is being developed under an NCI R25 grant for students at University of California Schools of Medicine (Los Angeles and San Francisco) and the Charles R. Drew University of Medicine and Science. Core competencies have been established and instructional material is being developed on topics such as the epidemiology of survival, risk assessment, treatment of late effects, psychosocial concerns, prevention strategies, and resources for cancer survivors (Box 5-2) (Stuber et al., 2003, 2004). Curricular materials include problem-based learning cases, multimedia web-based problems, a targeted preceptorship experience, and exercises to develop skills in behavior change

---

[5]The online database maintained by the American Association of Medical Colleges is called the Curriculum Management and Information Tool (CurrMit®). The database was searched using the following terms: Cancer AND (rehab OR quality of life OR late-effects OR late effect OR long-term effect OR long term effect OR patient surveillance OR follow-up OR follow up OR surviv OR chronic). The names of required courses and clerkships are available for all medical schools, but only 60 percent of schools have provided additional detail about the coursework.

BOX 5-2
Cancer as a Chronic Disease: Curriculum for Survivorship Required Objectives for Medical School Core Curriculum

Attitudes

1. Comfortable prescribing medications for pain control, including opioids
2. Comfortable asking new patients routinely about previous cancers
3. Willing to ask oncologists for consultation when appropriate
4. Considers general preventative issues as well as those related to cancer survivorship in cancer survivors

Knowledge

1. Understands that all cancer survivors are at increased risk for other cancers as well as recurrence of the original cancer, and need to avoid tobacco, eat right, and use sunscreen
2. Understands basic mechanisms of genetic contribution to risk of cancer
3. Understands common uses of the terms "cure", "disease free survival", and "cancer survivor"
4. Understands differences in cancer survivorship by gender, ethnicity and socio-economic status
5. Understands the variety of social consequences of cancer on survivors, including difficulty getting employment and insurance, stigma, and the impact on the family and friendships
6. Knows the essential elements to obtain about a cancer history, how to get information the patient can't give them, and how to interpret the health implications of the history
7. Understands consequences of cancer treatment for different developmental stages, including impact on growth, osteoporosis, learning, sexual function and fertility

Skills

1. Able to use key screening guidelines to identify people at higher risk for cancer
2. Able to provide appropriate and individualized recommendations for secondary prevention to cancer survivors regarding sunscreen, diet, obesity, exercise, alcohol, and tobacco
3. Able to tailor pain medication and other interventions for pain to the source and type as well as the severity of pain
4. Able to explain and help patients make decisions about a living will, do not resuscitate (DNR) orders, durable power of attorney, and advance health care directives
5. Able to give bad news about second malignancy or relapse, and to move to a palliative approach when appropriate without saying "there is nothing we can do"
6. Able to partner with patients in decision making, respecting what is important to the patient
7. Able to work as the primary care provider with a specialty team, providing continuity of care, and working with family as well as patient
8. Able to get current cancer information for cancer survivors at the appropriate reading level and language (e.g., from the Cancer Information Service and National Cancer Institute)

SOURCE: UCLA (2005b).

and risk assessment (Personal communication, L. Wilkerson, David Geffen School of Medicine at University of California–Los Angeles, January 13, 2005). A survey on survivorship knowledge and experience has been designed as a needs assessment or program evaluation tool. The survivorship curriculum and materials will be available through the UCLA Cancer Education Project's website (UCLA, 2005a) and the Health Education Assets Library (HEAL), an online, peer-reviewed health education repository (HEAL, 2005). As survivorship curricula and materials are developed, they can also be shared between medical schools through the MedEd Portal, a new online repository of education materials maintained by AAMC (2005b).

Graduate Medical Education

The curricula followed in graduate medical education is determined under the auspices of the American Council of Graduate Medical Education. According to a review of the curriculum for medical oncology, some of the 28 content areas listed are related to survivorship (e.g., knowledge of drug toxicity, rehabilitation, and psychosocial aspects of clinical management of the cancer patient), but no specific mention of cancer survivorship is made (Winn, 2002). The specific items to be included in the oncology fellowship training curriculum are not within the purview of the American Board of Internal Medicine and Accreditation Council for Graduate Medical Education. ASCO has assumed the task of creating a "Competence Comprising Curriculum" for medical oncology subspecialty training in 14 key areas, including supportive care and survivorship (Muss et al., 2005; ASCO, 2005a). For the primary care disciplines of internal medicine and family medicine, a review of curriculum guidelines found a lack of mention of cancer survivorship.

A review of selected general oncology and disease-specific medical textbooks found only one text that addressed cancer survivorship specifically (i.e., *Diseases of the Breast*, Harris et al., 2004) (Winn, 2000). Most of the other textbooks had certain survivorship issues represented, but there was relatively little discussion of practical clinical management issues. Several standard primary care and internal medicine textbooks were reviewed from the perspective of whether a primary care physician wishing to learn about the management of cancer survivors could readily obtain an overview of the entire area. The texts were not comprehensive or detailed enough in their coverage to serve as primary sources of information for the clinician seeking to effectively manage these patients. Available texts may, however, serve a purpose in highlighting some of the major problem areas of cancer survivorship and alerting the caregiver of the need to consult additional sources for more comprehensive information.

Some specialty texts were found that were directly related to survivorship care. The text *Cancer Patient Follow-Up* (Johnson and Virgo, 1997) provides a comprehensive review of follow-up practices. The major focus is on surveillance testing, but treatment complications and their management are also covered. This text provides an excellent source for clinicians interested in the scientific rationale for many survivor issues. Another resource is *Principles and Practice of Palliative Care and Supportive Oncology* (Berger et al., 2002). This text has two relevant chapters, "Long-term survivorship: Late effects" (Aziz, 2002), and "Psychosocial aspects of cancer survivorship" (Leigh and Clark, 2002). In addition, many of the chapters about specific supportive care issues, such as sexuality and reproduction or depression and anxiety, are pertinent to survivorship. Integrated discussions of these palliative and supportive care topics provide an excellent orientation for the clinician wanting to become grounded in survivorship.

A new certification program of the ABMS may provide opportunities for continuing education regarding survivorship care (ABMS, 2004b). Until recently, Board recertification testing occurred every 6, 7, or 10 years. A new program, called "Maintenance of Certification" (MOC), changed the specialty recertification process for physicians from periodic testing to a more continuous process. The new MOC program will require the assessment and improvement of practice performance by physician specialists. Examples of practice assessment and improvement approaches for MOC include, for internal medicine, Practice Improvement Modules in clinical preventive services and preventive cardiology, and, for pediatrics, web-based education improvement programs in pediatric asthma and attention deficit hyperactivity disorder. A module related to cancer survivorship could be developed to enhance specialists' knowledge of survivorship-related care.

Continuing Medical Education

For practicing clinicians, continuing medical education provides opportunities to gain skills in this relatively new area. There appears to be a demand for such education, at least among oncologists. According to a recent survey, more than 75 percent of medical oncologists reported that they provide some follow-up care for cancer survivors, but a significant proportion wanted additional training (ASCO, 2004).

Continuing medical education (CME) credits—attained through onsite meeting attendance, virtual meeting participation, or online CME venues—provide significant opportunities for clinicians to be exposed to issues related to survivorship. The Accreditation Council of Continuing Medical Education has accredited the major national societies to offer CME credit for certain sessions at their meetings. Examples of some recent CME opportunities at professional meetings are shown in Box 5-3.

BOX 5-3
Continuing Medical Education: Examples from Recent Professional Meetings

American Society of Clinical Oncology (2005 Annual Meeting)
- Cancer Survivorship: Long-Term Complications of Treatment
- Breast Cancer Survivorship: Long-Term Issues in Women with Breast Cancer
- Supportive Oncology: Complementary and Alternative Medicine
- Assessing and Teaching Humanistic and Spiritual Aspects of Cancer Care

Society of Gynecologic Oncologists (2005 Annual Meeting)
- Advances in Reproductive Health: Cancer and Conception
- Barriers to Sexual Health After Cancer: What Can Be Done?
- Ovarian Cancer Survivor's Course (for survivors and nurses)

The American Society for Therapeutic Radiology and Oncology (2004 meeting) raised awareness of cancer survivorship by creating a "Survivor Circle" exhibit in partnership with the Atlanta chapter of the American Cancer Society. Information on ACS support programs was featured (US Newswire, 2004).

American Association for Cancer Education (2004 Meetings)
- Integration of Cancer Survivorship Coursework into First Year Medical School Curriculum
- Quality of Life: Native American Cancer Education for Survivors
- Exploring the Needs of Cancer Patients and Their Family Caregivers Through a Training Workshop
- Does Diet Modification Have Potential to Reduce Cancer Suffering and Extend Life?
- Partners in Survival National Training Program: Training Minority Men to be Effective Caregivers for Women with Cancer

SOURCES: ASCO (2005c); SGO (2005); *Journal of Cancer Education* (2004).

In some cases, professional societies have, or are planning, continuing medical education opportunities for their specialty group.

Medical oncology To help oncologists better address the needs of cancer survivors, ASCO has formed a Survivorship Task Force to develop, implement, and manage ASCO survivorship programs related to physician education, survivorship guidelines, patient education, and research (ASCO, 2004). There are plans for the issuance of clinical practice guidelines on issues such as late effects and the development of a central online information resource on late and long-term effects of cancer and its treatment. At its 2005 annual meeting, ASCO examined prevention strategies for survivors at high risk for second cancers. ASCO also has a series of continuing education publications that are related to survivorship, for example, "Optimizing Cancer Care: The Importance of Symptom Management" and "Cancer Care in the Older Population" (ASCO, 2005d).

Primary care A comprehensive review of cancer survivorship is available through an American Academy of Family Physicians (AAFP) Home Study Self-Assessment monograph (Hamblin and Schifeling, 2001).[6] The following areas are covered in this 60-page monograph:

- Risk of recurrence or second malignancy
- Follow-up regimens for breast, colorectal, prostate, acute leukemia, lymphoma
- Late effects of treatment
- Evaluation of common problems in survivors, such as depression and anxiety, sexual dysfunction
- Diet, physical exercise, tobacco
- Complementary and alternative medicines
- Disability, discrimination, and related issues
- Internet resources

Approximately 6,200 physicians received this monograph in May 2001 as part of their subscription to the Home Study Self-Assessment program, but there are no plans for any other distribution (Personal communication, P. Dove, AAFP, March 9, 2005).

One state-based continuing education project directed at primary care providers is noteworthy: the development of a CME module on surveillance of cancer patients by the Physician Oncology Education Program (POEP) with support from the Texas Cancer Council. The module was first developed in 1999 as a slide set and short booklet describing the role of the primary care physician in caring for cancer patients following diagnosis and treatment (POEP, 1999). The POEP plans to revise the module as part of a web-based online CME program with support from a Small Business Innovation Research (SBIR) grant from NCI (Personal communication, G. Weiss, MD, POEP, April 22, 2004).

The American College of Physicians (ACP) has 48 online clinical problem-solving cases that provide CME credits upon their completion.

[6]The monograph contains pre-and post-test forms, and the user is qualified for up to five Category I CME credits.

Three of the cases are about cancer, and one of these involves a 52-year-old woman who seeks advice about follow-up cancer care. To complete the program, physicians use interactive software to review patient assessments, order tests, prescribe treatments, respond to outcomes, and receive expert feedback on decisions (ACP, 2005b).

Physical medicine and rehabilitation Topical self-directed study guides and examinations are published annually as a Medical Education Supplement to the *Archives of Physical Medicine and Rehabilitation.* These guides have included cancer rehabilitation as a focus (Roig et al., 2004; AAPM&R, 2005). CME credit for completion of the study guides may be obtained for up to 3 years from the date of publication.

Other Sources of Information on Cancer Survivorship

The ideal situation for a clinician who cares for cancer survivors would be to have immediate access to comprehensive clinical practice guidelines (CPGs) based on high-quality evidence where available that included a full range of recommendations for the many clinical decisions that might be encountered in the post-treatment phase of care (see discussion of CPGs in Chapter 3). As mentioned earlier, ASCO has plans for an online service to include information on late and long-term effects of cancer and its treatment. ASCO currently has guidelines available on its website on the post-treatment surveillance of individuals with breast and colorectal cancer for cancer recurrence (ASCO, 2005b). Guidelines on certain aspects of survivorship care are available online from other groups. For example, guidance on the management of cancer-related fatigue and psychosocial distress are available from the National Comprehensive Cancer Network (NCCN) (NCCN, 2005). The National Guidelines Clearinghouse is a searchable database of guidelines that includes guidelines for cancer patient follow-up when searched using the search terms "cancer" and "surveillance or follow-up" (AHRQ, 2004).

The NCI's PDQ (Physician Data Query) contains peer-reviewed summaries on supportive care, genetics services, and complementary and alternative medicine (NCI, 2005d). Although they are not formal CPGs, PDQ's supportive care summaries provide descriptions of the pathophysiology and treatment of common physical and psychosocial complications of cancer and its treatment (Box 5-4). PDQ cancer genetics summaries provide information about risk factors related to family history, major genes and syndromes associated with cancer, interventions specific to individuals at high risk, and the ethical, legal, and social issues related to cancer risk counseling and gene testing. PDQ also includes summaries of complementary and

BOX 5-4
Selected Examples of Survivorship-Related PDQ Summaries on Supportive Care (Coping with Cancer)

Symptoms
- Cardiopulmonary syndromes
- Fatigue
- Fever, sweats, and hot flashes
- Gastrointestinal complications
- Hypercalcemia
- Lymphedema
- Oral complications of chemotherapy and head/neck radiation
- Pain
- Pruritus (itching sensation)
- Radiation enteritis
- Sexuality and reproductive issues
- Sleep disorders

Psychosocial Issues
- Anxiety disorder
- Depression
- Normal adjustment, psychosocial distress, and the adjustment disorders
- Post-traumatic stress disorder

Lifestyle Issues
- Nutrition in cancer care
- Smoking cessation and continued risk in cancer patients
- Spirituality in cancer care
- Substance abuse issues in cancer
- Transitional care planning

SOURCE: NCI (2005c).

alternative treatments commonly used by cancer survivors. Summaries are available for both physicians and patients.

Journal review articles provide good opportunities for learning. Two issues of *Seminars in Oncology*, for example, focused on post-treatment surveillance for potentially curable malignancies (Doll et al., 2003) and late effects of treatment and survivorship issues in early-stage breast cancer (Shapiro and Winer, 2003). However, most such articles are based on expert opinion, due to a lack of high-quality evidence. Opinions of equally qualified experts often can conflict.

The *European Journal of Cancer Care* has a continuing professional education in oncology program, the Forum for Applied Cancer Education and Training (FACET) that includes a module called "After Treatment—Who Cares?" that addresses issues related to survivorship care (FACET, 2004).

Registered Nurses

Nursing represents the largest segment of the nation's health care workforce and has a significant role on the "front lines" of cancer care, both in hospitals and ambulatory settings (McCorkle et al., 1998; Ferrell et al., 2003). In 2000, an estimated 2.2 million registered nurses (RNs) were employed full- or part-time nationwide (Spratley et al., 2000). Relative to the number of RNs, there are relatively few with specialized training in oncology. Specialization in nursing is recognized through certification by the Oncology Nursing Certification Corporation (ONCC). As of early 2005, there were 19,132 basic-level Oncology Certified Nurses (OCNs®) and 1,514 Advanced Oncology Certified Nurses (AOCN®) (ONCC, 2005a). Some oncology nurse specialists have completed training as nurse practitioners, allowing them to assume more independent clinical roles (Mooney, 2000). In 2003, ONCC conducted a role delineation study of advanced practice nurses that identified significant differences between the work responsibilities of oncology clinical nurse specialists and nurse practitioners in oncology. Based on the results of that study, beginning in January 2005, two different advanced oncology nursing certifications became available: Advanced Oncology Certified Nurse Practitioner (AOCNP®) and Advanced Oncology Certified Clinical Nurse Specialist (AOCNS®). To be eligible for either certification, a nurse must have an RN license, a master's or higher degree in nursing, and a minimum of 500 hours of supervised clinical practice in oncology nursing; AOCNP® candidates must also have completed an accredited nurse practitioner program (ONCC, 2005b). Advanced practice nurses provide models for clinical practice, education, and advocacy. The professional society representing oncology nurses, the Oncology Nursing Society (ONS), has more than 32,000 registered nurses as members, and 127 members are enrolled in a survivorship special interest group (ONS, 2005) (Personal communication, D. Gutaj, Coordinator, ONS survivorship special interest group, January 23, 2005).

Information on the settings in which nurses practice suggests that the role of nursing in the provision of survivorship services may have lessened, in the sense that relatively few nurses work in ambulatory and community-based settings, the places where most cancer care is delivered. In 2000, only 9 percent of RNs worked in ambulatory settings, according to a large federally sponsored survey (Spratley et al., 2000). Substantially more oncology RNs (37 percent) work in ambulatory settings, according to a survey of the ONS membership conducted in 2000 (Lamkin et al., 2001, 2002).[7] Access to nurses in ambulatory care settings is limited by staff shortages that reduce the time available to assess or respond to other than acute care needs. Outpatients making cancer-related visits encounter nurses in just over one-quarter of visits, according to surveys of ambulatory care providers (see Chapter 4, Table 4-4). A belief that there are too few RNs specializing in oncology nursing in the United States and that RN staffing shortfalls will continue over the decade was reported by most of the oncologists, executives, and oncology RNs surveyed in 2000 about the adequacy of the nursing supply (Buerhaus et al., 2001). Executives who reported unfilled positions for oncology RNs said that the lack of qualified applicants was the largest reason for unfilled positions. Despite reported shortages, many oncologists' offices and some surgeons' offices have an oncology nurse, so that, for patients in these settings, the oncology nurse plays a critical role in survivorship care.

Education and Training

Undergraduate nursing education rarely includes didactic training in oncology, according to a review of the content of basic nursing education (McCorkle et al., 1998; Ferrell et al., 2003).[8] Nurses generally receive some exposure to cancer care through coursework related to surgical and medical care of chronic diseases. Cancer centers have worked with local nursing training programs to increase the number of students who rotate in oncology in an effort to attract students to oncology nursing positions upon graduation (Erikson, 2000).

Nurses with advanced training in oncology can assume important roles in providing survivorship care (see Chapter 4) but, even among nurses belonging to the ONS, there are relatively few with advanced training—only 11 percent reported having a certificate or degree as an advanced practice nurse[9] in a 2000 survey (Buerhaus et al., 2001). It is of some concern that a diminishing number of nursing graduate programs offer a special oncology focus. The number of programs offering an oncology specialty has decreased from approximately 45 programs in 1990 to only 26 programs in 2002 (Ferrell et al., 2003). Increased budgetary concerns

---

[7]A sample of members of the Oncology Nursing Society was surveyed. A limitation of this survey is the low response rate (40 percent).

[8]Relatively few RNs have a master's or doctoral degree—an estimated 10 percent in 2000, according to a federally sponsored study (Spratley et al., 2000). The highest level of preparation for most RNs was a diploma/associate degree (57 percent) or baccalaureate degree (33 percent).

[9]The following were defined as advanced practice nurses: nurse practitioner, certified nurse midwife, certified registered nurse anesthetist, or clinical nurse practitioner.

have led to the consolidation of specialty programs into more generalized tracks (e.g., chronic illness, medical-surgical). This finding holds important implications for the quality of care provided to cancer survivors. Generalized master's education tracks are less likely to provide adequate attention to the specific nursing care of cancer survivors. The preservation of oncology nursing as a specialty is central to efforts to assure quality cancer care, according to some nurse educators (Satryan, 2001).

A review of the curricula of available graduate nursing programs offering an oncology focus suggests that the survivorship content could be strengthened (Ferrell et al., 2003). Information gathered from 17 of these programs indicated that 11 of the 17 programs had curricula that covered quality-of-life and survivorship issues, 9 of the 17 programs had curricula that covered detection of recurrent and secondary cancers, and 3 of the 17 programs had curricula that covered rehabilitation services. Enhancing the survivorship-related content in these advanced training programs could generate more nurses with the training needed to assume active roles in survivorship care. Certified oncology nurses are expected to master cancer patient survivorship skills. A review of the examination content for certification as an oncology nurse suggested that survivorship issues were well represented (Ferrell et al., 2003). The authors of this review recommended that cancer centers encourage nurses to be certified in oncology. There appear to be limited incentives for nurses to obtain certification—only one-third of nurses working in oncology settings reported that nurses receive a salary increase or bonus for obtaining oncology nursing certification when surveyed in 2000 as part of a workforce survey (Lamkin et al., 2001).

Continuing Nursing Education

ONS provides opportunities for continuing education on cancer survivorship through its "Institutes of Learning" added to its annual congress. In addition, more than 200 chapters of ONS provide cancer education at the local level (Mooney, 2000). Strategies for effective nursing continuing education have been outlined and include a focus on participants' goals, examples of successes, inclusion of patients and families, and participatory learning (Ferrell et al., 2002).

The Nurse Oncology Education Program (NOEP) provides continuing education on cancer prevention, early detection, treatment, and survivorship to nursing professionals in Texas (NOEP, 2005). Continuing education credits are available through NOEP via workshops, online programs, and independent studies in print. The program is funded by the Texas Cancer Council and provided through the Texas Nurses Association and Foundation. Statewide surveys are conducted periodically to assess the continuing education needs of nurses (Meraviglia et al., 2003).

A continuing education supplement to the *American Journal of Nursing* on nursing and cancer survivorship will be published based on a symposium on long-term cancer survivorship at the University of Pennsylvania (Mason and Burke, 2005).

Other Sources of Information on Cancer Survivorship

- American Cancer Society has published *A Cancer Source Book for Nurses* that includes information on advances in symptom control and issues related to survivorship (Varricchio et al., 2004).
- Journal articles that describe the population of cancer survivors and review the roles of nurses in providing survivorship care are important sources of continuing education (Thaler-DeMers, 2001; Rowland et al., 2001) (see also Chapter 4 for a description of nursing roles in survivorship)

Rehabilitation Specialists

Rehabilitative care is multidisciplinary and may involve physicians trained in rehabilitation and physical medicine (physiatrists), nurses, and other specialists. In this section, three important professional groups that often provide rehabilitative care are described: physical therapists, occupational therapists, and speech and language pathologists. Of these three professional groups, physical therapists are the most commonly encountered providers of rehabilitation services.[10] An estimated 13 percent of cancer survivors report using the services of a physical therapist, occupational therapist, or other therapist in the past year (Hewitt et al., 2003). Such therapists are used more frequently (18 percent) among cancer survivors reporting one or more functional limitations.

Physical Therapists

Physical therapists (PTs) provide services that help restore function, improve mobility, relieve pain, and prevent or limit permanent physical disabilities of patients suffering from injuries or disease (BLS, 2004b). PTs also restore, maintain, and promote overall fitness and health. Cancer survivors may be referred to a physical therapist to manage late effects such as

[10]Most outpatient rehabilitation therapy services provided to Medicare beneficiaries (with and without a history of cancer) are provided by physical therapists (PTs) (Ciolek and Hwang, 2004). In 2002, 8 percent of beneficiaries used PT services, 2 percent used occupational therapy services, and 1 percent used speech-language pathology services.

lymphedema, pain, and fatigue. PT interventions for cancer survivors may include exercise, heat, therapeutic massage, gait training, and prosthetics to assist the patient in becoming as functional as possible (Mellette and Blunk, 1994). PTs focus on building lower body strength, dexterity, and flexibility. Nearly all hospital cancer programs provide PT services (see Chapter 4) and PT services may also be obtained through their independent practices. There were an estimated 37,000 PTs working in the United States as of 2002; however, the Oncology Section of the American Physical Therapy Association (APTA) has only about 600 members (Ries, 2004). Of the small number of physical therapists identified as specializing in oncology in the APTA database, most work in acute care hospitals and health systems, hospital-based outpatient facilities, private outpatient offices, or group practices (Personal communication, S. Miller, APTA, February 2, 2005).

The extent of coverage of cancer care in PT training programs is not well documented, but anecdotal evidence suggests that in many programs, oncology is integrated across the curriculum (Ries, 2004).[11] A survey of physical therapy programs conducted in the late 1990s shows that most physical therapy programs cover topics in lymphedema management (Augustine et al., 1998), and previous National Physical Therapy Examinations have included questions on the treatment of cancer patients (Personal communication, M. Lane, Federation of State Boards of Physical Therapy, February 15, 2005).

Continuing education opportunities are offered through the APTA as in-person training sessions and online audio/video or text-based courses. Some courses are cancer specific, such as a session at the 2005 annual meeting entitled "Exercise Training Guidelines for Individuals with Cancer: Endurance, Strength, Flexibility & Adherence" (Oncology Section, 2005). One course, "Physical Therapy Treatment for the Breast Cancer Patient" addresses functional limitations associated with the late effects of treatment (R^3 Programs, 2005). Other courses cover topics such as lymphedema, osteoporosis, and urinary incontinence, which, although not specific to cancer, may be relevant to cancer survivors (APTA, 2005b). The APTA publishes the journal *Physical Therapy*, which periodically publishes articles on cancer care. The comprehensive "Guide to Physical Therapist Practice," published in *Physical Therapy*, includes a section on lymphedema diagnosis and management (APTA, 2001). The Oncology Section of the APTA publishes its own journal, *Rehabilitation Oncology*, and has also produced a series of monographs on developing oncology rehabilitation programs and training program curriculums.

---

[11] In the United States, 80 training programs offer master's degrees in physical therapy, and 125 programs offer doctoral physical therapy degrees (APTA, 2005a).

Occupational Therapists

Occupational therapists (OTs) help people improve their ability to perform tasks in their daily living and working environments. They also help individuals develop, recover, or maintain daily living and work skills (BLS, 2004b). Cancer survivors may be referred to OTs for assistance with mobility impairments, pain, fatigue, shortness of breath, insomnia, auditory or visual impairment, and cognitive deficits (Penfold, 1996; COT, 2001). OTs can help by teaching various adaptive techniques, energy conservation, how to make the home or workplace more accessible, and how to use adaptive equipment (Mellette and Blunk, 1994). OTs focus on building upper body strength, dexterity, and flexibility. OTs work in cancer centers, community hospitals, ambulatory care settings, and independent practices (COT, 2001; BLS, 2004b). There were an estimated 111,151 certified OTs in the United States as of 2005, but virtually no information is available on the extent to which they provide cancer-related rehabilitation services.[12]

Speech-Language Pathologists

Speech-language pathologists, also known as speech therapists, are trained to treat problems with speech, voice, language, swallowing, and other related disorders (BLS, 2004c).[13] They often work with survivors of head and neck cancers who may develop speech or swallowing problems as a result of surgery or radiation. Speech-language pathologists may teach muscle exercises or head postures to help overcome swallowing problems, or modifications of mouth movements to help patients adapt to differences in size and shape of the mouth to speak clearly (ASHA, 2005a,b). Speech therapists typically meet with patients before surgery or radiation, to discuss possible changes in speech and swallowing, and after medical treatment, to assess and treat any problems that may have arisen.

Psychosocial and Mental Health Providers

Cancer may cause psychosocial distress, so referrals to social service and mental health professionals may be indicated. Psychosocial services may be provided by cancer caregivers, such as nurses, primary care physicians, surgeons, or oncologists, or by professionals with special training in social work, psychology, psychiatry, or pastoral counseling. Services might

---

[12]A bachelor's degree in occupational therapy is the minimum requirement for entry into the field, but beginning in 2007 a master's degree or higher will be required (BLS, 2004b).

[13]Nearly all states require that speech therapists have a master's degree and be licensed (BLS, 2004c).

be conceptualized as basic, that is, provided as part of routine care by sympathetic and supportive physicians, nurses, and clinical and hospital staff who come in contact with the cancer patient. Services might be more extensive, supplemented by others such as social workers, support groups, and clergy as needed and, for more serious problems, specifically trained mental health professionals such as psychiatrists, psychologists, and clinical social workers.

This section briefly describes the education and training of some of the most frequently encountered providers of psychosocial services and mentions sources of survivorship-related continuing education that are available within the various disciplines. Several sources of continuing education are available to the full range of psychosocial providers, and these are described following the specific offerings of the various disciplines.

Social Workers

Social workers assist cancer patients in several ways: by providing help with concrete services, such as assisting with insurance and benefits; by serving as case managers to coordinate care and help patients navigate health care systems; by leading peer support groups; and by referring patients and families to community services (Box 5-5).

Social workers are the primary providers of psychosocial services in hospitals and many cancer centers and are trained to facilitate patient and family adjustment to a cancer diagnosis, its treatment, and rehabilitation (Smith et al., 1998). Social workers may also refer cancer patients and family members who show signs of distress or who have significant family or social problems to psychologists or psychiatrists. In small oncology practices, social workers may be the only professionals available for handling psychosocial problems occurring with cancer. As more cancer patients survive and continue to work, some social workers are providing workplace consultations to help with the employment adjustments of survivors and their colleagues (Tolley, 1994).

Social work services have been strained in recent years by hospital cutbacks, in some cases leading to the elimination of entire departments of social work. Although there have been advances in psycho-oncology research of relevance to social workers assisting cancer survivors, reductions in staffing and increased caseloads have made it difficult for social workers to translate these findings into their practices (IASWR, 2003; NASW, 2003). As of 2003, there were an estimated 103,000 medical and public health social workers in the United States, most of them employed in hospitals (BLS, 2004a).

Most oncology social workers have a Master of Social Work (MSW) degree and receive training in chronic illness issues in graduate school.

BOX 5-5
Oncology Social Work: Scope of Practice

- Clinical Practice: Complete psychosocial assessments; develop multidisciplinary care plans; provide therapeutic interventions and case management; assist with financial, transportation, lodging, and other needs; advocate to remove barriers to care and address gaps in service; advance knowledge through research.

- Within Cancer Centers/Institutions: Provide education and consultation to professionals and staff regarding psychosocial and other factors affecting cancer care; collaborate in the delivery of psychosocial care, education, and research; develop programs and resources to address the needs of cancer survivors.

- Within the Community: Increase awareness of psychosocial needs of cancer survivors, families, and caregivers; collaborate with community agencies to remove barriers to care; collaborate in the development of special programs and resources to address community-based needs; consult with voluntary agencies to provide community education and develop programs.

- Within the Social Work Profession: Teach in the classroom or in clinical settings; supervise and evaluate practitioners; consult with colleagues; participate in research.

SOURCE: AOSW (2005).

There is no formal accreditation in oncology available for social workers. However, the Association of Oncology Social Work (AOSW), with a membership of nearly 1,000 social workers, defines oncology social workers' scope of practice (Box 5-4), sets standards of practice, and serves as an educational resource (AOSW, 2004) (Personal communication, L. Behar, Membership Chair, AOSW, July 2004). Psychiatric social workers who have additional training in psycho-oncology are particularly valuable as mental health professionals in oncology.

There are several continuing education opportunities for social workers. A web-based continuing education course, *Understanding Cancer: The Social Worker's Role*, is available through the National Association of Social Work and CancerCare, an organization providing psychosocial services (NASW, 2005b). The *Journal of Psychosocial Oncology* is the official journal of the AOSW and reports research findings and clinical observations relevant to the social workers involved in oncology. The book *Social Work in Oncology: Supporting Survivors, Families, and Caregivers* provides an overview of issues faced by social workers within various patient populations and practice settings (Lauria et al., 2001).

Psychologists

Psychologists are the mental health professionals who, after social workers, are most likely to be available for clinical consultation and management of psychosocial concerns in patients with cancer and their families.[14] They also represent the discipline that contributes predominantly to psycho-oncology research. As of 2005 there were approximately 90,200 U.S.-based members, fellows, and associates of the American Psychological Association (APA), the professional association that represents psychologists, of which nearly 3,000 belonged to the health division (Personal communication, K. Cooke, APA, April 25, 2005).

Undergraduate psychology programs do not routinely include training in psycho-oncology, except as it might occur in conjunction with clinical rotations. Some health psychology graduate programs have faculty members who do research in psycho-oncology, and graduate students in these programs can choose dissertations dealing with oncology issues. Psychology internships are not available in the specialized area of oncology. However, many 2-year post-doctoral fellowships exist that permit training in either research or clinical work alone, or a combination of both. A large number of members of the Society of Behavioral Medicine have their career emphasis in some area of psychosocial or behavioral oncology. They have made major contributions in cancer prevention, cancer control, and lifestyle change, such as smoking cessation.

The APA offers continuing education opportunities for psychologists, although cancer-related offerings are somewhat limited. Of the 60 continuing education courses offered at the 2005 APA meeting, only one deals with cancer (APA, 2005). Although psychologist-specific continuing education in cancer may be sparse, many continuing education offerings that are aimed at psychosocial care providers from other organizations are available, as discussed below.

Psychiatry

Psychiatrists with an interest in diagnosis and treatment of co-morbid psychological problems and psychiatric disorders are known as consultation-liaison psychiatrists. A subspecialty certification of psychiatry in the care of the medically ill has been established, with the first specialty examinations in psychosomatic medicine as a subspecialty to be adminis-

[14]Psychologists receive a PhD in clinical or health psychology or a PsyD, Doctorate of Psychology.

tered in 2005. Among the 1,000 U.S. psychiatrists who work primarily with the medically ill, approximately 100 identify oncology as a significant focus of their clinical work, and work with cancer patients either on a full-time basis or as a part of their clinical care or research. Control of symptoms that reduce quality of life, such as severe anxiety, depression, and delirium, often requires management with psychopharmacologic interventions and awareness of drug–drug interactions in the context of complex oncologic treatment.

Psychiatric residents must rotate for a period of time, after internship, through the inpatient and outpatient units, where they learn the common psychiatric disorders of chronically medically ill patients and their psychological and psychopharmacological management. Post-residency clinical fellowships of 1 or 2 years can be taken in psychiatric and psychosocial oncology at a few major academic cancer centers. There are several formal psycho-oncology training programs that offer fellowships to physicians (e.g., Memorial Sloan-Kettering Cancer Center, Mount Sinai Ruttenberg Cancer Center, Dana-Farber Cancer Institute, University of Pennsylvania).

Rehabilitation and Employment-Based Counseling

Master's-level counselors trained in specialized areas of counseling who work outside of oncology settings may be of assistance to cancer survivors. Rehabilitation counselors may help cancer survivors deal with the personal, social, and vocational effects of cancer-related disabilities. They may assist cancer survivors as they go back to work or reassess career options. Counseling may be available at worksites through corporate Employment Assistance Programs (EAPs). EAPs often employ social workers and other professional counselors who can provide short-term counseling and appropriate referrals to community resources. A demonstration project called the Individual Cancer Assistance Network (ICAN), sponsored by Bristol-Myers Squibb Foundation, trained 141 community-based counselors and EAP providers in Florida in a "face-to-face" and distance-learning program in psychosocial oncology. Efforts are underway to expand the program and use the core curriculum, developed by CancerCare, and the American Psychosocial Oncology Society (APOS), to train professionals who already have counseling skills to be oncology sensitive (Alter, 2005).

Marriage, Family, and Sex Counseling

Marriage and family therapists may work with individuals, couples, or families in dealing with cancer in the context of the family system. Marriage and family therapy is short-term, solution-focused therapy, and usually includes fewer sessions than individual therapy.[15] Sex counselors or therapists knowledgeable about the sexual side effects of cancer treatment (e.g., reduced libido, problems with sexual performance) can counsel individuals and their partners in both the psychological/psychosexual and practical issues arising from these difficulties.[16]

Pastoral Counseling

A diagnosis of cancer continues to be regarded as a threat to life, bringing the possibility of death into focus. Cancer survivors may seek assistance in coping with illness and its meaning from religious or spiritual counselors. Professional health care chaplains provide supportive spiritual care and may help educate the health care team on the relationship of religious and spiritual issues to aspects of clinical care (VandeCreek and Burton, 2001). Some of the 9,100 chaplains certified by the Association of Professional Chaplains (or other certifying organizations) work in hospitals, long-term care units, rehabilitation centers, hospices, or other specialized settings. Nearly all hospital cancer programs provide pastoral care (see Chapter 4). Pastoral care training and courses are available at some cancer centers (Roswell Park Cancer Institute, 2005), and certified chaplains may meet their continuing education requirements through such programs. The HealthCare Chaplaincy serving the New York metropolitan area is such a resource (The HealthCare Chaplaincy, 2005). Several journals cover the overlapping area of medicine and clergy (e.g., *Journal of Health Care Chaplaincy*, *Journal of Religion and Health*, *The Journal of Pastoral Care and Counseling*). Issues of *Psycho-Oncology* have been devoted to spiritual and religious aspects of psychosocial oncology (Russak et al., 1999) and the chaplain's experience in a cancer center (Flannelly et al., 2003).

Continuing Education Programs for Psychosocial Care Providers

A common source of continuing education for the multidisciplinary psychosocial providers described in this section is an online core curriculum in psychosocial oncology developed by APOS (APOS, 2005b). Lectures, accompanied by slides and a bibliography, are given by experts on topics

[15]Therapists have master's or doctoral degrees or other clinical post-graduate training. Certified marriage and family therapists can be located through the American Association for Marriage and Family Therapy on the web (AAMFT, 2005).

[16]Sexuality counselors, accredited by the American Association of Sex Educators, Counselors, and Therapists (AASECT), can be located through the Association (AASECT, 2004).

BOX 5-6
The American Psychosocial Oncology Society Online Education Program: Survivorship

Symptom Detection and Management
- Delirium
- Depression and Suicide
- Central Nervous System Effects of Drugs Used in Cancer Treatment
- Distress Management in Cancer: Standards and Clinical Practice Guidelines
- Cancer-Related Fatigue
- Substance Abuse in the Oncology Setting
- Anxiety and Adjustment Disorders
- Psychosocial Screening Goes Mainstream: A Prospective Problem-Solving System

Interventions
- Online Support Groups for Women with Breast Cancer: A Pilot Study of Effectiveness
- Maximizing Psychosocial Health & Making a Therapeutic Connection: Counseling Cancer Patients and Their Caregivers
- Cognitive and Behavioral Strategies for Cancer Patients
- Psychiatric Emergencies in the Oncology Setting

Population-Specific Issues
- Cancer Survivorship: Psychosocial Issues

Program Administration
- Establishing a Psychosocial Program: Challenges and Strategies

Introduction to Oncology
- Oncology for Psycho-Oncologists

SOURCE: APOS (2005b).

including survivorship (Box 5-6). The course provides a core of knowledge about psychosocial oncology that is relevant to many disciplines.

Professionals who complete the curriculum and examination are added to the APOS Referral Directory that will serve as a national registry of psychosocial oncologists. Founded in 1986, APOS is attempting to network all disciplines that provide psychosocial services to patients with cancer. Its goal is to become a nationally recognized organization that advocates for improvement of psychosocial care for these patients and their families. APOS also offers continuing education through its annual meetings. In addition to this opportunity available through APOS, continuing education opportunities in psycho-oncology are provided by several professional organizations: International Psycho-Oncology Society, Academy of Psychosomatic Medicine, Society of Behavioral Medicine, American Psychological Association, and American Psychiatric Association.

A textbook in psycho-oncology has provided comprehensive reviews of relevance to cancer survivorship (Holland and Rowland, 1989; Holland, 1998), and the journals *Psycho-Oncology* and *Psychosocial Oncology* provide relevant reviews of research of clinical relevance.

Clinical practice guidelines and standards have been developed by the NCCN to assist health care providers in the management of psychosocial distress among patients and families with cancer (see Chapter 3) (NCCN, 2004a).

Genetic Counseling

As knowledge of the genetic basis for some cancers has expanded and tests for genetic susceptibility to cancer have become available, genetic counseling and testing have become more important to cancer survivors and their families (see Chapter 4, Appendix D). In some cases, genetic services are provided directly by doctors or nurses, but patients are often referred to genetic counselors, master's-level trained professionals with expertise in medical genetics and counseling.[17] They provide risk assessment, help patients weigh the risks and benefits of genetic testing, interpret results of genetic tests, and review prevention, screening, and treatment options (NSGC, 2004). Genetic counselors also provide supportive counseling and refer patients to appropriate support services.

The National Society of Genetic Counselors regularly provides continuing education opportunities to members, including an annual meeting. The American College of Medical Genetics annual meeting also includes sessions of interest to cancer genetic counselors, as well as other medical professionals who are involved in genetic risk assessment or refer patients for genetic counseling. Continuing education in genetics is also available for oncology nurses and other health professionals who do cancer risk assessment and counseling, such as the "Advance Nurses' Training Course in Cancer Risk Counseling" developed at the Fox Chase Cancer Center with NCI support (NCI, 2005a). The *Journal of Genetic Counseling* and the journal *Genetics in Medicine* both publish articles relevant to the practice of cancer genetic counseling. Both ASCO and the NCCN have published guidelines on genetic testing, and several NCI PDQ publications address the genetics of breast, colorectal, prostate, and thyroid cancers (NCCN, 2004b; ASCO, 2005b; NCI, 2005d).

---

[17]There are 27 master's programs in genetic counseling in the United States and 3 in Canada that are accredited by the American Board of Genetic Counseling (ABGC) (ABGC, 2004a). Instruction in cancer genetics is required for accreditation, and many genetic counseling students have rotations in cancer genetics clinics (ABGC, 2004b).

SUPPORT FOR SURVIVORSHIP EDUCATION AND TRAINING PROGRAMS

Relatively few professionals are trained specifically to care for cancer survivors. It is therefore imperative that education and training programs be established to improve the cancer care workforce's ability to provide such care. Support for training professionals in survivorship is available from the NCI and from a few private voluntary organizations.

Federal

National Cancer Institute

NCI offers a number of training, career development, and education opportunties. The Cancer Education Grant Program (R25), for example, provides support to develop and sustain innovative educational approaches (NCI, 2005e). The program is flexible and can support short courses, the development of new curricula in academic institutions, national forums and seminar series, and hands-on workshop experiences for the continuing education of health care professionals, biomedical researchers, and the lay community. This funding mechanism is well suited to the education and training needs in the area of survivorship. For example, an NCI R25 grant is supporting the development of undergraduate medical school curricula in cancer survivorship as described above. Other recent R25 grants of relevance to cancer survivorship include those related to cancer genetics training for nurses and physicians, and cancer nursing training, including training that targets minority nurses and nurses working with minority groups (Box 5-7). Grants may not exceed $300,000 in direct costs for any single year. A plan for how the proposed education program will be evaluated is required.

SBIR grants are also available through NCI to support educational programs. For example, the online module on cancer survivorship described earlier is being developed by the program called POEP in Texas and is being supported through an SBIR grant.

Support for an individual's career development is also available through NCI. A variety of K grants are available to support scientists at all stages of their careers, from mentored researchers to senior scientists (NIH, 2005). These grants can be used by physicians, nurses, and other scientists to train for a career in survivorship research, or to support established survivorship researchers.

BOX 5-7
Examples of National Institutes of Health Program Education Grants Related to Cancer Survivorship

- Oncology Nursing PhD Using Distance Education Technology (R25-CA938313): To expand the scientific base for cancer prevention and control, including survivorship, by implementing and evaluating an innovative approach to preparing PhD oncology nurse scientists utilizing distance learning technology.

- Cancer as a Chronic Disease: Curriculum for Survivorship (R25-CA969753): Develop, implement, evaluate, and disseminate a coordinated 4-year multidisciplinary medical school curriculum on cancer as a chronic disease.

- Native American Cancer Education for Survivors (NACES) (R25-CA1019381): Implement and evaluate a culturally relevant quality-of-life education intervention designed to improve the lives of Native American breast cancer survivors.

- Essential Clinical Cancer Genetics Internet Curriculum (R25-CA092357): To produce a unique electronic-based cancer genetics medical school curriculum to help train students in medicine, nursing, genetic counseling, genetics and other related fields.

- Graduate Education in Oncology Nursing for Minorities (R25-CA056689): To provide training in advanced practice oncology nursing for minority students; expand clinical sites that provide students with opportunities to care for African-Americans, Hispanic, and Asian populations; and facilitate opportunities to mentor minority advanced practice oncology nurses after graduation.

SOURCE: NCI (2005b).

Private

American Cancer Society

The ACS provides several kinds of support for professional education and training for physicians, social workers, and nurses (Table 5-3). Although they are not specific to survivorship, all of the programs could enhance knowledge and skills related to survivorship. ACS also offers a number of fellowships that allow social workers to gain experience in palliative and end-of-life care.

Lance Armstrong Foundation

The Lance Armstrong Foundation supports a number of professional education programs (Table 5-4).

TABLE 5-3 Selected ACS Professional Education and Training Programs

Professional Group	Kind of Award	Amount of Award
Primary care physicians	Cancer Control Career Development Award	Awards are made for 3 years with progressive stipends of $50,000, $55,000, and $60,000 per year.
Social work	Doctoral Training Grant in Clinical Oncology Social Work	Awards are for up to 3 years with annual funding of $20,000 (trainee stipend of $15,000, and $5,000 for faculty/administrative support).
	Master's Training Grants in Clinical Oncology Social Work	Awarded to institutions to support the training of second-year master's-degree students to provide psychosocial services to persons with cancer and their families. The 1-year awards are for $12,000 (trainee stipend of $10,000, and $2,000 for faculty/administrative support).
Nurses	Doctoral Degree Scholarships in Cancer Nursing	Awarded to graduate students pursuing doctoral studies in the fields of cancer nursing research, education, administration, or clinical practice. Awards are for up to 4 years, with a stipend of $15,000 per year.
	Master's Degree Scholarships in Cancer Nursing	Awarded to graduate students pursuing master's degrees in cancer nursing. Awards are $10,000 annually for up to 2 years.

SOURCE: ACS (2005).

Susan G. Komen Breast Cancer Foundation

The Komen Foundation established a Professor of Survivorship Award in 1999 to advance research and awareness on the issues surrounding long-term survivorship of breast cancer. An award of $20,000 is made to two recipients a year (Komen Foundation, 2005).

TABLE 5-4 Professional Education Programs Supported by the Lance Armstrong Foundation

Project	Description
Cancer Survivorship Education Initiative for Texas Nurses, Nurse Oncology Education Program of the Texas Nurses Foundation (www.noeptexas.org)	The initiative, also funded by the Texas Cancer Council, aims to increase awareness among nurses of the unique psychological and physiologic problems faced by cancer survivors and to enable them to provide patients with accurate information, resources, and psychological support that will improve their quality of life. The initiative's educational module, which targets the state's practicing nurses and student nurses, includes a printed booklet, a PowerPoint presentation on CD (for use in presentations to nursing students or health professional groups), an audio CD, and a web-based independent study module. Four thousand Texas nurses will receive the booklet or audio CD, while additional nursing school faculty members will receive the booklet for presentation to nursing students.
Survivorship Professional Education Program, The Leukemia and Lymphoma Society (LLS) (www.lls.org)	The LLS, with the help of a 2003 LAF community grant, established the Survivorship Professional Education Program for oncology nurses and social workers who focus specifically on survivorship issues. The program educates participants on mind-body healing and integrative medicine options for patients during and beyond the treatment portion of their journey as cancer survivors.

SOURCE: LAF (2005).

The International Psycho-Oncology Society

The International Psycho-Oncology Society provides information about fellowship opportunities to social workers and others (IPOS, 2005) in addition to the information available from APOS (APOS, 2005a).

FINDINGS AND RECOMMENDATIONS

Few cancer care and primary care health professionals have had formal education and training regarding cancer survivorship. Needed are efforts to update: (1) undergraduate curricula for those in training; and (2) continuing education for practicing providers of survivorship care. Continuing education is needed across many disciplines, but in order to ensure the provision of quality survivorship care, it is especially important to reach (1) oncologists, hematologists, urologists, surgeons, and radiologists who initially treat cancer patients; (2) primary care physicians; (3) nurses; and (4) social workers and other providers of psychosocial services. To ensure the provision of comprehensive survivorship care, it is likely that additional health personnel will be needed, particularly nurses with advanced oncology training.

Many methods are being used to provide continuing education in survivorship (Table 5-5). Online resources are increasingly available and appear to be an attractive means of reaching many providers, but the effectiveness of this and other approaches need to be assessed. There appear to be few educational programs aimed at multiple provider audiences (e.g., APOS psycho-oncology online course), but it is likely that survivorship continuing education would lend itself to such an approach. The American Association

TABLE 5-5 Methods of Survivorship Continuing Education

Educational Approach	Example
1. Meeting on survivorship	• NCI/ACS cancer survivorship biennial conference
2. Session on survivorship at professional society meeting	• ASCO 2005 annual meeting session: Cancer Survivorship: Long-Term Complications of Treatment • SGO 2005 annual meeting session: Barriers to Sexual Health After Cancer: What Can Be Done?
3. Home study guides	• AAFP home study self-assessment cancer survivor monograph • American Academy of Physical Medicine and Rehabilitation self-directed study guides and examinations are published annually as a Medical Education Supplement to the *Archives of Physical Medicine and Rehabilitation*
4. Problem-based learning cases	• ACP online clinical problem-solving case on cancer follow-up
5. Online course directed to one specialty	• AOSW/CancerCare course, *Understanding Cancer: The Social Worker's Role*
6. Online course directed to multiple specialties	• APOS psycho-oncology course
7. Online repository of information, guidelines	• NCI's Physician Data Query summaries on supportive care, genetics services, and complementary and alternative medicine • AHRQ guideline clearinghouse

for Cancer Education (AACE) could play an important role. AACE is a multidisciplinary group that has included survivorship education in its annual meeting (AACE, 2005).

Limited support is available through public and private sources for survivorship-related education and training.

Recommendation 7: The National Cancer Institute (NCI), professional associations, and voluntary organizations should expand and coordinate their efforts to provide educational opportunities to health care providers to equip them to address the health care and quality of life issues facing cancer survivors.

Immediate steps to facilitate the development of programs include:

- Establish a clearinghouse of available sources of survivorship education and training (and guidelines), with opportunity for feedback.
- Appoint an interdisciplinary consortium to review available resources, identify promising approaches, develop new programs, and promote cost-effective approaches.
- Increase support of model formal training programs (undergraduate and graduate levels, continuing medical education) that could be adopted by others.

By specialty:

Physicians

1. Add more survivorship-related CME:
    - The American Board of Medical Specialties' new program, "Maintenance of Certification," will require continuous assurance of professional skills for board-certified physicians. The development of a module on cancer survivorship as part of this program could facilitate the assurance of competence for these and other specialty providers.
2. Improve online survivorship information aimed at health care providers:
    - Expand PDQ to include more information on survivorship care.
    - Centralize survivorship guidelines online.
    - Encourage the development and adoption of evidence-based guidelines.
    - Ease finding survivorship-related guidelines included in the Agency for Healthcare Research and Quality (AHRQ) sponsored guideline clearinghouse (e.g., add the term "survivorship" to the search engine to pick up surveillance guidelines for cancer).

3. Expand training opportunities to promote interdisciplinary, shared care.

Nurses

1. Increase survivorship content in undergraduate and graduate nursing programs.
2. Expand continuing education opportunities on survivorship for practicing nurses.
3. Increase the number of nursing schools that provide graduate training in oncology.
4. Increase the number of nurses who seek certification in oncology (incentives are needed).
5. Endorse activities of those working to ease the nursing shortage.

Social workers and other providers of psychosocial services

1. Support efforts of APOS to standardize and promote continuing education.
2. Endorse activities of those working to maintain social services in cancer programs.

It is important to verify the effectiveness of education programs because they may not always have the desired effect on practice. One such effort dealt withthe provision of survivorship care to residents in rural areas, which can be problematic, especially if they live far away from providers of cancer treatment. In an effort to improve the cancer care provided to rural residents in Minnesota, Michigan, and Wisconsin, investigators tested multimodal, multidisciplinary set of interventions among 18 communities randomized to be in either an intervention or control group (Elliott et al., 2001a,b, 2002, 2004). Among the study's interventions were efforts to involve community-based opinion leaders (physicians, nurses, and pharmacists), targeted education, quality improvement activities in rural hospitals and clinics, telecommunications via fax machines, clinical practice guidelines, and outreach oncology consultations. The interventions led to improvements in knowledge, but did not change practices, including appropriate post-treatment surveillance. Travel to health care was significantly reduced in the intervention communities, but there were no significant differences in satisfaction with care, economic barriers to care, or health-related quality of life.

REFERENCES

AACE (American Association of Cancer Education). 2005. *American Association of Cancer Education homepage*. [Online]. Available: http://www.aaceonline.com/index.asp [accessed July 27, 2005].

AAFP (American Academy of Family Physicians). 2005. *Facts About AAFP*. [Online] Available: http://www.aafp.org/x7637.xml [accessed August 12, 2005].

AAMC (Association of American Medical Colleges). 2005a. *Curriculum Management and Information Tool (CurrMIT)*. [Online]. Available: http://www.aamc.org/currmit [accessed January 21, 2005].

AAMC. 2005b. *MedEd Portal*. [Online]. Available: http://www.aamc.org/meded/mededportal/ [accessed April 25, 2005].

AAMFT (American Association for Marriage and Family Therapy). 2005. *TherapistLocator.net*. [Online]. Available: http://www.therapistlocator.net/ [accessed April 25, 2005].

AAPM&R (American Academy of Physical Medicine and Rehabilitation). 2005. *AAPM&R Self-Directed Physiatric Education Program*. [Online]. Available: http://www.aapmr.org/education/studygd.htm [accessed January 25, 2005].

AASECT (American Association of Sex Educators, Counselors and Therapists). 2004. *AASECT homepage*. [Online]. Available: http://www.aasect.org/ [accessed January 25, 2005].

ABGC (American Board of Genetic Counseling). 2003. *General Information*. [Online]. Available: http://www.abgc.net/genetics/abgc/about/intro.shtml [accessed May 17, 2005].

ABGC. 2004a. *Genetic Counseling Training Programs Accredited by the ABGC*. [Online]. Available: http://www.abgc.net/genetics/abgc/accred/tr-prog1.shtml [accessed December 13, 2004].

ABGC. 2004b. *Required Criteria for Graduate Programs in Genetic Counseling Seeking Accreditation by the American Board of Genetic Counseling*. [Online]. Available: http://www.abgc.net/genetics/abgc/accred/acc-03/2004_Required_AC_Criteria.pdf [accessed December 13, 2004].

ABIM (American Board of Internal Medicine). 2005. *Number of Diplomates*. [Online]. Available: http://www.abim.org/resources/dnum.shtm [accessed July 22, 2005].

ABMS (American Board of Medical Specialties). 2004a. *2004 Annual Report & Reference Handbook*. Evanston, IL: ABMS.

ABMS. 2004b. *Maintenance of Certification (MOC)*. [Online]. Available: http://www.abms.org/MOC.asp [accessed January 18, 2005].

ACP (American College of Physicians). 2005a. *About the American College of Physicians*. [Online]. Available: http://www.acponline.org/college/aboutacp/aboutacp.htm?hp [accessed June 21, 2005].

ACP. 2005b. *Clinical Problem Solving Cases*. [Online]. Available: http://cpsc.acponline.org/?in [accessed January 27, 2005].

ACS (American Cancer Society). 2005. *Index of Grants*. [Online]. Available: http://www.cancer.org/docroot/RES/RES_5_1.asp?sitearea=RES [accessed February 4, 2005].

AHRQ (Agency for Healthcare Research and Quality). 2004. *National Guideline Clearinghouse*. [Online]. Available: http://www.guideline.gov [accessed December 6, 2004].

Alter C. 2005 (January 27–29). *ICAN: The Individual Cancer Assistance Network*. Presentation at the Second Annual Meeting of the American Psychosocial Oncology Society, Phoenix, AZ.

American Society of Breast Surgeons. 2005. *American Society of Breast Surgeons homepage*. [Online]. Available: http://www.breastsurgeons.org [accessed January 12, 2005].

AOSW (Association of Oncology Social Work). 2004. *AOSW homepage*. [Online]. Available: http://www.aosw.org [accessed January 11, 2005].

AOSW. 2005. *Oncology Social Work Toolbox Scope of Practice in Oncology Social Work.* [Online]. Available: http://www.aosw.org/mission/scope.html [accessed January 11, 2005].

AOTA (American Occupational Therapy Assocation). 2005. *About AOTA.* [Online]. Available: http://www.aota.org/general/about.asp [accessed January 12, 2005].

APA (American Psychological Association). 2005. *Convention 2005.* [Online]. Available: https://cyberstore.apa.org/ceworkshops/index.cfm?action=keysearch [accessed April 22, 2005].

APOS (American Psychosocial Oncology Society). 2005a. *Fellowships in Psychosocial Oncology.* [Online]. Available: http://www.apos-society.org/professionals/career/fellowships.aspx [accessed January 11, 2005].

APOS. 2005b. *Webcasts—Online Continuing Education.* [Online]. Available: http://www.apos-society.org/professionals/meetings-ed/webcasts.aspx [accessed January 24, 2005].

APTA (American Physical Therapy Association). 2001. *Guide to Physical Therapist Practice.* 2nd ed. *Phys Ther* 81(1):9–746.

APTA. 2005a. *Number of PT and PTA Education Programs.* [Online]. Available: http://www.apta.org/Education/educatorinfo/program_numbers [accessed April 21, 2005].

APTA. 2005b. *Online Audio/Video Course Descriptions and Fees.* [Online]. Available: http://www.apta.org/Education/Continuing_Education/Online_AV_Courses/descripts_fees [accessed February 15, 2005].

ASCO (American Society of Clinical Oncology). 2004. *ASCO Announces New Task Force to Address Needs of Cancer Survivors.* [Online]. Available: http://www.asco.org/ac/1,1003,_12-002112-00_18-0036990,00.asp [accessed January 11, 2005].

ASCO. 2005a. *ASCO Publishes Updated Core Curriculum Online.* [Online]. Available: http://www.asco.org/ac/1,1003,_12-002144-00_18-0038375,00.asp [accessed February 28, 2005].

ASCO. 2005b. *Clinical Practice Guidelines.* [Online]. Available: http://www.asco.org/ac/1,1003,_12-002130-00_18-0010732,00.asp [accessed January 18, 2005].

ASCO. 2005c. *Online Pocket Program.* [Online]. Available: http://www.asco.org/ac/1,1003,_12-002553-00_18-0027976,00.asp. [accessed July 8, 2005].

ASCO. 2005d. *ASCO Curriculum Series.* [Online]. Available: http://www.asco.org/ac/1,1003,_12-002258-00_18-0026044-00_19-0026048-00_20-001,00.asp. [accessed July 12, 2005].

ASCO, AAMC to assess clinical oncology workforce. 2005. *The Cancer Letter* 31(17):5–6.

ASCRS (American Society of Colon and Rectal Surgeons). 2005. *About ASCRS.* [Online]. Available: http://www.fascrs.org/displaycommon.cfm?an=1 [accessed June 21, 2005].

ASHA (American Speech-Language-Hearing Association). 2005a. *Facts about Oral Cancer.* [Online]. Available: http://www.asha.org/public/speech/disorders/Facts-about-Oral-Cancer.htm [accessed April 28, 2005].

ASHA. 2005b. *Swallowing Problems After Head and Neck Cancer.* [Online]. Available: http://www.asha.org/public/speech/disorders/swallowing_probs.htm [accessed April 28, 2005].

ASTRO (American Society for Therapeutic Radiology and Oncology). 2002. *2002 Radiation Oncology Workforce Study.* Chicago, IL: Leever Research Services.

ASTRO. 2004. *Targeting Cancer Care.* Fairfax, VA: ASTRO.

AUA (American Urological Association). 2005. *Member Profile.* [Online]. Available: http://www.auanet.org/about/content/membersprofile.pdf [accessed April 14, 2005].

Augustine E, Corn M, Danoff J. 1998. Lymphedema management training for physical therapy students in the United States. *Cancer* 83(12 Suppl American):2869–2873.

Aziz N. 2002. Long-term survivorship: Late effects. 2nd ed. In: Berger AM, Portenoy RK, Weissman DE, eds. *Principles & Practice of Palliative Care and Supportive Oncology.* Philadelphia, PA: Lippincott Williams & Wilkins. Pp. 1019–1033.

Berger AM, Portenoy RK, Weissman DE, eds. 2002. *Principle and Practice of Palliative Care and Supportive Oncology.* 2nd ed. Philadelphia, PA: Lippincott Williams & Wilkins.

BLS (Bureau of Labor Statistics, U.S. Department of Labor). 2004a. *Occupational Employment and Wages, November 2003.* [Online]. Available: http://stats.bls.gov/oes/current/oes211022.htm [accessed January 11, 2005].

BLS. 2004b. *Occupational Outlook Handbook, 2004–05 Edition, Physical Therapists.* [Online]. Available: http://www.bls.gov/oco/ocos080.htm [accessed January 12, 2005].

BLS. 2004c. *Occupational Outlook Handbook, 2004–2005 Edition, Speech-Language Pathologists.* [Online]. Available: http://www.bls.gov/oco/ocos099.htm [accessed April 28, 2005].

Buerhaus P, Donelan K, DesRoches C, Lamkin L, Mallory G. 2001. State of the oncology nursing workforce: Problems and implications for strengthening the future. *Nursing Economics* 19:198–208.

Ciolek DE, Hwang W. 2004. *Outpatient Rehabilitation Services Payment System Evaluation: Final Project Report.* Columbia, MD: AdvanceMed, prepared for the Centers for Medicare and Medicaid Services.

COT (College of Occupational Therapists, The Specialist Section of Occupational Therapists in HIV/AIDS, Oncology, Palliative Care and Education). 2001. *Occupational Therapy Intervention in Cancer: Guidance for Professionals, Managers and Decision-Makers.* London, England: COT.

Doll DC, Shahab N, Wooldridge JE, eds. 2003. *Seminars in Oncology* 30(3). New York: W.B. Saunders.

Elliott TE, Elliott BA, Regal RR, Renier CM, Crouse BJ, Gangeness DE, Witrak MT, Jensen PB. 2001a. Lake Superior Rural Cancer Care Project, Part II: Provider knowledge. *Cancer Pract* 9(1):37–46.

Elliott TE, Elliott BA, Regal RR, Renier CM, Crouse BJ, Gangeness DE, Witrak MT, Jensen PB. 2001b. Lake Superior Rural Cancer Care Project, Part I: An interventional trial. *Cancer Pract* 9(1):27–36.

Elliott TE, Elliott BA, Regal RR, Renier CM, Haller IV, Crouse BJ, Witrak MT, Jensen PB. 2002. Lake Superior Rural Cancer Care Project, Part III: Provider practice. *Cancer Pract* 10(2):75–84.

Elliott TE, Elliott BA, Regal RR, Renier CM, Haller IV, Crouse BJ, Witrak MT, Jensen PB. 2004. Improving rural cancer patients' outcomes: A group-randomized trial. *J Rural Health* 20(1):26–35.

Emory University. 2004. *Ovarian Cancer Survivors Share Their Experiences With Medical Students.* [Online]. Available: http://whsc.emory.edu/press_releases2.cfm?announcement_id_seq=740. (accessed July 15, 2005).

Erikson J. 2000. The nursing shortage: What does it mean for oncology? *Oncology Times* 22(11):1, 38.

FACET. 2004. *Forum for Applied Cancer Education and Training.* [Online]. Available: http://www.blackwellpublishing.com/facet/default.asp?File=jul04 [accessed January 25, 2005].

Ferrell BR, Grant M, Barneman T, Juarez G, Virani R. 2002. Strategies for effective continuing education by oncology nurses. *Oncol Nurs Forum* 29(6):907–909.

Ferrell BR, Virani R, Smith S, Juarez G. 2003. The role of oncology nursing to ensure quality care for cancer survivors: A report commissioned by the National Cancer Policy Board and Institute of Medicine. *Oncol Nurs Forum* 30(1):E1–E11.

Flannelly KJ, Weaver AJ, Handzo GF. 2003. A three-year study of chaplains' professional activities at Memorial Sloan-Kettering Cancer Center in New York City. *Psychooncology* 12(8):760–768.

Hamblin JE, Schifeling DJ. 2001. *Cancer Survivors.* Monograph, Ed. No. 264, Home Study Self-Assessment Program. Leawood, KS: American Academy of Family Physicians.

Harris JR, Lippman ME, Morrow M, Osborne CK, eds. 2004. *Diseases of the Breast.* 3rd ed. New York: Lippincott, Williams & Wilkins.

HEAL. 2005. *HEAL National Digital Library.* [Online]. Available: http://www.healcentral.org/ [accessed July 15, 2005].

Hewitt M, Rowland JH, Yancik R. 2003. Cancer survivors in the United States: Age, health, and disability. *J Gerontol A Biol Sci Med Sci* 58(1):82–91.

Holland JC. 1998. *Psycho-Oncology.* New York: Oxford University Press.

Holland JC, Rowland J. 1989. *Handbook of Psychooncology: Psychological Care of the Patient with Cancer.* New York: Oxford University Press.

IASWR (Institute for the Advancement of Social Work Research). 2003. *Social Work's Contribution to Research on Cancer Prevention, Detection, Diagnosis, Treatment and Survivorship.* Washington, DC: IASWR.

IPOS (International Psycho-Oncology Society). 2005. *Fellowships.* [Online]. Available: http://www.ipos-society.org/professionals/career/fellowships.htm [accessed January 11, 2005].

Johnson FE, Virgo KS. 1997. *Cancer Patient Follow-Up.* St. Louis, MO: Mosby.

Journal of Cancer Education. 2004. Supplement to 19(4). Mahwah, NJ: Lawrence Earlbaum Associates.

Kennedy BJ. 1994. Future manpower needs in caring for an older cancer-patient population. *J Cancer Educ* 9(1):11–13.

Komen Foundation. 2005. *Professor of Survivorship Award.* [Online]. Available: http://www.komen.org/stellent/groups/public/@dallas/documents/-komen_site_documents/pos2005pdf.pdf [accessed February 3, 2005].

LAF (Lance Armstrong Foundation). 2005. *Survivorship Education or Support.* [Online]. Available: http://www.laf.org/Public_Health/Community_Program/2003_Participants.cfm#2 [accessed January 24, 2005].

Lamkin L, Rosiak J, Buerhaus P, Mallory G, Williams M. 2001. Oncology Nursing Society Workforce Survey. Part I: Perceptions of the nursing workforce environment and adequacy of nurse staffing in outpatient and inpatient oncology settings. *Oncol Nurs Forum* 28(10):1545–1552.

Lamkin L, Rosiak J, Buerhaus P, Mallory G, Williams M. 2002. Oncology Nursing Society Workforce Survey. Part II: Perceptions of the nursing workforce environment and adequacy of nurse staffing in outpatient and inpatient oncology settings. *Oncol Nurs Forum* 29(1):93–100.

Lauria MM, Clark EJ, Hermann JF, Stearns NM. 2001. *Social Work in Oncology: Supporting Survivors, Families, and Caregivers.* Atlanta, GA: American Cancer Society.

Leigh SA, Clark EJ. 2002. Psychosocial aspects of cancer survivorship. In: Berger AM, Portenoy RK, and Weissman DE, eds. *Principles & Practice of Palliative Care and Supportive Oncology.* 2nd ed. Philadelphia, PA: Lippincott Williams & Wilkins. Pp. 1034–1041.

Mason DJ, Burke KG. 2005 (April 28). American Journal of Nursing, University of Pennsylvania School of Nursing Letter to Maria Hewitt.

McCorkle R, Frank-Stromborg M, Pasacreta JV. 1998. Education of nurses in psycho-oncology. In: Holland JC, ed. *Psycho-Oncology.* New York, NY: Oxford University Press. Pp. 1069–1073.

Mellette SJ, Blunk KL. 1994. Cancer rehabilitation. *Semin Oncol* 21(6):779–782.

Meraviglia MG, McGuire C, Chesley DA. 2003. Nurses' needs for education on cancer and end-of-life care. *J Contin Educ Nurs* 34(3):122–127.

Mooney KH. 2000. Oncology nursing education: Peril and opportunities in the new century. *Semin Oncol Nurs* 16(1):25–34.

Muss HB, Von Roenn J, Damon LE, Deangelis LM, Flaherty LE, Harari PM, Kelly K, Kosty MP, Loscalzo MJ, Mennel R, Mitchell BS, Mortimer JE, Muggia F, Perez EA, Pisters PW, Saltz L, Schapira L, Sparano J. 2005. ACCO: ASCO core curriculum outline. *J Clin Oncol* 23(9):2049–2077.

NASW (National Association of Social Workers). 2003. *National Cancer Institute Special Project: Barriers of Translating Oncology Research to Social Work Practice.* Washington, DC: NASW.

NASW. 2005a. *About NASW.* [Online]. Available: http://www.socialworkers.org/nasw/default.asp [accessed May 6, 2005].

NASW. 2005b. *Welcome to NASW WebEd.* [Online]. Available: http://www.naswwebed.org/ [accessed January 11, 2005].

NCCN (National Comprehensive Cancer Network). 2004a. *Clinical Practice Guidelines in Oncology-v.1.2004. Distress Management.* [Online]. Available: http://www.nccn.org/physician_gls/f_guidelines.html [accessed 2004].

NCCN. 2004b. *Clinical Practice Guidelines in Oncology-v.1.2004. Genetic/Familial High-Risk Assessment: Breast and Ovarian.* [Online]. Available: http://www.nccn.org/professionals/physician_gls/PDF/genetics_screening.pdf [accessed 2004].

NCCN. 2005. *NCCN Clinical Practice Guidelines in Oncology Table of Contents.* [Online]. Available: http://www.nccn.org/professionals/physician_gls/f_guidelines.asp?button=I+Agree#care [accessed January 18, 2005].

NCI (National Cancer Institute). 1998. *The Cancer Journey: Issues for Survivors. A Training Program for Health Professionals.* Bethesda, MD: NCI.

NCI. 2000. *Your Health Care Team: Your Doctor Is Only the Beginning.* [Online]. Available: http://cis.nci.nih.gov/fact/8_10.htm [accessed January 11, 2005].

NCI. 2005a. *Advanced Cancer Risk Counseling Training for Nurses.* [Online]. Available: http://researchportfolio.cancer.gov/cgi-bin/abstract.pl?SID=324855&ProjectID=73395 [accessed January 14, 2005].

NCI. 2005b. *Cancer Research Portfolio.* [Online]. Available: http://researchportfolio.cancer.gov/ [accessed April 20, 2005].

NCI. 2005c. *PDQ Cancer Information Summaries: Supportive Care.* [Online]. Available: http://www.cancer.gov/cancertopics/pdq/supportivecare [accessed January 18, 2005].

NCI. 2005d. *Physician Data Query (PDQ).* [Online]. Available: http://www.cancer.gov/cancer_information/pdq/ [accessed January 18, 2005].

NCI. 2005e. *R25E Cancer Education Grant Program.* [Online]. Available: http://cancertraining.nci.nih.gov/cancerEd/cancered.html [accessed January 14, 2005].

NCI and ACS (National Cancer Institute and American Cancer Society). 2002 (June 2–4). *Cancer Survivorship: Resilience Across the Lifespan Program and Speaker Abstract Book.* Washington, DC: NCI.

NCI and ACS. 2004 (June 17–18). *Cancer Survivorship: Pathways to Health After Treatment Program Book.* Washington, DC: NCI.

NIH (National Institutes of Health). 2005. *K Kiosk—Information about NIH Career Development Awards.* [Online]. Available: http://grants.nih.gov/training/careerdevelopmentawards.htm [accessed April 20, 2005].

NOEP (Nurse Oncology Education Program). 2005. *NOEP homepage.* [Online]. Available: http://www.noeptexas.org/index.asp [accessed April 18, 2005].

NSGC (National Society of Genetic Counselors). 2004. *FAQs about Genetic Counselors and the NSGC*. [Online]. Available: http://www.nsgc.org/about/faq_about.asp [accessed December 13, 2004].

ONCC (Oncology Nursing Certification Corporation). 2005a. *About ONCC*. [Online]. Available: http://www.oncc.org/about/ [accessed January 18, 2005].

ONCC. 2005b. *Options in Advanced Oncology Nursing Certification: AOCNS—AOCNP—AOCN®*. [Online]. Available: http://www.oncc.org/publications/options.shtml [accessed April 19, 2005].

Oncology Section (APTA). 2005. *Exercise Training Guidelines for Individuals with Cancer: Endurance, Strength, Flexibility & Adherence*. [Online]. Available: http://www.oncologypt.org/nws/index.cfm#2 [accessed February 15, 2005].

ONS (Oncology Nursing Society). 2005. *ONS homepage*. [Online]. Available: http://www.ons.org [accessed April 21, 2005].

Penfold SL. 1996. The role of the occupational therapist in oncology. *Cancer Treat Rev* 22(1):75–81.

Plymale MA, Witzke DB, Sloan PA, Blue AV, Sloan DA. 1999. Cancer survivors as standardized patients: An innovative program integrating cancer survivors into structured clinical teaching. *J Cancer Educ* 14(2):67–71.

POEP (Physician Oncology Education Program). 1999. *Surveillance of Cancer Patients*. Austin, TX: Texas Cancer Council and Texas Medical Association.

R^3 Programs. 2005. *Physical Therapy Treatment for the Breast Cancer Patient*. [Online]. Available: http://www.r3programs.info/ [accessed May 5, 2005].

Ries E. 2004. A matter of survival. *PT Magazine* 12(11). [Online]. Available: http://www.apta.org/AM/Template.cfm?Section=Archives3&CONTENTID=8453&TEMPLATE=/CM/HTMLDisplay.cfm (accessed July 8, 2005).

Roig RL, Worsowicz GM, Stewart DG, Cifu DX. 2004. Geriatric rehabilitation. Physical medicine and rehabilitation interventions for common disabling disorders. *Arch Phys Med Rehabil* 85(7 Suppl 3):S12—S17; quiz S27–S30.

Roswell Park Cancer Institute. 2005. *Pastoral Care Courses*. [Online]. Available: http://www.roswellpark.org/document_2991.html [accessed January 26, 2005].

Rowland JH, Aziz N, Tesauro G, Feuer EJ. 2001. The changing face of cancer survivorship. *Semin Oncol Nurs* 17(4):236–240.

Russak SM, Lederberg M, Fitchett G, eds. 1999. Spiritual and religious beliefs and coping with cancer. *Psycho-Oncology*. 8(5). Hoboken, NJ: John Wiley & Sons.

Satryan MA. 2001. The oncology nursing shortage and its impact on cancer care services. *Oncology Issues* 16(1):21–23.

SGO (Society of Gynecologic Oncologists). 2005. *The Annual Meeting on Women's Cancer Advance Program*. [Online]. Available: http://www.sgo.org/meetings/2005Annual/SGOAdvanceProgram.pdf [accessed January 27, 2005].

Shapiro CL, Winer EP, eds. 2003. *Seminars in Oncology* 30(6). New York: W. B. Saunders.

Smith ED, Walsh-Burke K, Crusan C. 1998. Principles of training social workers in oncology. In: Holland JC, ed. *Psycho-Oncology*. New York: Oxford University Press.

Spratley E, Johnson A, Sochalski J, Fritz M, Spencer W. 2000. *The Registered Nurse Population: Finding From the National Sample Survey of Registered Nurses*. Rockville, MD: Health Resources and Services Administration.

Stuber ML, Guiton G, Wilkerson L. 2003. Cancer as a chronic illness: Competencies for a curriculum for medical students. *Journal of Cancer Education* 18:23.

Stuber ML, Wilkerson L, Go VLW. 2004. Integration of Cancer Survivorship Course Work Into First Year Medical Student Curriculum. Abstract presented at the American Association of Cancer Education Annual Meeting. *J Cancer Educ* 19(3):189–196.

Thaler-DeMers D. 2001. Intimacy issues: Sexuality, fertility, and relationships. *Semin Oncol Nurs* 17(4):255–262.

The HealthCare Chaplaincy. 2005. *The HealthCare Chaplaincy homepage.* [Online]. Available: http://www.healthcarechaplaincy.org/ [accessed February 18, 2005].

Tolley NS. 1994. Oncology social work, family systems theory, and workplace consultations. *Health Soc Work* 19(3):227–230.

UCLA. 2005a. *Cancer Education Projects.* [Online]. Available: http://www.medsch.ucla.edu/public/cancer/default.htm [accessed July 15, 2005].

UCLA. 2005b. *Cancer as a Chronic Disease: Curriculum for Survivorship Required Objectives for Medical School Core Curriculum.* [Online]. Available: http://www.medsch.ucla.edu/public/cancer/survivorship%20objectives.pdf [accessed July 15, 2005).

US Newswire. 2004. *American Society for Therapeutic Radiology and Oncology, American Cancer Society Join to Promote Cancer Survivorship.* [Online]. Available: http://www.highbeam.com/library/doc0.asp?DOCID=1G1:120166101&num=59&ctrlInfo=Round9d%3AProd1%3ASR%3AResult&ao= [accessed January 25, 2005].

VandeCreek L, Burton L, eds. 2001. *Professional Chaplaincy: Its Role and Importance in Healthcare.* New York: The Healthcare Chaplaincy.

Varricchio C, Ades T, Hinds P, Pierce M, Walker C, eds. 2004. *A Cancer Sourcebook for Nurses.* Atlanta, GA: American Cancer Society and Jones and Bartlett Publishers.

Winn R. 2002. *Cancer Survivorship: Professional Education and Training.* Background paper prepared for the National Cancer Policy Board. Unpublished.

6

Employment, Insurance, and Economic Issues

A history of cancer can have a significant impact on employment opportunities and may also affect the ability to obtain and retain health and life insurance. In addition, financial difficulties may arise because cancer survivors' health-related work limitations may necessitate a reduced work schedule. The economic burden of cancer can be compounded by high out-of-pocket expenses for prescription drugs, medical devices and supplies, and expenses related to co-insurance and copayments. These employment, insurance, and economic issues are not necessarily limited to the cancer survivor—they may extend to family members, limiting access to insurance and posing a financial burden. The extent of these socioeconomic problems and current legal remedies to address them are described in this chapter, as are potential programmatic, educational, legislative, and advocacy responses.[1] Selected federal and state programs are described that are relevant to cancer survivors, including the Medicare prescription drug program that will be implemented in 2006; a state Medicaid option available since 2000 to provide poor and uninsured women with coverage for treatment and follow-up of breast and cervical cancer; recent federal investments in state high-risk insurance pools that provide insurance coverage to people who cannot get insurance because of poor health; and federal income replacement programs through the Social Security Administration for individuals too disabled to work.

---

[1]This chapter is based, in part, on a background paper prepared in 2002 by Barbara Hoffman for the National Cancer Policy Board, *Policy Recommendations to Address the Employment and Insurance Concerns of Cancer Survivors.*

EMPLOYMENT

Impact of Cancer on Survivors' Employment Opportunities

There are an estimated 3.8 million working-age adults (ages 20 to 64) with a history of cancer as of 2002, and consequently more cancer survivors are in the workplace now than ever before, (NCI, 2005). The proportion of individuals with a history of cancer rises with age, from 1 percent among individuals ages 40 to 44 to 8 percent among those age 60 to 64 (see Chapter 2). Consequently, many employers have had to address issues related to the reintegration of workers following their treatment and the alteration of work schedules and environment to accommodate any lingering cancer-related impairments.

Most cancer survivors who worked before their diagnosis return to work following their treatment (Spelten et al., 2002). In fact, with the advent of effective interventions to curb the side effects of cancer therapies and an increased reliance on outpatient care, some individuals are able to work throughout their cancer treatment (Messner and Patterson, 2001). Retaining one's employment status has obvious financial benefits and is often also necessary for health insurance coverage, self-esteem, and social support (Voelker, 1999; Spelten et al., 2002). On the other hand, cancer may prompt retirement from an undesirable job or launch a search for a new career that is more satisfying personally, but less lucrative. Work after cancer must therefore be assessed in the context of an individual's priorities and values, rather than exclusively using social or economic metrics (Steiner et al., 2004).

Employers, supervisors, and co-workers may assume that persons with cancer are not able to perform job responsibilities as well as they did before the diagnosis. They may also perceive them as a poor risk for promotion. These misconceptions can lead to subtle or blatant discrimination in the workplace (Messner and Patterson, 2001). Cancer survivors have reported problems in the workplace that include dismissal, failure to hire, demotion, denial of promotion, undesirable transfer, denial of benefits, and hostility (NCCS and Amgen, undated; Fesko, 2001; Hoffman, 2004b). Studies conducted prior to the passage of comprehensive employment discrimination laws suggest that survivors of cancer encountered substantial employment obstacles (Mellette, 1985; Hoffman, 1989, 1991; Bordieri et al., 1990; Brown and Ming, 1992).

Federal and state laws passed in the early 1990s have helped to ease problems related to job discrimination. The most important is the Americans with Disabilities Act (ADA), which protects disabled workers. In addition, the Health Insurance Portability and Accountability Act (HIPAA) and the Consolidated Omnibus Budget Reconciliation Act (COBRA) have helped workers move from one job to another without loss of health insurance. Since the enactment of these laws (and their enforcement), employment practices have improved and employees have gained some protections (Hoffman, 1999). Common accommodations made for those living with illnesses include reduced and flexible schedules. Such flexibility is increasingly common in the workplace to meet the needs of employees with family responsibilities. However, providing flexibility in production or assembly line scheduling can be more difficult for "blue collar" workers (Voelker, 1999). Even with these new protections and improvements in employer practice, contemporary workers may lose employment because of cancer (Box 6-1).

To fully understand the impact of cancer on work outcomes, one would

BOX 6-1
Examples of Cancer-Related Job Loss

Allison Yowell, a seventh-grade teacher in a Virginia public school, was forced from her job when her Hodgkin's disease recurred. Although her prognosis was good, school officials notified her that she must resign, or face firing, because she had used all her sick days. As a recent hire, she was ineligible to request leave without pay. It was recommended that she resign before being terminated to avoid marring her teaching record. She submitted her resignation, but was reinstated only after adverse publicity regarding the case. Ms. Yowell, who wanted 4 months of leave without pay, couldn't take advantage of the federal Family and Medical Leave Act, which grants 12 unpaid weeks per year, because it applies only after an employee has worked a full year.

John Magenheimer, who had headed a research laboratory at a major company, was recovering from surgery, chemotherapy, and radiation treatment for cancer when he learned that his company had fired him and that his health, life, and dental insurance had been terminated. He and 180 other employees of the company who had been placed on long-term disability were fired. Most companies used to pay health benefits for the long-term disabled until they were 65, but as health insurance costs and the number of disabled employees have climbed, more companies are firing them. According to a survey of 723 companies in 2002, 27 percent had a policy to dismiss employees as soon as they went onto long-term disability and 24 percent dismissed them at a set time thereafter, usually 6 to 12 months. Only 15 percent of companies had a policy to keep the disabled on as employees with benefits until age 65. Mr. Magenheimer had the option of continuing his health insurance through a federal law known as COBRA, and as a disabled worker he could purchase Medicare coverage after 18 months. Both kinds of coverage cost thousands of dollars a year, which many disabled workers can ill afford.

SOURCES: Pereira (2003); Laris (2005a,b).

ideally have results from studies that had the following six characteristics (Steiner et al., 2004):

1. Inclusion of cancer survivors that represented the entire population of U.S. cancer survivors. Many studies are based on survivors followed at one cancer center, or who are from particular geographic areas. Their employment experience may not reflect that of the nation. Ideally, survivors would be selected for study from population-based cancer registries.
2. Designed to provide a prospective and longitudinal look at work outcomes so that both short-term and long-term work outcomes could be assessed and the dynamic nature of employment could be understood.
3. Include assessments of work, including information on the type, amount, content, physical demands, cognitive demands, and attitudes about work.
4. Include assessments of the impact of cancer on the economic status of the individual and the family.
5. Identify moderators of work return and work function, particularly those that are susceptible to intervention (e.g., availability of health insurance and disability benefits to offset lost income).
6. Include a cohort of survivors that is sufficiently large to allow multivariate statistical analysis and that provides information on important groups (e.g., minority groups, cancer types).

The committee reviewed the literature published in the past 10 years on the employment experience of U.S. cancer survivors who were studied in 1992, the year the ADA took effect, or later.[2] Most of the studies reviewed had some, but rarely all, of the ideal attributes just described. There are few prospective studies of cancer's effects on employment, but those that are available provide important insights into how interventions could be designed to assist cancer survivors.

In one prospective study, women with invasive breast cancer were less likely to work 6 months following diagnosis relative to a control sample of women. Breast cancer survivors who remained working worked fewer hours than women in the control group (Bradley et al., 2005a). At 12 months, however, many women who had stopped working had returned to work (Bradley, 2004). The nonemployment effect of breast cancer diagnosis and treatment at 6 months was twice as large for African-American women. Similar findings were evident among men with prostate cancer. Here, 28

[2]Studies of the experience of cancer survivors from other countries are excluded because differences in employment benefits and policies likely affect return-to-work behaviors.

percent of men were not employed 6 months following diagnosis but, at 12 and 18 months, survivors' employment was statistically not different from controls (Bradley, 2004). At 12 months, 26 percent of men with prostate cancer reported that cancer interfered with their ability to perform tasks that involved physical effort (Bradley et al., 2005b). Up to 16 percent of men said that they noticed changes in their ability to perform cognitive tasks (e.g., concentrate, keep up with others, learn new things). The implication of these findings is that interventions to assist survivors who stop working (e.g., income replacement programs, information about access to health insurance) are needed within 6 months of diagnosis. Workplace reintegration programs may be most needed through the year following diagnosis.

Nearly one out of five cancer survivors reported cancer-related limitations in ability to work when interviewed 1 to 5 years following their diagnosis as part of one of the largest cross-sectional studies to date (Short et al., 2005b). Nine percent were unable to work at all. Labor force participation dropped by 12 percentage points from diagnosis to follow-up and about two-thirds of survivors who quit working attributed the change to cancer. Other studies have found the drop in employment following cancer to be similar in magnitude. For example, a 10 percentage point greater decline in employment was noted among breast cancer survivors as compared to women without breast cancer (Bradley et al., 2002a,b).

The impact of cancer on employment has not been well studied across all types of cancer. However, work-related outcomes have been shown to be significantly worse for cancers of the central nervous system, hematologic cancers (Short et al., 2005b), and cancer of the head and neck. In one study, 52 percent of survivors of head and neck cancer who had worked before their diagnosis were disabled by their cancer treatment and could no longer work when assessed, on average, more than 4 to 5 years following their diagnosis (Taylor et al., 2004). Nearly three-quarters (74 percent) of survivors considered potentially cured of acute myelogenous leukemia (excluding those receiving allogenic marrow transplants) returned to full-time work according to a long-term follow-up study (median of 9.2 years from first or second complete remission) (de Lima et al., 1997). Less than a third of those who were not working cited physical limitation as the reason.

Other studies of cancer survivors have also shown that most cancer survivors continue to work, but that a minority have limitations that interfere with work. Of those working at the time of their initial diagnosis, 67 percent of survivors of lung, colorectal, breast, or prostate cancer were employed 5 to 7 years later when interviewed in 1999 (Bradley and Bednarek, 2002). Survivors in this study who stopped working did so because they retired (54 percent), were in poor health or disabled (24 percent), quit (4 percent), their business closed (9 percent), or for other reasons

TABLE 6-1 Limitations Imposed by Cancer and Its Treatment on Patients Currently Working

At least some of the time task requires:	Cancer Interfered with Work Performance (percentage)
Physical tasks	18
Lift heavy loads	26
Stoop, kneel, or crouch	14
Concentrate for long periods of time	12
Analyze data	11
Keep pace with others	22
Learn new things	14

SOURCE: Adapted from Bradley and Bednarek (2002).

(9 percent). Many employed survivors worked in excess of 40 hours per week, although some reported various degrees of disability that interfered with job performance. When work required lifting heavy loads, for example, 26 percent of subjects reported that cancer interfered with their performance (Table 6-1).

Other investigators point to the vulnerability of employees with jobs involving manual labor. In one study, type of occupation was the main determinant of whether individuals were employed after diagnosis. Although 76 percent of respondents indicated that they were working at the time of diagnosis and 82 percent said they wanted to work full- or part-time, only 56 percent were working at the time of the study (Rothstein et al., 1995). Laborers were most likely, and professionals least likely, to have some of their job duties reassigned upon their return to work.

Relatively few studies have examined the effect of cancer on income in the context of the family household. In one study that studied such effects, breast cancer survivors who were working at the time of their diagnosis experienced higher rates of functional impairment and significantly larger reductions in annual earnings over the 5-year study period than did working control subjects. These losses arose mostly from reduced work effort, not changes in pay rates. Changes in total household earnings were lower for survivors, suggesting the presence of family adjustments to the disease. However, no significant differences were detected between the groups in changes in total income or assets over the study period (Chirikos, 2001; Chirikos et al., 2002a,b). This study suggests that cancer can have an economic impact on the entire family, requiring compensatory employment behaviors on the part of family members to maintain earnings.

Analyses of national health surveys have provided some information on the effects of cancer on employment. According to analyses of the 2000 National Health Interview Survey (NHIS), cancer survivors were found to have poorer outcomes across all employment-related burden measures relative to matched control subjects (Yabroff et al., 2004). Cancer survivors were less likely than control subjects to have had a job in the past month. Furthermore, they were more likely to be unable to work because of health, more limited in the amount or kind of work because of a health problem, and had more days lost from work in the past year. The decrements in productivity were generally consistent across tumor sites. When analyzed by time since diagnosis, a higher percentage of survivors diagnosed in the past year also reported having jobs than survivors in any of the other time-since-diagnosis intervals. However, this group of survivors also had the most reported work loss days. This analysis included information on cancer survivors of all ages.[3] In an analysis of three years of NHIS data (1998 to 2000) limited to adults ages 18 to 64, nearly one in six individuals (17 percent) with a history of cancer reported that they were unable to work because of a physical, mental, or emotional problem (Hewitt et al., 2003). An additional 7.4 percent of cancer survivors were limited in the kind or amount of work they could do. This level of work limitation exceeded that of working-age individuals without a history of cancer (Figure 6-1). In an attempt to isolate cancer-related effects, investigators compared individuals reporting a history of cancer but no other chronic disease to individuals without a history of cancer or with no other chronic illness. Using multivariate analyses to control for potentially confounding factors (i.e., age, sex, race/ethnicity, educational attainment, health insurance status, and marital status), individuals with cancer but no other chronic disease were found to be three times more likely to be unable to work than individuals without a history of cancer and reporting no chronic illness. The likelihood of work limitation was much higher among cancer survivors who also reported comorbid chronic diseases (i.e., cardiovascular disease, diabetes, emphysema, ulcer, weak/failing kidneys, liver condition). They were 12 times more likely to be unable to work relative to those without cancer or other chronic illnesses.

The NHIS in 1992 included a supplement funded by the National Cancer Institute (NCI) with a section on issues related to cancer survivorship. Individuals who reported a recent history of cancer (within the past 10 years) were asked about changes in health or life insurance coverage and cancer-related problems with employment. Nearly one in five (18.2 percent) individuals who worked immediately before or after their cancer was

[3]Half (51 percent) of the sample were aged 65 and older.

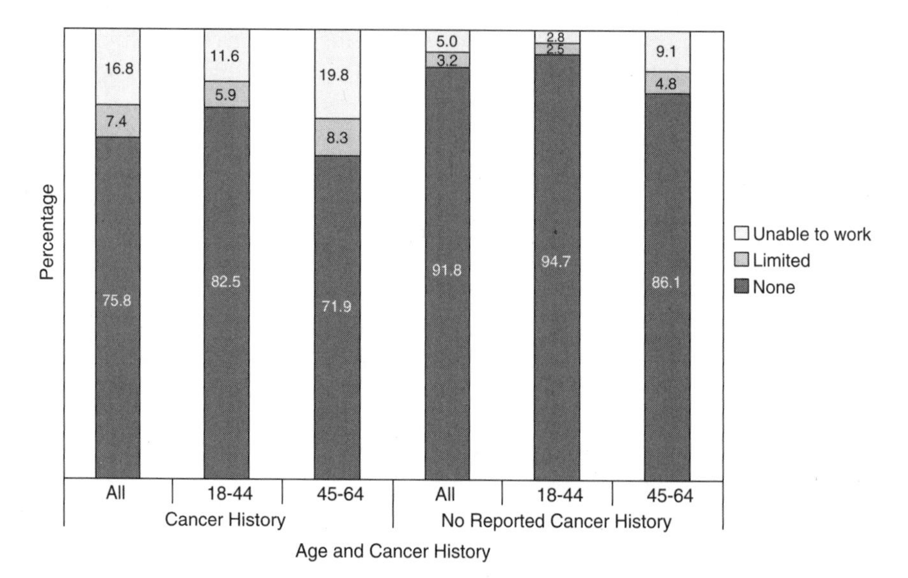

FIGURE 6-1 Work limitations by age and self-reported history of cancer, 1998–2000.
SOURCE: Hewitt et al. (2003).

diagnosed (but who were not self-employed) reported at least one of the following problems (Hewitt et al., 1999):

- Believed they could not take a new job because of a change in insurance related to cancer (13.2 percent).
- Believed they could not change jobs because of cancer (7.8 percent).
- Faced on-the-job problems from an employer or supervisor directly related to their cancer (4.5 percent).
- Refrained from applying for a new job because they did not want their medical records made public (4.4 percent).
- Were fired or laid off from their job because of their cancer (3.7 percent).

Kessler and colleagues, in an analysis of the MacArthur Foundation Midlife Development in the United States (MIDUS) survey, found 88 percent of employed people who develop cancer remain at work after receiving their diagnosis and during at least some part of their treatment (2001). Of all of the conditions examined, cancer had the highest reported prevalence of any 30-day work impairment. Two-thirds (66 percent) of those reporting cancer reported such impairment as compared to 48 percent of those with heart disease and 39 percent of those with arthritis.[4] An analysis of symptoms reported on the survey suggested that fatigue may have accounted for much of the impact of cancer on work impairment.

Whether or not cancer survivors disclose their diagnosis once they return to work has not been well researched. In one study of colorectal cancer patients who had been employed before their diagnosis, most (89 percent) returned to work and, of those returning to work, most disclosed their cancer history to employers (81 percent) and co-workers (85 percent) and did so for personal and work-related reasons (Sanchez and Richardson, 2004). Communication with physicians about work return decisions may have facilitated cancer history disclosure. Such high disclosure rates could be accounted for by the fact that anyone who requests a formal leave of absence from work must disclose their cancer diagnosis. Discussions with physicians about work return decisions should take place *prior* to the initiation of treatment because the acute effects of treatment may affect one's ability to work full time. Some patient's treatment decisions may be influenced by employment considerations.

From an employer's perspective, cancer represents a potential health and productivity burden. In addition to medical costs that may be borne by employers, there are concerns about absenteeism from work, disability program use, workers' compensation program costs, turnover, family medical leave, and on-the-job productivity losses. Consequently, the cost of cancer to employers greatly exceeds the cost of health insurance alone (Lee, 2004). Cancer accounts for about 10 percent of an employer's or insurer's annual medical claim costs, 10 percent of short-term disability claim costs, and 10 percent of long-term disability costs, according to a recent analysis (Pyenson and Zenner, 2002). One study that examined physical and mental health conditions contributing to employer health and productivity cost burden found that cancer ranked relatively low in burden relative to other chronic conditions such as heart conditions, diabetes mellitus, chronic obstructive pulmonary disease, low back disorders, trauma, sinusitis, and renal failure (Goetzel et al., 2003).[5] Other investigators found annual health care and disability costs for persons with cancer to be about five times

[4]Such high levels of impairment could be accounted for by the reporting timeframe—individuals were asked about chronic health conditions that they had experienced or been treated for in the past 12 months. Individuals could therefore have been reporting on their experiences during or shortly after treatment.

[5]These 1999 rankings took into account health care payments, absenteeism, and short-term disability and were based on a multiemployer database that links medical, prescription drug, absence, and short-term disability data.

higher than for their counterparts without cancer (Barnett et al., 2000).[6] Medical conditions not directly related to cancer accounted for about half of the total excess expenditures for patients with cancer. For example, infections, asthma, and dental procedures, although not immediately thought of as being associated with cancer, cost considerably more among cancer patients than controls.

In summary, a number of studies have been conducted to gauge the effect of cancer on employment. However, it is difficult to judge overall effects because these studies have:

- Included individuals with different types of cancer and survival probabilities;
- Assessed employment patterns at different lengths of time following treatment;
- Had relatively low participation rates, with healthier individuals enrolling in studies more readily than less healthy individuals;
- Examined employment at one point in time, possibly obscuring important transitions in and out of work over time;
- Been conducted in different parts of the country with varying employment patterns; and
- Had no control group or used control groups that may not have been well matched to subjects. Without adequate control subjects in such studies, it is difficult to distinguish declines in employment following cancer from those that might be expected for other reasons.

Information from the one prospective study that has been conducted indicates that employment is most affected in the period immediately following treatment, suggesting that programs, policies, and financial assistance are critical at this time. The type of occupation appears to be a key determinant of employment difficulties, with workers whose jobs involve physical labor most adversely affected. In terms of cancer site, cancers of the central nervous system, hematologic cancers, and head and neck cancer seem to be associated with poorer work outcomes. The finding from one of the largest cohort studies, that roughly 20 percent of people working at the time of their diagnosis face cancer-related work limitations 2 to 3 years later, is consistent with results of cross-sectional national survey research. This research suggests that cancer is one of several chronic conditions that markedly increase the likelihood of work-related disability.

[6]The costs of cancer to a major U.S. employer were estimated in an analysis of medical, pharmaceutical, and disability claims data from 1995 to 1997. Investigators found cancer accounting for 6.5 percent of the corporation's total health care cost.

Despite laws allowing portability of health insurance (see section on health insurance below), individuals with a history of cancer report in recent studies of being afraid to change jobs because of concerns about continuation of health insurance. More than 25 percent of cancer survivors in Short and colleagues' recent study expressed such fears (Short et al., 2005a). Most individuals returning to work appear to inform their supervisors and colleagues of their cancer for both personal and work-related reasons. Relatively few (5 percent) cancer survivors faced on-the-job problems from an employer or supervisor directly related to their cancer, according to survey research conducted in the early 1990s. However, at this time, 4 percent of cancer survivors employed before their diagnosis said they were fired or laid off from their jobs because of their cancer.

Population-based, prospective cohort studies with adequate control groups are needed to better understand the effects of cancer on employment and in order to observe transitions in and out of the work force over time following diagnosis. Also needed are studies of work-related outcomes other than employment status alone (e.g., full-time versus part-time, job mobility, limitations in ability to work) and systematic assessments of employment differences among cancer survivors, as well as between cancer survivors and noncancer control groups. Efforts to identify remediable risk factors and interventions to ameliorate the deleterious effects of cancer on employment are also needed. Investigators have proposed a conceptual model of work after cancer and have defined important work outcomes that should be monitored to improve our understanding of the relationships among cancer, quality of life, and work outcomes (Steiner et al., 2004).

Cancer Survivors' Current Employment Rights

Although cancer survivors do not have an unqualified right to obtain and retain employment, they do have the right to freedom from discrimination and to be treated according to their individual abilities. Four federal laws—the ADA, the Family and Medical Leave Act (FMLA), the Employee Retirement and Income Security Act (ERISA), and the Federal Rehabilitation Act—provide cancer survivors with some protection against employment discrimination.

Americans with Disabilities Act

The Americans with Disabilities Act of 1990 prohibits certain employers from discriminating against individuals with disabilities (see Box 6-2). A qualified individual with a disability is protected by the ADA if he or she can perform the essential functions of the job. Under the ADA, a disability is a major health impairment that substantially limits the ability to do

BOX 6-2
The Americans with Disabilities Act (ADA)

What is the ADA?

Title I of the Americans with Disabilities Act of 1990 prohibits private employers, state and local governments, employment agencies, and labor unions from discriminating against qualified individuals with disabilities in job application procedures, hiring, firing, advancement, compensation, job training, and other terms, conditions, and privileges of employment.

Who does the ADA cover?

The ADA covers employers with 15 or more employees, including state and local governments. It also applies to employment agencies and to labor organizations. The ADA's nondiscrimination standards also apply to federal-sector employees.

Who is considered disabled under the ADA?

An individual with a disability is a person who has a physical or mental impairment that substantially limits one or more major life activities; has a record of such an impairment; or is regarded as having such an impairment. A qualified employee or applicant with a disability is an individual who, with or without reasonable accommodation, can perform the essential functions of the job in question. Reasonable accommodation may include, but is not limited to:

- Making existing facilities used by employees readily accessible to and usable by persons with disabilities.
- Restructuring jobs, modifying work schedules, reassigning to a vacant position.
- Acquiring or modifying equipment or devices; adjusting or modifying examinations, training materials, or policies; and providing qualified readers or interpreters.

What is an employer required to do under the ADA?

An employer is required to make a reasonable accommodation to the known disability of a qualified applicant or employee if it would not impose an "undue hardship" on the operation of the employer's business. Undue hardship is defined as an action requiring significant difficulty or expense when considered in light of factors such as an employer's size, financial resources, and the nature and structure of its operation. An employer is not required to lower quality or production standards to make an accommodation, nor is an employer obligated to provide personal-use items such as glasses or hearing aids.

SOURCE: EEOC (2004b).

everyday activities, such as talking, caring for oneself, and getting to work. Some have the misperception that "hidden" disabilities such as cancer, AIDS, arthritis, and mental illness are not bona fide disabilities needing accommodation. The U.S. Department of Labor, however, explicitly states that such hidden disabilities, just like those that are visible, can result in functional limitations that substantially limit one or more of the major life activities (U.S. Department of Labor, 2000).

Cancer survivors, regardless of whether they are in treatment, in remission, or cured, are usually protected as persons with a disability because their cancer represents an impairment that substantially limits a major life activity. Federal courts and the Equal Employment Opportunities Commission (EEOC) usually consider cancer to be a disability under the ADA (Hoffman, 1999). Whether a cancer survivor is covered by the ADA is determined, however, on a case-by-case basis. Because the U.S. Supreme Court has not, to date, squarely addressed whether *all* cancer survivors are protected by the ADA, cancer survivors' rights under the law vary depending on the facts of the individual case and the court in which the case is heard.

Some courts have concluded that cancer survivors are "persons with a disability" as defined by the statute. Other courts, however, have placed cancer survivors in a "Catch-22" by concluding that a cancer survivor who is sufficiently healthy to work is not a person with a disability as defined by the ADA (Hoffman, 2000). In one case a woman with breast cancer was acknowledged to have experienced nausea, fatigue, swelling, inflammation, and pain resulting from her treatment, but the U.S. Court of Appeals for the Fifth Circuit found that she could nonetheless perform her essential job duties with accommodations (Ellison v. Software Spectrum Inc.). Although the Court of Appeals found that the woman's cancer affected her ability to work, it concluded that these limitations were not sufficient to render her a "person with a disability" as defined by the ADA. Other courts have followed the reasoning of the Fifth Circuit and rejected lawsuits by cancer survivors. In another case, a long-term survivor of non-Hodgkin's lymphoma, fired because his employer feared that future health insurance claims would cause his insurance costs to rise, was determined not to be covered under the ADA after his dismissal (Hirsch v. National Mall and Serv., Inc.). The court concluded that "the ADA was not truly meant to apply to this situation" because the claimant was discriminated against due to the costs of his cancer treatment, and not because of the cancer itself" (Hirsch, 989 F. Supp. 977, 980 [N.D. Ill. 1997]).

The ADA prohibits discrimination in most job-related activities such as hiring, firing, and the provision of benefits. In most cases, a prospective employer may not ask applicants if they have ever had cancer. An employer has the right to know only if an applicant is able to perform the essential

BOX 6-3
Examples of Accommodations of Individuals with Cancer

- An engineer working for a large industrial company had to undergo treatment for cancer during working hours. She was provided a flexible schedule in order to attend therapy and also continue to work full-time.
- A machine operator who was undergoing radiation therapy for cancer was accommodated by having his workstation moved. The move transferred the individual to an area of the plant where no radiation exposure existed.
- A warehouse worker whose job involved maintaining and delivering supplies was having difficulty with the physical demands of his job due to fatigue from cancer treatment. The individual was accommodated with a three-wheeled scooter to reduce walking. The warehouse was also rearranged to reduce climbing and reaching.
- A secretary with cancer was having difficulty working full-time due to fatigue. Her employer accommodated her by allowing her to work part-time and allowing her to take frequent rest breaks while working.
- A psychiatric nurse with cancer was experiencing difficulty dealing with job-related stress. He was accommodated with a temporary transfer and was referred to the employer's employee assistance program for emotional support and stress management tools.
- A lawyer with cancer was experiencing lapses in concentration due to the medication she was taking. Her employer accommodated her by giving her uninterrupted time to work. She was also allowed to work at home 2 days a week.

SOURCE: Job Accommodation Network (Loy and Batiste, 2004).

functions of the job. A job offer may be contingent on passing a relevant medical exam, provided that all prospective employees are subject to the same exam. An employer may ask detailed questions about health only after making a job offer.

Cancer survivors who need extra time or help to work are entitled to a "reasonable accommodation." Common accommodations for cancer survivors include changes in work hours or duties to accommodate medical appointments and treatment side effects (Box 6-3). An employer does not have to make changes that would impose an "undue hardship" on the business or other workers. "Undue hardship" refers to any accommodation that would be unduly costly, extensive, substantial, or disruptive, or that would fundamentally alter the nature or operation of the business. For example, an employer may replace a survivor who has to miss an extended period of work (e.g., 6 months or longer) that cannot be performed by a temporary employee.

Some employers express concerns about the costs of accommodations and whether accommodations interfere with typical work schedules and productivity (Roessler and Sumner, 1997). According to some estimates, the costs of accommodations for workers with disabilities needing special accommodations are typically very low; 71 percent of accommodations cost $500 or less, with 20 percent of those costing nothing (U.S. Department of Labor, 2004b).

Most employment discrimination laws protect only the employee. The ADA offers protection more responsive to survivors' needs because it also prohibits discrimination against family members. Employers may not discriminate against workers because of their relationship or association with a "disabled" person. Employers may not assume that an employee's job performance would be affected by the need to care for a family member who has cancer. An important exclusion of the Americans with Disabilities Act is contractual employees. Many people are "self-employed," but contract their services to large organizations that may terminate a survivor's contract without regard to the provisions of the ADA. Also excluded from ADA protection are those working for employers with fewer than 15 employees. Among private employees, an estimated 15 percent work for companies with fewer than 10 employees and an additional 11 percent work for companies with 10 to 19 employees (Bureau of Labor Statistics, 2005).[7]

The EEOC is charged with enforcing the ADA and other civil rights laws. During the 4-year period FY 2000–2003, the EEOC received 1,785 charges of cancer-related disability discrimination under the ADA, representing about 3 percent of all charges during this period (Table 6-2). The EEOC resolved 2,013 cancer-related disability discrimination charges,[8] with one-quarter (510/2,013) having outcomes favorable to charging parties or charges with meritorious allegations. The EEOC recovered $11 million in monetary benefits for 352 people (including charging parties and other aggrieved individuals). This amount does not include monetary benefits obtained through litigation.

Another source of information regarding the extent of cancer-related employment problems is the Job Accommodation Network (JAN), a service of the Office of Disability Employment Policy of the U.S. Department of Labor (U.S. Department of Labor, 2004c). JAN provides employers and other interested parties with information on job accommodations and employment opportunities and policies. In 2003, JAN handled 514 cases related to cancer (about 2 percent of their calls and e-mails). These came from

[7]Information was not available from published sources on the number of private-sector employees working in companies with fewer than 15 employees.

[8]The fact that there are more resolutions than charges is not unique to cancer cases and likely results from claims with multiple issues resulting in several resolutions.

TABLE 6-2 Resolution of Cancer-Related ADA Charges, FY 2000–2003

Number of charges for all disabilities/conditions	63,675
Cancer-related charges	1,785
Cancer-related resolutions	2,013
Merit resolutions[a]	510
People with monetary benefits	352
Total monetary benefit	$10,969,314

[a]Merit resolutions are charges with outcomes favorable to charging parties and/or charges with meritorious allegations. These include negotiated settlements, withdrawals with benefits, successful conciliations, and unsuccessful conciliations.
SOURCE: U.S. Equal Employment Opportunity Commission (EEOC, 2004a).

both employers and individuals. Most inquiries related to accommodations such as use of leave time and scheduling issues (Personal communication, A. Hirsh, JAN, June 14, 2004).

Family and Medical Leave Act

The Family and Medical Leave Act enacted in 1993 requires employers with at least 50 workers to provide certain benefits for serious medical illness, including cancer, for employees or dependents (U.S. Department of Labor, 2004a). The employee must have worked with his or her employer for at least 1 year. Box 6-4 shows a number of benefits of the statute.

The FMLA attempts to balance the needs of the employer and employee. It:

- Requires employees to make reasonable efforts to schedule foreseeable medical care so as to not unduly disrupt the workplace;
- Requires employees to give employers 30 days' notice of foreseeable medical leave, or as much notice as is practicable;
- Allows employers to require employees to provide certification of medical needs and allows employers to seek a second opinion, at the employer's expense, to corroborate medical need; and
- Permits employers to provide leave provisions more generous than those required by the FMLA.

BOX 6-4
Family and Medical Leave Act (FMLA) Benefits

- Provides 12 weeks of unpaid leave during any 12-month period (leave may be taken intermittently).
- Requires employers to continue to provide benefits, including health insurance coverage, during the leave period (employees must pay the employee contribution).
- Requires employers to restore employees to the same or equivalent position at the end of the leave period.
- Allows leave to care for a spouse, child, or parent who has a "serious health condition" such as cancer.
- Allows leave because a serious health condition renders the employee "unable to perform the functions of the position."
- Allows intermittent or reduced work schedule when "medically necessary." Under some circumstances, an employer may transfer the employee to a position with equivalent pay and benefits to accommodate the new work schedule.
- Allows employees to request to take FMLA leave in combination with other available leave or compensatory time off (referred to as "stacking" of leave).

SOURCE: U.S. Department of Labor (2004a).

The Employee Retirement and Income Security Act

The Employee Retirement and Income Security Act (ERISA) prohibits an employer from discriminating against an employee to prevent him or her from collecting benefits under an employee benefit plan. Employee benefit plans are defined broadly, and include any plan providing "medical, surgical, or hospital care benefits, or benefits in the event of sickness, accident, disability, death, or unemployment." Employers who offer group benefit packages to their employees are subject to ERISA. Some employers fear that the participation of a cancer survivor in a group medical plan will drain benefit funds or increase the employer's insurance premiums. An employer may violate ERISA if, upon learning of a worker's cancer history, it dismisses that worker to exclude him or her from a group health plan. An employer also may violate ERISA by encouraging a person with a cancer history to retire as a "disabled" employee. Most benefit plans define disability narrowly to include only the most debilitating conditions. Individuals with a cancer history often do not fit under such a definition and should not be compelled to so label themselves.

ERISA covers both participants (employees) and beneficiaries (spouses and children). Thus, if the employee is fired because his or her spouse has cancer, the employee may be entitled to file a claim. ERISA, however, is inapplicable to many victims of employment discrimination, including individuals who are denied a new job because of their medical status, employees who are subjected to differential treatment that does not affect their benefits, and employees whose compensation does not include benefits.

Federal Rehabilitation Act

The Federal Rehabilitation Act of 1973 is designed to promote equal employment opportunities for people with disabilities. Unlike the ADA, it is limited to employers of any size that receive money, equipment, or contracts from the federal government. Types of employers subject to the Act include schools, hospitals, defense contractors, and state and local governments. The Act does not apply to the military. The Federal Rehabilitation Act uses the same definition of "individual with a disability" as does the ADA. Also like the ADA, it requires employers to make reasonable accommodations to the physical or mental limitations of qualified individuals.

Executive Order

Unlike many private and state employees, federal employees are protected from genetic-based discrimination. An Executive Order issued in 2000 prohibits federal departments and agencies from making employment decisions about civilian federal employees based on protected genetic information (White House, 2000). The Order also prohibits federal employers from requiring genetic tests as a condition of being hired or receiving benefits.

Genetic nondiscrimination laws have also been enacted in most states. Discrimination in hiring, firing, or terms of employment based on the results of genetic tests is prohibited in 33 states, with many states also restricting the access of employers to genetic information (NCSL, 2005). Some states extend the protections to inherited characteristics, family history, the test results of family members, and information on receipt of genetic services.

State Employment Rights Laws

All states except Alabama and Mississippi have laws that prohibit discrimination against people with disabilities in public and private employment (Hoffman, 2002, 2004b).[9] Several states, such as New Jersey, cover

---

[9]Alabama and Mississippi laws, which have not been amended since the 1970s, cover only state employees.

BOX 6-5
Examples of State Initiatives on Leave Policies Benefiting Cancer Survivors

In Washington state, the "Sick Leave for Sick Families" bill was signed into law in 2002. The bill allows workers, public and private, to use sick leave and other paid leave to care for a child with a medical condition requiring treatment or supervision, or to care for a spouse, parent, parent-in-law, or grandparent who has a serious health condition or an emergency condition. Other states, such as Arizona and Hawaii, have also proposed this type of initiative.

In other states, such as California, New Jersey, and New York, lawmakers have introduced plans to extend temporary disability insurance benefits to workers who take family and medical leave. California signed S.B. 1661 into law in 2002, expanding the state's disability insurance program to provide up to 6 weeks of wage replacement benefits to workers who take time off to care for a seriously ill child, spouse, parent, or domestic partner, or to bond with a new child.

Another model under consideration in Illinois creates a cost-sharing fund, with contributions from the employer, employee, and state, and provides employees on leave with partial wage replacement. In Hawaii, Massachusetts, New Hampshire, and Washington, states have proposed establishing temporary disability Family Leave Insurance funds, financed by small payroll contributions by employers and/ or employees, which would help working families

SOURCE: Center on an Aging Society (2004).

all employers regardless of the number of employees. The laws in most states, however, cover only employers with a minimum number of employees. A few states, such as California and Vermont, expressly prohibit discrimination against cancer survivors.

Most state laws define "individual with a disability" much as it is defined in the ADA. Therefore, most survivors in those states would be considered "disabled" under those state discrimination laws. The rights of cancer survivors in states whose laws do not mirror the ADA vary depending on how those laws define the protected class.

Many states have leave laws similar to the federal FMLA in that they guarantee employees in the private sector unpaid leave for pregnancy, childbirth, and the adoption of a child (see Box 6-5). Some state laws provide employees with medical leave to address a serious illness, such as cancer. Several states provide coverage more extensive than the federal law.

State medical leave laws vary widely as to:

- How long an employee can take leave;
- Which employees may take leave (most states require an employee to have worked for a minimum period of time);

- Which employers must provide leave (a few states have leave laws that apply to employers of fewer than 50 employees);
- The definition of "family member" for whose illness an employee may take family medical leave;
- The type of illness that entitles an employee to medical leave;
- How much notice an employee must give prior to taking leave;
- Whether an employee continues to receive benefits while on leave and who pays for them;
- How the law is enforced (by state agency or through private lawsuit); and
- Provision and extent of replacement wages.

Programs to Ameliorate Employment Problems

Most employers treat cancer survivors fairly and legally. Some employers, however, erect unnecessary and sometimes illegal barriers to survivors' job opportunities (Hoffman, 1999, 2004b). Most personnel decisions are driven by economic factors, not by charitable or personal consideration. Employers may be motivated to fire an employee with cancer (or a history of cancer) because of concerns about increased costs due to insurance expenses and lost productivity or because of concerns about the psychological impact of a survivor's cancer history on other employees. Some employers may fail to revise their personnel policies to comply with new laws and, even among those with updated policies, employers may not train their personnel managers properly to comply with these laws. The interpretation of laws designed to prohibit discriminatory practices is sometimes unclear and is being resolved in the courts. Some employers and co-workers treat cancer survivors differently from other workers, in part because they have misconceptions about survivors' abilities to work during and after cancer treatment (NCCS and Amgen, undated). In an effort to educate employers regarding their responsibilities to employees with cancer, *Business and Health* published a special report, "Living, Coping, and Working with Cancer." A set of recommendations from a panel of health care and business experts convened by *Business and Health* is shown in Box 6-6.

Information, Support, and Referral

This section reviews sources of employment-related information, support, and referral available through employers, cancer voluntary organizations, consumer advocacy programs, and federal and state government programs. The next section reviews the provision of financial support (including health and disability insurance).

BOX 6-6
10 Tips for Employers

1. Know provisions of the Americans with Disabilities Act and the Family and Medical Leave Act. Make such information available to both managers and employees so that workers' rights are understood.
2. Be prepared to thoroughly explain how employee benefits and corporate policy apply to employees diagnosed with cancer.
3. Evaluate whether health plan benefit design provides for adequate treatment and supportive care for cancer patients.
4. Create a corporate culture that allows flextime, job restructuring, or other accommodations for cancer patients who can and want to continue working.
5. Sponsor "lunch and learn" sessions on health plan coverage of cancer therapies, new developments in cancer treatment, and the trend toward increased survivorship.
6. Educate managers to deal sensitively with employees who have cancer—for example, not making assumptions about a cancer patient's ability to perform job duties.
7. Educate managers about appropriate support for cancer patients and when referral to Human Resources or an employee benefits advocate is warranted.
8. Teach managers how to maintain a dialogue with employees being treated with cancer so that adjustments in workload or work schedules can be anticipated.
9. Allow employees to decide if or how they would like coworkers to be informed of their illness, and honor all requests for confidentiality.
10. Reassure coworkers who are concerned about their colleagues' status and what changes may take place in the department.

SOURCE: *Business and Health* Special Report (Voelker, 1999).

The role of employers Employers may provide information, support, and referral services of relevance to cancer survivors through onsite health programs or workplace intranets. Several employers offer their employees web-based personal health management tools allowing them to get information and identify resources (Blumklotz and Lansky, 2001). Toll-free medical decision support services are available to employees to help them make better informed health care purchasing decisions. Cancer questions and requests for information lead all other health care inquiries at some of these programs (Lee, 2004). To help employees balance their personal and professional lives, some companies have provided so-called "work-life" programs offering flexible work options, elder care programs, employee assistance programs (EAPs), and health care and wellness programs (Center on an Aging Society, 2004). Such programs are of benefit to individuals undergoing cancer treatment or in need of flexible scheduling upon a return to work. Leave policies may be prescribed by law (see earlier section on the

Family and Medical Leave Act and related state laws), but some employers provide benefits that exceed those mandated.

Many employers in the private and public sectors have formal or informal disability management and return-to-work programs (Bruyere, 2000). EAPs address productivity issues by helping employees identify and resolve personal concerns that may affect job performance, including issues related to health, marriage, family, substance abuse, stress, and legal problems (Employee Assistance Professionals Organization, 2004). EAPs may provide one-on-one assistance, employee training programs, and leadership consultations. An estimated 56 percent of companies with more than 100 employees provide EAPs that address work-life issues (FWI, 1998; Center on an Aging Society, 2004). In an effort to increase the availability of psychosocial support for cancer patients, the Individual Cancer Assistance Network project (funded by the Bristol-Myers Squibb Foundation) has trained master's-level counselors in EAPs and family service organizations located in Florida (Bristol-Myers Squibb, 2004; Alter, 2005).

It is important to note that employers cannot search records and then initiate contact with employees based on their health status, no matter how commendable their intentions (Lee, 2004). Such contact is prohibited by HIPAA.

Cancer voluntary organizations and consumer advocacy programs Several nonprofit cancer organizations provide education, counseling, and legal advice regarding employment to cancer survivors. The American Cancer Society (ACS) (2004a), the Lance Armstrong Foundation (LAF, 2004), the National Coalition for Cancer Survivorship (NCCS) (Hoffman, 2004a), and CancerCare (CancerCare, 2005), for example, provide information about employment concerns following a diagnosis of cancer.

A number of programs provide legal assistance to cancer survivors concerned about their employment and insurance rights (Box 6-7). For example, legal counseling and education and training for professionals and individuals with cancer are available through the Cancer Legal Resource Center, Western Law Center for Disability Rights. Supported in part by the California Division of ACS, callers to the ACS information line with legal questions are referred to the Center. In 2004 the Center served more than 3,000 callers and reached about 6,000 people through training and outreach. Approximately 13 percent of calls relate to employment, concerns about telling a new employer about cancer, expectations when going back to work, disclosure of cancer history when returning to work, and loss of a job (Schwerin, 2005). The Center serves individuals nationwide, and about half the people calling for assistance are from outside California.

CancerCare is a national nonprofit organization that provides free counseling (individual and group), education, information and referral, and

BOX 6-7
Examples of Programs Providing Legal Assistance to Cancer Survivors

The Cancer and ALS Legal Initiative of the Atlanta Legal Aid Society provides free legal assistance to low-income persons living with cancer in the metro Atlanta area.

Cancer Legal Resource Center provides information and educational outreach on cancer-related legal issues.

Cancer Legal Services Project of the Bar Association of San Francisco provides free services directly to low-income people with cancer.

Legal Advocacy for Cancer Patients at the Temple Legal Aid Office provides free attorney and advocate services to individuals in Philadelphia.

Legal Information Network for Cancer provides legal assistance to individuals with cancer in central Virginia and referrals to attorneys who provide services on a sliding-scale basis.

LegalHealth offers a comprehensive legal clinic onsite in New York area hospitals and at community-based organizations addressing the needs of chronically and seriously ill low-income New Yorkers. Training of doctors, social workers, and other medical professionals is also provided.

SOURCES: Legal Information Network for Cancer (2004); Bar Association of San Francisco (2004); New York Legal Assistance Group (2004); ABA (2004).

direct financial assistance to more than 90,000 people with cancer each year (Personal communication, C. Messner, CancerCare, September 22, 2004) (CancerCare, 2005).[10] Staff oncology social workers and case managers address issues related to employment through a program called "Cancer in the Workplace," where issues related to legal rights and reentering the workplace are discussed. CancerCare sponsors teleconferences regularly, including a series called "Strength for Caring: Living, Working, and Coping with Cancer" (Box 6-8). Some teleconferences are specifically for employers and are promoted through direct contact to companies and partnerships with other organizations. Human resources personnel are able to discuss employer responsibilities, accommodations, helping co-workers deal with colleagues with cancer, and how to interpret laws such as the FMLA and ADA. Teleconferences for patients and caregivers facilitate discussions on disclosure of cancer status to employers, physical examinations, and dealing with physical limitations at work. Caregiver rights under FMLA and ADA are also addressed.

[10]CancerCare's financial assistance program is described in the section below on survivors' insurance and financial concerns.

BOX 6-8
Teleconferences Addressing Workplace Issues Sponsored by CancerCare

- Strength for Caring: Living, Working, and Coping with Cancer Series
  —Part One: Critical Issues and Current Laws Affecting People with Cancer and Their Caregivers in the Workplace
  —Part Two: The Bereaved Caregiver in the Workplace
- Working While Undergoing Cancer Treatment: A Review of Your Legal Protections in the Workplace
- A Fresh Look at the Provisions of the Americans With Disabilities Act (ADA) and the Family and Medical Leave Act (FMLA)
- Employment Issues for People Living with Cancer and Their Caregivers
- Helping Caregivers in the Workplace: Resource Tips for Managers
- Knowing Your Rights: Practical Communication Tips With Your Health Maintenance Organization and Insurance Company

SOURCE: CancerCare (2004).

"Good Health for Life" is a program dedicated to getting cancer survivors back to work. Associated with Stanford University Medical Center, the program provides entrepreneurship resources for cancer survivors and educational programs for business and governments (Good Health for Life, 2004).

Federal and state government programs A number of education and referral programs offered by NCI address employment issues. For example, *Life After Cancer Treatment*, part of NCI's "Facing Forward Series" of publications, describes federal sources of information regarding employment rights, disability, and discrimination (NCI, 2002). Survivors concerned about employment issues are referred to fact sheets and other information provided by the EEOC, the federal agency that coordinates the investigation of employment discrimination. Other federal sources of information and referral include the U.S. Department of Justice, which provides information to assist persons with disabilities with legal issues, questions about the ADA, mediation services, and other employment issues. The U.S. Department of Labor's Office of Disability Employment Policy also provides information regarding discrimination, workplace accommodation, and legal rights. The Job Accommodation Network, a service of the U.S. Department of Labor, provides information on workplace accommodation to both employers and employees.

In addition to education and referral programs, 80 federally funded state vocational rehabilitation agencies employing more than 11,000 vocational counselors throughout the United States provide direct services to facilitate a return to work (Personal communication, J. Pepin, U.S. Department of Education, Office of Special Education and Rehabilitation, September 24, 2004). As of 2003, 2,191 individuals with cancer had completed rehabilitation at one of these agencies. Nearly 60 percent of these cancer survivors, upon completion of the rehabilitation program, were placed in a job and worked for at least 90 days (Personal communication, P. Nash, U.S. Department of Education, Office of Special Education and Rehabilitation, September 22, 2004). Individuals with a history of cancer represent less than 1 percent of those served by the federal/state rehabilitation system. It is unclear why so few persons with cancer complete rehabilitation programs—it may be that cancer survivors do not need, desire, or qualify for the services or, alternatively, that they are not referred to, or accepted by, such programs (Conti, 1990; Mundy et al., 1992). The programs are required to prioritize service delivery to those with severe disabilities, and cancer survivors may not always meet eligibility requirements.

In summary, a number of employer, consumer advocacy organizations, and governmental programs are available to provide information, counseling, and rehabilitation services to address employment-related concerns of cancer survivors. There is little information regarding the extent to which cancer survivors or their providers are aware of these services, or use them. There appears to be a patchwork of services, and it is unclear how accessible they are across the country, how comprehensive the services are, and whether they are meeting the needs of cancer survivors.

Financial Assistance

Private short- and long-term disability insurance and disability programs of the Social Security Administration can be important sources of income replacement for cancer survivors who have had extended times away from work or who are disabled and can no longer work. This section briefly reviews these programs. Sources of financial assistance for individuals' health-related expenditures are described in the next section of the chapter following a review of health insurance issues.

Short- and long-term disability insurance Private short- and long-term disability insurance can provide invaluable financial assistance to individuals who have exhausted their sick and annual leave at work. However, relatively few workers have employment-based disability benefits. In 2004, 39 percent of all workers in private industry had access to short-term disability benefits, other than paid sick leave, while 30 percent had access to long-term disability benefits. Access to these disability benefits is greater among higher wage earners and those working for large employers (Table

TABLE 6-3 Percentage of Workers with Access to Disability Insurance Benefits, by Selected Characteristics, Private Industry, 2004

Characteristic	Short-Term Disability Benefits	Long-Term Disability Benefits
All workers	39	30
Worker characteristics		
White-collar occupations	43	41
Blue-collar occupations	45	22
Service occupations	23	12
Full time	47	38
Part time	14	5
Union	67	30
Nonunion	36	30
Average wage <$15 per hour	29	17
Average wage ≥$15 per hour	55	48
Establishment characteristics		
Goods-producing	54	31
Service-producing	35	30
1-99 workers	28	19
100 workers or more	53	44

SOURCE: Bureau of Labor Statistics (2004).

6-3). Short-term disability programs are required by law in some states (e.g., New Jersey, New York).

Federal Social Security Administration programs Since 1974, the Supplemental Security Income (SSI) program has guaranteed a minimum level of income for needy aged, blind, or disabled individuals (SSA, 2004b). To be considered disabled, an individual must have a medically determinable physical or mental impairment that is expected to last (or has lasted) at least 12 continuous months or to result in death. For those aged 18 and older, the impairment must prevent him or her from doing any substantial gainful activity. The SSI program was designed to provide "assistance of last resort." It is means-tested and takes into account all income and resources that an individual has or can obtain. Generally, SSI recipients are immediately eligible for Medicaid. The program includes work incentives that

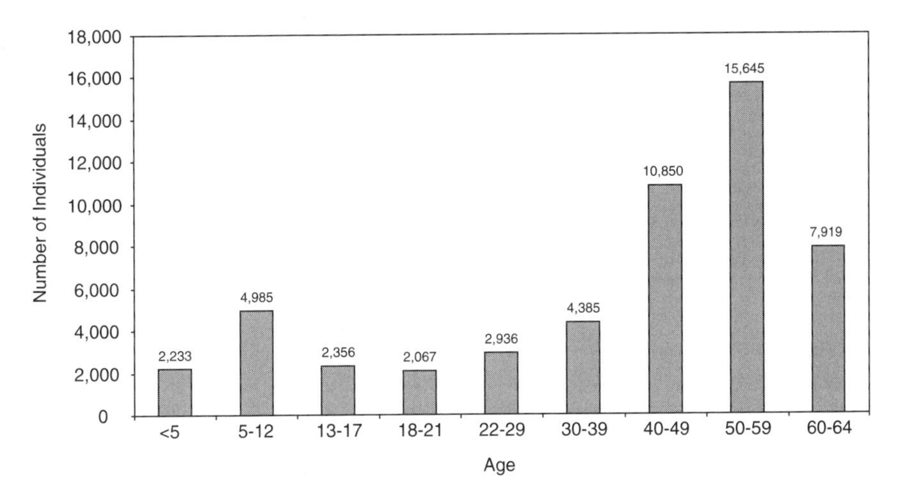

FIGURE 6-2 Number of SSI recipients eligible because of a cancer diagnosis, by age, December 2003. SOURCE: SSI Annual Statistical Report, 2003, Table 25 (SSA, 2004b).

enable recipients who are disabled to work and retain benefits and, in certain circumstances, extended Medicaid eligibility.

In December 2003, an estimated 53,376 individuals under age 65 were receiving SSI benefits because of a diagnosis of cancer. Cancer survivors represent only 1.1 percent of the total number of SSI recipients under age 65 (4.9 million) (Figure 6-2). Most SSI recipients under age 65 (58 percent) become eligible because of a mental disorder (SSA, 2004b). In December 2003, the average monthly federal SSI payment to beneficiaries with cancer was $404 (payment depends on income, and 45 states provide supplemental payments) (SSA, 2004b).

Social Security Disability Insurance (SSDI) is an insurance program that provides payments to persons with disabilities based on their history of Social Security-covered earnings. In contrast, the SSI program is a means-tested program that does not require prior participation in the labor force. The definition of disability and the process of determining disability are the same for both programs (IOM, 2002b). To be eligible, an individual must be unable to work at all, in any job, for at least 12 months or be in the terminal stages of illness. As of 2003, 160,986 disabled workers under age 65 were receiving SSDI payments because of cancer, representing 2.7 percent of all disabled workers receiving SSDI benefits (SSA, 2004a).

Summary: Employment Issues

It is difficult to gauge the extent of cancer-related employment problems, but recent evidence suggests that as many as 20 percent of survivors face work limitations 2 to 3 years after their diagnosis. Survivors appear to be most vulnerable in the immediate post-treatment period. A number of federal and state laws enacted in the 1990s provide some level of protection from employer discriminatory practices. However, these laws are not comprehensive and the courts continue to interpret the extent of protections provided to cancer survivors. A patchwork of educational, counseling, and referral sources is available. Unknown is whether cancer survivors are aware of their legal protections or of the services that are available to them. Limited financial assistance in the form of income replacement is available through the Social Security Administration to those who are poor and too disabled by cancer to work. Some individuals have some financial protection through short- and long-term disability programs, but these benefits tend to be offered by relatively few employers.

HEALTH INSURANCE

The Impact of Cancer on Health Insurance

Cancer care is very costly and represents one of the three most expensive conditions in the United States (Cohen and Krauss, 2003). Cancer-related medical expenditures in the United States totaled an estimated $48 billion in 2002 (AHRQ, 2004).[11] Although most cancer-related expenditures are for initial treatment, expenditures for continuing care are not insubstantial, especially for those cancers with good prognoses (Figure 6-3).

Most Americans have health insurance that provides coverage for most cancer-related care. However, the lack of health insurance for 42 million Americans has serious negative consequences and economic costs not only for the uninsured themselves, but also for their families, the communities they live in, and the nation as a whole (Cohen and Martinez, 2005; IOM, 2004a). The uninsured do not receive the care they need; they suffer from poorer health, and are more likely to die early than are those with coverage. Aside from the health consequences, even one uninsured person in a family can put the financial stability and health of the whole family at risk. Furthermore, a community's high uninsured rate can adversely affect the over-

[11]This estimate reflects spending only for medical care that was directly related to cancer. Cancer-related expenditures in 2002 were exceeded by expenditures for only two conditions, heart conditions ($68 billion) and trauma-related disorders ($56 billion).

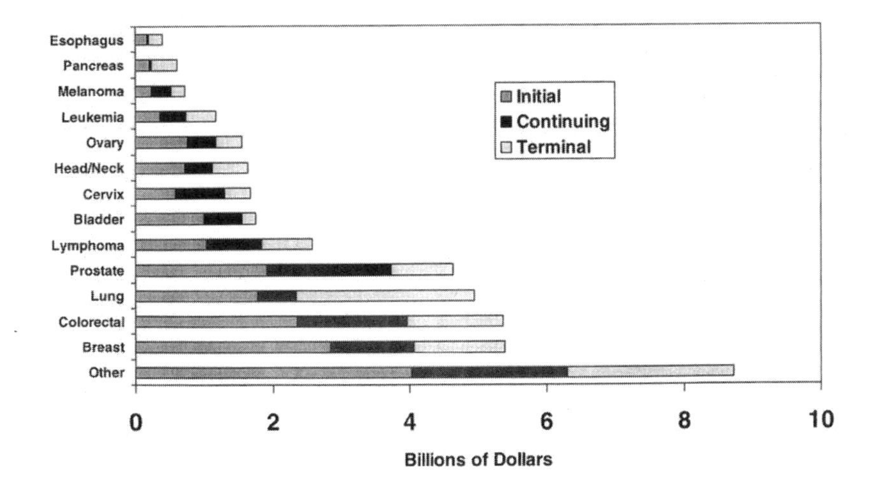

FIGURE 6-3 National U.S. Medicare expenditures in 1996 by cancer type and phase of care.
DATA SOURCE: SEER-Medicare database (Brown et al., 2002). Reprinted with permission from Lippincott, Williams & Wilkins. Brown ML, Riley GF, Schussler N, Etzioni R. 2002. Estimating health care costs related to cancer treatment from SEER-Medicare data. *Med Care* 40(8 Suppl):IV-104–IV-117.

all health status of *the com*munity and its health care institutions and providers, and the access of its residents to certain services. These are among the conclusions reached by the Institute of Medicine's (IOM's) Committee on the Consequences of Uninsurance in their 2004 report, *Insuring America's Health: Principles and Recommendations* (IOM, 2004a).

Many studies link lack of health insurance with poor cancer outcomes (Ayanian et al., 1993; Lee-Feldstein et al., 2000; Ferrante et al., 2000; Roetzheim et al., 2000a,b; Penson et al., 2001; IOM, 2001, 2002a). Access to health insurance has been found to influence the amount and quality of health care received, which in turn is likely related to survival. Three-year relative cancer survival was markedly poorer for those without health insurance as compared to the insured, according to one state's population-based study (Grann and Jacobson, 2003; McDavid et al., 2003). The link between insurance status and health outcomes is complex and confounded by socioeconomic status, race and ethnicity, and other factors. In one study, non-elderly cancer patients without insurance were found to be at risk for receiving inadequate cancer care, especially if they were Hispanic (Thorpe and Howard, 2003). Here, expenditures for uninsured patients under age 65 were nearly half (57 percent) that of privately insured patients over a 6-month period. Spending differences were believed to be due, in part or completely, to differences in use, suggesting that raising coverage rates would improve cancer treatment. These findings are consistent with other studies of the chronically ill that have compared those with and without health insurance and found the uninsured lack needed physician care and prescription medicines (Families USA, 2001).

To overcome such health disparities, the IOM Committee on the Consequences of Uninsurance envisioned an approach to health insurance that would promote better overall health for individuals, families, communities, and the nation by providing financial access for everyone to necessary, appropriate, and effective health services. The committee articulated five principles to guide the extension of coverage (Box 6-9) and recommended that the President and Congress develop a strategy to achieve universal insurance coverage and to establish a firm and explicit schedule to reach this goal by 2010. Many plans to reform the nations' health care insurance system have been proposed, and these principles are useful in assessing the relative merits of current proposals and in designing future strategies for extending coverage to everyone.

The IOM Committee on Cancer Survivorship agrees with the vision and implementation plan that has been put forth. Only through such an effort will cancer survivors, their families, and health care providers be able to fully focus on care and well-being without being burdened by financial worries. Although addressing national health care proposals to extend health insurance coverage to more Americans was not within the scope of the Committee on Cancer Survivorship's work, the committee wishes to highlight in this report the serious consequences of lack of insurance coverage to cancer survivors, their families, and their caregivers. The actions recommended in the IOM's insurance-focused work are endorsed by the Cancer Survivorship Committee.

BOX 6-9
Principles to Guide the Extension of Coverage

1. Health care coverage should be universal.
2. Health care coverage should be continuous.
3. Health care coverage should be affordable to individuals and families.
4. The health insurance strategy should be affordable and sustainable for society.
5. Health insurance should enhance health and well-being by promoting access to high-quality care that is effective, efficient, safe, timely, patient centered, and equitable.

SOURCE: IOM (2004a).

TABLE 6-4 People Without Health Insurance Coverage by Age, United States, 2004

Age	Percentage of the Population Uninsured
Total, all ages	14.6
Under 18	9.4
18 to 24	29.9
25 to 34	25.6
35 to 44	17.6
45 to 64	12.7

NOTE: The total number of uninsured for all age groups in 2004 was 42.1 million.
SOURCE: Cohen and Martinez (2005).

This section of the report begins with a description of the extent of the problem of lack of insurance coverage among cancer survivors and the limited remedies available to the uninsured who wish to gain health insurance coverage. Next, problems of cancer survivors with insurance are reviewed, including difficulties in maintaining health insurance coverage, gaining access to needed treatments and specialists, and paying health care out-of-pocket costs that stem from underinsurance (either due to insurance exclusions or benefit limits). In particular, the problem of paying for costly prescription medications is discussed. The limited number of programs to ameliorate financial hardships that result from uninsurance and underinsurance are described. Lastly, issues related to access to life insurance are briefly discussed.

As many as 15 percent of Americans lack health insurance (Table 6-4) and, for these individuals, cancer can be financially devastating. Among adults aged 45 to 64, an age when many develop cancer, 13 percent are uninsured. Adults aged 35 to 44 have even higher rates of being uninsured (18 percent). Vulnerability increases when measured over a longer timeframe. While 44 million Americans were uninsured in 2003, nearly twice that number, an estimated 84 million, were uninsured for at least 1 month over a 3-year period (Short et al., 2003). This, in part, reflects the dynamic nature of the population of the uninsured: About 2 million people become uninsured every month, while about the same number gain insurance (Short et al., 2003). Vulnerability also increases as health status declines. Research shows people in poor health are twice as likely to encounter a lengthy spell without health insurance compared to people in good health (Haley and Zuckerman, 2003).

The increase in the number of uninsured Americans in the past several years has been confined to adults, as public programs have expanded to offset the general decline in employer insurance for children. Among adults, loss of insurance can be traced to declines in employer-based insurance (DeNavas-Walt et al., 2004; Kaiser Family Foundation, 2004a). Employer-sponsored health insurance for retirees is also becoming less available, making it more difficult for survivors with significant health problems to retire early (American Benefits Council, 2004). Retirees are increasingly responsible for a larger share of the cost of their health care. Most uninsured adults had employer-based coverage prior to becoming uninsured. Several safety net laws and programs have been created to help people navigate coverage transitions and offer coverage to the uninsured. Although the protections offered by these laws and programs are important, they are incomplete. People with cancer can, and sometimes do, lose health insurance just when they need it most.

Much of the research that has documented insurance problems among cancer survivors was conducted prior to the enactment of laws to improve access to insurance coverage and protect consumers from some forms of discrimination. This literature documents instances of insurers refusing new applications, canceling or reducing policies, charging higher premiums, waiving or excluding preexisting conditions, or extending waiting periods for coverage (Kornblith, 1998; Guidry et al., 1998; Hoffman, 1999). Not much is known of the impact on contemporary cancer survivors of the relatively new federal and state laws that should facilitate obtaining and maintaining insurance coverage (Pollitz et al., 2000). What has been well documented are the very high costs associated with cancer and how such costs can serve as barriers to cancer care for both those with and those without health insurance (Guidry et al., 1998).

Cancer Survivors Who Are Uninsured

Virtually all (99 percent) cancer survivors aged 65 and older have health insurance coverage through the nation's Medicare program.[12] The problems the elderly have in coverage are discussed in the next section. With 39 percent of cancer survivors under age 65 and the potentially devastating impact of a cancer diagnosis on personal finances, the committee analyzed data from the National Health Interview Survey (NHIS) (2000 to 2003) to answer several questions about health insurance coverage among nonelderly cancer survivors (see Appendix 6A for details on the NHIS and the methods used to derive these estimates).

---

[12]This estimate is based on staff analyses of the National Health Interview Survey described in Table 6-5.

1. **How many nonelderly cancer survivors lack health insurance?** Among cancer survivors ages 25 to 64, 11 percent are uninsured (approximately 572,000 individuals) (Table 6-5).

2. **Which groups of cancer survivors are less likely to be insured?** Lacking health insurance is more common among younger survivors (ages 25 to 44) (19 percent) and Hispanic/Latino survivors (26 percent) (Table 6-5).

3. **To what extent do nonelderly cancer survivors rely on public health insurance programs?** An estimated 14 percent of non-elderly cancer survivors depend on Medicare or Medicaid for coverage. Lack of insurance and reliance on public insurance coverage increase with years since diagnosis. Rates of private insurance coverage are higher for survivors with breast and prostate cancer. This could reflect differences in age distribution (older individuals are more likely to have health insurance) or perhaps indicate that those with insurance are more likely to be screened and then survive their cancer (Table 6-5).

4. **How does the health insurance status of cancer survivors compare to that of the general population and to individuals with other chronic illnesses?** The uninsured rate among nonelderly cancer survivors is no higher than those seen in the general population (it is lower, 11.3 percent versus 16.3 percent). This may, in part, be explained by the older age distribution of cancer survivors and the general trend of increasing rates of insurance coverage with age (Table 6-4). It could also reflect greater efforts to maintain coverage by those with a chronic illness as compared to healthy individuals. Alternatively, it may be the case that individuals without health insurance and access to primary health care are not represented among cancer survivors (see Chapter 2). Lacking insurance is a problem of similar magnitude for cancer survivors (11.3 percent) and those with cardiovascular disease (12.1 percent) and diabetes (12.6 percent). People with other chronic conditions that are more prevalent in younger populations (e.g., diabetes) also exhibit higher coverage rates, however. This suggests people with chronic conditions may take on greater burdens and make more sacrifices, such as job lock, to get and keep coverage, compared to healthy individuals who can navigate insurance transitions with less difficulty and expense.

5. **To what extent does a lack of insurance coverage impede cancer survivors' access to care?** Among cancer survivors ages 25 to 64 and without health insurance, many report access problems due to concerns about cost—51 percent (291,000 individuals) report delays in obtaining medical care; 44 percent (250,000 individuals) report not getting needed care; and 31 percent (178,000 individuals) report not getting needed prescription medicine. Similar consequences of a lack of coverage have been documented among those with other chronic illnesses (Tu, 2004).

TABLE 6-5 Health Insurance Status of Cancer Survivors Ages 25 to 64, by Selected Characteristics, 2000–2003

	Estimated Population	
Characteristic	In Millions	%
Total	5.0	100.0
Age		
25–44	1.5	30.6
45–64	3.5	69.4
Sex		
Male	1.5	29.8
Female	3.5	70.2
Race/ethnicity		
White, non-Hispanic	4.3	85.3
Hispanic	0.3	5.2
Black, non-Hispanic	0.4	7.1
Other	0.1	2.3
Years since diagnosis		
<2	0.8	16.6
2–4	1.2	23.7
5–9	1.1	21.3
10–19	1.2	24.0
20+	0.7	14.5
Age at interview, age at diagnosis		
25–44, <45	1.5	30.7
45–64, <45	1.5	29.0
45–64, 45–64	2.0	40.3
Cancer type		
Female breast	1.0	19.4
Female reproductive[a]	1.5	29.7
Prostate	0.2	4.7
Colorectal	0.3	5.9
Other	2.0	40.3
Has other chronic disease		
Yes	1.8	35.1
No	3.3	64.9
Self-reported health status		
Excellent/very good	2.1	41.5
Good	1.5	30.5
Fair/poor	1.4	28.0

NOTE: — indicates too few cases for reliable estimate. The NHIS estimate of the number of cancer survivors ages 25 to 64 (5 million) is somewhat higher than that estimated from surveillance data (4 million). This could be explained if there is overreporting of a cancer history among those ages 25 to 64 and interviewed for the NHIS.

Health Insurance Status (percentage distribution)				
Medicare	Medicaid	Private	Other Coverage	**Uninsured**
7.4	6.8	70.6	3.9	11.3
3.5	9.2	65.3	3.6	18.5
9.1	5.8	72.9	4.1	8.2
10.5	5.1	70.9	5.2	8.3
6.0	7.6	70.5	3.4	12.6
7.1	5.8	73.2	4.0	10.0
—	10.2	56.4	—	25.8
10.0	14.1	56.0	—	15.0
—	—	52.5	—	—
—	6.4	76.0	—	7.9
6.3	6.5	75.2	—	9.5
8.3	7.1	68.7	4.3	11.5
8.8	7.2	67.1	—	13.1
7.6	7.1	66.3	—	14.7
3.3	9.3	65.3	3.5	18.6
7.9	6.3	71.4	3.4	11.0
9.9	5.5	74.3	4.4	5.9
6.3	5.1	80.2	—	5.4
4.9	10.6	61.8	4.0	18.7
—	—	80.0	—	—
—	—	72.0	—	—
9.4	5.5	71.1	3.8	10.2
15.2	11.2	56.2	5.3	12.1
3.1	4.5	78.3	3.2	10.9
—	—	84.2	2.6	10.2
4.0	5.6	74.6	3.7	12.1
20.1	15.9	45.6	6.2	12.1

[a]Female reproductive cancer includes cancer of the cervix, uterus, and ovary.
SOURCE: NHIS tabulations, committee staff. See Appendix 6A for a description of the NHIS and the methods used to derive these estimates.

These estimates of health insurance coverage among cancer survivors are based on a national survey and have limitations. First, the results pertain only to the adult civilian noninstitutionalized household population and not to cancer survivors who reside in institutions (e.g., hospices or nursing homes). The NHIS interviews rely on self-reports of cancer, and such reports tend to underestimate cancer prevalence (Hewitt et al., 1999; Desai et al., 2001). Furthermore, the survey is cross-sectional and does not capture the dynamic nature of insurance coverage status.

What are the options for the estimated 572,000 cancer survivors under age 65 who lack health insurance, but wish to obtain coverage? A safety net of sorts exists, but there are many barriers to coverage that is simultaneously available, affordable, and adequate.

Limited access to public insurance coverage Medicaid, the leading safety net program for health insurance coverage, is not available to millions of uninsured poor Americans. Only certain categories of people are eligible for Medicaid: children, parents of dependent children, pregnant women, the elderly, and the disabled. In many states, adults who fit one of these eligibility categories also must have income far below the federal poverty level in order to qualify for Medicaid coverage. If individuals are uninsured and have income above Medicaid eligibility levels, medical expenses related to cancer may force them to "spend down" to become eligible for Medicaid—that is, to deplete their assets until they meet income eligibility criteria. This option is not available in all states, however, and in states where there is a "spend-down" option, individuals still need to meet other eligibility categories (i.e., be a child, parent of a dependent child, disabled, or elderly). The Medicaid spend-down option, therefore, is far from a comprehensive safety net for the uninsured who are seriously ill. Those too disabled to work and under age 65 may qualify for Medicaid (if very poor and eligible for SSI disability benefits) or Medicare (if eligible for SSDI benefits, and disabled for a period of 2 years) (Kaiser Family Foundation, 2001, 2004e). For those who do qualify for Medicaid, coverage may be transient (i.e., change from month-to-month) so that once an individual's condition improves, he or she may no longer qualify for Medicaid coverage. Furthermore, those who "spend down" their assets may only qualify for Medicaid in months with high medical expenses.

Some women who are uninsured and poor may become eligible for Medicaid if they are diagnosed with breast or cervical cancer through the Centers for Disease Control and Prevention (CDC) National Breast and Cervical Cancer Early Detection Program. Breast and cervical cancer screening is available to low-income, uninsured, and underserved women through this program. All states have also accepted the option, available since 2000, to provide Medicaid coverage for women diagnosed with cancer through this program so that they have access to treatment (CDC, 2004; CMS, 2004b). Medicaid coverage is not limited to treatment of breast and cervical cancer. However, the coverage ends when a woman's course of treatment is completed (CMS, 2004d). The scope and duration of Medicaid coverage under this program needs to be clarified because evidence suggests there is confusion about what services are covered and for how long (e.g., coverage of Tamoxifen therapy, which is typically prescribed for 5 years) (Kenny et al., 2004). In terms of access to this gateway for coverage for treatment, CDC's early detection program is severely limited—the program reaches fewer than 15 percent of women who are eligible for screening by virtue of their income, age, and insurance status (CDC, 2005). In addition, once enrolled in Medicaid, women in some states may encounter other limits on covered benefits. In Texas, for example, Medicaid covers only three prescription drugs per month.

Limited access to private insurance Individuals who are uninsured, without access to group coverage, and not eligible for public programs may try to purchase private health insurance on an individual basis, but for those with a history of cancer, such coverage may be unavailable, very costly, or restrictive. Common circumstances that lead people to seek individually purchased health insurance include self-employment, early retirement, working part-time, divorce or widowhood, or "aging off" a parent's policy (Pollitz et al., 2001). An estimated 17 million individuals had individually purchased health insurance coverage in 2002 (Williams and Fuchs, 2004). One in four adults have a need for individual health insurance at some point over a 3-year period (Duchon et al., 2001). The barriers to obtaining private individual coverage can be categorized as those of availability, affordability, and adequacy (referred to as "the three A's") (Box 6-10).

The three "A's" barriers facing cancer survivors in the individual health insurance market are well illustrated by a study commissioned by the Kaiser Family Foundation. As part of this study, 19 insurance companies and health maintenance organizations (HMOs) in eight markets around the country were asked to consider for coverage (using rates in effect in 2000) hypothetical applicants with different health histories (Pollitz et al., 2001). One of the scenarios was for a 48-year-old, 7-year breast cancer survivor. Insurers reviewing the "applicants" determined whether or not they would be offered coverage and on what terms. The application made on behalf of the breast cancer survivor was rejected 43 percent of the time (i.e., in 26 of 60 applications filed for this case). Of the 34 offers of coverage received, 18 had limits on benefits covered. Most often the policies had riders excluding coverage for her treated breast, her implant, or cancer of any type. Eighteen offers imposed a premium surcharge, ranging from 40 to 100 percent (including 13 that were accompanied by some other benefit restriction). A

BOX 6-10
Barriers Faced by the Uninsured in Obtaining Private Individual Insurance—"The Three A's"

Availability barriers
- Individual insurance is medically underwritten in most states

Affordability barriers
- Premium surcharges for substandard risks
- Age rating
- Premium subsidies are rare

Adequacy barriers
- Preexisting condition exclusions, often permanent
- Limited coverage for pharmaceuticals and other key benefits
- High cost sharing

SOURCE: Pollitz (2004).

unmodified offer for coverage was made only 18 percent of the time (11 of 60 applications). The average annual premium for this hypothetical applicant was $3,912, with a range from $1,464 to $16,344 per year.

In the 1990s, states enacted individual market reforms to make coverage more available and affordable, especially for higher risk people (Williams and Fuchs, 2004). New York, for example, requires all individual-market health insurance to be sold on a guaranteed-issue, community-rated basis—which means no resident can be turned down or charged more due to their health status, age, or gender (Pollitz et al., 2001; Georgetown University Health Policy Institute, 2004). Some states have also restricted the extent to which premium rates can vary based on health status and/or age. Florida law prohibits insurers from denying coverage or imposing exclusion riders based on breast cancer if treatment ended more than 2 years prior to application. Florida does not prohibit premium rate-ups for breast cancer survivors.

More than half of the states operate high-risk insurance pools to help provide coverage to individuals with serious medical conditions who have been denied private health insurance in the individual market (Achman and Chollet, 2001; Abbe, 2005). These risk pools, however, typically do not provide coverage that is available, affordable, and adequate (Box 6-11). Relatively few people are covered by state high-risk pools; 172,000 people as of 2003 (U.S. DHHS, 2003c), representing a very small share (2 percent) of individual market participants in those states. To improve access to such coverage, the federal government for the first time provided assistance to

BOX 6-11
Limitations of State High-Risk Pools

Availability barriers

- Lack of public awareness/marketing
- Eligibility barriers
- Application delays or limits (e.g., waiting lists or program closures to new applicants)

Affordability barriers

- Premiums are typically set at 150–200 percent of standard rates
- Age rating increases the cost further for older individuals
- Subsidies are rare and modest

Adequacy barriers

- Preexisting conditions excluded in most states. Although high-risk pools are designed to provide coverage for people with serious or chronic illnesses, they often limit access by imposing waiting and "look-back" periods for preexisting conditions to reduce adverse selection. Enrollees who were diagnosed with a condition during a look-back period (typically 6 months before enrolling in the pool) are not covered for treatment of that condition during a specified waiting period after coverage (typically 6 months or a year) (Achman and Chollet, 2001).
- High deductibles, cost sharing, limited annual or lifetime benefits
- Limits on prescription drugs and/or other key benefits

SOURCE: Pollitz (2004).

states in support of high-risk pools under the Trade Act of 2002. In 2002, $20 million was appropriated to help states create high-risk pools and $80 million was appropriated over 2 years to offset a portion of losses incurred by states from operating high-risk pools (U.S. DHHS, 2002, 2003a,b,c). These grant programs expired at the end of 2004. In the 109th Congress, legislation has been introduced to reauthorize $15 million in seed grants for fiscal years 2005 and 2006 for states launching high-risk insurance pools and to provide $75 million in grants for fiscal years 2005 through 2009 for states that currently operate high-risk pools (State High Risk, 2004, 2005; Kaiser Family Foundation, 2004c).

Comprehensive state reforms of the individual market that were made in the 1990s increased the availability of coverage for higher risk people, according to a recent assessment of their impact (Williams and Fuchs, 2004). However, while premiums for higher risk people decreased, coverage became less affordable, on average. States with comprehensive reforms experienced a decrease in coverage rates overall because people with lower risks left the market due to the higher price they faced for individual insurance, although coverage increased for people who were older and in poorer health. This problem might be alleviated if tax credits or other assistance to individual buyers reduce the effective premium to the point where insurance remains attractive to low-risk people (Merlis, 2005).

Relatively little is known directly of the experience of individuals with a history of cancer who lack health insurance. A recent study in California of the uninsured population's access to specialty care found the safety net to be inadequate (Felt-Lisk et al., 2004). Nearly one-third (32 percent) of medical directors of the state's federally qualified health centers (FQHCs) in 2002–2003 indicated that uninsured patients have difficulty obtaining oncology care "often" or "always." Obtaining neurology, endocrinology, and allergy/immunology care were much more problematic. One-half of the FQHC medical directors reported that access to specialty care in general had gotten worse in the past 2 years. Hospitals were found to be the major source of specialty care for the uninsured. That chronic symptoms or conditions were not well managed or treated on a timely basis were among the findings from focus groups held among uninsured individuals with a range of chronic conditions requiring specialty care services. In other research, community health centers were found to be able to provide primary care and other services to most of their uninsured patients, but were limited in their ability to provide diagnostic, specialty, and behavioral health services. Uninsured patients often failed to receive additional services for which they were referred (Gusmano et al., 2002).

Cancer Survivors with Health Insurance

Cancer survivors with health insurance coverage may have problems maintaining their coverage following a cancer diagnosis. In addition, those with coverage may find it is inadequate to pay for all of the care and services they need. Sometimes, it is unclear whether an insurance policy covers recommended treatments. For example, insurers may challenge claims for interventions designed to prevent or ameliorate late effects of cancer because of interpretations of what constitutes accepted and appropriate care. In some cases, states have mandated that insurers cover survivorship-related services such as breast prostheses and lymphedema therapy. Federal law mandates coverage for reconstructive surgery and these survivorship-related services in health plans that cover mastectomy.

Maintaining health insurance coverage For cancer survivors who lose their jobs, the federal law known as COBRA mandates that they can keep the health insurance they had through their employer for 18 months.[13] Some

---

[13]The Consolidated Omnibus Budget Reconciliation Act of 1986 (Pub. L. No. 99–272) requires employers to offer group medical coverage to employees and their dependents who otherwise would have lost their group coverage due to qualifying events. Employers with

states have enacted "mini" COBRA laws similar to the federal law to provide individuals with extended coverage. Although the survivor, and not the former employer, must pay for the continued coverage, the rate may not exceed by more than 2 percent the rate set for the survivor's former co-workers. Not all employees are aware of COBRA benefits and roughly one in five persons who are eligible for coverage claim it, although some studies suggest take-up is higher among individuals who are older and have health problems (Gruber and Madrian, 1993).

Many cancer survivors (and family members who hold the family's health insurance policy) avoid changing jobs because they fear losing health insurance and other employment-related benefits. In one study, more than one-quarter (27 percent) of cancer survivors reported this sense of "job lock" (Short et al., 2005a). Congress tried to remedy this problem in 1996, enacting the Health Insurance Portability and Accountability Act (HIPAA)[14] to improve the portability and continuity of health insurance coverage in private insurance markets and among employer-sponsored group health plans.

For people changing jobs, HIPAA added important protections. It prohibited employers and insurers from conditioning eligibility for health benefits on health status. In addition, it limited the imposition of preexisting condition exclusion periods and required credit to be given for continuous prior coverage. However, federal law does not require employers to offer health benefits nor, for the most part, does it require minimum standards for what must be covered under job-based health plans. As a result, cancer survivors who change jobs may still find the next job does not offer coverage, or offers a plan that does not cover all the health services and providers a cancer survivor may need.

HIPAA also limits the ability of insurers in the individual market to deny or limit coverage because of preexisting conditions such as cancer. This protection applies to people who are "HIPAA eligible," that is, who have left job-based coverage, exhausted COBRA, and meet other requirements. However, the increased cost of premiums for portable insurance products and difficulties in implementing and enforcing the law have limited the value of these protections for consumers (GAO, 1997, 2000, 2001). Some of the limitations of HIPAA's protections are outlined in Box 6-12.

---

more than 20 employees are required to make continued insurance coverage available to employees (and their covered spouses and dependents) who quit, are terminated, or work reduced hours. Coverage must extend to spouses and dependent children who would otherwise lose coverage due to the death, divorce, legal separation, or Medicare eligibility of a covered worker, and to children who attain the age of majority and lose dependent status.

[14]HIPAA was signed into law as Pub. L. No. 104–191 on August 21, 1996.

BOX 6-12
Limitations of Individual Market Protections Under the Health Insurance Portability and Accountability Act

Availability barriers

- Eligibility usually requires election/exhaustion of COBRA benefits
- Public awareness: As of 2005, group health plans and group health insurance issuers are required to give workers a statement about their rights under the law

Affordability barriers

- Dramatic premium surcharges in many states
- No premium subsidies

Adequacy barriers

- No benefit standard in most states

SOURCE: Pollitz (2004).

Foremost among these is the HIPAA eligibility requirement that individuals have elected and exhausted COBRA benefits and the high costs associated with premiums.[15]

Inadequate health insurance coverage Consumer cost sharing has increased greatly in recent years, placing a larger financial burden on those with insurance. Employers are asking employees to pay more for health care through higher contributions and deductibles, lower subsidies for dependent coverage, and numerous benefit changes that increase spending at the point of care (Goff, 2004). Out-of-pocket spending for medical services increases with the number of chronic conditions a person has, and large out-of-pocket expenditures can limit access to care, affect health status and quality of life, and leave insufficient income for other necessities (Hwang et al., 2001).

According to analyses of the 2001–2002 Medical Expenditure Panel Survey (MEPS), health-related out-of-pocket expenditures made by those reporting health effects of cancer are high, averaging $1,267 annually for those ages 25 to 64 (13.5 percent of total expenditures) and $1,456 annually (12.5 percent of total expenditures) for those aged 65 and older (Figures 6-4 and 6-5) (see Appendix 6A for a description of MEPS and the

[15]HIPAA does not require exhaustion of COBRA benefits in all circumstances. For example, if a man is dependent on his wife's employer for health insurance and the wife quits work because of breast cancer and loses coverage, the husband may seek health insurance (if offered) through his employer for himself and his wife

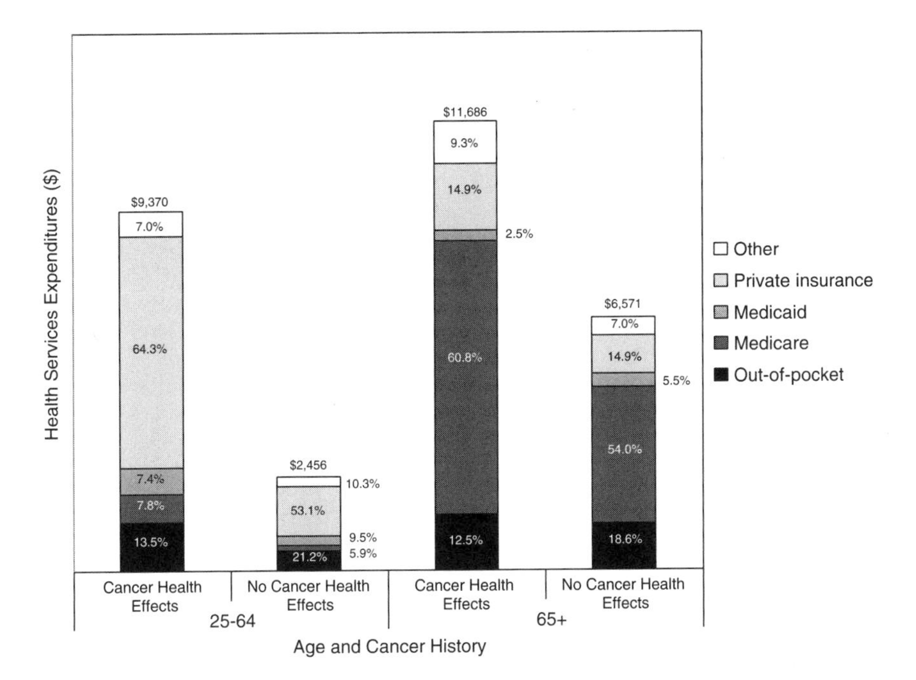

FIGURE 6-4 Sources of payment for health services expenditures among people reporting cancer-related health effects, by age, 2001–2002. The "cancer health effects" group does not necessarily include all cancer survivors; cancer survivors who do not experience adverse cancer-related health effects would not be included. Expenditures include both spending for care directly related to cancer and spending for other medical care unrelated to cancer (see Appendix 6A for a description of the Medical Expenditure Panel Survey and the methods used to derive these estimates). SOURCE: Special tabulations of MEPS (Friedland, 2005).

methods used to derive these estimates). These expenditures are significantly higher than those made by individuals who do not report health effects of cancer ($520 among those ages 25 to 64 and $1,221 for those aged 65 and older) (Figure 6-5).

These expenditures represent a considerable burden, especially for those with low incomes. In 1998, health-related out-of-pocket spending among those with a cancer history represented 9 percent of income for those with an annual family income under $20,000 and about 1 percent for those with an annual family income of $55,000 or more (Center on an Aging Society, 2002).

The experiences of cancer survivors who are poor and privately insured are likely similar to individuals with other chronic illnesses. Between 2001

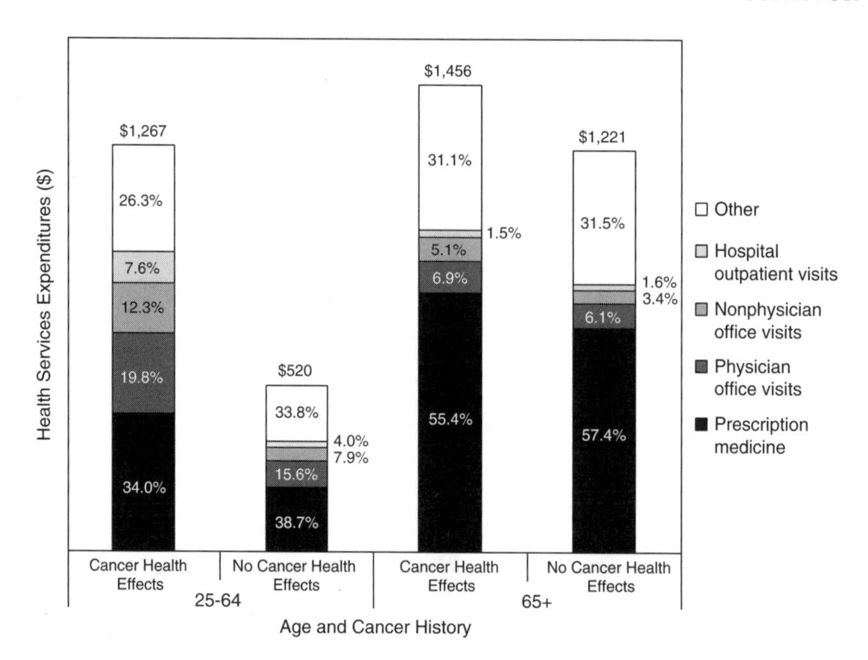

FIGURE 6-5 Average annual out-of-pocket expenditures among people reporting cancer-related health effects, by age, 2001–2002. The "cancer health effects" group does not necessarily include all cancer survivors; cancer survivors who do not experience adverse cancer-related health effects would not be included. Expenditures include both spending for care directly related to cancer and spending for other medical care unrelated to cancer (see Appendix 6A for a description of the Medical Expenditure Panel Survey and the methods used to derive these estimates).
SOURCE: Special tabulations of the Medical Expenditure Panel Survey (MEPS), Friedland (2005).

and 2003, the proportion of low-income, chronically ill people with private insurance who spent more than 5 percent of their income on out-of-pocket health care costs grew from 28 percent to 42 percent (Tu, 2004). In 2003, 12.3 million people aged 18–64 with chronic conditions,[16] lived in families with problems paying medical bills (Tu, 2004). Among families with medical bill problems, nearly two-thirds report having difficulty paying for other basic necessities—rent, mortgage payments, transportation, or food—as a

[16]For purposes of this study, chronic conditions included asthma, arthritis, diabetes, chronic obstructive pulmonary disease, heart disease, hypertension, cancer, benign prostate enlargement, abnormal uterine bleeding, and depression (Tu, 2004).

result of medical debt (May and Cunningham, 2004). About half of the 1.5 million American families that filed for bankruptcy in 2001 did so because of medical costs and, among these, about 10 percent reported that the cost of cancer care bankrupted them (i.e., an estimated 75,000 individuals) (Himmelstein et al., 2005). A new bankruptcy law will make it more difficult for such individuals to regain their financial footing. Under the old law, people who filed for bankruptcy under Chapter 7 were allowed to erase their debt and start fresh. The new measure makes is less likely that debtors—particularly those who earn more than their state's median income level—will qualify for Chapter 7. Instead, they will have to file under Chapter 13, which requires paying off some or all debt over a designated period of time (Fleck, 2005).

Some cancer survivors with health insurance lack coverage for needed care. In one study of the insurance experience of cancer survivors, 20 of 60 subjects reported that their insurer refused to pay for some aspect of care, including wigs, referrals, out-of-state consultations, antidepressant drugs, and basic supplies (Calhoun and Bennett, 2003). Cancer survivors may have coverage for a needed service (e.g., psychological counseling), but find that the specialists needed to deliver it, for example, a psychologist or social worker trained in oncology, may not be available within their plan's network of providers (IOM, 2004b). Others may face financial hardship paying for services that are explicitly not covered by their policies. Of particular concern for cancer survivors are the costs of expensive drugs used as adjuvant therapies. In a study of men who had transferred from non-Veterans Affairs (VA) hospitals to the VA system for prostate care, the most common reason (reported by 35 percent of men) for transferring care was the high out-of-pocket costs associated with hormonal therapies, primarily oral nonsteroidal antiandrogens (Calhoun and Bennett, 2003).

Some types of coverage for services needed by cancer survivors are mandated by the federal government. The Women's Health and Cancer Rights Act of 1998, for example, is a federal law that requires group health plans or health insurance issuers that cover mastectomies to pay for related services, including reconstruction and surgery to achieve symmetry between the breasts, prostheses, and management of complications resulting from a mastectomy (including lymphedema). This federal law covers those plans not currently covered by state law and sets a minimum standard for women in all states (ACS, 2001; CMS, 2004e).

Every state regulates policies sold by insurance companies in the state. These laws vary significantly. Some states require insurance policies to cover off-label chemotherapy, minimum hospital stays for cancer surgery, and benefits for certain types of cancer treatment and screening. Information on private insurers' policies regarding coverage of post-treatment interventions of potential benefit to cancer survivors is scant. For services related to breast cancer care, 29 states had mandates for coverage of post-mastectomy prosthetic devices for women with breast cancer and 19 states had mandated coverage for post-mastectomy lymphedema therapy as of 2004 (NCI, 2004b). These state mandates, however, do not affect most individuals (54 percent) with employer-based private insurance because of their enrollment in self-insured plans.[17] Such plans are not subject to state health insurance regulation, including regulation relating to mandated benefits and consumer protection (Claxton et al., 2004).

Health insurers have not yet made policies relating to certain cancer-related services of potential benefit to cancer survivors. For example, health insurance coverage of prophylactic mastectomy and oophorectomy varied in one study, with only 44 percent of private plans surveyed having specific policies for coverage of prophylactic mastectomy for patients with a strong family history of breast cancer and 20 percent having a policy for coverage of prophylactic oophorectomy under any clinical circumstance (Kuerer et al., 2000).

Medicare coverage issues The majority of cancer survivors are protected from some elements of insurance discrimination and financial burden because they have Medicare coverage by virtue of being aged 65 and older (61 percent of cancer survivors are aged 65 and older). Because of gaps in Medicare's coverage, however, the elderly spent an estimated 22 percent of their income, on average, for health care services and premiums in 2003 (Caplan and Brangan, 2004). Most individuals covered by Medicare have supplemental insurance through employer-sponsored benefits, Medigap policies, or Medicaid (Kaiser Family Foundation, 2004e).[18] Even with this extent of coverage, however, out-of-pocket expenditures are high. Elderly cancer survivors who report cancer-related health effects had out-of-pocket expenditures that were on average $1,456 as compared to $1,221 among the elderly not reporting cancer-related health effects in 2001–2002 (Figure 6-5). Much of the out-of-pocket expenditures were accounted for by prescription medications which, at the time, Medicare did not cover. Nonelderly cancer survivors face substantially greater incremental out-of-

---

[17]Unlike commercial insurance plans that employers purchase to provide health insurance as a benefit for their employees, self-insured plans are funds set aside by employers to reimburse employees for their allowable medical expenses. Generally, large employer groups or unions find it to their benefit to self-insure, while smaller employer groups choose to finance employee health benefits through commercial insurers.

[18]In 2001, of noninstitutionalized beneficiaries: 34 percent had employer-sponsored benefits; 23 percent owned a Medigap policy; 12 percent were covered under Medicaid; and 18 percent were enrolled in Medicare+Choice plans (Kaiser Family Foundation, 2004e).

pocket expenditures (either because many lack insurance or are underinsured, or because fewer people without cancer have other significant conditions).

In an assessment of 1995 expenditures among cancer survivors aged 70 and older, out-of-pocket spending represented roughly one-quarter of yearly income for those in the bottom income quartile (Langa et al., 2004). Insurance programs that fill Medicare's gaps are important, but even those with supplemental coverage through Medigap policies and retiree health benefits can lack coverage for some out-of-pocket costs. Nearly one-quarter (23 percent) of Medicare beneficiaries, for example, own a Medigap policy, but only 7 percent of all beneficiaries had drug coverage from Medigap (Kaiser Family Foundation, 2004e).

Because so many cancer survivors have health insurance coverage through the federal Medicare program by virtue of their age, its coverage policies are of particular interest. Coverage may vary by the type of Medicare plan in which a survivor may be enrolled. Most Medicare beneficiaries' care is provided through the traditional fee-for-service program. Only 11 percent of beneficiaries are covered by so-called "Senior Advantage Programs" that are managed care plans, primarily HMOs (Kaiser Family Foundation, 2004d). Medicare covers more than 41 million Americans: 35 million seniors and 6 million nonelderly people with disabilities. Medicare consists of four parts (Kaiser Family Foundation, 2004e):

- **Part A**, the Hospital Insurance program, covers inpatient hospital, skilled nursing facility, hospice, and home health care.
- **Part B**, Supplementary Medical Insurance, covers physician and outpatient hospital care, laboratory tests, medical supplies, and home health (the monthly Part B premium is $78.20 in 2005).
- **Part C** refers to managed care plans, referred to as Medicare Advantage (formerly called Medicare+Choice).
- **Part D** refers to the outpatient prescription drug benefit that will be fully implemented in 2006, enacted under the Medicare Prescription Drug, Improvement, and Modernization Act of 2003. The Congressional Budget Office estimates the average monthly Part D premium will be $35 in 2006, although premiums are expected to vary across plans.

The new prescription drug benefit provided by Medicare is of particular interest to cancer survivors because some of the recommended adjuvant and other therapies are extremely costly and currently not covered by Medicare (Marcus, 2004). For example, Tamoxifen, which is prescribed for many women with breast cancer for a period of 5 years following primary treatment, costs an estimated $1,642 annually. Gleevec, a recently approved drug that must be taken indefinitely to treat individuals with chronic myel-

TABLE 6-6 Annual Costs for Cancer Drugs Commonly Administered to Cancer Survivors

Disease	Compound Name (Brand Name) Description of Drug	Annual Estimated Retail Cost[a]
Breast cancer (Stages II to IV)	Letrozole (Femara®) belongs to the family of drugs called nonsteroidal aromatase inhibitors. Letrozole is used to decrease estrogen production and suppress the growth of estrogen-dependent tumors.	$2,843
	Exemestane (Aromasin®) is used to decrease estrogen production and suppress the growth of estrogen-dependent tumors.	$2,827
	Anastrozole (Arimidex®) is a nonsteroidal aromatase inhibitor used to decrease estrogen production and suppress the growth of estrogen-dependent tumors.	$2,700
	Tamoxifen (Nolvadex®) belongs to the family of drugs called antiestrogens and blocks the effects of the hormone estrogen in the breast. It is used to treat breast cancer, and to prevent it in women who are at a high risk of developing breast cancer.	$1,642
	Toremifene (Fareston®) is an antiestrogen that may help control some cancers from growing, and it may delay or reduce the risk of cancer recurrence.	$1,411
Cutaneous T cell lymphoma	Bexarotene (Targretin®) is used to decrease the growth of some types of cancer cells. It belongs to the family of drugs called retinoids. Also called LGD1069.	$61,320
Chronic myelogenous leukemia	Imatinib Mesylate (Gleevec®) inhibits the growth of certain cancers by interfering with an enzyme controlling cell proliferation. Also called STI571.	$45,952

TABLE 6-6 Continued

Disease	Compound Name (Brand Name) Description of Drug	Annual Estimated Retail Cost[a]
Multiple myeloma	Thalidomide (Thalomid®) belongs to the family of drugs called angiogenesis inhibitors. It prevents the growth of new blood vessels into a solid tumor.	$24,098
Gastrointestinal stromal tumor	Imatinib Mesylate (Gleevec®) inhibits the growth of certain cancers by interfering with a portion of the protein produced by the bcr/abl oncogene. Also called STI571.	$45,952

NOTE: Descriptions of drugs adapted from NCI Cancer Dictionary (NCI, 2004a).

[a]The estimated annual retail cost is based on 100 percent of Average Wholesale Price (AWP) from the March 2004 Redbook for a typical dosage; actual retail price for an individual may be more or less.

SOURCES: CMS (2004a).

ogenous leukemia and gastrointestinal stromal tumors, costs $45,952 per year (Table 6-6). These estimates represent annual retail costs, and the extent to which individuals bear the cost depends largely on their insurance policy drug coverage. How Medicare pays for cancer drugs administered in physicians' offices is a subject of great controversy. However, this report focuses on payment issues related primarily to commonly used oral drugs that are now excluded under Medicare's traditional benefit (Part B). Oral and self-administered drugs have not been covered under Medicare and so the cost of many cancer survivors' adjuvant therapy drugs has to be paid for through other means.

Until the Part D prescription drug benefit goes into effect in 2006, beneficiaries can sign up for a federally approved drug discount card, with some low-income beneficiaries receiving a $600 subsidy to help pay drug costs, although relatively few have done so. As of January 2006, beneficiaries will be able to opt for private Part D insurance coverage. Under the standard benefits of such plans, beneficiaries would pay (Kaiser Family Foundation, 2004e):

- The first $250 in drug costs (annual deductible);
- 25 percent of total drug costs between $250 and $2,250;
- 100 percent of drug costs between $2,250 and $5,100 in total drug costs (the $2,850 gap or "hole in the doughnut"), equivalent to a $3,600 out-of-pocket limit; and

- The greater of $2 for generics, $5 for brand drugs, or 5 percent coinsurance after reaching the $3,600 out-of-pocket limit ($5,100 catastrophic threshold).

More generous coverage will be available to those who are poor. About 14 million beneficiaries with limited assets and annual incomes would have 85 to 95 percent of their prescription drug costs covered under Medicare (Kaiser Family Foundation, 2004b,f). Part D premiums and deductibles are to be waived for beneficiaries who are eligible for both Medicare and Medicaid and would require copayments of $1 to $3 per prescription.

A pilot program announced in June 2004 provides prescription drug coverage to 500,000 Medicare beneficiaries with certain serious illnesses, including cancer, until 2006, when the Part D Medicare drug benefit will go into effect (CMS, 2004c). The program provides generous coverage for many of the oral drugs used by cancer survivors (the nine drugs described in Table 6-6 and altretamine [Hexalen] and gefitinib [Iressa]). As of mid-September 2004, fewer than 7,000 individuals had applied to participate in the program. The low levels of participation may be attributed to a lack of awareness of the program on the part of physicians and patients or difficulties in applying to the program (Kaiser Family Foundation, 2004a).

Managed care issues Many people receive care through a managed care plan offered either by a private insurer, Medicaid, or other provider (e.g., military services). Improved access to primary care and coordination of care are potential benefits of managed care plans. There are, however, potential disadvantages within managed care plans for adults with chronic illnesses who need specialized complex care. Under fee-for-service arrangements, individuals with chronic or disabling conditions generally are able to receive specialty care through tertiary care centers and specialty clinics, and from specialty providers. Fully capitated managed care plans may control the use of specialists, especially those outside of their plans' networks. For example, there are anecdotal reports of insurers denying coverage for treatment of lymphedema because the plan does not include a certified lymphedema specialist (Parker-Pope, 2004).

Increasingly, mental health services are being provided by managed behavioral health organizations under separate contracts between the payor and a behavioral health provider. These so-called "carve-out" managed behavioral health care arrangements allow payors to isolate mental health services from overall insurance risk and have mental health care services managed separately from general health care. Some efforts have been made to reintegrate these carve-outs back into health plans in an effort to better coordinate medical and psychosocial care, but there are still hundreds of large corporations that have a behavioral health manager independent of their health insurer (Lee, 2004). This separation is generally acceptable for physically healthy individuals. However, it is highly disadvantageous to patients with a life-threatening or chronic illness who require psychiatric/psychological consultation for related mental disorders. The separation of care delivery can lead to fragmentation of services across medical and behavioral health providers (IOM, 2004b).

Programs Providing Financial Assistance to Help Pay for Care and Other Services

Limited financial assistance is available through government, charitable, and other programs to those who cannot pay for their cancer-related care. These programs and services cannot substitute for adequate insurance coverage for cancer care, but they can ease the financial burden somewhat for small numbers of individuals in need.

A federal program called the Hill-Burton Free Care Program provides limited free or reduced-cost medical services through obligated facilities (mostly hospitals). In exchange for federal funds for construction and modernization, facilities agree to provide a reasonable volume of services to persons unable to pay. Applicants for assistance must meet income eligibility requirements, and assistance may be denied once a facility has given out its required amount of free care (HRSA, 2004).

Many charitable organizations provide free services, financial assistance, or information on getting financial aid to individuals with cancer who lack the means to pay for their care and related expenses:

- The American Cancer Society offers services that can offset some patient costs. The volunteer-based Road to Recovery program, for example, provides transportation for breast cancer patients to and from medical appointments and treatments (ACS, 2004b). The ACS is building "Hope Lodges" near cancer centers where housing and transportation during treatment are available. The extent of ACS services varies from state to state. Not all units offer the same services.
- CancerCare, a nonprofit, voluntary agency, provides, on a limited basis, financial assistance for treatment-related expenses (e.g., transportation, child care, home care, pain medication) (CancerCare, 2003).
- The Leukemia and Lymphoma Society offers financial aid to patients who have leukemia, non-Hodgkin's lymphoma, Hodgkin's disease, or multiple myeloma.
- AVONCares Program provides limited financial assistance for women with breast cancer for transportation, child care, and home care services (CancerCare, 2003).

• Some states support care for the poor and uninsured. Maryland, for example, has a state-funded program (not Medicaid) that provides free treatment for low-income, uninsured women with breast cancer (Pollitz et al., 2004).

• Sharing Hope, a program started by the advocacy organization Fertile Hope, offers cancer patients significant price reductions for sperm banking and egg or embryo freezing through participating reproductive service providers (Fertile Hope, 2005). The Lance Armstrong Foundation is providing funding for the administration of the Sharing Hope program.

Many pharmaceutical companies have patient assistance programs to help individuals with expensive prescription drugs. These programs have stringent eligibility requirements and do not provide comprehensive coverage. In addition, applications for assistance and renewals may be considered on a case-by-case basis and can be time consuming for physicians and their patients. Such programs are vital to cancer survivors; however, they are often limited because of the costly nature of the drugs prescribed for cancer survivors (Table 6-6). The ACS call center links people to pharmaceutical companies that provide financial assistance and helps them with the paperwork.

The National Coalition for Cancer Survivorship, in collaboration with the Oncology Nursing Society, Association of Oncology Social Work, and National Association of Social Workers, has developed a *Cancer Survival Toolbox* that addresses health insurance and financial resources (NCCS, 2004). The NCCS also publishes *What Cancer Survivors Need to Know About Health Insurance*, which describes types of health insurance, legal issues, and information sources (Calder and Pollitz, 2002). A number of other organizations provide comprehensive consumer information related to health insurance (CancerCare, 2003; ACS, 2004a).

The Patient Advocate Foundation is a national nonprofit organization that serves as a liaison between patients and their insurer, employer, and/or creditors to resolve insurance, job retention, and/or debt crisis matters relative to their diagnosis through case managers, doctors, and attorneys. Mediation is provided to assure access to care, maintenance of employment, and preservation of financial stability. The Foundation also provides financial assistance to patients who meet certain qualifications to help them pay for prescriptions and/or treatments. A search by state and type of service needed is available at its website (PAF, 2005).

In summary, very limited financial assistance is available to cancer survivors who are uninsured or underinsured. Evidence suggests such cancer survivors may be financially strained paying for needed care out of pocket, and may delay or forego needed care when they cannot pay. Some of the care provided to such individuals may be uncompensated care borne by physicians and hospitals. The goal of anyone with a history of cancer is to use available means to gain access to health insurance. For the estimated 75,000 individuals facing bankruptcy as a result of cancer-related medical bills, a newly enacted bankruptcy law will make it more difficult for them to get out of debt.

LIFE INSURANCE

Obtaining life insurance coverage may be difficult for survivors of cancer. Because life insurance plans are based on an actuarial risk of death (or survival), the cancer history is often taken into account because it increases the potential risk of death at an earlier age (Lemaire et al., 2000). Some life insurance companies will not insure cancer survivors, and others will charge very high premiums. After 5 years without treatment, some survivors may qualify for standard rates (Lankford, 2002).

Group life insurance (through employment) is a possible solution because a health history is not usually required for such plans. Table 6-7 shows that in 2003, only half of workers in private industry have access to life insurance through their employer (Bureau of Labor Statistics, 2004). Those who have full-time employment are higher wage earners, and those working in large establishments were more likely to have access to life insurance at work.

FINDINGS AND RECOMMENDATIONS

Most working cancer patients require some kind of accommodation to work throughout treatment, and some experience difficulties at work after treatment. Estimates of the impact of cancer on employment vary, but one large recent study showed that one of five individuals who had worked at the time of diagnosis had cancer-related limitations in ability to work 1 to 5 years later. Half of those with limitations were unable to work at all. Cancer-related work limitations appear to be most pronounced in the first 6 months following diagnosis. Many individuals who leave work during treatment are able to return to work a year or two later. Cancer survivors whose jobs involve physical labor are especially likely to have difficulty returning to work following treatment for cancer.

All survivors are at risk of experiencing subtle, although not necessarily blatant, employment discrimination. Federal laws enacted in the 1990s have offered cancer survivors some protections from discriminatory practices such as firing or denial of benefits because of cancer. Such laws have clarified the responsibilities of employers to accommodate workers returning to work with health-related limitations. The most important of these laws, the ADA, continues to be interpreted by the courts and, while protec-

TABLE 6-7 Percentage of Workers with Access to Life Insurance Benefits, by Selected Characteristics, Private Industry, 2003

Characteristic	Life Insurance
All workers	50
Worker characteristics	
White-collar occupations	56
Blue-collar occupations	53
Service occupations	29
Full time	62
Part time	11
Union	63
Nonunion	49
Average wage <$15 per hour	40
Average wage ≥$15 per hour	65
Establishment characteristics	
Goods-producing	61
Service-producing	47
1-99 workers	36
100 workers or more	66

SOURCE: Bureau of Labor Statistics (2004).

tions cover disabled cancer survivors, some survivors have not been fully protected from job loss and access to accommodations for cancer-related work limitations. Successful resolutions on the part of cancer survivors who have filed formal complaints against employers suggest that not all employers have yet fully complied with the law.

Opportunities exist for employers to assist cancer survivors through disability management and return-to-work programs. In addition, information and support can be provided to employees facing cancer through employer-sponsored health programs, workplace intranets, work-life programs, and employee assistance programs. Many employment-related services are available to cancer survivors through public and private voluntary and advocacy organizations, including education, counseling, support, legal advice, vocational rehabilitation, and referral. Limited financial assistance is available as income replacement for cancer survivors who have extended times away from work or who are disabled and can no longer work. Resources available include private short- and long-term disability insurance, available to a minority of employees as a benefit of employment, and income support through the Social Security Administration to those who are disabled.

Recommendation 8: Employers, legal advocates, health care providers, sponsors of support services, and government agencies should act to eliminate discrimination and minimize adverse effects of cancer on employment, while supporting cancer survivors with short-term and long-term limitations in ability to work.

- Cancer professionals, advocacy organizations, and the National Cancer Institute and other government agencies should continue to educate employers and the public about the successes achieved in cancer treatment, the improved prospects for survival, and the continuing productivity of most patients who are treated for cancer.
- Public and private sponsors of services to support cancer survivors and their families should finance programs offering education, counseling, support, legal advice, vocational rehabilitation, and referral for survivors who want to work.
- Providers who care for cancer survivors should become familiar with the employment rights that apply to survivors who want to work and make available information about employment rights and programs that provide counseling, legal services, and referral.
- Providers should routinely ask patients who are cancer survivors if they have physical or mental health problems that are affecting their work, with the goal of improving symptoms and referring patients for rehabilitative and other services.
- Employers should implement programs to assist cancer survivors. Examples include short- and long-term disability insurance, return-to-work programs, wellness programs, accommodation of special needs, and employee assistance programs.
- Cancer survivors should tell their physicians when health problems are affecting them at work. Survivors should educate themselves about their employment rights and contact support organizations for assistance and referrals when needed.

The health insurance issues facing cancer survivors bring into sharp focus the gaps and limitations of health insurance in the United States. All Americans are at risk of becoming a cancer survivor and finding themselves without access to adequate and affordable health insurance. Cancer survivors, like other Americans with serious, chronic health conditions, face significant barriers to coverage because of their health status. In particular, access to individual health insurance may be denied to residents in many states if they have a history of cancer. Cancer survivors may also face surcharged premiums for coverage because of their cancer history, depending on where they live and what type of coverage they seek. The improvements in the care of cancer survivors envisioned by the committee can not be achieved without health insurance that is accessible, adequate, and affordable.

Health insurance provides protection from the very high costs of cancer care. Most cancer survivors have health insurance through the federal Medicare program because they are aged 65 and older. Nevertheless, more than 4 million cancer survivors are under the age of 65. Eleven percent of cancer survivors ages 25 to 64 (approximately 572,000 individuals) are uninsured, and for these individuals, the costs of cancer care can be financially devastating. These younger uninsured cancer survivors report problems in access to care due to concerns about cost—51 percent report delays in obtaining medical care; 44 percent report not getting needed care; and 31 percent report not getting needed prescription medicine. The financial problems posed by cancer loom larger, because even those with health insurance can have trouble paying for prescription drugs and other types of care.

Some evidence indicates that individuals without health insurance have worse cancer outcomes because they receive less appropriate care. Even for those with health insurance, however, out-of-pocket expenditures for cancer care can be high. According to the committee's analyses of the 2001–2002 Medical Expenditure Panel Survey, health-related out-of-pocket expenditures made by those reporting health effects of cancer are high, averaging $1,267 annually for those ages 25 to 64 (13.5 percent of total expenditures) and $1,456 annually (12.5 percent of total expenditures) for those aged 65 and older. These expenditures are significantly higher than those of individuals without a history of cancer.

Since 2000, most states have provided Medicaid coverage to poor and uninsured women who are diagnosed with breast or cervical cancer through the Centers for Disease Control and Prevention's (CDC's) state-based screening programs. Such coverage affords women treatment and follow-up services. The screening program currently serves only 15 percent of the low-income, uninsured women it is intended to serve, so this is not an avenue for many women to ultimately get coverage for their breast or cervical cancer.

State reforms of the individual health insurance market have improved access to coverage among those with chronic health conditions; however, there is evidence that the increased premiums have led some who had individual coverage to forego insurance. High-risk pools are available in most states as insurers of last resort for those ineligible for public or private insurance programs. However, costs of coverage are high and many have limited benefits. The federal government for the first time in 2002 has provided support to assist states with the losses incurred by high-risk pool programs.

HIPAA and COBRA provide some assurance of continuation of insurance coverage if individuals move from one job to another. Cancer survivors, however, continue to have fears regarding maintenance of health insurance—more than one-quarter of survivors expressed concerns about job lock, according to a recent study of cancer survivors' employment-related experiences.

Some benefits needed by cancer survivors have been mandated by the federal government or by states. Women who have had mastectomies, for example, are entitled to reconstruction, prostheses, and care for complications, including lymphedema. Many cancer survivors, however, lack coverage for oral adjuvant therapies that can be very expensive. Medicare's prescription drug plan will go into effect in 2006 and provide some coverage for drugs currently not covered by the program (orally administered cancer drugs). Until then, a pilot program has provided generous prescription drug coverage to cancer survivors in need of these drugs. Relatively few cancer survivors, however, have signed up for this program.

Very limited direct financial assistance is available through the government or voluntary organizations to offset the high costs of cancer care for those who are uninsured or underinsured. The Hill-Burton Free Care Program provides some care, and voluntary organizations sometimes provide assistance for transportation, medicine, and medical supplies. Pharmaceutical companies have patient assistance programs to help individuals with prescription drug costs, but they provide limited assistance and the application process can be onerous. The goal for those without insurance is to gain access to it through available means, for example, through a high-risk insurance pool.

The IOM Committee on the Consequences of Uninsurance, in its 2004 report, *Insuring America's Health*, recommended that the President and Congress develop a strategy to achieve universal insurance coverage and to establish a firm and explicit schedule to reach this goal by 2010 (IOM, 2004a). Only through such efforts will cancer survivors, their families, and health care providers be able to fully focus on care and well-being without being burdened by financial worries. Consistent with this goal, the IOM Committee on Cancer Survivorship recommends the following steps that can be taken between now and 2010 to strengthen health security for cancer survivors.

Recommendation 9: Federal and state policy makers should act to ensure that all cancer survivors have access to adequate and affordable health insurance. Insurers and payors of health care should recognize survivorship care as an essential part of cancer care and design benefits,

payment policies, and reimbursement mechanisms to facilitate coverage for evidence-based aspects of care.

Cancer survivors, like all Americans, may encounter spells when no health insurance is available to them. Most uninsured Americans are not eligible for job-based health benefits (even though the vast majority are in working families) or for Medicaid (even though the vast majority have low incomes). In addition, cancer survivors, like other Americans with serious, chronic health conditions, face other barriers to coverage because of their health status. In particular, access to individual health insurance may be denied to residents in many states if they have a history of cancer. Policy makers should act to ensure that cancer survivors and others with serious chronic health conditions can obtain health insurance that is adequate and affordable. For example, federal funding could support improvements in state high-risk pools—such as premium subsidies, lower cost-sharing options, expanded coverage for prescription drugs, and elimination of preexisting condition exclusion periods. This could help such programs better serve the needs of cancer survivors (as well as people with other serious and chronic health conditions). COBRA, HIPAA, and other programs that guarantee availability of coverage could also be expanded to include premium subsidies.

Because federal legislation generally covers only federal programs such as Medicare and Medicaid, many insurance reforms must be addressed at the state level. Health insurance reforms to expand access to individuals with chronic health conditions must be considered. Whether states pursue reforms through private markets, public programs, or some other means, the goal must be to ensure that all people have access to affordable, adequate health coverage, and furthermore, that the ability to obtain and maintain such coverage is not dependent on health status.

Policy makers can also improve other existing programs aimed at improving health insurance coverage of cancer survivors. In 2000, Congress established a new eligibility category option in Medicaid for uninsured women with breast and cervical cancer. However, only women screened through CDC-funded programs are eligible for this Medicaid coverage and CDC-funded programs today reach less than 15 percent of the program-eligible population. Policy makers could strengthen and build on this program first by ensuring that more eligible women with breast and cervical cancer are reached by it, and second by expanding screening services and Medicaid eligibility to include other cancer patients and survivors who have no other coverage options.

All health insurance in the United States—including Medicare, Medicaid, employer-sponsored group health plans, and individually purchased policies—should cover effective cancer survivorship care. National coverage standards should be promulgated for effective cancer survivorship care, and must include interventions for which there is good evidence of effectiveness (e.g., certain post-treatment surveillance strategies, treatments for late effects, management of symptoms, rehabilitative services). Importantly, coverage standards should include the development of a post-treatment survivorship care plan (see Chapter 3, Recommendation 2). National coverage standards should evolve with the development of clinical guidelines and evidence-based research into quality and effectiveness, and provide adequate reimbursement for quality care provided by cancer centers as well as specialists and primary care providers in communities. The application of cost-sharing requirements to cancer survivorship care must be limited so that financial barriers do not deter access to covered services. Congress has already taken preliminary steps to assure adequacy of some cancer survivorship care. The Women's Health and Cancer Rights Act requires health insurance to cover reconstructive surgery, prostheses, and care for complications following mastectomy, including lymphedema. This model could be expanded to assure minimum federal standards for all cancer survivorship care under all health insurance.

APPENDIX 6A
DESCRIPTION OF THE NATIONAL HEALTH INTERVIEW SURVEY AND THE MEDICAL EXPENDITURE PANEL SURVEY AND THE METHODS USED TO DERIVE ESTIMATES OF INSURANCE COVERAGE AND MEDICAL EXPENDITURES PRESENTED IN THE CHAPTER

NATIONAL HEALTH INTERVIEW SURVEY (NHIS)

Information on the health insurance status of cancer survivors ages 25 to 64 is based on analyses of 4 years of NHIS data (2000 through 2003) (NCHS, 2002, 2003a,b, 2004). The NHIS is a multipurpose health survey conducted by the National Center for Health Statistics, Centers for Disease Control and Prevention. The NHIS is the principal source of information on the health of the civilian, noninstitutionalized, household population of the United States. Analyses were limited to the adult sample component of the survey. Sample sizes and response rates for the sample adult component are shown by year in Table 6A-1.

Computer-assisted personal interviews are conducted in the homes of respondents. The data collected in the NHIS are obtained through a complex sample design involving stratification, clustering, and multistage sampling. African Americans and Hispanics/Latinos are oversampled. All pro-

TABLE 6A-1 NHIS Sample Size and Response Rates, 2000–2003

Year	Sample Size	Response Rate (%)
2000	32,374	72.1
2001	33,326	73.8
2002	31,044	74.3
2003	30,852	74.2

SOURCES: NCHS (2002, 2003a,b, 2004).

portions and population counts (average annual) presented are weighted to provide national estimates.

History of cancer Respondents were asked "Have you ever been told by a doctor or other health professional that you had cancer or a malignancy of any kind?" If the respondent reports a history of cancer, he/she is asked the site of the cancer (the interviewer asked about 30 possible cancer sites) and the age when he/she was first diagnosed with that type of cancer (up to three cancer sites/types could be reported). In these analyses, cancer survivors include respondents who reported ever having a diagnosis of cancer, regardless of whether they had symptoms of cancer at the time of the survey. The current cancer status (i.e., active disease or remission) was not ascertained in the interview. A total of 3,150 sample adults ages 25 to 64 reported a history of cancer (excluding nonmelanoma skin cancers).

Insurance status Individuals with more than one type of insurance were coded as having coverage by Medicare, Medicaid, private, or other type of health insurance, in that order. Other coverage includes state-sponsored health plans, other government programs, and military coverage (includes VA, TRICARE, and CHAMP-VA). The uninsured are persons who did not report having health care coverage at the time of the interview under private health insurance (from employer or workplace, purchased directly, or through a state, local government, or community program), Medicare, Medicaid, Children's Health Insurance Program, a state-sponsored health plan, other government programs, or military health plan.

Number of years since diagnosis Years since diagnosis was calculated from the reported age at interview and age at first diagnosis. When more than one cancer was reported, years since the first diagnosis (excluding superficial skin cancer) were used to calculate years since diagnosis. In a few instances, a correction was made for respondents who provided years since diagnosis instead of age at diagnosis.

MEDICAL EXPENDITURE PANEL SURVEY (MEPS)

Information on cancer-related medical expenditures is based on analyses of 2 years of data from MEPS, 2001–2002. MEPS is co-sponsored by the Agency for Healthcare Research and Quality (AHRQ) and the National Center for Health Statistics (AHRQ, 2005). The household component of MEPS is a nationally representative survey of the U.S. civilian noninstitutionalized population that collects medical expenditure data at both the person and household levels.

The sample for the household component of MEPS was selected from respondents to the NHIS. MEPS is a panel survey, and data are collected through a precontact interview that is followed by a series of five rounds of interviews over 2 years. Two calendar years of medical expenditure and utilization data are collected from each household and captured using computer-assisted personal interviewing.

A history of cancer is not directly asked about as part of MEPS. Instead, the respondent is asked, "We're interested in learning about health problems that may have bothered you since [date]." A history of cancer would be identified if the respondent identified cancer as a condition that had bothered him or her during the reference period. A cancer history would also be identified if a person sought care for cancer, had a bed day or disability day attributable to cancer, or took a prescription medicine for cancer (Personal communication, K. Beauregard, AHRQ, March 2, 2005). Medical conditions reported during the interview were coded using International Classification of Disease, 9th Revision, Clinical Modification (ICD-9-CM) codes. For analyses presented in this chapter, individuals reporting superficial skin cancer were excluded. MEPS may not identify individuals with a history of cancer if they do not have symptoms, are not seeking care for cancer, or are not taking cancer-related prescription medicines.

Expenditures in MEPS refer to payments for health care services. These expenditures are defined as the sum of direct payments for care provided during the year, including out-of-pocket payments and payments by private insurance, Medicaid, Medicare, and other sources. Payments for over-the-counter drugs, alternative care services, and phone contacts with medical providers are not included in MEPS total expenditure estimates. Expenditure data are from a sample of medical and pharmaceutical providers that provided care and medicines to individuals interviewed for the survey. These data from providers are used to improve the overall quality of expenditure data.

In addition to expenditures for total health services, expenses are classified into eight broad types of services and equipment: hospital inpatient, emergency room, outpatient services, medical provider visits, prescribed medicines, dental services, home health services, and other medical equipment and services. These categories are described below:

Hospital inpatient services—This category includes room and board and all hospital diagnostic and laboratory expenses associated with the basic facility charge and payments for separately billed physician inpatient services.

Emergency room (ER) services—This category includes hospital diagnostic and laboratory expenses associated with the ER facility charge and payments for separately billed inpatient services.

Outpatient services—This category includes outpatient diagnostic and laboratory expenses associated with the basic facility charge and payments for separately billed inpatient services.

Medical provider visits—This category covers expenses for visits to a medical provider seen in an office-based setting.

Prescribed medicines—This category includes expenses for all prescribed medications that were initially purchased or otherwise obtained during the calendar year as well as any refills.

Dental services—This category covers expenses for any type of dental care provider, including general dentists, dental hygienists, dental technicians, dental surgeons, orthodontists, endodontists, and periodontists.

Home health services—This category includes expenses for care provided by home health agencies and independent home health providers. Agency providers accounted for most of the expenses in this category.

Other medical equipment and services—This category includes expenses for eyeglasses, contact lenses, ambulance services, orthopedic items, hearing devices, prostheses, bathroom aids, medical equipment, disposable supplies, and other miscellaneous items or services that were obtained, purchased, or rented during the year.

Source-of-Payment Categories

Estimates of sources of payment are classified as follows:

- Out of pocket by user or family.
- Private insurance—Includes payments made by insurance plans covering hospital and medical care (excluding payments from Medicare, Medicaid, and other public sources). Payments from Medigap plans or CHAMPUS and CHAMPVA (Armed Forces-related coverage) are included. Payments from plans that provide coverage for a single service only, such as dental or vision coverage, are not included.
- Medicare—A federally financed health insurance plan for the elderly, persons receiving Social Security disability payments, and most persons with end-stage renal disease. Medicare Part A, which provides hospital insurance, is automatically given to those who are eligible for Social Secu-

rity. Medicare Part B provides supplementary medical insurance that pays for medical expenses and can be purchased for a monthly premium.

- Medicaid—A means-tested government program jointly financed by federal and state funds that provides health care to those who are eligible. Program eligibility criteria vary significantly by state, but the program is designed to provide health coverage to families and individuals who are unable to afford necessary medical care.
- Other public programs—Includes payments from the Department of Veterans Affairs (excluding CHAMPVA); other federal sources (Indian Health Service, military treatment facilities, and other care provided by the federal government); various state and local sources (community and neighborhood clinics, state and local health departments, and state programs other than Medicaid); and Medicaid payments reported for people who were not enrolled in the Medicaid program at any time during the year.
- Other sources—Includes payments from Workers Compensation; other unclassified sources (automobile, homeowner's, or liability insurance, and other miscellaneous or unknown sources); and other private insurance (any type of private insurance payments reported for people without private health insurance coverage during the year as defined in MEPS).

REFERENCES

ABA (American Bar Association). 2004. *Breast Cancer Pro Bono Legal Referral Services.* [Online]. Available: http://www.abanet.org/women/probono.html [accessed September 24, 2004].

Abbe B (CA, Inc.). 2005. *Overview—State High Risk Health Insurance Pools Today.* [Online]. Available: http://www.selfemployedcountry.org/riskpools/overview.html [accessed April 27, 2005].

Achman L, Chollet D (Mathematica Policy Research, Inc.). 2001. *Insuring the Uninsurable: An Overview of State High-Risk Health Insurance Pools.* New York, NY: Commonwealth Fund.

ACS (American Cancer Society). 2001. *Women's Health and Cancer Rights Act.* [Online]. Available: http://www.cancer.org/docroot/MIT/content/MIT_3_2X.asp [accessed September 22, 2004].

ACS. 2004a. *Financial Guidance for Cancer Survivors and Their Families: Off Treatment.* Atlanta, GA: ACS.

ACS. 2004b. *Reach to Recovery.* [Online]. Available: http://www.cancer.org/docroot/ESN/content/ESN_3_1x_Reach_to_Recovery_5.asp?sitearea=SHR [accessed September 27, 2004].

AHRQ (Agency for Healthcare Research and Quality). 2004. *Total Number of People Accounting for Expenditures (deduplicated) by Site of Service: United States, 2002. Medical Expenditure Panel Survey Household Component Data.* [Online]. Available: http://www.meps.ahrq.gov/MEPSNet/TC/TC15.asp?File=HCFY2002&Table=HCFY2002_CNDXP [accessed March 1, 2005].

AHRQ. 2005. *Overview of the MEPS Website.* [Online]. Available: http://www.ahrq.gov/data/mepsweb.htm [accessed April 15, 2005].

Alter C. 2005 (January 27–29). *ICAN: The Individual Cancer Assistance Network.* Presentation at the Second Annual Meeting of the American Psychosocial Oncology Society, Phoenix, AZ.

American Benefits Council. 2004. *Safe and Sound: A Ten-Year Plan for Promoting Personal Financial Security, An Employer Perspective.* Washington, DC: American Benefits Council.

Ayanian JZ, Kohler BA, Abe T, Epstein AM. 1993. The relation between health insurance coverage and clinical outcomes among women with breast cancer. *N Engl J Med* 329(5):326–331.

Bar Association of San Francisco. 2004. *Bar Association of San Francisco homepage.* [Online]. Available: http://www.sfbar.org/ [accessed September 24, 2004].

Barnett A, Birnbaum H, Cremieux PY, Fendrick AM, Slavin M. 2000. The costs of cancer to a major employer in the United States: A case-control analysis. *Am J Manag Care* 6(11):1243–1251.

Blumklotz A, Lansky DJ. 2001. *Health Care Communications for Employees With Chronic Conditions.* Washington, DC: National Health Care Purchasing Institute.

Bordieri JE, Drehmer DE, Taricone PF. 1990. Personnel selection bias for job applicants with cancer. *Journal of Applied Social Psychology* 20(3):244–253.

Bradley C. 2004 (June 16–18). *Labor Market Outcomes of Cancer Survivors.* Presentation at the National Cancer Institute and American Cancer Society Meeting, Cancer Survivorship: Pathways to Health After Treatment, Washington, DC.

Bradley CJ, Bednarek HL. 2002. Employment patterns of long-term cancer survivors. *Psychooncology* 11(3):188–198.

Bradley CJ, Bednarek HL, Neumark D. 2002a. Breast cancer survival, work, and earnings. *J Health Econ* 21(5):757–779.

Bradley CJ, Bednarek HL, Neumark D. 2002b. Breast cancer and women's labor supply. *Health Serv Res* 37(5):1309–1328.

Bradley CJ, Neumark D, Bednarek HL, Schenk M. 2005a. Short-term effects of breast cancer on labor market attachment: Results from a longitudinal study. *J Health Econ* 24(1):137–160.

Bradley CJ, Neumark D, Luo Z, Bednarek HL, Schenk M. 2005b. Employment outcomes of men treated for prostate cancer. *J Natl Cancer Inst* 97(13):958–965.

Bristol-Myers Squibb. 2004. *Creating a Legacy of Hope: Corporate Social Responsibility at Bristol-Myers Squibb.* New York, NY: Bristol-Myers Squibb.

Brown HG, Ming TS. 1992. Vocational rehabilitation of cancer patients. *Semin Oncol Nurs* 8(3):202–211.

Brown ML, Riley GF, Schussler N, Etzioni R. 2002. Estimating health care costs related to cancer treatment from SEER-Medicare data. *Med Care* 40(8 Suppl): IV-104–IV-117.

Bruyere SM. 2000. *Disability Employment Policies and Practices in Private and Federal Sector Organizations.* Ithaca, NY: Cornell University.

Bureau of Labor Statistics. 2004. *National Compensation Survey: Employee Benefits in Private Industry in the United States, March 2004.* Washington, DC: U.S. Department of Labor.

Bureau of Labor Statistics. 2005. *Private industry by supersector and size of establishment: Establishments and employment, first quarter 2003, by State.* [Online]. Available: http://www.bls.gov/cew/ew03table4.pdf [accessed July 18, 2005].

Calder KJ, Pollitz K. 2002. *What Cancer Survivors Need to Know About Health Insurance.* Silver Spring, MD: National Coalition for Cancer Survivorship.

Calhoun EA, Bennett CL. 2003. Evaluating the total costs of cancer. The Northwestern University Costs of Cancer Program. *Oncology (Huntingt)* 17(1):109–114; discussion 119–121.

CancerCare. 2003. *Financial Needs: CancerCare's Financial Assistance Programs.* [Online]. Available: http://www.cancercare.org/FinancialNeeds/FinancialNeedsList.cfm?c=387 [accessed September 19, 2004].

CancerCare. 2004. *Cancer in the Workplace.* [Online]. Available: http://www.cancercare.org/TelephoneEducationWorkshopArchive/TelephoneEducationWorkshop ArchiveList.cfm?c=408 [accessed September 23, 2004].

CancerCare. 2005. *CancerCare homepage.* [Online]. Available: http://www.cancercare.org [accessed May 11, 2005].

Caplan C, Brangan N. 2004. *Out-of-Pocket Spending on Health Care by Medicare Beneficiaries Age 65 and Older in 2003. Public Policy Institute Data Digest.* Washington, DC: AARP Public Policy Institute.

CDC (Centers for Disease Control and Prevention). 2004. *Breast and Cervical Cancer Prevention and Treatment Act of 2000.* [Online]. Available: http://www.cdc.gov/cancer/nbccedp/law106-354.htm [accessed September 22, 2004].

CDC. 2005. *NBCCEDP Screening Program Summaries.* [Online]. Available: http://www.cdc.gov/cancer/nbccedp/sps/index.htm#2 [accessed April 26, 2005].

Center on an Aging Society. 2002. *Cancer: A major national concern.* Challenges for the 21st Century: Chronic and Disabling Conditions Series. No. 4. Washington, DC: Georgetown University.

Center on an Aging Society. 2004. *Workers affected by chronic conditions: How can workplace policies and programs help?* Challenges for the 21st Century: Chronic and Disabling Conditions Series. No. 7. Washington, DC: Georgetown University.

Chirikos TN. 2001. Economic impact of the growing population of breast cancer survivors. *Cancer Control* 8(2):177–183.

Chirikos TN, Russell-Jacobs A, Cantor AB. 2002a. Indirect economic effects of long-term breast cancer survival. *Cancer Pract* 10(5):248–255.

Chirikos TN, Russell-Jacobs A, Jacobsen PB. 2002b. Functional impairment and the economic consequences of female breast cancer. *Women Health* 36(1):1–20.

Claxton G, Gil I, Finder B, Holve E, Gabel J, Pickreign J, Whitmore H, Hawkins S, Fahlman C. 2004. *Employer Health Benefits 2004 Annual Survey.* Menlo Park, CA and Chicago, IL: Henry J. Kaiser Family Foundation and Health Research and Educational Trust.

CMS (Centers for Medicare and Medicaid Services). 2004a. *Beneficiary Fact Sheet (External Use).* [Online]. Available: http://www.cms.hhs.gov/researchers/demos/FctSht_Benefic_REVISED_COSTS_070104.pdf [accessed May 10, 2005].

CMS. 2004b. *Breast and Cervical Cancer Prevention and Treatment Activity Map.* [Online]. Available: http://www.cms.hhs.gov/bccpt/bccptmap.asp [accessed February 17, 2005].

CMS. 2004c. *The Medicare Replacement Drug Demonstration.* [Online]. Available: http://www.cms.hhs.gov/researchers/demos/drugcoveragedemo.asp [accessed September 24, 2004].

CMS. 2004d. *SHO Letter.* [Online]. Available: http://www.cms.hhs.gov/states/letters/sho01041.asp [accessed February 17, 2005].

CMS. 2004e. *The Women's Health and Cancer Rights Act.* [Online]. Available: http://www.cms.hhs.gov/hipaa/hipaa1/content/whcra.asp [accessed September 22, 2004].

Cohen JW, Krauss NA. 2003. Spending and service use among people with the fifteen most costly medical conditions, 1997. *Health Aff (Millwood)* 22(2):129–138.

Cohen RA, Martinez ME. 2005. *Health Insurance Coverage: Estimates from the National Health Interview Survey, 2004.* [Online]. Available: http://www.cdc.gov/nchs/nhis.htm [accessed July 19, 2005].

Conti JV. 1990. Cancer rehabilitation: Why can't we get out of first gear? *Journal of Rehabilitation* 56(4):19–22.

de Lima M, Strom SS, Keating M, Kantarjian H, Pierce S, O'Brien S, Freireich E, Estey E. 1997. Implications of potential cure in acute myelogenous leukemia: Development of subsequent cancer and return to work. *Blood* 90(12):4719–4724.

DeNavas-Walt C, Proctor BD, Mills RJ (U.S. Census Bureau). 2004. *Income, Poverty, and Health Insurance Coverage in the United States: 2003.* Current Population Reports, Pp. 60–226. Washington, DC: U.S. Census Bureau.

Desai MM, Bruce ML, Desai RA, Druss BG. 2001. Validity of self-reported cancer history: A comparison of health interview data and cancer registry records. *Am J Epidemiol* 153(3):299–306.

Duchon L, Schoen C, Doty MM, Davis K, Strumpf E, Bruegman S. 2001. *Security Matters: How Instability in Health Insurance Puts U.S. Workers at Risk.* Washington, DC: The Commonwealth Fund.

EEOC (U.S. Equal Employment Opportunity Commission). 2004a. *Americans with Disabilities Act of 1990 (ADA) Charges FY 1992–FY 2003.* [Online]. Available: http://www.eeoc.gov/stats/ada-charges.html [accessed June 1, 2004].

EEOC. 2004b. *Disability Discrimination.* [Online]. Available: http://www.eeoc.gov/types/ada.html [accessed June 1, 2004].

Employee Assistance Professionals Organization. 2004. *Employee Assistance Professionals Organization.* [Online]. Available: http://www.eapassn.org [accessed September 20, 2004].

Families USA. 2001. *Getting Less Care: The Uninsured With Chronic Health Conditions.* Washington, DC: Families USA.

Felt-Lisk S, McHugh M, Thomas M. 2004. *Examining Access to Specialty Care for California's Uninsured: Full Report.* Oakland, CA: California HealthCare Foundation.

Ferrante JM, Gonzalez EC, Roetzheim RG, Pal N, Woodard L. 2000. Clinical and demographic predictors of late-stage cervical cancer. *Arch Fam Med* 9(5):439–445.

Fertile Hope. 2005. *Financial Assistance.* [Online]. Available: http://www.fertilehope.org/resources/assistance.cfm [accessed February 20, 2005].

Fesko SL. 2001. Workplace experiences of individuals who are HIV+ and individuals with cancer. *Rehabil Couns Bull* 45(1):2–11.

Fleck C. 2005. Throw me a lifeline: The new bankruptcy law could sink families with big medical bills. *AARP Bulletin* (May):28.

Friedland R (Georgetown Center on an Aging Society). 2005. Special analysis of the Medical Expenditure Panel Survey (MEPS). Commissioned by the IOM Committee on Cancer Survivorship. Unpublished.

FWI (Families and Work Institute). 1998. *Business Work-Life Study.* [Online]. Available: http://www.familiesandwork.org/summary/worklife.pdf [accessed April 27, 2005].

GAO (General Accounting Office). 1997. *The Health Insurance Portability and Accountability Act of 1996: Early Implementation Concerns.* Washington, DC: GAO.

GAO. 2000. *Implementation of HIPAA: Progress Slow in Enforcing Federal Standards in Nonconforming States.* Washington, DC: GAO.

GAO. 2001. *Private Health Insurance: Federal Role in Enforcing New Standards Continues to Evolve.* Washington, DC: GAO.

Georgetown University Health Policy Institute. 2004. *Summary of Key Consumer Protections in Individual Health Insurance Markets.* Washington, DC: Georgetown University.

Goetzel RZ, Hawkins K, Ozminkowski RJ, Wang S. 2003. The health and productivity cost burden of the "top 10" physical and mental health conditions affecting six large U.S. employers in 1999. *J Occup Environ Med* 45(1):5–14.

Goff V. 2004. *Consumer Cost Sharing in Private Health Insurance: On the Threshold of Change. NHPF Issue Brief* No. 798. Washington, DC: National Health Policy Forum.

Good Health for Life. 2004. *Good Health for Life homepage.* [Online]. Available: http://www.ghfl.org/ [accessed September 20, 2004].

Grann VR, Jacobson JS. 2003. Health insurance and cancer survival. *Arch Intern Med* 163(18):2123–2124.

Gruber J, Madrian BC. 1993. *Health Insurance and Early Retirement: Evidence From the Availability of Continuation Coverage.* NBER Working Paper Series, Working Paper No. 4594. Cambridge, MA: National Bureau of Economic Research.

Guidry JJ, Aday LA, Zhang D, Winn RJ. 1998. Cost considerations as potential barriers to cancer treatment. *Cancer Pract* 6(3):182–187.

Gusmano MK, Fairbrother G, Park H. 2002. Exploring the limits of the safety net: Community health centers and care for the uninsured. *Health Aff (Millwood)* 21(6):188–194.

Haley J, Zuckerman S. 2003. *Is Lack of Coverage a Short- or Long-Term Condition? Report to the Kaiser Family Foundation Commission on Medicaid and the Uninsured.* Washington, DC: Kaiser Family Foundation.

Hewitt M, Breen N, Devesa S. 1999. Cancer prevalence and survivorship issues: Analyses of the 1992 National Health Interview Survey. *J Natl Cancer Inst* 91(17):1480–1486.

Hewitt M, Rowland JH, Yancik R. 2003. Cancer survivors in the United States: Age, health, and disability. *J Gerontol A Biol Sci Med Sci* 58(1):82–91.

Himmelstein DU, Warren E, Thorne D, Woolhandler S. 2005. MarketWatch: Illness and injury as contributors to bankruptcy. *Health Aff (Millwood)* [Online]. Available: http://content.healthaffairs.org/cgi/reprint/hlthaff.w5.63v1?maxtoshow=&HITS=10&hits=10&RESULTFORMAT=&author1=himmelstein&fulltext=bankruptcy&andorexactfulltext=and&searchid=1121117324126_3699&stored_search=&FIRSTINDEX=0&resourcetype=1&journalcode=healthaff [accessed July 11, 2005].

Hoffman B. 1989. Cancer survivors at work: Job problems and illegal discrimination. *Oncol Nurs Forum* 16(1):39–43.

Hoffman B. 1991. Employment discrimination: Another hurdle for cancer survivors. *Cancer Invest* 9(5):589–595.

Hoffman B. 1999. Cancer survivors' employment and insurance rights: A primer for oncologists. *Oncology (Huntingt)* 13(6):841–846; discussion 846, 849, 852.

Hoffman B. 2000. Between a disability and a hard place: The cancer survivors' Catch-22 of proving disability status under the Americans with Disabilities Act. *Maryland Law Review* 59(2):352–439.

Hoffman B. 2002. *Policy Recommendations to Address the Employment and Insurance Concerns of Cancer Survivors.* Background paper commissioned by the IOM. Unpublished.

Hoffman B. 2004a. *A Cancer Survivor's Almanac: Charting Your Journey.* 3rd ed. Hoboken, NJ: John Wiley & Sons.

Hoffman B. 2004b. Working it out: Your employment rights. In: Hoffman B, ed. *A Cancer Survivor's Almanac: Charting Your Journey.* 3rd ed. Hoboken, NJ: John Wiley & Sons. Pp. 242–269.

HRSA (Health Resources and Services Administration). 2004. *Health Resources and Services Administration homepage.* [Online]. Available: http://www.hrsa.gov [accessed September 22, 2004].

Hwang W, Weller W, Ireys H, Anderson G. 2001. Out-of-pocket medical spending for care of chronic conditions. *Health Aff (Millwood)* 20(6):267–278.

IOM (Institute of Medicine). 2001. *Coverage Matters: Insurance and Health Care.* Washington, DC: National Academy Press.

IOM. 2002a. *Care Without Coverage: Too Little, Too Late.* Washington, DC: The National Academies Press.

IOM. 2002b. *The Dynamics of Disability: Measuring and Monitoring Disability for Social Security Programs.* Wunderlich GS, Rice DP, Amado NL, eds. Washington, DC: The National Academies Press.

IOM. 2004a. *Insuring America's Health: Principles and Recommendations.* Washington, DC: The National Academies Press.

IOM. 2004b. *Meeting Psychosocial Needs of Women with Breast Cancer.* Hewitt M, Herdman R, Holland J, eds. Washington, DC: The National Academies Press.

Kaiser Family Foundation. 2001. *Medicaid's Role for the Disabled Population Under Age 65.* Washington, DC: Kaiser Family Foundation.

Kaiser Family Foundation. 2004a. *The Economic Downturn and Changes in Health Insurance Coverage, 2000–2003* [Online]. Available at: http://www.kff.org/uninsured/7174.cfm (accessed July 11, 2005).

Kaiser Family Foundation. 2004b. *Kaiser Daily Health Policy Report: Bush Administration Releases Proposed Rules for Medicare Prescription Drug Benefit.* [Online]. Available: http://www.kaisernetwork.org/daily_reports/rep_index.cfm?DR_ID=24978 [accessed July 27, 2004].

Kaiser Family Foundation. 2004c. *Kaiser Daily Health Policy Report: Senate Committee Approves Bill to Help States Create High-Risk Health Insurance Pools.* [Online]. Available: http://www.kaisernetwork.org/daily_reports/print_report.cfm?DR_ID=25896&dr_cat+3 [accessed September 23, 2004].

Kaiser Family Foundation. 2004d. *Medicare Advantage Fact Sheet.* Menlo Park, CA: Kaiser Family Foundation.

Kaiser Family Foundation. 2004e. *Medicare at a Glance Fact Sheet.* Menlo Park, CA: Kaiser Family Foundation.

Kaiser Family Foundation. 2004f. *The Medicare Prescription Drug Law Fact Sheet.* Menlo Park, CA: Kaiser Family Foundation.

Kenny KA, Blake SC, Maloy K, Ranji UR, Salganicoff A (George Washington University School of Public Health and Health Services and the Henry J. Kaiser Family Foundation). 2004. *Hearing Their Voices: Lessons From the Breast and Cervical Cancer Prevention and Treatment Act.* Menlo Park, CA: Kaiser Family Foundation.

Kessler RC, Greenberg PE, Mickelson KD, Meneades LM, Wang PS. 2001. The effects of chronic medical conditions on work loss and work cutback. *J Occup Environ Med* 43(3):218–225.

Kornblith AB. 1998. Psychosocial adaptation of cancer survivors. In: Holland JC, ed. *Psycho-Oncology.* New York, NY: Oxford University Press.

Kuerer HM, Hwang ES, Anthony JP, Dudley RA, Crawford B, Aubry WM, Esserman LJ. 2000. Current national health insurance coverage policies for breast and ovarian cancer prophylactic surgery. *Ann Surg Oncol* 7(5):325–332.

LAF (Lance Armstrong Foundation). 2004. *LiveStrong.* [Online]. Available: http://www.livestrong.org [accessed September 20, 2004].

Langa KM, Fendrick AM, Chernew ME, Kabeto MU, Paisley KL, Hayman JA. 2004. Out-of-pocket health-care expenditures among older Americans with cancer. *Value Health* 7(2):186–194.

Lankford K. 2002. Covering a Survivor. *Kiplinger's Personal Finance* 56(3):108.

Laris M. 2005a (January 10). Loudoun teacher with cancer forced out. *The Washington Post.* P. B3.

Laris M. 2005b (January 13). Teacher with cancer is offered her job back. *The Washington Post.* P. B1.

Lee FC. 2004. Employer-based disease management programs in cancer. *Dis Manage Health Outcomes* 12(1):9–17.

Lee-Feldstein A, Feldstein PJ, Buchmueller T, Katterhagen G. 2000. The relationship of HMOs, health insurance, and delivery systems to breast cancer outcomes. *Med Care* 38(7):705–718.

Legal Information Network for Cancer. 2004. *LINC homepage*. [Online]. Available: http://www.cancerlinc.org/ [accessed September 24, 2004].

Lemaire J, Subramanian K, Armstrong K, Asch DA. 2000. Pricing term insurance in the presence of a family history of breast or ovarian cancer. *North American Actuarial Journal* 4(2):75–87.

Loy B, Batiste LC. 2004. *Accommodating People with Cancer*. [Online]. Available: http://www.jan.wvu.edu/media/Cancer.html [accessed June 1, 2004].

Marcus AD. 2004 (September 7). Price becomes factor in cancer treatment. *The Wall Street Journal*. P. D1.

May JH, Cunningham PJ. 2004. *Tough Trade-Offs: Medical Bills, Family Finances, and Access to Care*. Issue Brief No. 85. Washington, DC: Center for Studying Health System Change.

McDavid K, Tucker TC, Sloggett A, Coleman MP. 2003. Cancer survival in Kentucky and health insurance coverage. *Arch Intern Med* 163(18):2135–2144.

Mellette SJ. 1985. The cancer patient at work. *CA Cancer J Clin* 35(6):360–373.

Merlis M. 2005. *Fundamentals of Underwriting in the Nongroup Health Insurance Market: Access to Coverage and Options for Reform*. NHPF Background Paper. Washington, DC: National Health Policy Forum.

Messner C, Patterson D. 2001. The challenge of cancer in the workplace. *Cancer Pract* 9(1):50–51.

Mundy RR, Moore SC, Mundy GD. 1992. A missing link: Rehabilitation counseling for persons with cancer. *Journal of Rehabilitation* 58(2):47–49.

NCCS (National Coalition for Cancer Survivorship). 2004. *Cancer Survival Toolbox*. Silver Spring, MD: NCCS.

NCCS and Amgen. Undated. *Cancer in the Workplace Survey Highlights*. Silver Spring, MD: NCCS.

NCHS (National Center for Health Statistics). 2002. *2000 National Health Interview Survey (NHIS) Public Use Data Release*. Hyattsville, MD: NCHS.

NCHS. 2003a. *2001 National Health Interview Survey (NHIS) Public Use Data Release*. Hyattsville, MD: NCHS.

NCHS. 2003b. *2002 National Health Interview Survey (NHIS) Public Use Data Release*. Hyattsville, MD: NCHS.

NCHS. 2004. *2003 National Health Interview Survey (NHIS) Public Use Data Release*. Hyattsville, MD: NCHS.

NCI. 2002. *Facing Forward: Life After Cancer Treatment*. Bethesda, MD. NCI.

NCI (National Cancer Institute). 2004a. *Dictionary of Cancer Terms*. [Online]. Available: http://www.nci.nih.gov/templates/db_alpha.aspx?expand=A [accessed September 24, 2004].

NCI. 2004b. *Fact Sheet: Breast Cancer*. Bethesda, MD. NCI.

NCI. 2005. *Estimated U.S. Cancer Prevalence*. [Online]. Available: http://cancercontrol.cancer.gov/ocs/prevalence/prevalence.html [accessed July 29, 2005].

NCSL (National Conference of State Legislatures). 2005. *State Genetics Employment Laws*. [Online]. Available: http://www.ncsl.org/programs/health/genetics/ndiscrim.htm [accessed June 15, 2005].

New York Legal Assistance Group. 2004. *NYLAG homepage*. [Online]. Available: http://nylag.org/ [accessed September 24, 2004].

PAF (Patient Advocate Foundation). 2005. *Report Search*. [Online]. Available: http://www.patientadvocate.org/report.php [accessed February 20, 2005].

Parker-Pope T. 2004 (June 1). Efforts mount to combat lymphedema, a devastating side effect of cancer care. *The Wall Street Journal.* P. D1.

Penson DF, Stoddard ML, Pasta DJ, Lubeck DP, Flanders SC, Litwin MS. 2001. The association between socioeconomic status, health insurance coverage, and quality of life in men with prostate cancer. *J Clin Epidemiol* 54(4):350–358.

Pereira J. 2003 (July 14). To save on healthcare costs, firms fire disabled workers. *The Wall Street Journal.* P. A1.

Pollitz K. 2004 (October 27–28). *Health Insurance Problems for People with Serious and Chronic Illnesses.* Presentation at the meeting of the IOM Committee on Cancer Survivorship, Irvine, CA.

Pollitz K, Lewis S, Kofman M, Bangit E, Lucia K, Libster J. 2004. *A Consumer's Guide to Getting and Keeping Health Insurance in Maryland.* Washington, DC: Georgetown University Health Policy Institute.

Pollitz K, Sorian R, Thomas K (Georgetown University Institute for Health Care Research and Policy and K.A. Thomas and Associates). 2001. *How Accessible Is Individual Health Insurance for Consumers in Less-Than-Perfect Health?* Menlo Park, CA: Kaiser Family Foundation.

Pollitz K, Tapay N, Hadley E, Specht J. 2000. Early experience with 'new federalism' in health insurance regulation. *Health Aff (Millwood)* 19(4):7–22.

Pyenson B, Zenner PA. 2002. *The Cost of Cancer to the Worksite.* New York, NY: Milliman USA, Inc.

Roessler R, Sumner G. 1997. Employer opinions about accommodating employees with chronic illnesses. *Journal of Applied Rehabilitation Counseling* 28(3):29–34.

Roetzheim RG, Gonzalez EC, Ferrante JM, Pal N, Van Durme DJ, Krischer JP. 2000a. Effects of health insurance and race on breast carcinoma treatments and outcomes. *Cancer* 89(11):2202–2213.

Roetzheim RG, Pal N, Gonzalez EC, Ferrante JM, Van Durme DJ, Krischer JP. 2000b. Effects of health insurance and race on colorectal cancer treatments and outcomes. *Am J Public Health* 90(11):1746–1754.

Rothstein MA, Kennedy K, Ritchie KJ, Pyle K. 1995. Are cancer patients subject to employment discrimination? *Oncology (Huntingt)* 9(12):1303–1306; discussion 1311–1312, 1315.

Sanchez KM, Richardson JL. 2004 (June 16–18). *Cancer History Disclosure in the Workplace.* Presentation at the NCI and ACS Cancer Survivorship: Pathways to Health After Treatment meeting, Washington, DC.

Schwerin B. 2005 (January 27–28). *The Cancer Legal Resource Center—Assistance for Cancer-Related Legal Issues.* Presentation at the Annual Conference of the American Psychosocial Oncology Society, Phoenix, AZ.

Short PF, Graefe DR, Schoen C. 2003. *Churn, Churn, Churn: How Instability of Health Insurance Shapes America's Uninsured Problem.* Washington, DC: The Commonwealth Fund Issue Brief.

Short PF, Vasey J, Markowski M, Zabora J, Harper G, Rybka W. 2005a. *Quality of Life in a Large Cohort of Adult Cancer Survivors.* Penn State Population Research Institute Working Paper 2005–01. [Online]. Available: http://www.pop.psu.edu/general/pubs/working_papers/psu-pri/wp0501.pdf [accessed April 13, 2005].

Short PF, Vasey JJ, Tunceli K. 2005b. Employment pathways in a large cohort of adult cancer survivors. *Cancer* 103(6):1292–1301.

Spelten ER, Sprangers MA, Verbeek JH. 2002. Factors reported to influence the return to work of cancer survivors: A literature review. *Psychooncology* 11(2):124–131.

SSA (Social Security Administration). 2004a. *Annual Statistical Report on the Social Security Disability Insurance Program.* Washington, DC: SSA.

SSA. 2004b. *SSI Annual Statistical Report, 2003*. Washington DC: SSA.

State High Risk. 2004. *State High Risk Pool Funding Extension Act of 2004 (Introduced in Senate)*. [Online]. Available: http://thomas.loc.gov/cgi-bin/query/z?c108:S.2283: [accessed October 5, 2004].

State High Risk. 2005. *State High Risk Pool Funding Extension Act of 2005 (Reported in Senate)*. [Online]. Available: http://thomas.loc.gov/cgi-bin/query/D?c109:1:./temp/~c109zOUpsl: [accessed April 14, 2005].

Steiner JF, Cavender TA, Main DS, Bradley CJ. 2004. Assessing the impact of cancer on work outcomes: What are the research needs? *Cancer* 101(8):1703–1711.

Taylor JC, Terrell JE, Ronis DL, Fowler KE, Bishop C, Lambert MT, Myers LL, Duffy SA, Bradford CR, Chepeha DB, Hogikyan ND, Prince ME, Teknos TN, Wolf GT. 2004. Disability in patients with head and neck cancer. *Arch Otolaryngol Head Neck Surg* 130(6):764–769.

Thorpe KE, Howard D. 2003. Health insurance and spending among cancer patients. *Health Aff (Millwood)* (Suppl): W3-189–198 [Online]. Available: http://content.healthaffairs.org/cgi/reprint/hlthaff.w3.189v1 (accessed July 11, 2005).

Tu HT. 2004. *Rising Health Costs, Medical Debt and Chronic Conditions*. Issue Brief No. 88. Washington, DC: Center for Studying Health System Change.

U.S. Department of Labor. 2000. *Accommodating Employees with Hidden Disabilities*. [Online]. Available: http://www.dol.gov/odep/pubs/ek00/hiddenemp.htm [accessed June 7, 2004].

U.S. Department of Labor. 2004a. *Fact Sheet #28: The Family and Medical Leave Act of 1993*. [Online]. Available: http://www.dol.gov/esa/regs/compliance/whd/printpage.asp?REF=whdfs28.htm [accessed September 16, 2004].

U.S. Department of Labor. 2004b. *Low Cost Accommodation Solutions*. [Online]. Available: http://www.jan.wvu.edu/media/LowCostSolutions.html [accessed September 15, 2004].

U.S. Department of Labor. 2004c. *What is JAN?* [Online]. Available: http://www.jan.wvu.edu/english/whatis.htm [accessed June 4, 2004].

U.S. DHHS (U.S. Department of Health and Human Services). 2002. *HHS to Help States Create High-Risk Pools to Increase Access to Health Coverage*. [Online]. Available: http://www.hhs.gov/news/press/2002pres/20021126a.html [accessed January 31, 2003].

U.S. DHHS. 2003a. *HHS Awards $690,000 to Maryland to Promote High-Risk Pools to Cover Uninsured Residents*. [Online]. Available: http://www.hhs.gov/news/press/2003pres/20030430b.html [accessed September 2004].

U.S. DHHS. 2003b. *HHS to Award $80 Million to States to Offset Costs of Insurance for Residents Too Sick for Conventional Coverage*. [Online]. Available: http://www.hhs.gov/news/press/2003pres/20030428.html [accessed September 2004].

U.S. DHHS. 2003c. *HHS Awards Nearly $30 Million to States to Offset Costs of Insurance for Residents Too Sick for Conventional Coverage*. [Online]. Available: http://www.hhs.gov/news/press/2003pres/20031217a.html [accessed September 2004].

Voelker R, ed. 1999. *Living, Coping, and Working with Cancer. Business and Health*. Vol. 3. Montvale, NJ: Medical Economics Company.

White House. 2000. *Executive Order to Prohibit Discrimination in Federal Employment Based on Genetic Testing*. [Online]. Available: http://www.opm.gov/pressrel/2000/genetic_eo.htm [accessed September 16, 2004].

Williams CH, Fuchs BC (Robert Wood Johnson Foundation). 2004. *Expanding the Individual Health Insurance Market: Lessons From the State Reforms of the 1990s*. The Synthesis Project, Policy Brief No. 4. Princeton, NJ: Robert Wood Johnson Foundation.

Yabroff KR, Lawrence WF, Clauser S, Davis WW, Brown ML. 2004. Burden of illness in cancer survivors: Findings from a population-based national sample. *J Natl Cancer Inst* 96(17):1322–1330.

7

Research

The emergence of survivorship research represents a change in focus for cancer research—from a focus largely on cure to one including longer term issues of morbidity and the quality of life of cancer survivors (Aziz, 2002, 2004). This chapter describes survivorship research in terms of its scope, methodologies for its conduct, the challenges it poses to investigators, and available sources of support. The chapter concludes with the committee's identification of priority areas for research and recommendations for improving what we know about cancer survivors and their health care.

SURVIVORSHIP RESEARCH

The goal of survivorship research is to understand, and thereby reduce, the adverse effects of cancer diagnosis and treatment and to optimize outcomes for cancer survivors and their families (Aziz, 2002, 2004). Treatment effects, follow-up care, economic sequelae, health disparities, and family and caregiver issues are among the domains of survivorship research (Table 7-1). Survivorship research has in the past decade evolved from small, single-investigator, hypothesis-generating studies relying on convenience samples to interdisciplinary, rigorous tests of interventions through clinical trials. Research efforts have also broadened to begin to examine issues of concern to the full range of cancer survivors, with attention to ethnic and racial minorities, the elderly, rural residents, and those with rare cancers (Aziz, 2004). As Table 7-1 illustrates, a variety of research methods, both qualitative and quantitative, can be applied to this field. The increased

TABLE 7-1 Domains of Cancer Survivorship Research

Survivorship Research Domain	Definition and Potential Research Foci
Descriptive and analytic research	Documenting for diverse cancer sites the prevalence and incidence of physiologic and psychosocial late effects, second cancers, and their associated risk factors Determining physiologic outcomes of interest, including late and long-term medical effects such as cardiac or endocrine dysfunction, premature menopause, and the effects of other comorbidities on these adverse outcomes Measuring psychosocial outcomes of interest, including the longitudinal evaluation of survivors' quality of life, coping and resilience, and spiritual growth
Intervention research	Examining strategies that can prevent or diminish adverse physiologic or psychosocial sequelae of cancer survivorship Elucidating the impact of specific interventions (psychosocial, behavioral, or medical) on subsequent health outcomes or health practices
Examination of survivorship sequelae for understudied cancer sites	Examining the physiologic, psychosocial, and economic outcomes among survivors of colorectal, head and neck, hematologic, lung, or other understudied sites
Follow-up care and surveillance	Elucidating whether the timely introduction of optimal treatment strategies can prevent or control late effects Evaluating the effectiveness of follow-up care clinics/programs in detecting recurrence of the index cancer, detecting new primary cancers, and preventing or ameliorating long-term effects of cancer and its treatment, thereby increasing duration of life and quality of life Evaluating alternative surveillance strategies and models of follow-up care for cancer survivors that take into account cultural expectations, patient preference, insurance status, and other factors Developing a consistent, standardized model of service delivery for cancer-related follow-up care across cancer centers and community oncology practices Assessing optimal quality, content, frequency, setting, and provider of follow-up care for survivors
Economic sequelae	Examining the economic effects of cancer for the survivor and family and the health and quality of life outcomes resulting from diverse patterns of care and service delivery settings

Continued

TABLE 7-1 Continued

Survivorship Research Domain	Definition and Potential Research Foci
Health disparities	Elucidating similarities and differences in the survivorship experience across diverse diagnostic, race, ethnic, gender, and socioeconomic groups Examining the potential role of ethnicity in influencing the quality and length of survival from cancer
Family and caregiver issues	Exploring the impact of cancer diagnosis in a loved one on the family and the impact of family and caregivers on survivors
Instrument development	Developing instruments capable of collecting valid data on survivorship outcomes, specifically for survivors beyond the acute cancer treatment period Developing/testing tools to evaluate long-term survivorship outcomes that (1) are sensitive to change, (2) include domains of relevance to long-term survivorship, and (3) will permit comparison of survivors to groups of individuals without a cancer history and/or with other chronic diseases over time Identifying criteria or cutoff scores for qualifying a change in function as being clinically significant

SOURCE: Adapted from Aziz and Rowland (2003).

sophistication and breadth of survivorship research can be traced largely to a prioritization by the National Cancer Institute (NCI) of survivorship research and the establishment in 1996 of the NCI's Office of Cancer Survivorship (NCI Director, 2002, 2003; Aziz, 2004). Trends in research publications indicate an increased level of activity within this relatively new discipline (Figure 7-1).

Despite the apparent growth in research productivity, the volume of cancer survivorship research is dwarfed by research aimed at cancer treatment (Figure 7-2). The recent emergence of the discipline and the modest levels of research support relative to that available for treatment-related research (see discussion below) may explain some of the difference in research activity. Inherent challenges of the research itself—for example, the need for extended periods of follow-up—may also account for the observed differences (see discussion below).

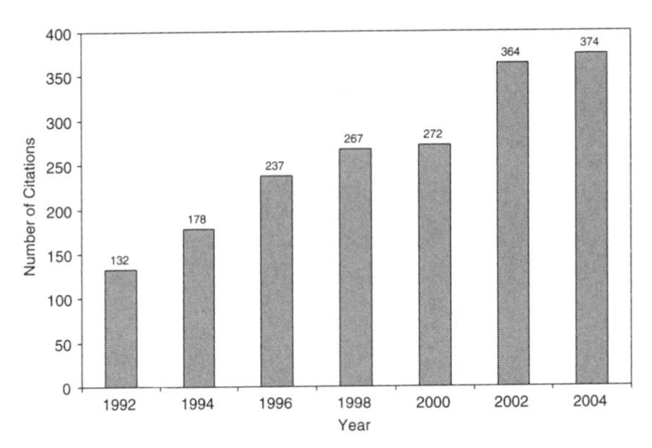

FIGURE 7-1 PubMed citations for adult cancer survivorship research, 1992–2004.

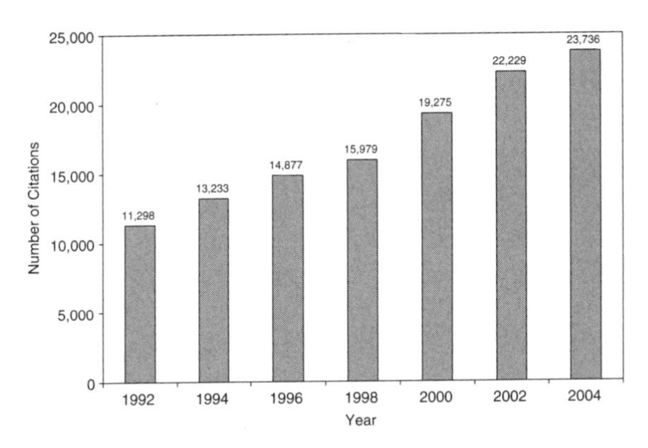

FIGURE 7-2 PubMed citations for adult cancer treatment research, 1992–2004.

NOTE: The National Library of Medicine's PubMed database includes citations from MedLine, HealthStar, and other bibliographic databases. The database stores information about individual citations, including index terms used to characterize each article (articles are indexed according to a dictionary of medical subject headings called MeSH terms). Citations were identified using the MeSH terms "neoplasms" and "survivors," and keywords (e.g., survivor, survivorship, late effects, long-term effects), excluding citations categorized under the MeSH terms "child," "adolescent," "infant," "child, preschool," or "pediatrics." The MeSH heading "survivors" refers to "persons who have experienced a prolonged survival after serious disease or who continue to live with a usually life-threatening condition as well as family members, significant others, or individuals surviving traumatic life events" (NLM, 2004). Citations were limited to those pertaining to "humans" and published in English. There would be an underestimate of survivorship-related citations if the "survivors" MeSH term was not applied by abstractors to the citations or if the title and abstracts of articles varied in their inclusion of keywords.
SOURCE: National Library of Medicine's PubMed database (NLM, 2005).

MECHANISMS FOR CONDUCTING RESEARCH

Survivorship-related research is often conducted through several mechanisms—clinical trials, cohort studies and analyses of cancer registries, administrative data, and surveys. This section of the chapter briefly describes these research mechanisms. The next section of the chapter enumerates some of the challenges investigators face in conducting survivorship research.

Clinical Trials

Much has been learned about the late effects of cancer treatment through long-term follow-up of participants enrolled in clinical trials of cancer treatments (Fairclough et al., 1999; Ganz et al., 2003b). In addition, clinical trials are conducted to test interventions to prevent treatment late effects among survivors of adult cancer and to test treatments for late effects (Table 7-2). Many of these survivorship-related trials are supported by the NCI through its Clinical Trials Cooperative Group Program, whose purpose is to develop and conduct large-scale trials in multi-institutional settings. There are currently 12 NCI-supported Cooperative Groups, 11 for adult malignancies and 1 for childhood cancer. This program involves more than 1,700 institutions and enrolls more than 22,000 new patients into cancer treatment clinical trials each year (NCI, 2003b).

Cancer clinical trials in the United States have focused on primary treatment, with relatively few trials examining supportive care, and none examining surveillance strategies (Table 7-3). An analysis of NCI-sponsored clinical trials on symptom management from 1987 to 2004 found relatively few trials with a primary end point related to late effects (e.g., hot flashes, cognitive function, osteoporosis) (Buchanan et al., 2005). Most such trials were focused on immediate symptoms of treatment (e.g., cachexia, pain). Relatively few clinical trials have assessed the appropriateness of follow-up strategies for individuals with cancer, and most of them have been conducted in Europe (see Chapter 3).

Cohort Studies

Cohort studies assess the experience of a group of individuals with a common characteristic, for example, a cancer diagnosis or a particular type of treatment. The cohort may be identified currently and followed up prospectively, or identified retrospectively with subsequent evaluation of health status. Cohorts of individuals with cancer diagnoses have been identified from cancer registries and asked to participate in special studies. Four examples of this approach include the American Cancer Society's (ACS's)

Study of Cancer Survivors, the NCI's Prostate Cancer Outcomes Study, the Cancer of the Prostate Strategic Urologic Research Endeavor (CaPSURE), and studies of the NCI-sponsored Cancer Care Outcomes Research and Surveillance (CanCORS) Consortium. Cohorts may also be identified from patients treated at cancer centers. Two examples of such efforts are the long-term follow-up experience of individuals with Hodgkin's disease who were treated at Stanford University Medical Center in California and a collaborative study of a cohort of survivors of childhood cancer. Although survivors of childhood cancer are not the focus of this study,[1] the cohort study of childhood cancer is described here because it can possibly serve as a model for a comparable study of adult cancer survivors.

ACS Study of Cancer Survivors

The ACS's intramural Behavioral Research Center is conducting two surveys of cancer survivors. The first is the Study of Cancer Survivors–I (SCS–I), a longitudinal study of quality of life of adult cancer survivors. Participating survivors complete questionnaires at 1, 2, 5, and 10 years after diagnosis, allowing a comparison of changes over time and an assessment of the long-term impact of cancer on survivors. The study's sample includes adults diagnosed with 1 of 10 common cancers (breast, prostate, lung, colorectal, bladder, non-Hodgkin's lymphoma, cutaneous melanoma, kidney, ovarian, and uterine). SCS-I also includes a family caregiver research component to explore the impact of the family's involvement in cancer care on the quality of life of the cancer survivor and the caregiver.

The second survey of cancer survivors is the Study of Cancer Survivors–II (SCS–II), a national cross-sectional study of 2-, 5-, and 10-year cancer survivors that also focuses on quality of life. Survivors of breast, prostate, colorectal, bladder, cutaneous melanoma, and uterine cancer are participating in this study. The results will provide a basis for advocacy and planning by the ACS as well as by other health organizations and agencies.

The participants in both studies are selected with the cooperation of state cancer registries from the lists they maintain of people diagnosed with cancer. As of 2005, nearly 10,000 participants had been enrolled in the combined studies. Preliminary analyses of the cross-sectional data have provided information on the quality of life problems faced by survivors. The SCS–II study is expected to complete accrual of participants in the spring of 2005, while SCS–I will continue for several years.

---

[1]For more information on survivors of childhood cancer, see the IOM report *Childhood Cancer Survivorship: Improving Care and Quality of Life* (IOM, 2003a).

TABLE 7-2 Examples of Clinical Trials of Relevance to Survivors of Adult Cancers

Topic	Trial	Sponsor	Phase[a]
Preventing the late effects of treatment			
Sense of taste	Zinc sulfate in preventing loss of sense of taste in patients undergoing radiation therapy for head and neck cancer	North Central Cancer Treatment Cooperative Group	III
Bone loss	Zoledronate, calcium, and vitamin D in preventing bone loss in women receiving adjuvant chemotherapy for breast cancer	Cancer and Leukemia Cooperative Group B	III
Ovarian failure	Goserelin in preventing ovarian failure in women receiving adjuvant chemotherapy for breast cancer	Southwest Oncology Cooperative Group	III
Lymphedema	Fibrin sealant in decreasing lymphedema following surgery to remove lymph nodes in patients with cancer of the vulva	Gynecologic Oncology Cooperative Group	III
Treating or ameliorating late effects			
Peripheral neuropathy	Amifostine in treating peripheral neuropathy in patients who have received chemotherapy for gynecologic malignancy	Gynecologic Oncology Cooperative Group	III
Depression	Sertraline compared with hypericum perforatum (St. John's Wort) in treating mild to moderate depression in patients with cancer	Comprehensive Cancer Center of Wake Forest University	III

Neurocognitive function	Donepezil and EGb761 in improving neurocognitive function in patients who have previously undergone radiation therapy for primary brain tumor or brain metastases	Comprehensive Cancer Center of Wake Forest University	II
Hot flashes	Randomized study of gabapentin for the management of hot flashes in patients with prostate cancer	North Central Cancer Treatment Cooperative Group	III
Sleep	Valeriana officinalis (Valerian) for improving sleep in patients with cancer receiving adjuvant therapy	North Central Cancer Treatment Cooperative Group	III
Sexual function	Low-dose testosterone in improving libido in post-menopausal female cancer survivors	North Central Cancer Treatment Cooperative Group	III
Fatigue	Randomized study of levocarnitine (L-carnitine) for the management of fatigue in cancer patients	Eastern Cooperative Oncology Group	III
Pain	Acupuncture for neck and shoulder pain following neck surgery in cancer patients	National Center for Complementary and Alternative Medicine	III
Lymphedema	Pycnogenol for the treatment of lymphedema of the arm in breast cancer survivors	National Center for Complementary and Alternative Medicine	II

[a]Phase I clinical trials generally enroll few people and evaluate how an intervention should be administered (e.g., for drugs, if by mouth, injected into the blood, or injected into the muscle) and the safety of the intervention. Phase II clinical trials continue to test the safety of the intervention, and begin to evaluate how well the intervention works. Phase III clinical trials tend to be large tests of an intervention in comparison to the current standard, usually through random assignment of participants to the standard group or the new group.
SOURCE: NCI (2004d).

TABLE 7-3 Cancer Clinical Trials

Type of Trial	Number of Trials
Treatment	1,891
Supportive Care	197
Diagnostic	75
Prevention	70
Genetics	33
Screening	23
Total	2,183

SOURCE: NCI (2004d).
NOTE: Clinical trials may be categorized as more than one type (e.g., treatment, supportive care, etc.) The total represents the total number of trials, irrespective of the type of trial.

The Prostate Cancer Outcomes Study

The Prostate Cancer Outcomes Study examined health and quality of life outcomes after prostatectomy or radiotherapy for prostate cancer (Potosky et al., 2000; Potosky et al., 2004; Johnson et al., 2004). For this study, a socioeconomically heterogeneous cohort of more than 1,500 newly diagnosed prostate cancer patients treated in community medical practices was selected from six Surveillance, Epidemiology, and End Results (SEER) cancer registries. Men selected for the study were asked to complete and mail back questionnaires that covered disease-specific and general quality of life, and satisfaction and regret about treatment decisions. Surveys were completed at 6 months and 1, 2, and 5 years after diagnosis. Outpatient medical records were abstracted to obtain information on prostate-specific antigen (PSA) values, Gleason score,[2] and details of initial treatment. At 2 and at 5 years of follow-up, important differences in urinary, bowel, and sexual functions were identified by treatment group and by race/ethnicity. This NCI-supported special study is estimated to have cost $7.5 million over the 10-year study period.

[2]A Gleason score is obtained through a system of grading prostate cancer cells based on how they look under a microscope. Gleason scores range from 2 to 10 and indicate how likely it is that a tumor will spread. A low Gleason score means the cancer cells are similar to normal prostate cells and are less likely to spread; a high Gleason score means the cancer cells are very different from normal and are more likely to spread.

Cancer of the Prostate Strategic Urologic Research Endeavor

CaPSURE is an industry-supported national disease registry of more than 11,000 men with prostate cancer accrued at 31 primarily community-based sites across the United States (Cooperberg et al., 2004; CaPSURE, 2005b). The disease registry was founded in 1995. Since then investigators have used it to assess disease management trends, resource utilization, and health and quality of life outcomes (Box 7-1).

At each practice site all men with biopsy-proven prostate cancer are invited to join CaPSURE. Clinical information is collected at baseline and each time the patient returns for care. At each clinic visit, the treating urologist completes a progress record, including current disease status, new prostate or unrelated diagnoses, disease signs and symptoms, and changes in medications. At enrollment each patient completes a questionnaire addressing sociodemographic parameters, comorbidities, and health-related quality of life. Every 6 months thereafter patients are asked to complete a follow-up questionnaire to report on their quality of life, health care utilization, and since 1999 their level of satisfaction with care and degree of fear of cancer recurrence. Patients are followed until death or study withdrawal.

Cancer Care Outcomes Research and Surveillance

The CanCORS Consortium involves eight teams of investigators from around the United States who evaluate the quality of cancer care delivered

BOX 7-1
Selected Recent Publications from Research Conducted Using the CaPSURE Database

- Predicting quality of life after radical prostatectomy: Results from CaPSURE (Hu et al., 2004)
- Longitudinal assessment of changes in sexual function and bother in patients treated with external beam radiotherapy or brachytherapy, with and without neoadjuvant androgen ablation: Data from CaPSURE (Speight et al., 2004)
- Watchful waiting and health related quality of life for patients with localized prostate cancer: Data from CaPSURE (Arredondo et al., 2004)
- Bowel function and bother after treatment for early stage prostate cancer: A longitudinal quality of life analysis from CaPSURE (Litwin et al., 2004)
- Health related quality of life patterns in patients treated with interstitial prostate brachytherapy for localized prostate cancer: Data from CaPSURE (Downs et al., 2003)
- Fear of cancer recurrence in patients undergoing definitive treatment for prostate cancer: Results from CaPSURE (Mehta et al., 2003)

SOURCE: CaPSURE (2005a).

and assess outcomes for approximately 10,000 newly diagnosed patients with lung and colorectal cancer (Ayanian et al., 2004) (Personal communication, A. Potosky, NCI, March 7, 2005). Individuals with cancer identified through cancer registries are being assessed at 4 to 6 months and at 13 months as part of this study sponsored by the NCI and the Department of Veterans Affairs (VA). Longer term follow-up will be possible if additional grant funding is forthcoming. A caregiver supplement is being administered at some sites. CanCORS grantees will receive a total of approximately $34 million over the 5-year study period. The two principal research aims of the consortium are to: (1) determine how the characteristics and beliefs of cancer patients and providers, and the characteristics of health care organizations, influence treatments and outcomes, spanning the continuum of cancer care from diagnosis to recovery or death; and (2) evaluate the effects of specific therapies on patients' survival, quality of life, and satisfaction with care, supplementing rather than substituting for data from randomized clinical trials (Ayanian et al., 2004).

The Stanford Hodgkin's Disease Experience

Between 1960 and 1999, more than 3,000 patients with Hodgkin's disease were seen, treated, and followed at Stanford University Medical Center (Personal communication, S. Donaldson, Stanford University, January 17, 2005) (Donaldson et al., 1999). This cohort includes patients of all ages and stages of disease and has provided information on the survival, mortality, and morbidity experience related to Hodgkin's disease over four decades. Evidence of the high risk of cardiovascular late effects of treatment for Hodgkin's disease emerged in the early 1990s from a special study of the Stanford cohort. Subsequent modifications in patient management and treatment have contributed to a reduction in this serious late effect. Evaluations of the risk of second cancers among this cohort have provided female cancer survivors of Hodgkin's disease and their clinicians with information on the high risk of post-radiation breast cancer and the need for close surveillance with mammography. The Stanford follow-up program has not had core financial support. The cost of long-term follow-up is substantial and has only been partly offset by grant support. Payment for special studies, tests, and examinations has depended on unstable support.

The Childhood Cancer Survivor Study (CCSS)

Survivors of childhood cancer face both short- and long-term adverse outcomes as a result of their cancer and its treatment. In the early 1990s, studies of the late effects of childhood cancer were typically limited in

BOX 7-2
Selected Recent Publications from Research Conducted Using the Childhood Cancer Survivor Study

- Psychological outcomes in long-term survivors of childhood brain cancer: A report from the Childhood Cancer Survivor Study (Zebrack et al., 2004)
- Multiple risk behaviors among smokers in the childhood cancer survivors study cohort (Butterfield et al., 2004)
- Health care of young adult survivors of childhood cancer: A report from the Childhood Cancer Survivor Study (Oeffinger et al., 2004)
- The cancer screening practices of adult survivors of childhood cancer: A report from the Childhood Cancer Survivor Study (Yeazel et al., 2004)
- Smoking among participants in the childhood cancer survivors cohort: The Partnership for Health Study (Emmons et al., 2003)
- Health status of adult long-term survivors of childhood cancer: A report from the Childhood Cancer Survivor Study (Hudson et al., 2003)

SOURCE: University of Minnesota Cancer Center (2002).

sample size, duration of follow-up, and rigor (e.g., low participation rates, high rates of loss to follow-up, lack of appropriate comparison populations, imprecise assessment or quantification of cancer-related treatments). To address these limitations, the Childhood Cancer Survivor Study was established with support from the NCI in 1993 (University of Minnesota Cancer Center, 2002; Robison et al., 2002). The CCSS consortium consists of 26 participating clinical centers in the United States and Canada. A cohort of more than 14,000 5-year survivors of childhood and adolescent cancer has been assembled.

Study participants have completed a baseline and two comprehensive self-administered questionnaires and consented to release their medical records and to be contacted in the future. Nearly 4,000 siblings have been identified to serve as a control group. CCSS investigators have examined issues related to late effects, quality of life, health-related behaviors, and patterns of medical care use in an attempt to develop prevention strategies and to assess follow-up needs (Box 7-2).

In addition to continuing to collect follow-up data from participants, the study is collecting biologic materials, including tumor specimens from participants who develop subsequent cancers; buccal (cheek) cells from all participants, including siblings, as a source of genomic DNA; and peripheral blood samples from a subset of survivors to establish cell lines as a source of genomic DNA and RNA. These materials will be used to evaluate the role of genetics in the occurrence of cancer and long-term adverse outcomes among survivors (University of Minnesota Cancer Center, 2002). Proposals to utilize the CCSS cohort can be submitted by any investigator, whether or not they have been directly involved with the study. Proposals that require direct contact with cohort members or that use banked biological materials require additional review.

Educational activities for study participants include access to the study website, a semi-annual newsletter, informational brochures targeted to subgroups at risk for particular late effects, and contact with investigators through e-mail and a toll-free telephone number. Intervention studies may also provide educational opportunities. For example, a smoking cessation study being conducted in the CCSS cohort is using a peer counseling approach that may have broad application to the cohort.

The CCSS investigators have described the far-reaching significance of its study for participants, health care providers, and scientists (University of Minnesota Cancer Center, 2002):

- For study participants, the CCSS can improve their understanding of the consequences of their disease and treatment and their ability to make informed choices regarding health behaviors.
- For current and future cancer patients, the study can help lead to improvements in treatment protocols that will minimize adverse health effects of therapy.
- For physicians involved with the care of children with malignant disease, knowledge of late effects of therapy is critical to the design and choice of optimal cancer treatment regimens.
- For health care providers and planners, the study offers the first opportunity to quantitatively assess the impact of long-term cancer survivorship on the delivery of care.
- For epidemiologists and biologists, the CCSS is a resource to investigate current and emerging questions regarding consequences of therapy, genetic associations, disease processes and causation, and the quality of life of survivors.

Cancer Registries, Administrative Data, and Surveys

A great deal has been learned about the delivery of cancer care from studies that link two or more complementary data sources. The linkage of cancer registry data to insurance claims databases, for example, has provided evidence of significant geographic variations in care (IOM, 2000). Registry data contain useful measures of severity of cancer (e.g., cancer stage) and date of diagnosis, but may lack complete information on treatment and outcomes. Claims-based data may lack certain diagnostic information, but include detailed information on the cost and use of medical services. Linkages between these two types of data sources allow the evaluation of large, relatively unbiased population-based samples of patients. Claims data are routinely collected, usually in a computer-readable format, and are therefore relatively easily and inexpensively accessible. However, there are limitations associated with claims data. Claims data are not collected for research, and coding misspecification and errors are common. Moreover, although registries can accurately document presenting cancer stage, they are less reliable for capturing recurrence. Consequently, algorithms that rely on information from claims must be used to identify cancer-free survivors—individuals who have survived their treatment, and have not had their cancer recur.

SEER-Medicare Linked Data

One of the most fruitful linkages for cancer care assessment is that of the SEER cancer registries to claims records in Medicare's administrative database (Potosky et al., 1993; Warren et al., 2002). This is a collaborative effort of the NCI, the SEER registries, and the Centers for Medicare and Medicaid Services (CMS) to create a large population-based source of information for cancer-related epidemiologic and health services research. The SEER-Medicare data offer an opportunity to examine patterns of care prior to the diagnosis of cancer, during the period of initial diagnosis, and during long-term follow-up. Topics that can be addressed with the linked database include patterns of care for specific cancers, health care disparities, and the costs of care. Important findings on the quality of survivorship care have come from analyses of the SEER-Medicare data (Nattinger et al., 2002). Examples of recent survivorship research conducted with SEER-Medicare are shown in Box 7-3.

The linkage of the SEER-Medicare data was first completed in 1991 and is updated every 3 years. The most recent linkage in 2002 included the registries that were part of the SEER program as of 1999. These registries are located in 11 geographic areas, representing 14 percent of the U.S. population. With the 2005 linkage, the SEER-Medicare data will include the four expansion registries, and will then represent 26 percent of the U.S. population (NCI, 2004a).[3] The Medicare utilization data (claims) cover stays in institutions (i.e., hospitals and skilled nursing facilities), physician and lab services, hospital outpatient visits, and home health and hospice

[3]The database includes claims for beneficiaries receiving fee-for-service care, but most studies require exclusion of individuals cared for in health maintenance organizations. A control sample of individuals who do not have cancer is available so that comparisons can be made, for example, on health care costs for individuals with and without cancer.

BOX 7-3
Selected Survivorship Research Based on SEER-Medicare Data

Morbidity

- Favorable cardiac risk among elderly breast carcinoma survivors (Lamont et al., 2003)
- Low risk of hip fracture among elderly breast cancer survivors (Lamont and Lauderdale, 2003)
- Variations in morbidity after radical prostatectomy (Begg et al., 2002)
- Risk of fracture after androgen deprivation for prostate cancer (Shahinian et al., 2005)

Patterns of Care

- Under use of necessary care among cancer survivors (Earle and Neville, 2004)
- Geographic and patient variation in receipt of surveillance procedures after local excision of cutaneous melanoma (Barzilai et al., 2004)
- Adherence to surveillance among patients with superficial bladder cancer (Schrag et al., 2003)
- Racial differences in the receipt of bowel surveillance following potentially curative colorectal cancer surgery (Ellison et al., 2003)
- Quality of non-breast cancer health maintenance among elderly breast cancer survivors (Earle et al., 2003)
- The prevalence of patients with colorectal carcinoma under care in the U.S. (Mariotto et al., 2003)
- Bowel surveillance patterns after a diagnosis of colorectal cancer in Medicare beneficiaries (Knopf et al., 2001)
- Patterns of endoscopic follow-up after surgery for nonmetastatic colorectal cancer (Cooper et al., 2000)
- Underutilization of mammography in older breast cancer survivors (Schapira et al., 2000)
- Geographic and patient variation among Medicare beneficiaries in the use of follow-up testing after surgery for nonmetastatic colorectal carcinoma (Cooper et al., 1999)

Costs of Care

- Lifetime cancer-attributable cost of care for long-term survivors of colorectal cancer (Ramsey et al., 2002)
- Obtaining long-term disease specific costs of care: Application to Medicare enrollees diagnosed with colorectal cancer (Brown et al., 1999)

Methodologic Studies

- Identifying cancer relapse using SEER-Medicare data (Earle et al., 2002)

SOURCE: NCI (2004f).

use. Information on noncovered services such as prescription drugs and long-term care is not yet available. The linkage was first completed in 1991 and has been updated most recently in 2003 (NCI, 2004e). The annual cost of maintaining the linked SEER-Medicare database is approximately $500,000.

State and Local Cancer Registries

State cancer registry data have also been linked to administrative records to assess survivorship care. For example, investigators linked state cancer registry data to health insurance claims from Blue Cross/Blue Shield of Virginia to assess adherence to standards of care for women with breast cancer (Hillner et al., 1997). More than three-quarters (79 percent) of women get a follow-up mammogram within the first 18 months postoperatively, according to this study. State cancer registries have also been linked to Medicaid data to examine the experience of Medicaid enrollees diagnosed with cancer (Bradley et al., 2003).

Other survivorship research has relied on hospital cancer registries to identify cohorts of individuals to follow prospectively (Pakilit et al., 2001; Ganz et al., 2002, 2003a). The American Society of Clinical Oncology's National Initiative on Cancer Care Quality (NICCQ) identified subjects by using the National Cancer Data Base, a national registry of incident cancer cases, and its network of hospital cancer registries.[4] Included in the study were a few measures related to the quality of survivorship care (e.g., receipt of tamoxifen for 5 years for certain women with breast cancer, receipt of counseling about the need for first-degree relatives of certain patients with colorectal cancer to undergo screening for this type of cancer) (Schneider et al., 2004).

NCI's Cancer Research Network (CRN)

Some studies of cancer survivorship, including those based on SEER-Medicare data, exclude members of managed care organizations because such plans often do not have to report encounter data (e.g., individual claims for visits or services) to Medicare. Such plans insure approximately

[4]The National Cancer Data Base (NCDB) is a nationwide, facility-based oncology dataset that captures 75 percent of all newly diagnosed cancer cases in the United States annually. It holds information on more than 15 million cases of reported cancer diagnoses from 1985 to 2002, and continues to grow. The NCDB is supported by the American Cancer Society and the American College of Surgeons Commission on Cancer (Winchester et al., 2004; ACoS, 2004).

15 percent of the Medicare-eligible population and cover the majority of commercially insured Americans. The Cancer Research Network, an initiative of the NCI, encourages the expansion of collaborative cancer research among health care provider organizations that are oriented to community care and have access to large, stable, and diverse patient populations. Collaborating investigators are able to take advantage of existing integrated databases that can provide patient-level information relevant to research studies on cancer control and to cancer-related population studies. Beginning in 1999, the NCI funded the CRN—a consortium of large, not-for-profit, research-oriented health maintenance organizations (HMOs). The CRN, now cooperatively funded by the Agency for Healthcare Research and Quality (AHRQ), includes 11 HMOs nationwide that provide care for nearly 9 million enrollees. The proportion of HMO enrollees diagnosed with cancer who remain enrolled and available for CRN research projects is high. Retention rates of enrollees diagnosed with cancer within five of the CRN HMOs was 96 percent at 1 year and 84 percent at 5 years following diagnosis (Field et al., 2004). CRN investigators have proposed to study long-term survivors of colorectal cancer to assess the interrelationship among aspects of their initial care and subsequent physical, functional, and psychological outcomes (NCI, 2004b). CRN is also conducting a study, with a grant from the National Institutes of Health (NIH), of patient-oriented outcomes among women who have had prophylactic mastectomy. Although evidence suggests that a substantial reduction in breast cancer risk occurs after prophylactic mastectomy, its effect on other patient-oriented outcomes is unclear. This study will address this deficiency by gathering information from women identified for an ongoing study of the efficacy of prophylactic mastectomy in six HMO community-based populations across the United States (NCI, 2005a). A cancer survivorship group and a quality of cancer care special interest group have been convened within CRN to develop research proposals, and there are plans to survey cancer patients about their care experiences, particularly care coordination (Geiger, 2004) (Personal communication, S. Green, Group Health Cooperative, March 5, 2005). Core CRN support (excluding affiliated individual investigator awards, supplements, and other funding mechanisms) is $20 million over 4 years, 2003 to 2007 (Personal communication, S. Green, Group Health Cooperative, March 5, 2005).

Federal Health Surveys and Data

The results from federally sponsored surveys and other data collection activities provide national estimates of health indicators such as the prevalence of health conditions, the use of health care services, and health care expenditures. Such surveys have been invaluable in estimating the prevalence of cancer risk behaviors (e.g., smoking), use of preventive health services (e.g., mammography), and use of supportive care services (e.g., mental health services). Federal surveys conducted of individuals are often very large, including members of as many as 50,000 households. With the prevalence of cancer estimated to be 3.5 percent, a sufficiently large, nationally representative sample of cancer survivors may be identified for study through such surveys.

In 1992 the NCI included a cancer survivorship section in the National Health Interview Survey (NHIS) to obtain population-based estimates on aspects of the medical, insurance, and employment experiences of cancer survivors (Hewitt et al., 1999). Subsequent analyses of the NHIS have provided estimates of health status, health service use, and burden of illness among cancer survivors (Hewitt and Rowland, 2002; Hewitt et al., 2003; Yabroff et al., 2004). The Medical Expenditure Panel Survey has been used to estimate health insurance and spending among cancer patients (Center on an Aging Society, 2002; Thorpe and Howard, 2003). These household surveys exclude residents of institutions and therefore miss individuals with cancer who are in nursing homes, hospices, or other facilities. There are also limitations in self-reports of cancer. Evidence suggests, for example, that some individuals do not accurately report the occurrence of cancer or the type of cancer diagnosed (Chambers et al., 1976; Bergmann et al., 1998).

Summary

Investigators have used a number of research mechanisms to learn about the health and quality of life of cancer survivors. Information about patterns of care and the quality of survivorship care have been forthcoming from existing data resources such as cancer registries linked to administrative records. Long-term prospective studies of cancer survivors have been conducted based on samples drawn from cancer registries and from cancer centers. There are examples of survivorship studies being incorporated into the NCI's cooperative group system treatment trials, but opportunities to use this infrastructure to further survivorship research have not been fully realized. No clinical trials of adequate design and sufficient size to judge the appropriateness of surveillance strategies for cancer survivors have been conducted in the United States.

CHALLENGES OF SURVIVORSHIP RESEARCH

Survivorship research is by nature challenging (Ganz, 2003). Late effects may not emerge for decades, necessitating prolonged follow-up. In addition, the constant evolution of diagnostic tests and cancer treatments, although desirable, means that studies of late effects must be ongoing. A frustration for patients is that research on the late effects of therapies they are considering may not be available to them when they are making treatment decisions. Cancer is predominantly a disease of the elderly, so another challenge to survivorship researchers is to design studies that can isolate the effects of cancer and its treatment from the symptoms and disabilities expected from normal aging and the onset of comorbid conditions. Some of the specific challenges of survivorship research are highlighted below, including those related to long-term follow-up and the need to accrue large and diverse patient populations. In addition, some administrative issues are described that are faced by researchers in general, but are of particular concern to survivorship investigators, including those related to informed consent and assuring privacy of medical records.

Long-Term Follow-up

Because ongoing surveillance is needed to identify late effects, survivorship researchers often need to follow individuals for lengthy periods. During follow-up, participants may move, change doctors or health plans, tire of being a research subject, or become too sick to answer questions or submit to examinations. When research subjects are "lost to follow-up," investigators' ability to reach conclusions about the significance of symptoms that may have been identified during the follow-up period are diminished (Sears et al., 2003). Investigators have reported particular difficulties in collecting quality of life data in longitudinal studies of clinical trial participants (Moinpour and Lovato, 1998; Bernhard et al., 1998). Most research has focused on the early survivorship period (within 2 years of diagnosis) despite the increasing number of cancer survivors living 5 years or more after a cancer diagnosis (Aziz and Rowland, 2003). Research studies with extended follow-up periods are needed to identify recurrent cancer, new primary cancers, and the many late effects that have long latency periods.

Long-term follow-up is labor intensive, and studies of late effects can be very expensive. Biomedical tests to document physiological and functional impairments (cardiac and pulmonary tests, cognitive functioning and brain imaging studies) are expensive, but are necessary to detect subclinical disease that can put patients at risk. Even periodic assessments of quality of life following cancer treatment can be expensive. In one study, conducted in 1995, quality of life assessments added approximately $7,000 to the average monthly direct cost of a clinical trial (Moinpour, 1996). One of the major reasons for this is keeping track of patients.

Researchers have called for the establishment of mechanisms to facilitate monitoring of the late effects of new therapies (Gotay, 2004). Information about late effects would be much easier to obtain if patients agreed to long-term follow-up and monitoring when they entered a treatment trial and if investigators maintained current contact information as part of the treatment protocol.

Accruing Large and Heterogeneous Study Cohorts Through Multiple Institutions

Another inherent challenge for survivorship investigation is the need to study large numbers of individuals who will survive their cancers for many years. Study sample sizes must also be large enough to include individuals who will manifest unusual late effects and individuals who may have been exposed to unique treatments. In addition, the ability to detect interactions of cancer treatments with underlying comorbid conditions depends on studies with large and heterogeneous populations. Inclusion of individuals from ethnic minorities and medically underserved groups is also needed to identify health disparities and interventions to reduce them (Aziz and Rowland, 2002).

One mechanism to accrue large numbers of cancer survivors who represent the diversity of the United States is to conduct multi-institution collaborative research. Such efforts, while advantageous in terms of study design, can be costly and hard to administer. An area of particular concern is the process of gaining institutional review board (IRB) approval for research studies. In one study of IRB processes in a multisite mailed survey, investigators found that IRBs had different requirements that affected the consistency of project protocols (e.g., agreement on centralized data collection with outside firms; allowance for cash incentives for participation; requirement for active or passive physician consent before contacting subjects) (Greene and Geiger, 2004). Incorporating site-specific IRB requirements into project planning and potentially streamlining, centralizing, and reaching reciprocity agreements were recommended by investigators, especially for lower risk studies. Recognizing that IRBs are overloaded and underfunded, central or lead review boards have been recommended for multisite studies to reduce the redundancy of reviews and variability of approvals and/or required modifications to study design (IOM, 2003b).

Case Ascertainment Through Cancer Registries

Survivorship studies that enroll individuals identified through population-based cancer registries are advantageous because inferences from study results often can be generalized to the population at large. In contrast, results of studies based on convenience samples may be misleading because of biases in selection (e.g., if only healthy survivors volunteer to be studied). A barrier to the timely conduct of cancer registry-based studies is the lack of rapid case ascertainment mechanisms to identify cases early enough to administer surveys or examinations within one year of diagnosis. Registries are an attractive means of identifying subjects for research but, in some areas, registries restrict access to individuals in the registry because of their involvement in other research studies. Shortages of resources and staff within the registries further hamper the conduct of research. Additional support for population-based cancer registries would not only improve their primary epidemiologic function, but would also improve survivorship research opportunities (IOM, 2000). With advances in information technology, it is likely that in the next decade cancer surveillance will be expanded to include quality of care measures and patient-centered outcomes (Hiatt, 2005).

Informed Consent

Adherence to legal requirements for human subject protection through informed consent can be labor intensive and contribute to problems in achieving high rates of participation among potential study subjects. As part of the ACS study of cancer survivors described above, investigators notified all physicians caring for potential study subjects of the study and obtained their consent to contact patients. In some states, investigators were able to inform physicians of the study and their plans to contact patients unless told not to do so. In contrast to this "passive consent" approach, other states required that physicians provide "active consent" in order to contact potential subjects. Physician restrictions on investigator access to patients, coupled with patient refusal to enter the study, resulted in participation rates that varied widely across the 14 states involved in the study (from 20 to 60 percent). The relatively low participation rates have led to concerns about the representativeness of the enrolled cohort of cancer survivors (Yates, 2004).

Assuring Privacy of Medical Records

Another potential barrier to the conduct of clinical and health services research has emerged with the passage of privacy provisions of the Health Insurance Portability and Accountability Act of 1996 (HIPAA).[5] Under HIPAA, a federal Privacy Rule established new responsibilities for health

[5]Pub. L. No. 104–191, § 264, 110 Stat. 1936, 2033.

care providers, health plans, and other entities to protect the confidentiality of an individual's health information (Box 7-4). Compliance with provisions of the Act was required by April 2003. Many investigators have subsequently concluded that HIPAA is having a deleterious impact on the conduct of clinical, epidemiologic, and health services research (Hiatt, 2003; Gunn et al., 2004; GAO, 2004; Raghavan, 2005).

HIPAA's Privacy Rule has fundamentally changed the way researchers obtain health data (Gunn et al., 2004). Researchers must use one of three options to gain access to protected health information: obtain patient authorization; obtain a waiver of authorization by having their research protocol reviewed and approved by an IRB or privacy board; or use a limited dataset with direct identifiers removed. Researchers may seek health information without authorization if the data do not identify an individual and there is no reasonable basis to believe it could be used to identify an individual.

An ad hoc subcommittee of the National Cancer Advisory Board (NCAB) solicited comments from NCI-affiliated comprehensive and clinical cancer centers, cooperative groups, and Specialized Programs of Research Excellence (SPOREs) to assess the impact of HIPAA on oncology clinical research (Ramirez and Niederhuber, 2003; NCAB, 2003). The Association of American Medical Colleges (AAMC) has also solicited information on research activities that have been affected by the new HIPAA privacy regulations (AAMC, 2004). Consistent findings on HIPAA's impact from the AAMC and NCAB surveys emerged (Ehringhaus, 2004):

1. The informed consent process is negatively affected (e.g., subjects are overwhelmed/confused by added length to consent form).
2. Recruitment is impaired or prevented (e.g., obtaining information from other providers has become more difficult).
3. Subject selection bias is introduced (e.g., complexity of the authorization form intimidates some potential participants, introducing potential biases).
4. Research processes are hindered (e.g., there is a burden of documentation, paperwork).
5. Research costs are increased (e.g., study resources are diverted to compliance).
6. Shifts in the direction of research are required (e.g., there are delays in gaining access to data, and some data are inaccessible).
7. Difficulties arise in collaborations (e.g., some providers no longer provide data; it is difficult to get agreement in multisite trials).
8. There are inconsistent interpretations of HIPAA requirements.

BOX 7-4
HIPAA's Privacy Rule

What Does HIPAA's Privacy Rule Address?

The Privacy Rule addresses the use and disclosure of individuals' health information and establishes individuals' rights to obtain and control access to this information. Specifically, the rule covers "protected health information," defined as individually identifiable health information that is transmitted or maintained in any form. It applies to "covered entities," defined as health plans, health care clearinghouses, and health care providers that transmit information electronically with respect to certain transactions. The protections under the Privacy Rule do not preempt state privacy laws that are more stringent.

What Are Permissible Uses and Disclosures of Health Information Under HIPAA?

Under the Privacy Rule, a covered entity may use and disclose an individual's protected health information without obtaining the individual's authorization when the information is used for treatment, payment, or health care operations. Protected health information may also be disclosed without an individual's authorization for such purposes as certain public health and law enforcement activities, and judicial and administrative proceedings, provided certain conditions are met. In addition, an individual's authorization is not required for disclosures for research purposes if a waiver of authorization, under defined criteria, is obtained from an institutional review board (IRB) or a privacy board.[1] Except where the rule specifically allows or requires a use of disclosure without an authorization, the individual's written authorization must be obtained. The Privacy Rule allows covered entities to use their discretion in deciding whether to disclose protected health information for many types of disclosures, such as those to family and friends, public health authorities, and health researchers.[2]

What Individual Privacy Rights Does the Privacy Rule Confer?

The Privacy Rule provides the following:

- *Access to and amendment of health information:* Individuals have the right to inspect and copy their protected health information and to request amendments of their records.

The AAMC and NCAB have recommended that certain provisions of the Privacy Rule be amended to reverse these unintended consequences to medical research. Specifically, these groups recommend that some of the accounting of disclosure requirements be eliminated, that authorization and waiver processes be refashioned, and that standards for deidentification of records be relaxed (Ramirez and Niederhuber, 2003; Ehringhaus, 2004).

In summary, survivorship research has inherent challenges that include the difficulties and costs of following research subjects for lengthy periods and the need for large and diverse study populations. Additional challenges, not unique to survivorship research but which impact its conduct, are

- *Notice of privacy practices:* Individuals generally have a right to written notice of the uses and disclosures of their health information.
- *Accounting for disclosures:* Individuals generally have the right to request and receive a listing of disclosures of their protected health information that is shared with others for purposes other than treatment, payment, or health care operations.
- *Complaints:* Complaints regarding compliance to the Privacy Rule may be filed with the Secretary of Health and Human Services.

What Are the Responsibilities of Health Care Providers, Health Plans, and Clearinghouses?

- *Develop policies and procedures for protecting health information*
- *Limit information used and disclosed to the minimum necessary*
- *Account for disclosures of protected health information:* On request, covered entities must provide individuals with an accounting of disclosures of their protected health information made in the preceding 6 years. This requirement applies to most disclosures other than those for treatment, payment, or operations purposes, including those that are mandated by law (e.g., certain disclosures to public health entities).
- *Ensure that "downstream users" protect the privacy of health information by implementing business associate agreements:* Covered entities must enter into a contract or other written agreement with any business associates with which they share protected health information for various purposes.

---

[1]An IRB is a board, committee, or other group established in accordance with applicable federal regulations and formally designated by an institution to review human subject research. A privacy board is a review body that may be established to act on research requests under the Privacy Rule in place of using an IRB. Before issuing waivers, these boards must determine, among other things, that the use or disclosure of protected health information involves no more than a minimal risk to the privacy of the individuals (GAO, 2004)

[2]Physicians are required to report new cancer cases to cancer registries according to state regulations. Physicians and hospitals are also permitted to provide follow-up and treatment information to hospital cancer registries without patient authorization (NAACCR, 2003).

SOURCE: GAO (2004).

administrative complexities associated with multi-institutional research and emerging problems associated with the implementation of the privacy provisions of HIPAA.

STATUS OF SURVIVORSHIP RESEARCH

The committee, in an effort to understand how resources for research are applied to questions regarding cancer survivorship, undertook a review of topics of investigation and levels of research spending. Such a review provides only a snapshot as of 2005, but it does give an indication of the prominence and priority of survivorship within the field of cancer research, and a sense of the emphasis on different areas within cancer survivorship research. This assessment aided the committee as they considered ways in which a research program could be structured in the future to better respond to the needs of cancer survivors. There is no one comprehensive source of information on research support and, as part of its review, the committee relied on the following sources:

- Descriptions of NIH-sponsored survivorship research compiled by the NCI's Office of Cancer Survivorship
- Listings of research projects in the CRISP (Computer Retrieval of Information on Scientific Projects), a searchable database of federally funded biomedical research projects conducted at universities, hospitals, and other research institutions[6]
- Contacts with organization representatives (e.g., ACS, Lance Armstrong Foundation, Centers for Disease Control and Prevention [CDC])
- Review of each organization's website.

The committee's review of research support is limited to federal agencies, primarily the National Institutes of Health and selected private organizations and foundations (i.e., ACS, Lance Armstrong Foundation, Susan G. Komen Foundation). Although these organizations are not the only sponsors of research on cancer survivorship, they represent the major funding sources for such research. Excluded from this review was research supported by health plans, insurers, pharmaceutical companies, and other private organizations. Much of the research done in those settings is proprietary.

Federal Research Support

The level of dedicated NIH support for cancer survivorship research has grown from $2 to $22 million from 1998 to 2004, signaling a growing

[6]CRISP is a biomedical database system containing information on research projects and programs supported by the Department of Health and Human Services. Most of the research falls within the broad category of extramural projects, grants, contracts, and cooperative agreements conducted primarily by universities, hospitals, and other research institutions, and funded by NIH and other government agencies (e.g., Centers for Disease Control and Prevention, Food and Drug Administration, Health Resources and Services Administration, Agency for Healthcare Research and Quality). CRISP also contains information on the intramural programs of NIH and Food and Drug Administration (NIH, 2004a).

interest in the area (Figures 7-3 and 7-4).[7] While the increase in support has been substantial, survivorship research support represents a tiny fraction of support for treatment-related research, estimated at more than $1 billion in 2003 (NCI, 2003a). Cancer survivorship research is conducted throughout the institutes of NIH (e.g., National Institute on Aging, National Institute of Nursing Research, National Institute of Mental Health, National Center for Complementary and Alternative Medicine). Within the NCI, several Divisions have ongoing survivorship-related activities (e.g., Division of Cancer Prevention, Division of Cancer Control and Population Sciences, Division of Cancer Treatment and Diagnosis, and the Training Branch). The locus of cancer survivorship research at the federal level is the NCI's Office of Cancer Survivorship.

National Cancer Institute, Office of Cancer Survivorship

The NCI's Office of Cancer Survivorship was established in 1996 to support research on the physical, psychosocial, and economic consequences of cancer among survivors (of all ages), their families, and caregivers (NCI, undated). The Office of Cancer Survivorship supports research related to:

- The identification, prevention, and amelioration of the late effects of cancer and its treatment;
- Follow-up care and surveillance of cancer survivors and their family members;
- Optimization of health after cancer treatment; and
- Communication to health care professionals, cancer survivors and their families, and the public regarding survivorship issues.

The Office of Cancer Survivorship has led a modest level of survivorship-specific grant initiatives since its inception, and has been successful in efforts to incorporate consideration of survivorship issues into diverse NCI-supported funding mechanisms (e.g., program announcements

[7]For these estimates, survivorship research was defined as that which focused on the health and life of a person with a history of cancer beyond the acute diagnosis and treatment phase. Studies that examined newly diagnosed survivors or those in active treatment were included in the estimates if follow-up lasted at least 2 months or longer post-treatment. Studies addressing recurrence or end-of-life research were not included in these estimates. Estimates include research conducted among survivors of both childhood and adult cancers (NCI, 2005b). These estimates of dedicated NIH support for cancer survivorship do not capture all survivorship research, for example, that conducted through the Clinical Trials Cooperative Groups Program.

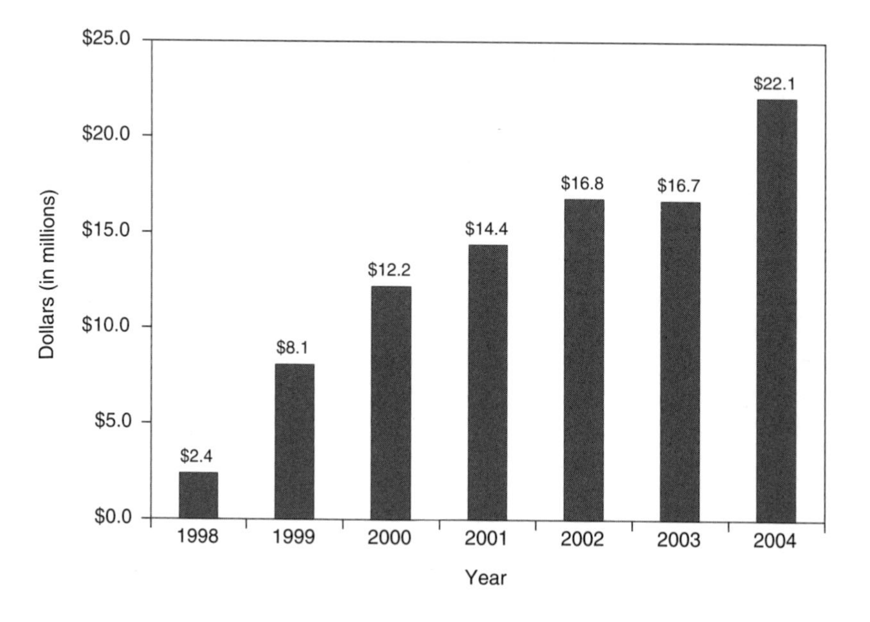

FIGURE 7-3 NIH cancer survivorship grant support ($ millions), by year
SOURCE: NCI (2004c).

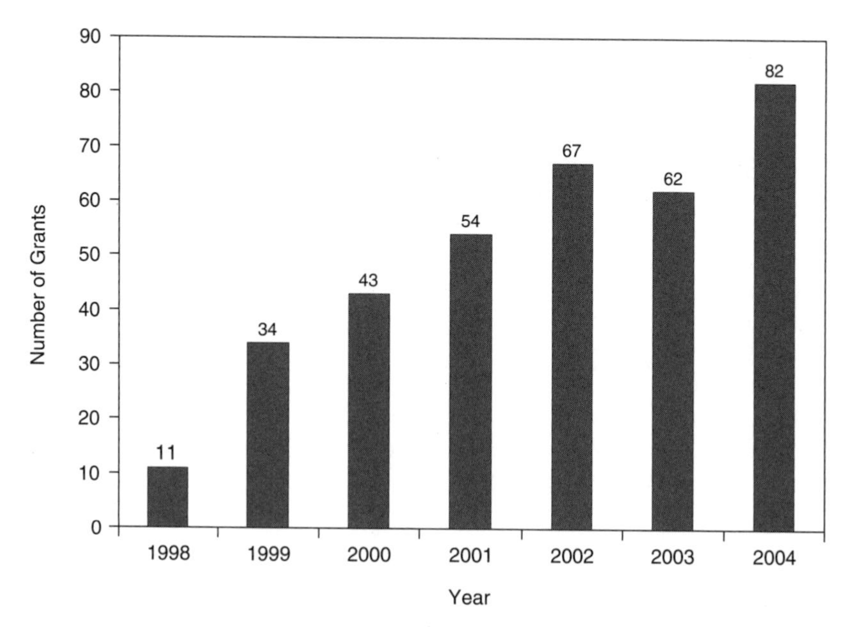

FIGURE 7-4 Number of cancer survivorship grants awarded by NIH, by year
SOURCE: (NCI, 2004c).

for R03 and R21 applications),[8] as well as several trans-NIH program initiatives. In terms of its own research portfolio, the Office of Cancer Survivorship awarded its first formally solicited research grants in 1997, totaling $4 million over 2 years (NCI, 1998). In 1998, the Office of Cancer Suvivorship awarded another $15 million over 5 years in response to its Long-Term Cancer Survivors Request for Applications (RFA). The Office of Cancer Survivorship awarded $1 million in 2000 to support supplements to comprehensive cancer centers (P30s) to conduct pilot or exploratory research on issues related to the functioning of family members of survivors. In 2001, using a similar mechanism, the Office of Cancer Survivorship awarded an additional $1 million to support pilot research on issues faced by minority and underserved cancer survivors. A reissuance of the original Long-Term Cancer Survivors RFA was announced in 2003 and 17 new grants were awarded[9] with $6 million over 5 years (with co-funding from the CDC and the National Institute on Aging) (Aziz, 2002, 2004; Rowland, 2004). Over its lifetime, the Office of Cancer Survivorship has controlled and distributed about $28 million to support cancer survivorship research. With limited resources of its own, the Office of Cancer Survivorship has actively encouraged investigators to utilize a number of existing support mechanisms that are relevant to cancer survivorship research (Box 7-5).

Health services research has been a somewhat less well-developed area of survivorship research. Two new NCI-supported research initiatives will provide much needed information about late effects among, and the care received by, cancer survivors (Aziz, 2004):

- Follow-up Care Use by Survivors (FOCUS)—This population-based study of 1,600 survivors of breast, prostate, colorectal, and gynecologic cancer will examine the self-reported prevalence of long-term and late effects of cancer treatment, aspects of follow-up care (frequency, content, setting, experiences, and perceived quality and purpose), knowledge of late effects of cancer treatment, screening and health behaviors, and attitudes toward and practices regarding cancer follow-up care.
- Experiences of Care and Health Outcomes Among Survivors of NHL (ECHOS-NHL)—The quality of follow-up care provided to adult survivors of aggressive non-Hodgkin's lymphoma will be assessed along with related health outcomes.

[8]R03s are small research grants and R21s are exploratory/development grants (NIH, 2004d).

[9]A total of 125 applications were received, signifying an active interest on the part of researchers in this area of research.

BOX 7-5
Examples of National Institutes of Health (NIH) Program Funding Opportunities Related to Cancer Survivorship

- Decision Making in Cancer: Single-Event Decisions (PA-05-017): To support research to enhance understanding of decision-making processes related to cancer prevention, detection, treatment, survivorship, or end-of-life care.

- Research Partnerships for Improving Functional Outcomes (PAR-04-077): To support basic, applied, and translational multidisciplinary research that addresses biological, behavioral, medical, and/or psychosocial research problems related to rehabilitation or health maintenance for acute or chronic disease.

- Physical Activity and Obesity Across Chronic Diseases (PA-01-017): Research to include studies to test intervention approaches that incorporate physical activity during and after cancer treatment.

- Testing Interventions to Improve Adherence to Pharmacological Treatment Regimens (RFA OD-00-006): Research on adherence to post-treatment interventions, including those administered to prevent/minimize cancer recurrence and prevent post-treatment toxicities.

- Mind-Body Research Centers (Specialized Center Grants-P50): NIH supported five research centers from 1999 to 2004 to investigate the links between stress and health, including a center for psycho-oncology research.

SOURCES: NIH (2004b,c).

A physician survey to learn more about cancer control practices is planned in 2006–2007. Questions will be included to ascertain physicians' follow-up care recommendations and practices for cancer survivors (Personal communication, J. Rowland, Office of Cancer Survivorship, NCI, April 12, 2005).

An important opportunity to disseminate research findings is provided by a biennial conference on cancer survivorship co-sponsored by the NCI and the ACS. The meeting also provides a forum for interdisciplinary dialogue, sessions for professional education and training, and networking opportunities for new investigators (NCI and ACS, 2004).

Department of Defense (DoD)

Beginning in FY 1992, the U.S. Congress directed DoD to manage several appropriations for an extramural grant program directed toward specific research initiatives. The U.S. Army Medical Research and Materiel Command established the office of the Congressionally Directed Medical

Research Programs (CDMRP) to administer these funds. Between FY 1992 and 2004, $1.65 billion has been appropriated by Congress to DoD for research on breast cancer (DoD, 2004a). In addition, $10.3 million has been generated in sales of the U.S. Postal Service's first-class stamp (Pub. L. No. 105–41, Stamp Out Breast Cancer Act [H.R. 1585]). Since 1997, Congress has appropriated money to fund peer-reviewed research for prostate cancer ($565 million appropriated to date), ovarian cancer ($81 million), and chronic myelogenous leukemia ($13.5 million). The CDMRP attempts to identify gaps in funding and provide award opportunities that will enhance program research objectives without duplicating existing funding opportunities. A number of funded research projects are related to cancer survivorship, including those focused on quality of life and symptom management (DoD, 2004b). Training grants are available through CDMRP and have include those related to psycho-oncology.

Agency for Healthcare Research and Quality

AHRQ has published evidence reports on the management of cancer symptoms (i.e., pain, depression, and fatigue) and the effectiveness of behavioral interventions to modify physical activity behaviors in cancer patients and survivors (AHRQ, 2002b, 2004a). Additional syntheses related to survivorship may be forthcoming because cancer is among the 10 top conditions affecting Medicare beneficiaries and therefore, the subject of a new AHRQ initiative. State-of-the art information about the effectiveness of interventions for these conditions will be developed, including reviews of prescription drugs. Funding for the initiative was authorized by the Medicare Prescription Drug, Improvement, and Modernization Act of 2003. Systematic reviews and syntheses of the scientific literature will focus on the evidence of outcomes, comparative clinical effectiveness, and appropriateness of health care items such as pharmaceuticals and health care services, including the manner in which they are organized, managed, and delivered (AHRQ, 2004b).

Two large research networks supported by AHRQ could provide opportunities for survivorship research. The Primary Care Practice-based Research Networks (PBRNs) provide opportunities to examine care within primary care settings. Together, the 19 PBRNs provide access to more than 5,000 primary care providers and nearly 7 million patients across the United States (AHRQ, 2001). Among the research that has been conducted within PBRNs is a study of the coordination between referring physicians and specialists (Forrest et al., 2000). The Integrated Delivery System Research Network (IDSRN) is a model of field-based research that links researchers with large health care systems to conduct research (AHRQ, 2002a). As a group, the IDSRN provides health services in a wide variety of organizational care settings to more than 55 million Americans. IDSRN partners collect and maintain administrative, claims, encounter, and other data on large populations that are clinically, demographically, and geographically diverse. From 2000 to 2004, AHRQ has provided nearly $20 million for 75 projects. One of these projects is analyzing ways to improve communication and care monitoring among providers collaborating on care within different care settings. The PBRN and IDSRN have not yet been used to investigate survivorship issues directly, but both networks could be valuable resources for such research.

Centers for Disease Control and Prevention

The CDC has recognized cancer survivorship as one of the many chronic conditions for which a public health approach is needed. Evaluation of survivorship services and research on preventive interventions were among the recommendations in the report co-sponsored by CDC and the Lance Armstrong Foundation, *A National Action Plan for Cancer Survivorship: Advancing Public Health Strategies*. To further this report's recommendations, the CDC has supported state efforts to develop comprehensive cancer control plans that incorporate initiatives to meet the needs of cancer survivors (see Chapter 4). The CDC oversees the National Program of Cancer Registries (NPCR) and is supporting a study in New York state to assess the feasibility of using existing data sources to collect the follow-up data needed for basic survival analysis in a statewide cancer registry. Another study will measure and explore differences in cancer survival among cancer patients in Europe, Canada, and the United States (CONCORD Study) (CDC, 2003). CDC is in the process of developing an agencywide research agenda that will include a focus on public health interventions to further reduce the risk factors associated with the leading causes of death and illness, including heart disease, cancer, and diabetes (CDC, 2005).

Private Research Support

Private philanthropic organizations have been major sponsors of cancer research. This section of the report reviews the research activity of two national sponsors of survivorship-related research on all types of cancer, the ACS and the Lance Armstrong Foundation, and a foundation that supports research related to breast cancer.[10]

[10] Foundations that restrict support to certain states or local areas were excluded from this review. Many private foundations provide support for research, and the description of private foundation support here is meant to be illustrative, and not to be considered comprehensive.

American Cancer Society

The ACS is the largest nongovernmental source of cancer research funding in the United States and supports psychosocial and behavioral research. In FY 2003–2004, approximately 17 percent of the total research program was devoted to these areas. The Society's intramural research program includes a Behavioral Research Center, which is conducting two large population-based surveys of cancer survivors (described above). The ACS Behavioral Research Center is also analyzing data on health-related quality of life of cancer survivors who are Medicare beneficiaries enrolled in managed care plans. The data are from the Medicare Beneficiary Survey, a national survey conducted for the Department of Health and Human Services' Centers for Medicare and Medicaid Services. Survivorship-related grants that are active through ACS's extramural program are shown in Box 7-6. The total level of support for these grants is approximately $4 million.

Lance Armstrong Foundation (LAF)

The mission of the Lance Armstrong Foundation is to enhance the length and quality of life of those living with, through, and beyond cancer with activities targeted to cancer survivorship. LAF was founded in 1997 by cancer survivor and champion cyclist Lance Armstrong. By 2005, LAF had awarded more than $9.7 million for 75 grants on the study of testicular cancer and survivorship issues (LAF, 2004, 2005). Survivorship-related awards in 2003 include those related to the effects of physical activity on relieving chronic fatigue and other late effects, educational interventions to reduce breast cancer among Hodgkin's disease survivors, and long-term follow-up of survivors of Hodgkin's lymphoma enrolled in trials conducted by the European Organization for Research and Treatment of Cancer (EORTC) Lymphoma Group (LAF, 2004). Awards made in 2004 include those to study follow-up care for African-American breast cancer survivors, the impact of exercise in lymphoma survivors, and the fertility of women following chemotherapy for early breast cancer. Other initiatives will focus on chemotherapy-induced peripheral neuropathy and the psychological late effects of cancer (LAF, 2005).

LAF has received support from CDC to disseminate programs to improve cancer survivorship among African Americans, American Indians, Alaskan Natives, Spanish speakers, and rural Americans. LAF plans to develop and disseminate culturally relevant and linguistically appropriate materials for these groups (CDC, 2004).

BOX 7-6
Active American Cancer Society Cancer Survivorship Grants (Adults)

- Two psychosocial programs will be compared, one with an educational focus and the other a spiritual focus. The programs' effects on physical, emotional, social, and spiritual well-being will be assessed among cancer patients who are medically underserved and members of minority populations.

- Problems faced by younger breast cancer survivors and their partners will be identified and compared to those of older survivors, and a control group of women (acquaintances of the breast cancer survivors).

- Assessments will be made of the impact of various treatments for prostate cancer on the quality of life of poor white and African-American survivors.

- Comparison of treatment for chronic myelogenous leukemia on thinking and memory will be made in an effort to develop strategies to improve quality of life after cancer treatment.

- An assessment will be made of how quality of social support resources affects adjustment among lesbians with breast cancer.

- A longitudinal study will attempt to distinguish between cause and effect in the search for meaning in life, benefit finding, and quality of life for individuals diagnosed with lung or colorectal cancer.

SOURCE: Personal communication, B. Teschendorf, ACS, February 23, 2005.

Susan G. Komen Foundation

The Susan G. Komen Foundation is dedicated to eradicating breast cancer through research and education. Since its inception in 1982, it has awarded over $144 million through more than 1,000 research grants. In 2003–2004, the Foundation supported five survivorship-related research grants totaling approximately $1.25 million (Komen Foundation, 2004). The projects supported by the grants explore topics such as memory problems, osteoporosis, and other long-term treatment effects; characteristics and needs of Hispanic breast cancer survivors; and outcomes in women diagnosed with breast cancer during pregnancy.

Summary

Federal investments in cancer survivorship research have been relatively modest. The NCI's Office of Cancer Survivorship, the federal locus for cancer survivorship research, has distributed an estimated $28 million in research funds to date. The Office of Cancer Survivorship oversees a small grant portfolio and leverages resources from other parts of NIH to encourage survivorship research. Additional support for clinical survivorship research has been available through the NCI's Clinical Trials Cooperative Group Program, but the level of such support, while difficult to gauge, appears to be low. These groups represent important opportunities to evaluate the consequences of contemporary cancer treatments. CDC's new focus on survivorship and public health and AHRQ's focus on cancer among Medicare beneficiaries could lead to increased research support related to cancer survivorship. Other federal support is available for survivorship research through the DoD's extramural grant programs. In terms of private resources for research, the ACS has invested in large survivorship cohort studies; the Lance Armstrong Foundation is building on its portfolio of survivorship research; and other private foundations are supporting research on survivorship issues relevant to their constituencies.

FINDINGS AND RECOMMENDATIONS

In summary, cancer survivorship research has emerged as a unique area of inquiry covering areas such as clinical late effects, psychosocial adjustment, and quality of care. The field is by nature interdisciplinary and includes investigators in nursing, clinical medicine, epidemiology, and health services research. Within the past decade, a focus for federally sponsored research has been organized within the NCI. Findings from this research have informed much of this report. Investigators have used several mechanisms to conduct survivorship research, including focus groups and other qualitative methods, clinical trials, cohort studies, cancer registries, administrative data, and surveys. Among the challenges to conducting survivorship research are the difficulties and costs associated with long-term follow-up, the complexities of accruing sufficient sample sizes through multi-institutional research endeavors, changes in treatment and the latency to recognition of late effects, and emerging problems associated with compliance with HIPAA. Survivorship research is funded at relatively modest levels within both public and private sectors, especially as contrasted to levels of support for treatment-related research.

Recommendation 10: The National Cancer Institute (NCI), Centers for Disease Control and Prevention (CDC), Agency for Healthcare Research and Quality (AHRQ), Centers for Medicare and Medicaid Services (CMS), Department of Veterans Affairs (VA), private voluntary organizations such as the American Cancer Society (ACS), and private

health insurers and plans should increase their support of survivorship research and expand mechanisms for its conduct. New research initiatives focused on cancer patient follow-up are urgently needed to guide effective survivorship care.

Research is especially needed to improve understanding of:

- Mechanisms of late effects experienced by cancer survivors
- How to identify and intervene to alleviate symptoms and improve function
- The prevalence and risk of late effects (prospective, long-term follow-up studies are needed)
- The cost-effectiveness of alternative models of survivorship care and community-based psychosocial services
  - —Post-treatment surveillance strategies and interventions (large clinical trials are needed)
  - —Survivors' and caregivers' attitudes and preferences regarding outcomes and survivorship care
  - —Needs of racial/ethnic groups, residents of rural areas, and other potentially underserved groups
  - —Supportive care and rehabilitation programs
- Interventions to improve quality of life
  - —Family and caregiver needs and access to supportive services
  - —Mechanisms to reduce financial burdens of survivorship care (e.g., the new Medicare prescription drug benefit should be carefully monitored to evaluate its impact, especially how private plan formularies cover cancer drugs)
  - —Employer programs to meet return-to-work needs
  - —Approaches to improve health insurance coverage
  - —Legal protections afforded cancer survivors through the Americans with Disabilities Act, Family and Medical Leave Act, HIPAA, and other laws
- Survivorship research methods
  - —Barriers to participation
  - —Impact of HIPAA
  - —Methods to overcome challenges of survivorship research (e.g., methods to adjust for bias introduced by nonparticipation; methods to minimize loss to follow-up)

To conduct research in these priority areas, large study populations are needed that represent the diversity of cancer survivors in terms of their type of cancer and treatment as well as their sociodemographic and health care characteristics. Existing research mechanisms need to be fully utilized and expanded to provide opportunities for cancer survivorship research:

NCI Cooperative Groups—More long-term follow-up studies need to be conducted of individuals enrolled in clinical trials.

SPOREs (P50) or Research Program Projects (P01)—Extramural research mechanisms could be used to support focused research efforts on survivorship. Such mechanisms facilitate interdisciplinary collaboration and take advantage of services and infrastructure available through core institutional support.

NCI-sponsored special studies—Additional survivorship special studies are needed that are based on population-based cancer registries.

National surveys—Refinements to ongoing national surveys (e.g., the Medical Expenditure Panel Survey) and supplements to others (e.g., National Health Interview Survey) could help capture information on survivorship.

Population-based cancer registries—The SEER Program and the NPCR should begin to collect data on cancer recurrence among survivors as an outcome measure. State and regional registries should also develop mechanisms to obtain comorbidity data that can be used to enhance analyses of short-term and long-term outcomes among cancer survivors. Measures of socioeconomic status (e.g., income, education, health insurance status) would assist health services researchers as they assess health care disparities in cancer care and outcomes. These additional data and measures could be obtained through existing linkages with Medicare claims in the SEER-Medicare database, new linkages with electronic data from health plans and provider networks, or an expansion of data elements that are routinely reported by hospitals and physicians to cancer registries. Opportunities should be sought to link data from cancer registries to other administrative databases (e.g., private insurance claims, Medicaid data).

Health services research resources—The follow-up period of ongoing cancer health services research studies (e.g., CanCORS) should be extended to yield more information on long-term survivorship.

Research networks—Investigators should be encouraged to use existing research networks (e.g., CRN, PBRN, IDSRN) to conduct cancer survivorship research.

Longitudinal studies—Longitudinal studies such as the Nurses' Health Study and the Physician's Health Study provide opportunities to assess survivorship issues.

In addition to harnessing these existing mechanisms, the committee recommends that federal and private research sponsors support a large new research initiative on cancer patient follow-up. Answers to the following basic questions about survivorship care are needed: How frequently should patients be evaluated following their primary cancer therapy? What tests should be included in the follow-up regimen? Who should provide follow-up care? A call for such research was made in the Institute of Medicine's 1999 *Ensuring Quality Cancer Care* report, but it has not yet been conducted (IOM, 1999). In some cases large clinical trials will be needed to answer these questions. There is renewed interest in designing affordable and relatively simple practical trials, registries, and other real-world prospective studies to answer the many such clinical questions (Tunis, 2005).

During follow-up, the ability to detect cancer recurrence and late effects is usually of great concern to survivors and providers alike. The modalities used for detection are numerous and may be very costly. Cancer patient follow-up typically lasts indefinitely or at least for many years after primary therapy. There is significant and sometimes dramatic variation in follow-up practices (see Chapter 4) and associated costs (Johnson and Virgo, 1997). Much of this variability is currently felt to stem from a lack of high-quality evidence supporting any particular strategy. Gathering such evidence by means of well-designed clinical trials of alternative follow-up strategies is expensive, in part because such trials must incorporate many years of surveillance.

The committee concludes that improvements in cancer survivors' care and quality of life depend on a much expanded research effort.

REFERENCES

AAMC (American Association of Medical Colleges). 2004. *Welcome to the AAMC Project to Monitor and Document the Effects of HIPAA on Research*. [Online]. Available: http://services.aamc.org/easurvey/survey/login.cfm [accessed December 9, 2004].

ACoS (American College of Surgeons). 2004. *What is the NCDB?* [Online]. Available: http://www.facs.org/cancer/ncdb/ncdbabout.html [accessed February 23, 2005].

AHRQ (Agency for Healthcare Research and Quality). 2001. *Primary Care Practice-based Research Networks*. Rockville, MD: AHRQ.

AHRQ. 2002a. *Integrated Delivery System Research Network (IDSRN): Field Partnerships to Conduct and Use Research*. Fact Sheet. AHRQ Publication No. 03-P00. [Online]. Available: http://www.ahrq.gov/research/idsrn.htm [accessed April 1, 2005].

AHRQ. 2002b. *Management of Cancer Symptoms: Pain, Depression, and Fatigue*. Summary, Evidence Report/Technology Assessment: Number 61. AHRQ Publication No. 02-E031. [Online]. Available: http://www.ahrq.gov/clinic/epcsums/csympsum.htm [accessed December 21, 2004].

AHRQ. 2004a. *Effectiveness of Behavioral Interventions to Modify Physical Activity Behaviors in General Populations and Cancer Patients and Survivors*. Evidence Report/Technology Assessment 102. Rockville, MD: AHRQ.

AHRQ. 2004b. *List of Priority Conditions for Research under Medicare Modernization Act Released. Press Release*. [Online]. Available: http://www.ahrq.gov/news/press/pr2004/mmapr.htm [accessed December 17, 2004].

Arredondo SA, Downs TM, Lubeck DP, Pasta DJ, Silva SJ, Wallace KL, Carroll PR. 2004. Watchful waiting and health related quality of life for patients with localized prostate cancer: Data from CaPSURE. *J Urol* 172(5 Pt 1):1830–1834.

Ayanian JZ, Chrischilles EA, Fletcher RH, Fouad MN, Harrington DP, Kahn KL, Kiefe CI, Lipscomb J, Malin JL, Potosky AL, Provenzale DT, Sandler RS, van Ryn M, Wallace RB, Weeks JC, West DW. 2004. Understanding cancer treatment and outcomes: The Cancer Care Outcomes Research and Surveillance Consortium. *J Clin Oncol* 22(15):2992–2996.

Aziz N. 2004 (July 26–27). *The Art and Science of Cancer Survivorship in the New Millennium: An Integral Concept Underlying Quality Care.* Presentation at the Meeting of the IOM Committee on Cancer Survivorship, Woods Hole, MA.

Aziz NM. 2002. Cancer survivorship research: Challenge and opportunity. *J Nutr* 132(11 Suppl):3494S–3503S.

Aziz NM, Rowland JH. 2002. Cancer survivorship research among ethnic minority and medically underserved groups. *Oncol Nurs Forum* 29(5):789–801.

Aziz NM, Rowland JH. 2003. Trends and advances in cancer survivorship research: Challenge and opportunity. *Semin Radiat Oncol* 13(3):248–266.

Barzilai DA, Cooper KD, Neuhauser D, Rimm AA, Cooper GS. 2004. Geographic and patient variation in receipt of surveillance procedures after local excision of cutaneous melanoma. *J Invest Dermatol* 122(2):246–255.

Begg CB, Riedel ER, Bach PB, Kattan MW, Schrag D, Warren JL, Scardino PT. 2002. Variations in morbidity after radical prostatectomy. *N Engl J Med* 346(15):1138–1144.

Bergmann MM, Byers T, Freedman DS, Mokdad A. 1998. Validity of self-reported diagnoses leading to hospitalization: A comparison of self-reports with hospital records in a prospective study of American adults. *Am J Epidemiol* 147(10):969–977.

Bernhard J, Cella DF, Coates AS, Fallowfield L, Ganz PA, Moinpour CM, Mosconi P, Osoba D, Simes J, Hurny C. 1998. Missing quality of life data in cancer clinical trials: Serious problems and challenges. *Stat Med* 17(5–7):517–532.

Bradley CJ, Given CW, Roberts C. 2003. Late stage cancers in a Medicaid-insured population. *Med Care* 41(6):722–728.

Brown ML, Riley GF, Potosky AL, Etzioni RD. 1999. Obtaining long-term disease specific costs of care: Application to Medicare enrollees diagnosed with colorectal cancer. *Med Care* 37(12):1249–1259.

Buchanan DR, O'Mara AM, Kelaghan JW, Minasian LM. 2005. Quality-of-life assessment in the symptom management trials of the National Cancer Institute-supported community clinical oncology program. *J Clin Oncol* 23(3):591–598.

Butterfield RM, Park ER, Puleo E, Mertens A, Gritz ER, Li FP, Emmons K. 2004. Multiple risk behaviors among smokers in the Childhood Cancer Survivor Study cohort. *Psychooncology* 13(9):619–629.

CaPSURE. 2005a. *Publications.* [Online]. Available: http://www.capsure.net/pub/pub.aspx [accessed January 24, 2005].

CaPSURE. 2005b. *What is CaPSURE?* [Online]. Available: http://www.capsure.net [accessed January 19, 2005].

CDC (Centers for Disease Control and Prevention). 2003. *Science in Brief: Cancer Registries.* National Program of Cancer Registries Research and Evaluation Activities. Atlanta, GA: CDC.

CDC. 2004. *Lance Armstrong Foundation.* [Online]. Available: http://www.cdc.gov/cancer/partners/fp_laf.htm [accessed March 17, 2004].

CDC. 2005. *CDC Announces First Ever Agency-wide Research Agenda.* [Online]. Available: http://www.cdc.gov/od/oc/media/pressrel/r050303.htm [accessed April 14, 2005].

Center on an Aging Society. 2002. *Cancer: A Major National Concern.* Challenges for the 21st Century: Chronic and Disabling Conditions Series. Number 4. Washington, DC: Georgetown University.

Chambers LW, Spitzer WO, Hill GB, Helliwell BE. 1976. Underreporting of cancer in medical surveys: A source of systematic error in cancer research. *Am J Epidemiol* 104(2):141–145.

Cooper GS, Yuan Z, Chak A, Rimm AA. 1999. Geographic and patient variation among Medicare beneficiaries in the use of follow-up testing after surgery for nonmetastatic colorectal carcinoma. *Cancer* 85(10):2124–2131.

Cooper GS, Yuan Z, Chak A, Rimm AA. 2000. Patterns of endoscopic follow-up after surgery for nonmetastatic colorectal cancer. *Gastrointest Endosc* 52(1):33–38.

Cooperberg MR, Broering JM, Litwin MS, Lubeck DP, Mehta SS, Henning JM, Carroll PR. 2004. The contemporary management of prostate cancer in the United States: Lessons from the Cancer of the Prostate Strategic Urologic Research Endeavor (CaPSURE), a national disease registry. *J Urol* 171(4):1393–1401.

DoD (Department of Defense). 2004a. *Congressionally Directed Medical Research Programs: Breast Cancer*. [Online]. Available: http://cdmrp.army.mil/bcrp/ [accessed December 21, 2004].

DoD. 2004b. *Congressionally Directed Medical Research Programs: Search Awards*. [Online]. Available: http://cdmrp.army.mil/scripts/search.asp [accessed December 21, 2004].

Donaldson SS, Hancock SL, Hoppe RT. 1999. The Janeway lecture. Hodgkin's disease—finding the balance between cure and late effects. *Cancer J Sci Am* 5(6):325–333.

Downs TM, Sadetsky N, Pasta DJ, Grossfeld GD, Kane CJ, Mehta SS, Carroll PR, Lubeck DP. 2003. Health related quality of life patterns in patients treated with interstitial prostate brachytherapy for localized prostate cancer—data from CaPSURE. *J Urol* 170(5):1822–1827.

Earle CC, Burstein HJ, Winer EP, Weeks JC. 2003. Quality of non-breast cancer health maintenance among elderly breast cancer survivors. *J Clin Oncol* 21(8):1447–1451.

Earle CC, Nattinger AB, Potosky AL, Lang K, Mallick R, Berger M, Warren JL. 2002. Identifying cancer relapse using SEER-Medicare data. *Med Care* 40(8 Suppl):IV-75–81.

Earle CC, Neville BA. 2004. Under use of necessary care among cancer survivors. *Cancer* 101(8):1712–1719.

Ehringhaus, JD. 2004. *AAMC Project to Document the Effects of HIPAA on Research*. [Online]. Available: http://www.hhs.gov/ohrp/sachrp/mtgings/mtg03-04/hipaaamc_files/frame.htm [accessed December 17, 2004].

Ellison GL, Warren JL, Knopf KB, and Brown ML. 2003. Racial differences in the receipt of bowel surveillance following potentially curative colorectal cancer surgery. *Health Serv Res* 38(6 Pt 2):1885–1903.

Emmons KM, Butterfield RM, Puleo E, Park ER, Mertens A, Gritz ER, Lahti M, Li FP. 2003. Smoking among participants in the childhood cancer survivors cohort: The Partnership for Health Study. *J Clin Oncol* 21(2):189–196.

Fairclough DL, Fetting JH, Cella D, Wonson W, Moinpour CM. 1999. Quality of life and quality adjusted survival for breast cancer patients receiving adjuvant therapy. Eastern Cooperative Oncology Group (ECOG). *Qual Life Res* 8(8):723–731.

Field TS, Cernieux J, Buist D, Geiger A, Lamerato L, Hart G, Bachman D, Krajenta R, Greene S, Hornbrook MC, Ansell G, Herrinton L, Reed G. 2004. Retention of enrollees following a cancer diagnosis within health maintenance organizations in the Cancer Research Network. *J Natl Cancer Inst* 96(2):148–152.

Forrest CB, Glade GB, Baker AE, Bocian A, von Schrader S, Starfield B. 2000. Coordination of specialty referrals and physician satisfaction with referral care. *Arch Pediatr Adolesc Med* 154(5):499–506.

Ganz PA. 2003. Why and how to study the fate of cancer survivors: Observations from the clinic and the research laboratory. *Eur J Cancer* 39(15):2136–2141.

Ganz PA, Desmond KA, Leedham B, Rowland JH, Meyerowitz BE, Belin TR. 2002. Quality of life in long-term, disease-free survivors of breast cancer: A follow-up study. *J Natl Cancer Inst* 94(1):39–49.

Ganz PA, Greendale GA, Petersen L, Kahn B, Bower JE. 2003a. Breast cancer in younger women: Reproductive and late health effects of treatment. *J Clin Oncol* 21(22):4184–4193.

Ganz PA, Moinpour CM, Pauler DK, Kornblith AB, Gaynor ER, Balcerzak SP, Gatti GS, Erba HP, McCoy S, Press OW, Fisher RI. 2003b. Health status and quality of life in patients with early-stage Hodgkin's disease treated on Southwest Oncology Group Study 9133. *J Clin Oncol* 21(18):3512–3519.

GAO (General Accounting Office). 2004. *Health Information: First-Year Experiences Under the Federal Privacy Rule*. Washington, DC: GAO.

Geiger A. 2004. Scientific interest group profile: Survivorship. *CRN Connection* 5(5):2.

Gotay C. 2004. *Shortening the Timeline for New Cancer Treatments*. Background paper commissioned for the IOM. Unpublished.

Greene SM, Geiger AM. 2004. *Impact of Different IRB Processes in a Multi-Site Mailed Survey*. [Online]. Available: http://crn.cancer.gov/dissemination/impact_irb_survey.pdf [accessed December 15, 2004].

Gunn PP, Fremont AM, Bottrell M, Shugarman LR, Galegher J, Bikson T. 2004. The Health Insurance Portability and Accountability Act Privacy Rule: A practical guide for researchers. *Med Care* 42(4):321–327.

Hewitt M, Breen N, Devesa S. 1999. Cancer prevalence and survivorship issues: Analyses of the 1992 National Health Interview Survey. *J Natl Cancer Inst* 91(17):1480–1486.

Hewitt M, Rowland JH. 2002. Mental health service use among adult cancer survivors: Analyses of the National Health Interview Survey. *J Clin Oncol* 20(23):4581–4590.

Hewitt M, Rowland JH, Yancik R. 2003. Cancer survivors in the United States: Age, health, and disability. *J Gerontol A Biol Sci Med Sci* 58(1):82–91.

Hiatt R. 2005 (October 27–28). *Cancer Survivorship: Improving Care and Quality of Life*. Presentation at the meeting of the IOM Committee on Cancer Survivorship, Irvine, CA.

Hiatt RA. 2003. HIPAA: The end of epidemiology, or a new social contract? *Epidemiology* 14(6):637–639.

Hillner BE, McDonald MK, Penberthy L, Desch CE, Smith TJ, Maddux P, Glasheen WP, Retchin SM. 1997. Measuring standards of care for early breast cancer in an insured population. *J Clin Oncol* 15(4):1401–1408.

Hu JC, Elkin EP, Pasta DJ, Lubeck DP, Kattan MW, Carroll PR, Litwin MS. 2004. Predicting quality of life after radical prostatectomy: Results from CaPSURE. *J Urol* 171(2 Pt 1):703–707; discussion 707–708.

Hudson MM, Mertens AC, Yasui Y, Hobbie W, Chen H, Gurney JG, Yeazel M, Recklitis CJ, Marina N, Robison LR, Oeffinger KC. 2003. Health status of adult long-term survivors of childhood cancer: A report from the Childhood Cancer Survivor Study. *JAMA* 290(12):1583–1592.

IOM (Institute of Medicine). 1999. *Ensuring Quality Cancer Care*. Hewitt M, Simone JV, eds. Washington, DC: National Academy Press.

IOM. 2000. *Enhancing Data Systems to Improve the Quality of Cancer Care*. Hewitt M, Simone JV, eds. Washington, DC: National Academy Press.

IOM. 2003a. *Childhood Cancer Survivorship: Improving Care and Quality of Life*. Hewitt M, Weiner SL, Simone JV, eds. Washington, DC: The National Academies Press.

IOM. 2003b. *Responsible Research: A Systems Approach to Protecting Research Participants*. Federman DD, Hanna KE, Lyman Rodriguez L, eds.. Washington, DC: The National Academies Press.

Johnson FE, Virgo, KS. 1997. *Cancer Patient Follow-Up*. St. Louis, MO: Mosby.

Johnson TK, Gilliland FD, Hoffman RM, Deapen D, Penson DF, Stanford JL, Albertsen PC, Hamilton AS. 2004. Racial/ethnic differences in functional outcomes in the 5 years after diagnosis of localized prostate cancer. *J Clin Oncol* 22(20):4193–4201.

Knopf KB, Warren JL, Feuer EJ, Brown ML. 2001. Bowel surveillance patterns after a diagnosis of colorectal cancer in Medicare beneficiaries. *Gastrointest Endosc* 54(5):563–571.

Komen Foundation. 2004. *Population Specific Research*. [Online]. Available: http://www.komen.org/grants/awards/04awardswcso.asp?id=1&nodeId=567 [accessed February 24, 2005].

LAF (Lance Armstrong Foundation). 2004. *2004 Overview— Individual Grant Awards*. Austin, TX: LAF.

LAF. 2005. *Lance Armstrong Foundation Awards $3.3 Million in Research Grants*. [Online]. Available: http://www.laf.org/News_Events/News/pr-20050201.cfm [accessed March 6, 2005].

Lamont EB, Christakis NA, Lauderdale DS. 2003. Favorable cardiac risk among elderly breast carcinoma survivors. *Cancer* 98(1):2–10.

Lamont EB, Lauderdale DS. 2003. Low risk of hip fracture among elderly breast cancer survivors. *Ann Epidemiol* 13(10):698–703.

Litwin MS, Sadetsky N, Pasta DJ, Lubeck DP. 2004. Bowel function and bother after treatment for early stage prostate cancer: A longitudinal quality of life analysis from CaPSURE. *J Urol* 172(2):515–519.

Mariotto A, Warren JL, Knopf KB, Feuer EJ. 2003. The prevalence of patients with colorectal carcinoma under care in the U.S. *Cancer* 98(6):1253–1261.

Mehta SS, Lubeck DP, Pasta DJ, Litwin MS. 2003. Fear of cancer recurrence in patients undergoing definitive treatment for prostate cancer: Results from CaPSURE. *J Urol* 170(5):1931–1933.

Moinpour CM. 1996. Costs of quality-of-life research in Southwest Oncology Group trials. *J Natl Cancer Inst Monogr* (20):11–6.

Moinpour CM, Lovato LC. 1998. Ensuring the quality of quality of life data: The Southwest Oncology Group experience. *Stat Med* 17(5–7):641–651.

NAACCR (North American Assocation of Central Cancer Registries) 2003. *Frequently Asked Questions and Answers About Cancer Reporting and the HIPAA Privacy Rule*. Springfield, IL: NAACCR.

Nattinger AB, Schapira MM, Warren JL, Earle CC. 2002. Methodological issues in the use of administrative claims data to study surveillance after cancer treatment. *Med Care* 40(8 Suppl):IV-69–74.

NCAB (National Cancer Advisory Board). 2003. *Summary of Meeting, September 9–10, 2003*. Bethesda, MD: NIH.

NCI (National Cancer Institute). 1998. *NCI Awards $15 Million to Study Cancer Survivors*. [Online]. Available: http://www.cancer.gov/newscenter/15million [accessed January 10, 2005].

NCI. 2003a. *Fact Book, National Cancer Institute*. Bethesda, MD: NCI.

NCI. 2003b. *NCI's Clinical Trials Cooperative Group Program*. [Online]. Available: http://cis.nci.nih.gov/fact/1_4.htm [accessed December 14, 2004].

NCI. 2004a. *About SEER*. [Online]. Available: http://seer.cancer.gov/about/ [accessed December 13, 2004].

NCI. 2004b. *Cancer Research Network: Overview of Survivorship Research*. [Online]. Available: http://crn.cancer.gov/areas/survivorship/ [accessed December 15, 2004].

NCI. 2004c. *Funding History for Cancer Survivorship Research*. [Online]. Available: http://dccps.nci.nih.gov/overview/proghistory.jsp?progid=6 [accessed December 20, 2004].

NCI. 2004d. *Search for Clinical Trials: Advanced.* [Online]. Available: http://www.nci.nih.gov/Search/SearchClinicalTrialsAdvanced.aspx [accessed December 16, 2004].

NCI. 2004e. *SEER-Medicare: How the SEER & Medicare Data are Linked.* [Online]. Available: http://healthservices.cancer.gov/seermedicare/overview/linked.html [accessed December 14, 2004].

NCI. 2004f. *SEER-Medicare: Publications (Sorted by Author).* [Online]. Available: http://healthservices.cancer.gov/seermedicare/overview/publications.html [accessed December 13, 2004].

NCI. 2005a. *Program Testing Early Cancer Treatment and Screening (PROTECTS).* [Online]. Available: http://crn.cancer.gov/areas/treatment/protects.html. (accessed July 14, 2005).

NCI. 2005b. *About Survivorship Research: OCS Chart Analysis for FY04.* [Online]. Available: http://dccps.nci.nih.gov/ocs/ocs_chart_analysis04.html (accessed April 15, 2005).

NCI. Undated. *Facts About Office of Cancer Survivorship, National Cancer Institute.* Bethesda, MD: NCI.

NCI and ACS (National Cancer Institute and American Cancer Society). 2004 (June 16–18). *Cancer Survivorship: Pathways to Health After Treatment Program Book.* 2nd biennial ACS and NCI Cancer Survivorship Research Conference. Washington, DC: NCI.

NCI Director. 2002. *The Nation's Investment in Cancer Research: A Plan and Budget Proposal for Fiscal Year 2004.* Bethesda, MD: NCI.

NCI Director. 2003. *The Nation's Investment in Cancer Research: A Plan and Budget Proposal for Fiscal Year 2005.* Bethesda, MD: NCI.

NIH (National Institutes of Health). 2004a. *ERA Commons, Computer Retrieval of Information on Scientific Projects.* [Online]. Available: http://crisp.cit.nih.gov/ [accessed December 17, 2004].

NIH. 2004b. *Grants & Funding Opportunities.* [Online]. Available: http://grants.nih.gov [accessed December 21, 2004].

NIH. 2004c. *Office of Behavioral and Social Sciences homepage.* [Online]. Available: http://obssr.od.nih.gov/ [accessed December 21, 2004].

NIH. 2004d. *Activity Codes, Organization Codes, and Definitions Used in Extramural Programs.* Rockville, MD: NIH.

NLM (National Library of Medicine). 2004. *MeSH.* [Online]. Available: http://www.ncbi.nlm.nih.gov/entrez/query.fcgi?db=MeSH&term= [accessed December 17, 2004].

NLM. 2005. *PubMed.* [Online]. Available: http://www.pubmed.gov [accessed June 22, 2005].

Oeffinger KC, Mertens AC, Hudson MM, Gurney JG, Casillas J, Chen H, Whitton J, Yeazel M, Yasui Y, Robison LL. 2004. Health care of young adult survivors of childhood cancer: A report from the Childhood Cancer Survivor Study. *Ann Fam Med* 2(1):61–70.

Pakilit AT, Kahn BA, Petersen L, Abraham LS, Greendale GA, Ganz PA. 2001. Making effective use of tumor registries for cancer survivorship research. *Cancer* 92(5):1305–1314.

Potosky AL, Davis WW, Hoffman RM, Stanford JL, Stephenson RA, Penson DF, Harlan LC. 2004. Five-year outcomes after prostatectomy or radiotherapy for prostate cancer: The Prostate Cancer Outcomes Study. *J Natl Cancer Inst* 96(18):1358–1367.

Potosky AL, Legler J, Albertsen PC, Stanford JL, Gilliland FD, Hamilton AS, Eley JW, Stephenson RA, Harlan LC. 2000. Health outcomes after prostatectomy or radiotherapy for prostate cancer: Results from the Prostate Cancer Outcomes Study. *J Natl Cancer Inst* 92(19):1582–1592.

Potosky AL, Riley GF, Lubitz JD, Mentnech RM, Kessler LG. 1993. Potential for cancer related health services research using a linked Medicare-tumor registry database. *Med Care* 31(8):732–748.

Raghavan D. Hidden by HIPAA: The costs of cure. 2005. *Journal of Clinical Oncology* 23 (16):3663-3665.

Ramirez AG, Niederhuber JE. 2003 (November 5). Letter to The Honorable Tommy G. Thompson, Secretary of Health and Human Services. Washington, DC.

Ramsey SD, Berry K, Etzioni R. 2002. Lifetime cancer-attributable cost of care for long term survivors of colorectal cancer. *Am J Gastroenterol* 97(2):440–445.

Robison LL, Mertens AC, Boice JD, Breslow NE, Donaldson SS, Green DM, Li FP, Meadows AT, Mulvihill JJ, Neglia JP, Nesbit ME, Packer RJ, Potter JD, Sklar CA, Smith MA, Stovall M, Strong LC, Yasui Y, Zeltzer LK. 2002. Study design and cohort characteristics of the Childhood Cancer Survivor Study: A multi-institutional collaborative project. *Med Pediatr Oncol* 38(4):229–239.

Rowland J. 2004. Cancer survivorship: Activities and research looking beyond the cure. *NCI Cancer Bulletin* 1(26):1–2.

Schapira MM, McAuliffe TL, Nattinger AB. 2000. Underutilization of mammography in older breast cancer survivors. *Med Care* 38(3):281–289.

Schneider EC, Epstein AM, Malin JL, Kahn KL, Emanuel EJ. 2004. Developing a system to assess the quality of cancer care: ASCO's national initiative on cancer care quality. *J Clin Oncol* 22(15):2985–2991.

Schrag D, Hsieh LJ, Rabbani F, Bach PB, Herr H, Begg CB. 2003. Adherence to surveillance among patients with superficial bladder cancer. *J Natl Cancer Inst* 95(8):588–597.

Sears SR, Stanton AL, Kwan L, Krupnick JL, Rowland JH, Meyerowitz BE, Ganz PA. 2003. Recruitment and retention challenges in breast cancer survivorship research: Results from a multisite, randomized intervention trial in women with early stage breast cancer. *Cancer Epidemiol Biomarkers Prev* 12(10):1087–1090.

Shahinian VB, Kuo YF, Freeman JL, Goodwin JS. 2005. Risk of fracture after androgen deprivation for prostate cancer. *N Engl J Med* 352(2):154–164.

Speight JL, Elkin EP, Pasta DJ, Silva S, Lubeck DP, Carroll PR, Litwin MS. 2004. Longitudinal assessment of changes in sexual function and bother in patients treated with external beam radiotherapy or brachytherapy, with and without neoadjuvant androgen ablation: Data from CaPSURE. *Int J Radiat Oncol Biol Phys* 60(4):1066–1075.

Thorpe KE, Howard D. 2003. Health insurance and spending among cancer patients. *Health Aff (Millwood)* (Suppl):W3-189–198. [Online]. Available: http://content.healthaffairs.org/cgi/reprint/hlthaff.w3.189v1 (accessed July 11, 2005).

Tunis SR. 2005. A clinical research strategy to support shared decision making. *Health Aff (Millwood)* 24(1):180–184.

University of Minnesota Cancer Center. 2002. *Long-term Follow-Up Study*. [Online]. Available: http://www.cancer.umn.edu/ltfu [accessed December 14, 2004].

Warren JL, Klabunde CN, Schrag D, Bach PB, Riley GF. 2002. Overview of the SEER-Medicare data: Content, research applications, and generalizability to the United States elderly population. *Med Care* 40(8 Suppl):IV-3–18.

Winchester DP, Stewart AK, Bura C, Jones RS. 2004. The National Cancer Data Base: A clinical surveillance and quality improvement tool. *J Surg Oncol* 85(1):1–3.

Yabroff KR, Lawrence WF, Clauser S, Davis WW, Brown ML. 2004. Burden of illness in cancer survivors: Findings from a population-based national sample. *J Natl Cancer Inst* 96(17):1322–1330.

Yates J. 2004 (July 26–27). *American Cancer Society – Survivorship Programs*. Presentation at the meeting of the IOM Committee on Cancer Survivorship, Woods Hole, MA.

Yeazel MW, Oeffinger KC, Gurney JG, Mertens AC, Hudson MM, Emmons KM, Chen H, Robison LL. 2004. The cancer screening practices of adult survivors of childhood cancer: A report from the Childhood Cancer Survivor Study. *Cancer* 100(3):631–640.

Zebrack BJ, Gurney JG, Oeffinger K, Whitton J, Packer RJ, Mertens A, Turk N, Castleberry R, Dreyer Z, Robison LL, Zeltzer LK. 2004. Psychological outcomes in long-term survivors of childhood brain cancer: A report from the Childhood Cancer Survivor Study. *J Clin Oncol* 22(6):999–100.

Glossary

adjuvant therapy—treatment given after the primary treatment to increase the chances of survival. Adjuvant therapy may include chemotherapy, radiation therapy, hormone therapy, or biological therapy.

allogenic marrow transplant—bone marrow transplant in which the donor marrow is obtained from a person who is not an identical twin and then given to the patient.

ambulatory care—the use of outpatient facilities—doctors' offices, home care, outpatient hospital clinics and day-care facilities—to provide care without the need for hospitalization. Often refers to any care outside a hospital.

amenorrhea—abnormal suppression or absence of menstruation.

atherosclerosis—a form of arteriosclerosis in which the arteries become clogged by the buildup of fatty substances, which eventually reduces the flow of blood to the tissues. These fatty substances, called plaque, are made up largely of cholesterol.

autonomic neuropathy—a disease of the non-voluntary, non-sensory nervous system affecting mostly the internal organs such as the bladder muscles, the cardiovascular system, the digestive tract, and the genital organs.

axillary dissection—surgery to remove lymph nodes found in the armpit region. Also called axillary lymph node dissection.

axillary lymph nodes—lymph nodes in the armpit region.

BRCA mutations—BRCA genes normally help suppress cell growth. When damaged (mutated), a person is at a higher risk of developing breast, ovarian, or prostate cancer.

cachexia—loss of body weight and muscle mass, and weakness that may occur in patients with cancer, AIDS, or other chronic diseases.
chemoprevention—the use of natural or laboratory-made substances to prevent cancer.
chemotherapy—the treatment of disease by means of chemicals that have a specific toxic effect on the disease-producing microorganisms (antibiotics) or that selectively destroy cancerous tissue (anticancer therapy).
chronic condition—a condition that is continuous or persistent over an extended period of time. A chronic condition is one that is longstanding, and not easily or quickly resolved.
clinical practice guidelines—systematically defined statements to assist practitioner and patient decisions about appropriate health care for specific clinical circumstances.
clinical trial—a formal study carried out according to a prospectively defined protocol that is intended to discover or verify the safety and effectiveness of procedures or interventions in humans.
cohort study—a research study that compares a particular outcome (such as lung cancer) in groups of individuals who are alike in many ways but differ by a certain characteristic (for example, female nurses who smoke compared with those who do not smoke).
colonoscopy—an examination of the inside of the colon using a thin, lighted tube, called a colonoscope, inserted into the rectum. Samples of tissues may be collected for examination under a microscope.
colostomy—an opening into the colon from the outside of the body. A colostomy provides a new path for waste material to leave the body after part of the colon has been removed.
comorbid conditions—disorders or syndromes occurring at the same time in the same patient.
comorbidity—refers to the co-occurrence of two or more disorders or syndromes (not symptoms) in the same patient.

dental caries—tooth decay.

edema—swelling caused by excess fluid in body tissues.
end-of-life care—care provided during the period of time in which an individual copes with declining health from an ultimately terminal illness.
endoscopy—the use of a thin, lighted tube (called an endoscope) to examine the inside of the body.
enterostomal nurses—nurses that specialize in the care of ostomies. They help patients adjust to an ostomy and learn to manage it.

epidemiology—science concerned with defining and explaining the interrelationships of factors that determine disease frequency and distribution.
estradiol—a form of the hormone estrogen.
etiology—the cause or origin of disease.
evidence-based—based on systematically reviewed clinical research findings.
exogenous—originating outside the body.

fibrosis—the growth of fibrous tissue.
first-degree relatives—genetically-related parents, children, and full siblings.

gene therapy—treatment that alters a gene. In studies of gene therapy for cancer, researchers are trying to improve the body's natural ability to fight the disease or to make the cancer cells more sensitive to other kinds of therapy.
genetic testing—analyzing DNA to look for a genetic alteration that may indicate an increased risk for developing a specific disease or disorder.
grade—the grade of a tumor depends on how abnormal the cancer cells look under a microscope and how quickly the tumor is likely to grow and spread. Grading systems are different for each type of cancer.

hematologic cancers—a cancer of the blood or bone marrow, such as leukemia or lymphoma. Also called hematologic malignancy.
hemicolectomy—surgical removal of the right or left side of the colon.
hepatic—of or relating to the liver.
hormonal status—the presence or absence of hormone receptors on the surface of cancer cells.
hormonal therapy—treatment that adds, blocks, or removes hormones. To slow or stop the growth of certain cancers (such as prostate and breast cancer), synthetic hormones or other drugs may be given to block the body's natural hormones. Sometimes surgery is needed to remove the gland that makes a certain hormone. Also called hormone therapy, hormone treatment, or endocrine therapy.
hypothyroidism—too little thyroid hormone. Symptoms include weight gain, constipation, dry skin, and sensitivity to the cold. Also called underactive thyroid.

incident cases—the number of newly diagnosed cancer cases.
intestinal stricture—abnormal narrowing of the intestines.
invasive cancer—cancer that has spread beyond the layer of tissue in which it developed and is growing into surrounding, healthy tissues. Also called infiltrating cancer.

ischemia—a decrease in the blood supply to a bodily organ, tissue, or part caused by constriction or obstruction of the blood vessels.

late effects—side effects of cancer treatment that appear months or years after treatment has ended. Late effects include physical and mental problems and second cancers.

latent disease—a condition that is present but not active or causing symptoms.

longitudinal study—study that follows subjects for an extended period of time.

lumpectomy—surgery to remove the tumor and a small amount of normal tissue around it.

lymphedema—a condition in which excess fluid collects in tissue and causes swelling. It may occur in the arm or leg after lymph vessels or lymph nodes in the underarm or groin are removed or treated with radiation.

malabsorption syndrome—a group of symptoms such as gas, bloating, abdominal pain, and diarrhea resulting from the body's inability to properly absorb nutrients.

mantle irradiation—radiation to areas above the diaphragm.

marker—a diagnostic indication that disease may develop.

mastectomy—surgery to remove the breast (or as much of the breast tissue as possible).

metastases—the spread of cancer from one part of the body to another. A tumor formed by cells that have spread is called a "metastatic tumor" or a "metastasis." The metastatic tumor contains cells that are like those in the original (primary) tumor. The plural form of metastasis is metastases.

morbidity—a disease or the incidence of disease within a population. Morbidity also refers to adverse effects caused by a treatment.

motility—rhythmic contractions of smooth muscle that move food along the digestive tract. Motility disorders can cause either slow contractions (hypomotility), rapid contractions (hypermotility), or both.

myelodysplasia—abnormal bone marrow cells that may lead to myelogenous leukemia.

myocardial infarction—the death of heart muscle from the sudden blockage of a coronary artery. Commonly known as a heart attack.

neoplasm—an abnormal mass of tissue that results when cells divide more than they should or do not die when they should. Tumors may be benign (not cancerous), or malignant (cancerous). Also called tumor.

neuropathic pain—pain which is the result of nervous system injury or malfunction, which may not have any external cause.

nuclear grade—an evaluation of the size and shape of the nucleus in tumor cells and the percentage of tumor cells that are in the process of dividing or growing. Cancers with low nuclear grade grow and spread less quickly than cancers with high nuclear grade.

oncology—the study of cancer.

oophorectomy—surgical removal of the ovaries.

ophthalmology—branch of medicine that deals with the anatomy, functions, pathology, and treatment of the eye.

orthotist—professional who specializes in mechanical devices to support or supplement weakened or abnormal joints or limbs.

osteopenia—decreased calcification, decreased density, or reduced mass of bone.

ostomy—an operation to create an opening (a stoma) from an area inside the body to the outside. Colostomy and urostomy are types of ostomies.

palliative care—treatment of symptoms associated with the effects of cancer and its treatment.

peripheral neuropathy—a condition of the nervous system that causes numbness, tingling, burning or weakness. It usually begins in the hands or feet, and can be caused by certain anticancer drugs.

physiatrists—a physician specializing in physical medicine and rehabilitation.

polypectomy—surgery to remove a polyp.

prevalent cases—the number of people who are alive and have ever had a diagnosis of cancer.

primary cancer—original cancer.

primary care provider—provider who manages a person's health care over time. A primary care provider is able to give a wide range of care, including prevention and treatment, can discuss cancer treatment choices, and can refer a patient to a specialist.

primary treatment—Primary treatment consists of the therapeutic interventions provided with the intention to cure cancer. In clinical situations in which the treatment of recurrent disease may be curative, the therapeutic approaches may be viewed as "primary treatment" which if successful will be followed by a phase of post-treatment survivorship.

prostate-specific antigen (PSA)—a substance produced by the prostate that may be found in an increased amount in the blood of men who have prostate cancer, benign prostatic hyperplasia, or infection or inflammation of the prostate.

psychosocial services—services relating to the psychological, social, behavioral, and spiritual aspects of cancer, including education, prevention, and treatment of problems in those areas.

pulmonary—having to do with the lungs.

quality measure—quantitative indicators that reflect the degree to which care is consistent with the best available, evidence-based clinical standards.

quality of care—the degree to which health services for individuals and populations increase the likelihood of desired health outcomes and are consistent with current professional knowledge.

quality of life—the overall enjoyment of life. Many clinical trials assess the effects of cancer and its treatment on the quality of life. These studies measure aspects of an individual's sense of well-being and ability to carry out various activities.

radiotherapy—the use of high-energy radiation from x rays, gamma rays, neutrons, and other sources to kill cancer cells and shrink tumors. Radiation may come from a machine outside the body (external-beam radiation therapy), or it may come from radioactive material placed in the body near cancer cells (internal radiation therapy, implant radiation, or brachytherapy). Systemic radiotherapy uses a radioactive substance, such as a radiolabeled monoclonal antibody, that circulates throughout the body. Also called radiation therapy.

recurrence—cancer that has returned after a period of time during which the cancer could not be detected. The cancer may come back to the same place as the original (primary) tumor or to another place in the body. Also called recurrent cancer.

relapse—the return of signs and symptoms of cancer after a period of improvement.

relative survival rate—a specific measurement of survival. For cancer, the rate is calculated by adjusting the survival rate to remove all causes of death except cancer. The rate is determined at specific time intervals, such as 2 years and 5 years after diagnosis.

remission—a decrease in or disappearance of signs and symptoms of cancer. In partial remission, some, but not all, signs and symptoms of cancer have disappeared. In complete remission, all signs and symptoms of cancer have disappeared, although cancer still may be in the body.

renal—of or relating to the kidneys.

resection—a procedure that uses surgery to remove tissue or part or all of an organ.

senescence—the process of growing old; aging.

sentinel lymph node biopsy—removal and examination of the sentinel node(s) (the first lymph node(s) to which cancer cells are likely to spread from a primary tumor). To identify the sentinel lymph node(s), the surgeon injects a radioactive substance, blue dye, or both near the tumor. The surgeon then uses a scanner to find the sentinel lymph node(s) containing the radioactive substance or looks for the lymph node(s) stained with dye. The surgeon then removes the sentinel node(s) to check for the presence of cancer cells.

sepsis—the presence of bacteria or their toxins in the blood or tissues.

sigmoidoscopy—inspection of the lower colon using a thin, lighted tube called a sigmoidoscope. Samples of tissue or cells may be collected for examination under a microscope. Also called proctosigmoidoscopy.

stage—the extent of a cancer in the body. Staging is usually based on the size of the tumor, whether lymph nodes contain cancer, and whether the cancer has spread from the original site to other parts of the body.

stem cell transplantation—a method of replacing immature blood-forming cells that were destroyed by cancer treatment. The stem cells are given to the person after treatment to help the bone marrow recover and continue producing healthy blood cells.

Surveillance, Epidemiology, and End Results (SEER) Program—a program of the National Cancer Institute that collects and publishes cancer incidence and survival data from 14 population-based cancer registries and three supplemental registries covering approximately 26 percent of the U.S. population.

survivor—an individual is considered a cancer survivor from the time of cancer diagnosis through the balance of his or her life, according to the National Coalition for Cancer Survivorship and the NCI Office of Cancer Survivorship. Family members, friends, and caregivers are also impacted by the survivorship experience and are therefore included in this definition. In this report, the committee chose to focus on cancer survivors who are in the post-treatment phase.

survivorship care—as defined in this report, survivorship care is a distinct phase of care for cancer survivors that includes four components: (1) prevention and detection of new cancers and recurrent cancer; (2) surveillance for cancer spread, recurrence, or second cancers; (3) intervention for consequences of cancer and its treatment; and (4) coordination between specialists and primary care providers to ensure that all of the survivor's health needs are met.

survivorship research—cancer survivorship research encompasses the physical, psychosocial, and economic sequelae of cancer diagnosis and its treatment among both pediatric and adult survivors of cancer. It also includes within its domain, issues related to health care delivery, access, and follow-up care, as they relate to survivors. Survivorship research focuses on the health and life of a person with a history of cancer beyond the acute diagnosis and treatment phase. It seeks to both prevent and control adverse cancer diagnosis and treatment-related outcomes such as late effects of treatment, second cancers, and poor quality of life, to provide a knowledge base regarding optimal follow-up care and surveillance of cancers, and to optimize health after cancer treatment (from OCS).

syndrome—a set of symptoms or conditions that occur together and suggest the presence of a certain disease or an increased chance of developing the disease.

third-party payors—entities that pay for health care, but are not the direct recipient of care. Includes insurers, employers, and the local, state, and federal governments (through Medicare, Medicaid, and other programs).

thrombosis—the formation or presence of a blood clot inside a blood vessel.

toxicity—a measure of the degree to which something is toxic or poisonous.

transplantation—the replacement of tissue with tissue from the person's own body or from another person.

Index

A

D

E

F

G

H

I

J

K

L

M

N

O

P

Q

R

S

T

U

V

W

Y

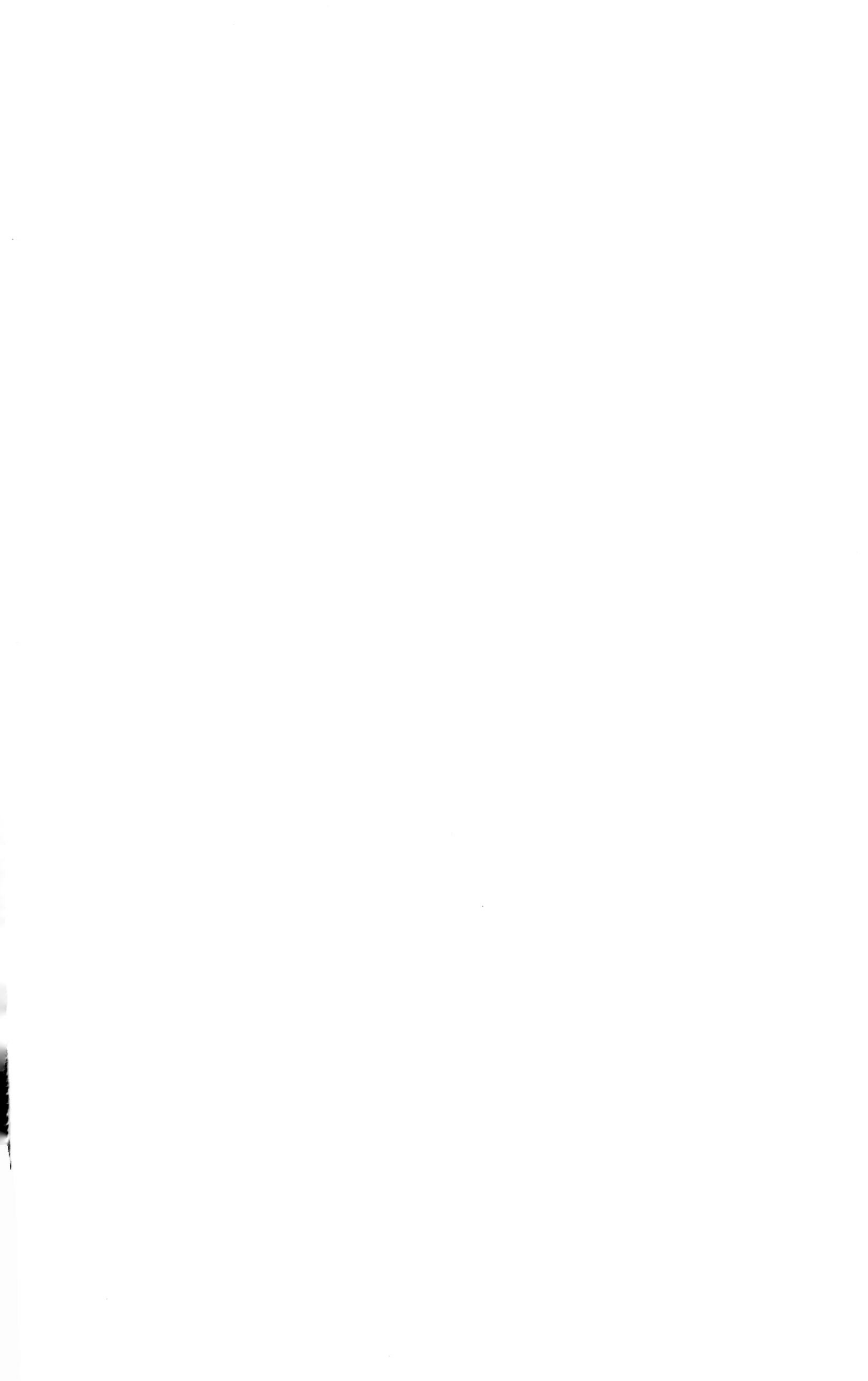